Ocular Surface Disease: Cornea, Conjunctiva and Tear Film

Content Strategist: *Russell Gabbedy*
Content Development Specialist: *Sharon Nash*
Content Coordinator: *Trinity Hutton*
Project Manager: *Sruthi Viswam*
Design: *Christian Bilbow*
Illustration Manager: *Jennifer Rose*
Illustrator: *Richard Tibbitts*
Marketing Manager(s) (UK/USA): *Gaynor Jones/Shaun Miller*
Cover design by Steven Osborne, University of California, Davis Eye Center

Ocular Surface Disease: Cornea, Conjunctiva and Tear Film

Edward J. Holland MD

Director of Cornea
Cincinnati Eye Institute
Professor of Ophthalmology
University of Cincinnati
Cincinnati, Ohio, USA

Mark J. Mannis MD FACS

Professor and Chair
Department of Ophthalmology & Vision Science
UC Davis Health System Eye Center
University of California, Davis
Sacramento, CA, USA

W. Barry Lee MD FACS

Cornea, External Disease, & Refractive Surgery
Eye Consultants of Atlanta/Piedmont Hospital
Medical Director, Georgia Eye Bank
Atlanta, GA, USA

For additional online content visit expertconsult.com

ELSEVIER
SAUNDERS

London, New York, Oxford, Philadelphia, St Louis, Sydney, Toronto

SAUNDERS is an imprint of Elsevier Inc.

ISBN: 978-1-4557-2876-3
Ebook ISBN: 978-1-4557-5623-0

Printed in China
Last digit is the print number: 9 8 7 6 5 4 3 2 1

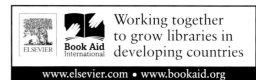

Contents

Video Contents

Total video running time approximately 21 minutes

Preface

The slaying of a beautiful hypothesis is both the tragedy as well as the great joy of scientific discovery. Since our last book on the subject of the ocular surface, many beautiful hypotheses have gone by the wayside, and there have likewise been a succession of brilliant revelations (aka 'ugly facts'). Indeed, what we have learned about the structure and function of the ocular surface has both broadened the range of therapeutic options we now employ and has raised numerous new questions that need to be asked about this very complex surface on which ocular function is so dependent.

Three decades ago, we barely understood the concept of the "stem cell"; two decades ago we began to understand where these stem cells reside on the ocular surface; and only in the past decade have we learned how to nurture or replace these vital pluripotential units that differentiate into surfaces as radically different as the corneal and conjunctival epithelia.

A decade ago, dry eye was understood primarily as aqueous tear deficiency. We now know that there are major differences in the categories of tear dysfunction, and we are aware of crucially important neural feedback mechanisms that link inflammatory activity on the ocular surface to lacrimal gland function. We have begun to understand the array of inflammatory mechanisms at the ocular surface and how to modulate these mechanisms for the good of the patient. And we now understand, with much greater clarity, the important role of the lid and its multiple functions for the health of the ocular surface.

From these revelations and the parsing of disease entities into their component effects on the cornea and conjunctiva, we view the ocular surface as both an expanding mystery as well as a gradually unraveling story of how the eye interacts with adjacent tissues and with the environment to which it is exposed.

In this volume, we have attempted to gather the current state of our understanding of surface physiology in health and disease. In collaboration with a group of world-renowned experts, we have sought to organize the therapeutic state-of-the-art in order to assist the practitioner in effective decision-making in the management of external eye disease. But in a field changing this rapidly, there will be new discoveries even as this book goes to press. And, therein, lies the excitement.

Edward J. Holland

Mark J. Mannis

W. Barry Lee

Contributors

Guillermo Amescua MD
Assistant Professor of Clinical Ophthalmology
Bascom Palmer Eye Institute
University of Miami-Miller School of Medicine
Miami, FL, USA

Andrea Y. Ang MPH FRANZCO
Consultant Corneal Surgeon
Centre for Ophthalmology and Visual Science
University of Western Australia
Lions Eye Institute
Perth, WA, Australia

Björn Bachmann MD
Cornea, Ocular Surface & Cataract Surgery Specialist
Department of Ophthalmology
Friedrich-Alexander-Universität Erlangen-Nürnberg
Erlangen, Germany

Alireza Baradaran-Rafii MD
Associate Professor of Ophthalmology
Department of Ophthalmology
Cornea & Refractive Surgery Service
Labbafinejad Medical Center
Shahid Beheshti University of Medical Sciences
Tehran, Iran

Priti Batta MD
Attending Staff Physician
New York Eye & Ear Infirmary
New York, NY, USA

Joseph M. Biber MD
Private Practitioner
Private Practice
Horizon Eye Care
Charlotte, NC, USA

Jay C. Bradley MD
Cornea, External Disease, Cataract & Refractive Surgery
    Specialist
University of Illinois Eye and Ear Infirmary
West Texas Eye Associates
Lubbock, TX, USA

Clara C. Chan MD FRCSC
Instructor
Department of Ophthalmology and Vision Sciences
University of Toronto
Toronto, Ontario, Canada

James Chodosh MD MPH
David G. Cogan Professor of Ophthalmology
Massachusetts Eye and Ear Infirmary
Harvard Medical School
Boston, MA, USA

Jessica Chow MD
Assistant professor of ophthalmology
Yale Eye CenterYale
University school of medicine
New Haven, CT, USA

Jeanie J Y Chui MBBS PhD
Postdoctoral Scientist
Department of Ophthalmology
Prince of Wales Hospital
Randwick, NSW, Australia

Jessica Ciralsky MD
Assistant Professor of Ophthalmology
Department of Ophthalmology
Weill Cornell
San Diego, CA, USA

Kathryn A. Colby MD PhD
Associate Professor of Ophthalmology
Harvard Medical School
Surgeon in Ophthalmology
Massachusetts Eye and Ear Infimary
Boston, MA, USA

Byron T. Cook III MD
Chief Resident
Department of Ophthalmology
University of Kentucky College of Medicine
Lexington, KY, USA

Minas T. Coroneo BSc (Med) MB BS MSc (Syd) MD MS (UNSW) FRACS FRANZCO
Professor & Chairman
Department of Ophthalmology
University of New South Wales
Randwick, NSW, Australia

Alexandra Z. Crawford MBChB BA
Research Fellow
Ophthalmology Department
University of Auckland
Auckland, New Zealand

Richard S. Davidson MD
Associate Professor & Vice Chair for Quality and Clinical
    Affairs
Cataract, Cornea, and Refractive Surgery
University of Colorado Eye Center
University of Colorado School of Medicine
Aurora, Colorado, USA

Sheraz M. Daya MD FACP FACS FRCS(Ed) FRCOphth
Chairman & Medical Director
Centre for Sight
East Grinstead, UK

Denise de Freitas MD
Associate Professor of Ophthalmology
Department of Ophthalmology
Paulista Medical School
Federal University of São Paulo
São Paulo, SP, Brazil

Ali R. Djalilian MD
Associate Professor
Illinois Eye and Ear Infirmary
Department of Ophthalmology and Visual Sciences
University of Illinois at Chicago
Chicago, IL, USA

Ana G. Alzaga Fernandez MD
Assistant Professor of Ophthalmology
Department of Ophthalmology
Weill Cornell Medical College
New York, NY, USA

J. Brian Foster MD
Corneal, Cataract & Refractive Surgeon
Private Practice
The Eye Associates
Bradenton/Sarasota, FL, USA

Gary N. Foulks MD FACS
Emeritus Professor of Ophthalmology
Department of Ophthalmology and Vision Science
University of Louisville School of Medicine
Louisville, KY, USA

Elham Ghahari MD
Clinical Fellow in Glaucoma
Department of Ophthalmology
Labbafinejad Medical Center
Shahid Beheshti University of Medical Science
Tehran, Iran
Corneal Research Fellowship
Univeristy of Illinois at Chicago
Chicago, IL, USA

David Goldman MD
Assistant Professor of Clinical Ophthalmology
Bascom Palmer Eye Institute
University of Miami
Palm Beach Gardens, FL, USA

Jose Alvaro Pereira Gomes MD PhD
Associate Professor & Director
Anterior Segment & Ocular Surface Advanced Center (CASO)
Department of Ophthalmology
Federal University of Sao Paulo (UNIFESP/EPM)
Sao Paulo, SP, Brazil

Enrique O. Graue Hernandez MD
Head
Cornea & Refractive Surgery
Instituto de Oftalmología Fundación Conde de Valenciana.
Mexico City, Mexico

Darren G. Gregory MD
Associate Professor of Ophthalmology
Department of Ophthalmology
University of Colorado School of Medicine
Denver, CO, USA

Mark A. Greiner MD
Assistant Professor
Cornea & External Diseases/Refractive Surgery
University of Iowa Hospitals & Clinics
Department of Ophthalmology & Visual Sciences
Iowa City, IA, USA

Pedram Hamrah MD
Assistant Professor of Ophthalmology
Department of Ophthalmology
Massachusetts Eye & Ear Infirmary
Harvard Medical
Boston, MA, USA

Thomas M. Harvey MD
Partner
Chippewa Valley Eye Clinic
Eau Claire, WI, USA

Edward J. Holland MD
Director of Cornea
Cincinnati Eye Institute
Professor of Ophthalmology
University of Cincinnati
Cincinnati, Ohio, USA

Deborah S. Jacobs MD
Medical Director
Boston Foundation for Sight
Needham, MA, USA
Assistant Clinical Professor of Ophthalmology
Harvard Medical School
Massachusetts Eye and Ear
Boston, MA, USA

Bennie H. Jeng MD MS
Professor of Ophthalmology
UCSF Department of Ophthalmology & Proctor Foundation
Co-Director, UCSF Cornea Service
Chief, Department of Ophthalmology, San Francisco General Hospital
San Francisco, CA, USA

Lynette K. Johns OD FAAO
Senior Optometrist
Boston Foundation for Sight
Adjunct Clinical Faculty
The New England College of Optometry
Boston, MA, USA

Carol L. Karp MD
Professor of Ophthalmology
Bascom Palmer Eye Institute
University of Miami School of Medicine
Miami, FL, USA

Douglas G. Katz MD
Associate Professor
Department of Ophthalmology
University of Kentucky
Lexington, KY, USA

Amy T. Kelmenson MD
Cornea, Ocular Surface & Refractive Surgery Fellow
Department of Ophthalmology
Tufts New England Eye Center
Boston, MA, USA

Friedrich E. Kruse MD
Professor of Ophthalmology, Chairman
Department of Ophthalmology
Friedrich-Alexander-Universität Erlangen-Nürnberg
Erlangen, Germany

Judy Y.F. Ku MBChB FRANZCO
Cornea, External Diseases & Refractive Surgery Fellow
Department of Ophthalmology
University of Toronto
Toronto Western Hospital
Toronto, ON, Canada

Hong-Gam Le BA
Clinical Research Assistant
Research
Boston Foundation for Sight
Needham, MA, USA

W. Barry Lee MD FACS
Cornea, External Disease, & Refractive Surgery
Eye Consultants of Atlanta Piedmont Hospital
Medical Director, Georgia Eye Bank & Piedmont Eye
  Surgery Center
Atlanta, GA, USA

Michael A. Lemp MD
Clinical Professor of Ophthalmology
Georgetown University
Centre for Sight
Lake Wales, FL, USA

Jennifer Y. Li MD
Assistant Professor
Department of Ophthalmology & Vision Science
UC Davis Health System Eye Center
University of California, Davis
Sacramento, CA, USA

Lily Koo Lin MD
Assistant Professor
Department of Ophthalmology & Vision Science
University of California Davis Medical Center
Sacramento, CA, USA

Douglas A.M. Lyall MRCOphth
Specialty Registrar
Department of Ophthalmology
University Hospital Ayr
Ayr, Scotland, UK

Marian Macsai MD
Chief, Division of Ophthalmology
NorthShore University HealthSystem
Professor of Ophthalmology
University of Chicago Pritzker School of Medicine
Glenview, IL, USA

Mark J. Mannis MD FACS
Professor and Chair
Department of Ophthalmology & Vision Science
UC Davis Health System Eye Center
University of California, Davis
Sacramento, CA, USA

Kenneth C. Mathys MD
Adjunct Clinical Professor of Ophthalmology
University of North Carolina School of Medicine
Charlotte, NC USA

Charles N.J. McGhee, MB PhD FRCS FRCOphth FRANZCO
Maurice Paykel Professor & Chair of Ophthalmology
Director, New Zealand National Eye Centre
Department of Ophthalmology
Faculty of Medical & Health Sciences
University of Auckland
Auckland, New Zealand

Johannes Menzel-Severing MD MSc
Research Fellow
Department of Ophthalmology
Friedrich-Alexander-Universität Erlangen-Nürnberg
Erlangen, Germany

Shahzad Ihsan Mian MD
Associate Chair, Education
Terry J. Bergstrom Professor
Associate Professor
Department of Ophthalmology & Visual Sciences
University of Michigan
Ann Arbor, MI , USA

Gioconda Mojica MD
Cornea, External Disease & Refractive Surgery Fellow
Department of Ophthalmology
University of Minnesota
Minneapolis, MN, USA

Takahiro Nakamura MD PhD
Associate Professor
Research Center for Inflammation and Regenerative
  Medicine
Faculty of Life & Medical Sciences
Doshisha University
Kyoto, Japan

Alejandro Navas MD MSc
Associate Professor of Ophthalmology
Department of Cornea & Refractive Surgery
Institute of Ophthalmology Conde de Valenciana
Mexico City, Mexico

Kristiana D. Neff MD
Partner
Cornea, Cataract & External Disease
Carolina Cataract & Laser Center
Ladson, SC, USA

Florentino E. Palmon MD
Medical Director
Southwest Florida Eye Care
Fort Myers, FL, USA

Gregory Robert Nettune MD MPH
Cornea, Refractive Surgery & External Disease Fellow
Department of Ophthalmology
Cullen Eye Institute, Baylor College of Medicine
Houston, TX, USA

Lisa M. Nijm MD JD
Assistant Clinical Professor of Ophthalmology
Department of Ophthalmology and Visual Sciences
University of Illinois Eye and Ear Infirmary
Chicago, IL, USA

Florentino E. Palmon MD
Medical Director
Southwest Florida Eye Care
Fort Myers, FL, USA

Ravi Patel MD MBA
Fellow
Corneal, External Disease and Refractive Surgery
Bascom Palmer Eye Institute
University of Miami
Palm Beach Gardens, FL, USA

Dipika V. Patel PhD MRCOphth
Associate Professor of Ophthalmology
Department of Ophthalmology
University of Auckland
Auckland, New Zealand

Victor L. Perez MD
Associate Professor and Director Ocular Surface Center
Ophthalmology, Microbiology and Immunology
Bascom Palmer Eye Institute
University of Miami Miller School of Medicine
Miami, FL, USA

Stephen C. Pflugfelder MD
Professor and Director
Ocular Surface Center
Department of Ophthalmology
Baylor College of Medicine
Houston, TX, USA

Patricia A. Ple-plakon MD
Ophthalmology Resident
Department of Ophthalmology and Visual Sciences
University of Michigan
Ann Arbor, MI, USA

Naresh Polisetti PhD
Post-Doctoral Fellow
Department of Ophthalmology
Friedrich-Alexander-Universität Erlangen-Nürnberg
Erlangen, Germany

Christina R. Prescott MD PhD
Assistant Professor of Ophthalmology
Wilmer Eye Institute
Johns Hopkins University School of Medicine
Baltimore MD, USA

Michael B. Raizman MD
Associate Professor of Ophthalmology
Ophthalmic Consultants of Boston
Department of Ophthalmology
Tufts University School of Medicine
Boston, MA, USA

Arturo Ramirez-Miranda MD
Assistant Professor of Ophthalmology
Department of Cornea & Refractive Surgery
Instituto de Oftalmología Fundacion Conde de Valenciana
   IAP. UNAM
Mexico City, Mexico

Naveen K. Rao MD
Fellow in Cornea, External Disease, and Anterior Segment
   Surgery
Tufts Medical Center/New England Eye Center and
   Ophthalmic Consultants of Boston
Boston, MA, USA

Shawn C. Richards MD
Cornea/Refractive Surgery Fellow
Department of Ophthalmology
University of Colorado - Denver
Aurora, CO, USA

David S. Rootman MD FRCSC
Associate Professor
Department of Ophthalmology and Vision Sciences
University of Toronto
Toronto Western Hospital of the University Health
   Network
Toronto, ON, Canada

Afsun Şahin MD
Assistant Professor of Ophthalmology
Department of Ophthalmology
Eskisehir Osmangazi University Medical School
Eskisehir, Turkey

Ursula Schlötzer-Schrehardt PhD
Associate Professor
Department of Ophthalmology
Friedrich-Alexander-Universität Erlangen-Nürnberg
Erlangen, Germany

Gary S. Schwartz MD
Adjunct Associate Professor
Department of Ophthalmology
University of Minnesota
Stillwater, MN, USA

Anita N. Shukla MD
Clinical Fellow, Cornea & Refractive Surgery
Department of Ophthalmology
Massachusetts Eye & Ear Infirmary
Boston, MA, USA

Heather M. Skeens MD
Cornea, Cataract, and Refractive Surgery
WV Eye Consultants
Charleston, WV, USA

Abraham Solomon MD
Associate Professor of Ophthalmology
Cornea & Refractive Surgery Service
Department of Ophthalmology
Hadassah-Hebrew University Medical Center
Jerusalem, Israel

Sathish Srinivasan FRCSEd FRCOphth
Consultant Corneal Surgeon
Department of Ophthalmology
University Hospital Ayr
Ayr, Scotland, UK

J. Stuart Tims MD
Private Practice
Cornea, Cataract & Refractive Surgery Division
Vistar Eye Center
Roanoke, VA, USA

Julie H. Tsai MD
Assistant Professor
Department of Ophthalmology
Albany Medical College
Albany, NY, USA

Elmer Yuchen Tu MD
Associate Professor of Clinical Ophthalmology
Department of Ophthalmology and Visual Sciences
University of Illinois Eye and Ear Infirmary Chicago
Chicago, IL, USA

Woodford S. Van Meter MD
Professor of Ophthalmology
Department of Ophthalmology
University of Kentucky Medical School
Lexington, KY, USA

Ana Carolina Vieira MD
Post-graduation Student
Federal University of São Paulo, Brazil
Professor of Ophthalmology
State University of Rio de Janeiro
São Paulo, Brazil

Tais Hitomi Wakamatsu MD PhD
Postdoctoral Researcher
Ophthalmology Department
Federal University of São Paulo (UNIFESP)
São Paulo Hospital (HSP)
São Paulo, Brazil

Steven J. Wiffen FRANZCO FRACS
Associate Professor
Centre for Ophthalmology and Visual Science
University of Western Australia
Nedlands, WA, Australia

Fasika A. Woreta MD
Cornea Fellow
Bascom Palmer Eye Institute
Miller School of Medicine
University of Miami
Miami, FL, USA

Sonia N. Yeung MD PhD FRCSC
Assistant Professor
Department of Ophthalmology & Visual Sciences
University of British Columbia
Vancouver, BC, Canada

To
My wife, Lynette for her love, support and guidance
Our children, Colson, Kelsey and Natalie who balance
our lives
–**Edward J. Holland**

To
Judith and our wonderful children, Gabriel, Tova, Avi,
Tara, and Elliott
–**Mark J. Mannis**

To
My wife, Michelle, for her unconditional love and
constant support;
Our children, Ashton, Aidan, and Addy, who remind us
of the importance of family;
My parents, Bill and Bonnie, and sister, Barbara, for
their love and guidance through the years.
–**W. Barry Lee**

Acknowledgements

The production of a text relies on creative, factual and up to date writing all completed in a timely fashion together with a production team that will work with the demands and quirks of the editors and contributors. First of all, we would like to thank the contributing authors whose research and clinical skills provided the latest information to our readers. We appreciate their knowledge and expertise as well as their respect of the tight production schedule. We would also like to thank the team at Elsevier who agreed to take on this project and who worked with us at every step of the way to make this text as good as possible. Russell Gabbedy and Sharon Nash, who headed up the Elsevier team, were a pleasure to work with. In addition, we thank our administrative assistants, Megan Redmond, Roberto Quant, and Suzan Benton, who were invaluable in keeping us organized and on time. We thank Steven Osborne for his beautiful cover design. And finally and most importantly, we thank our families who have supported us and given us the time to complete this book.

PART 1

FUNDAMENTALS

1 *Historical Concepts of Ocular Surface Disease*

W. BARRY LEE and MARK J. MANNIS

Introduction

The ocular surface is the interface between the functioning eye and our environment. This surface provides anatomic, physiologic, and immunologic protection and comprises the palpebral and bulbar conjunctival epithelium, the corneoscleral limbus, the corneal epithelium, and the tear film. While these structures represent the anatomical ocular surface, adnexal structures including the anterior lamellae of the eyelids, eyelashes, meibomian glands, and the lacrimal system are essential for appropriate protection and function of the ocular surface.

The ocular surface functions to maintain optical clarity of the cornea, serves as a refractive surface for accurate projection of light through the ocular media, and provides protection of the structures of the eye against microbes, trauma, and toxins. Creation of an unstable ocular surface from trauma or disease can compromise the integrity of any one of these protective functions and can lead to various forms of corneal and conjunctival dysfunction, broadly ranging from a mild corneal abrasion to severe stem cell loss, decreased vision, and ultimate blindness in the most severe disease. While the health and function of all these structures is imperative for a stable ocular surface, the most important key to anatomic and functional ocular surface stability remains the corneal epithelial stem cells. Our understanding of ocular surface disorders and stem cell physiology has undergone substantial evolution over the last three decades, with remarkable advancements in both corneal epithelial stem cell research as well as medical and surgical techniques for support and restoration of the ocular surface.

Ocular Surface Disease: Advances in Diagnosis & Medical Management

Disorders of the ocular surface include a variety of conditions. Some of the more common conditions encountered in practice include dry eye disease, blepharitis, ocular allergies and pterygia. In addition, less common but more challenging conditions include limbal stem cell deficiency, and ocular surface disease (OSD) from systemic disease (Fig. 1.1). As our understanding of OSD has expanded, the availability of advanced diagnostic tools, medical and surgical therapeutic options, and treatment algorithms for various conditions has enhanced success with OSD. There are classic diagnostic tools for diagnosis of OSD, such as

impression cytology, Schirmer testing, tear break-up time, and vital dye staining of the cornea and conjunctiva. These remain valuable tools, however, new diagnostic devices have emerged (Fig. 1.2). Devices, such as tear osmolarity analysis, matrix metalloproteinase-9 analysis, rapid antigen detection for various ocular infectious diseases, and comprehensive analysis of the tear film and lipid are just some of the new diagnostic devices available. Additional advanced

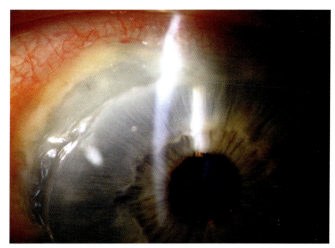

Figure 1.1 Slit lamp photograph of a patient with severe peripheral ulcerative keratitis from rheumatoid arthritis.

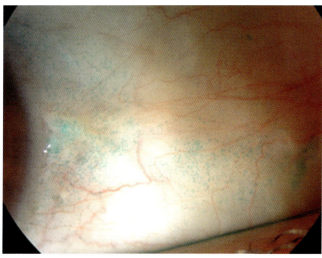

Figure 1.2 A slit lamp photograph demonstrating lissamine green staining of the interpalpebral bulbar conjunctiva in a patient with mild symptoms from dry eye disease.

diagnostic tools include confocal microscopy, optical coherence tomography (OCT) of the anterior segment, and Scheimpflug imaging of the cornea for advanced diagnosis of various OSD states.[1,2] Confocal microscopy enables a detailed investigation of the tarsal and palpebral conjunctiva, central and peripheral cornea, tear film, and eyelids, while affording evaluation of the ocular surface at the cellular level. The device has been particularly useful as a diagnostic tool for cases of atypical keratitis and as a tool to detect phenotypic alterations of the conjunctival epithelium in dry eye disease.[1–3]

Two of the most common OSD challenges remain dry eye disease and blepharitis. Our knowledge of both of these conditions has expanded over the last few decades with both clinical and basic science research to support the key role of inflammation as a major factor in the development of symptoms and clinical findings of these diseases. The combination of factors leading to dry eye states, often referred to as 'dysfunctional tear syndrome,' refers to the compilation of lid margin disease, altered tear film composition, decreased tear volume, diminished corneal sensation, and the presence of anti-inflammatory factors in the tear film.[4] The International Dry Eye Workshop (DEWS) included a panel of international ocular surface disease experts challenged to update and review new concepts of dry eye disease. The group developed current concepts of dry eye disease including definition and classification, diagnosis, epidemiology, treatment and management, and research. A fundamental change in our understanding of dry eye is evident in its current definition: 'Dry eye is a multifactorial disease of the tears and ocular surface that results in symptoms of discomfort, visual disturbance, and tear film instability with potential damage to the ocular surface. It is accompanied by increased osmolarity of the tear film and inflammation of the ocular surface.'[4] DEWS provided levels of disease severity with regard to symptoms and signs of dry eye followed by evidence and consensus-based treatment recommendations for dry eye treatment based on new research linking dry eye disease to inflammation.[4] Similarly, the Meibomian Gland Workshop involved a panel of international experts challenged to expand our understanding of meibomian gland disease (MGD) (Fig. 1.3). The group

developed a contemporary definition and classification of MGD, reviewed methods of diagnosis and evaluation, developed recommendations for the management and therapy of MGD, and presented recommendations for study designs and future research in MGD.[5] The treatment recommendations from these workshops have afforded a better understanding of the underlying pathology of dry eye disease, dysfunctional tear syndrome and blepharitis.

With expanded diagnostic tools and a better understanding of the pathophysiology of various forms of OSD, we have seen an explosion of new therapeutic strategies from novel medication classes to new therapeutic devices. In the past, treatment options for various conditions, such as dry eye disease were limited to environmental modifications, artificial tears, and punctal plugs. Current medical treatment advances for OSD include new topical and oral therapies for allergic eye disease, limbal stem cell deficiency, and dysfunctional tear syndrome. Topical nonsteroidal anti-inflammatory agents, cyclosporine A, mast cell stabilizer/antihistamine agents, and various new formulations of corticosteroids can aid in difficult inflammatory eye conditions, such as severe atopic keratoconjunctivitis and dysfunctional tear syndrome. Medical management of limbal stem cell deficiency includes therapeutic agents from topical vitamin A formulations to autologous serum, various topical growth factors, oral omega 3 fatty acid supplementation, and topical vascular endothelial growth factor (VEGF) inhibitors to counteract corneal neovascularization. In addition, new therapeutic devices, such as meibomian gland probing, intense pulse light therapy, and LipiFlow® can be additive to topical and oral medication regimens for relief of signs and symptoms of various types of OSD.[5]

Origins of the Surgical Management of Severe Ocular Surface Disease

An early concept for the surgical treatment of ocular surface disease (OSD) appeared in 1940 with use of amniotic membrane for the repair of conjunctival defects and symblepharon by De Rotth.[6] In 1951, Hartman suggested the use of a free conjunctival graft for correction of pterygium, pseudopterygium, and symblepharon.[7] This report suggested the benefit of using conjunctiva for grafting procedures and introduced the notion of harvesting conjunctiva from the contralateral eye in selected cases for the surgical treatment of unilateral disease.[7] While Jose Barraquer is credited as the first surgeon to describe stem cell transplant techniques in ocular surface chemical burns,[8] Thoft's description of conjunctival transplantation for monocular chemical burns stands as the basis for the contemporary understanding of ocular surface disease and its treatment.[9] Thoft employed autologous 'conjunctival transplantation' for the treatment of five cases involving unilateral chemical burns of the cornea. The technique required a complete lamellar keratectomy with removal of the epithelium and pannus formation on the corneal surface followed by 360 degrees of limbal conjunctival resection. Four conjunctival grafts were next harvested from the four bulbar conjunctival quadrants in the uninvolved eye, and each graft was fixated to an analogous quadrant of the

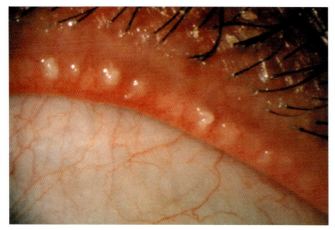

Figure 1.3 High-magnification slit lamp view of severe meibomian gland inspissation in advanced meibomian gland dysfunction.

diseased eye and secured with sutures.[9] The autologous conjunctival graft has stood the test of time and remains the procedure of choice for unilateral stem cell disease as well as contemporary pterygium surgery.

Thoft later described the first allograft procedure, which he termed 'keratoepithelioplasty,' in patients with bilateral OSD. This procedure laid the groundwork for contemporary limbal stem cell transplantation techniques (Fig. 1.4).[10] Keratoepithelioplasty employed four lenticules which included epithelium and a thin layer of stroma harvested from the peripheral cornea of a donor globe. Each lenticule was secured at the corneoscleral limbus of the surface-damaged eye in each of the four quadrants.[10] While kerato-epithelioplasty was the first attempt at transplantation of corneal epithelial stem cells in patients with severe bilateral OSD, neither the origin and location of the corneal limbal stem cells nor their functional physiology were clearly understood at that time.

Corneal Stem Cell Theory and Early Clinical Applications

Corneal epithelial stem cells are the progenitor cells and the source of epithelial regeneration after demise or loss of the corneal epithelium. Throughout the body, adult stem cells are found in limited numbers with long life spans, slow cell cycling capabilities, and less differentiation.[11–15] Despite these characteristics, they do possess the ability to regenerate and repair tissue after injury. Upon activation, stem cells produce progeny, referred to as 'transient amplifying cells' that are responsible for proliferation, differentiation and migration in response to normal physiologic renewal or repair after injury. Daughter cells, in contrast, have short life spans, rapid cell cycling, and high mitotic activity. After epithelial injury, transient amplifying cells migrate centripetally from the limbus and vertically from the basal epithelial layers forward to promote epithelial renewal.[15–19] This process of epithelial cell migration is critical in maintenance of the corneal epithelial mass and its ability to regenerate after injury. The limbus serves as a functional 'barrier,' preventing encroachment of the conjunctival epithelium onto the cornea during normal homeostasis.[19] When this barrier function is impaired, conjunctival epithelium together with blood vessels and fibrous tissue encroach onto the cornea (Fig. 1.5). Loss of this barrier function is one of the first signs in corneal epithelial stem cell deficiency and may result in significant abnormality of the ocular surface.

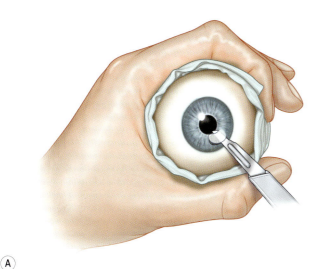

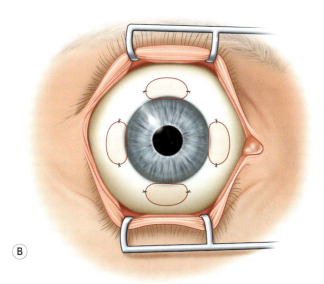

Figure 1.4 Keratoepithelioplasty as described by Thoft. **(A)** Four lenticules are harvested from a donor globe. **(B)** The lenticules are secured to the diseased corneoscleral limbus in equidistant positions. (Reprinted with permission from Albert & Jakobiec's Principles and Practice of Ophthalmology, Saunders 2008;871–80. Figure 65.4.)

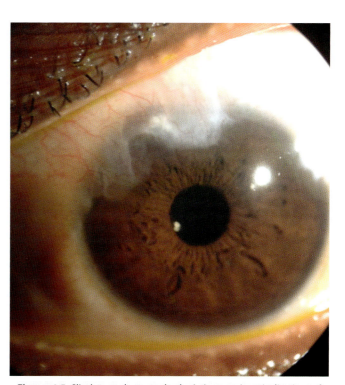

Figure 1.5 Slit lamp photograph depicting conjunctivalization of the cornea related to an alkaline chemical burn. The picture demonstrates loss of the barrier function of the limbus, typical of stem cell deficiency.

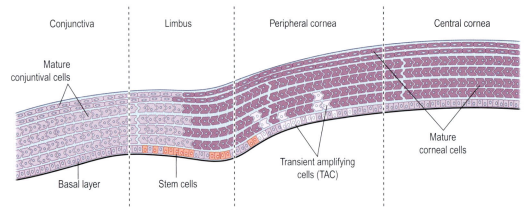

Figure 1.6 A schematic depicting the anatomic location of corneal epithelial stem cells, transient amplifying cells, and mature epithelial cells within the cornea.

While several surgical advancements had been made in the treatment of OSD in the late twentieth century, the pivotal breakthrough occurred with the understanding of the anatomic location and function of the limbal stem cells. Our knowledge of corneal epithelial stem cell location and function is relatively new, having been elaborated over the last three decades. One of the most important initial observations of stem cell presence and function was the observation by Friedenwald that the corneal epithelium regenerated fully after total de-epithelialization.[20] In the 1970s and 1980s, researchers determined that the palisades of Vogt were the location of corneal epithelial stem cells.[21,22] While additional research supported the palisades of Vogt as the anatomic location of corneal epithelial stem cells, several studies have co-located these stem cells in the limbal basal epithelium by identification of cornea-specific keratins (Fig. 1.6).[23–26] Other laboratories provided evidence that stem cells reside at the limbus using tritiated thymidine incorporation into limbal basal cells, demonstrating higher rates of mitotic activity, as well a senhanced cell culture growth from limbal basal epithelium.[27,28] Moreover, other studies demonstrated that limbal stem cells are less differentiated than epithelial cells found elsewhere in the cornea and that stem cells, as well as transient amplifying cells (TAC), constitute the proliferating cells of the epithelium that are responsible for repair after injury.[29,30]

With clarification of the location and function of corneal stem cells, Kenyon and Tseng[31] were the first to provide clinical translational applications of stem cell theory. In 1989, they modified Thoft's original procedure to include limbal stem cells in the conjunctival transplantation procedure. This represented the first programmatic clinical use of transplanted limbal stem cells for severe OSD and represents the initiation of true stem cell autografting techniques (Fig. 1.7).[31]

In 1994, Tsai and Tseng[32] modified Thoft's keratoepithelioplasty technique and called it 'allograft limbal transplantation,' using a donor whole globe to provide a keratolimbal graft for the treatment of severe OSD. The cadaveric keratolimbal ring was divided into three equal pieces and was transferred to the recipient eye. The authors employed oral cyclosporine in additional to topical immunosuppression for postoperative treatment. This represented the first keratolimbal allograft (KLAL) with adjunct systemic immunosuppression in limbal stem cell transplant for treatment of severe OSD. Tsubota and colleagues[33] further modified the KLAL procedure and were the first to report use of stored corneoscleral rims for stem cell transplantation in OSD. The concept of stored tissue for ocular surface reconstruction engendered new considerations in eye banking that established the groundwork for modified procedures in tissue procurement and delivery for transplant.

Kwitko and colleagues[34] developed the concept of using living-related ocular tissue as allografts for the treatment of bilateral OSD in 1995. They described a technique referred to as 'allograft conjunctival transplantation' in which harvested conjunctival tissue (not limbal tissue) was obtained from siblings or a parent and transplanted to the recipient eye of the affected relative. Kenyon and Rapoza[35] expanded this concept to include conjunctival and limbal tissue in a technique similar to Kenyon's earlier report of limbal autografting. However, their procedure utilized donor tissue from a living relative rather than the contralateral eye. This technique formed the basis for using living-related limbal tissue for transplantation to a relative with bilateral severe OSD, in which the contralateral eye cannot be used for limbal autografting techniques. Topical and systemic immunosuppression were employed as adjuncts in all of the living-related allograft cases.[35]

Ocular Surface Disease: Contemporary Advances in Surgical Management

A major landmark in the surgical treatment of OSD occurred with the development of a uniform classification system to describe the variety of proposed surgical techniques for restoration of the ocular surface. Holland and colleagues developed a nomenclature that included a standardization of surgical techniques based on the donor and the tissue transplanted with corresponding acronyms. In addition, the nomenclature was linked to treatment algorithms for the implementation of specific techniques based on the severity and laterality of OSD.[36–39] Moreover, in conjunction with corneal surgeons interested in ocular surface disease, the eye banking system developed eye banking

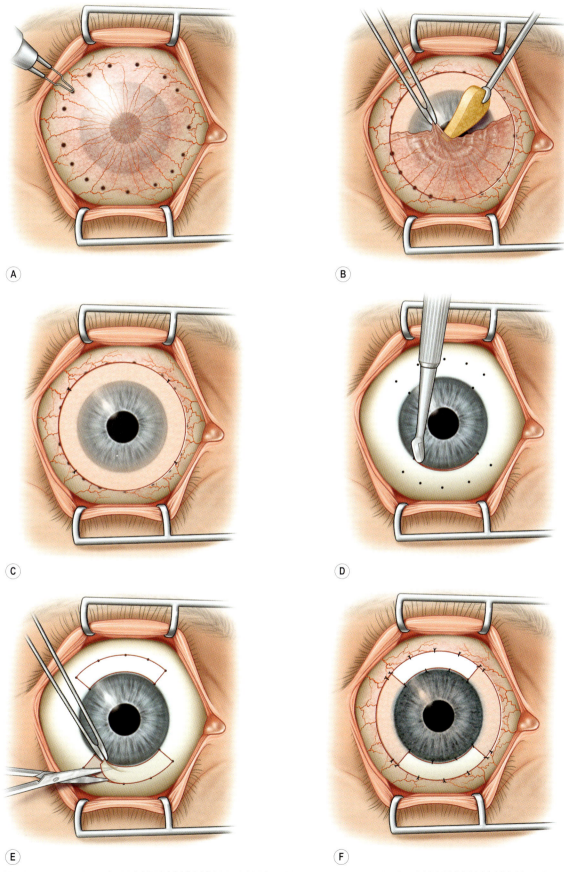

Figure 1.7 A depiction of the original description of limbal allografting from Kenyon and Tseng. (Reproduced with permission form Kenyon KR, Tseng SCG. Limbal autograft transplantation for ocular surface disorders. Ophthalmology 1989;96:709–23.)

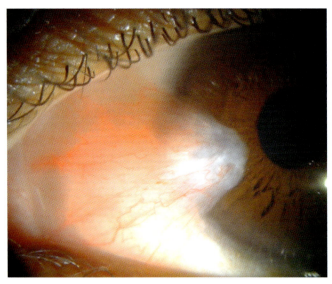

Figure 1.8 A slit lamp photograph demonstrating a recurrent pterygium.

criteria and the establishment of procurement and tissue processing regimens specific to the delivery of corneoscleral limbal tissue to surgeons treating OSD.[37] Further advances in eye banking protocols for the harvesting and delivery of limbal tissue for transplantation followed the development of surgical treatment classifications for OSD.

Pterygium surgery represents one of the most common examples of an OSD that requires surgical intervention for a cure (Fig. 1.8). This is hardly surprising given the relatively recent understanding of its pathophysiology that demonstrates a localized stem cell dysfunction in combination with genetic factors and inflammation play a key role in its development. A recent review of the surgical treatment of pterygia demonstrated a wide variety of surgical approaches exist, owing to the difficulty in curing this condition.[40] The review recommendations reported that the bare sclera excision of pterygium results in a significantly higher recurrence rate than excision accompanied by use of certain adjuvants. Additional adjuvants utilized in pterygium surgery include amniotic membrane, conjunctival autografts, fibrin glue for graft adherence, and antifibrotic agents, such as mitomycin C. Conjunctival or limbal autograft was superior to amniotic membrane graft surgery in reducing the rate of pterygium recurrence in the review of adjunvants.[40] Advanced surgical techniques corroborate the findings of the review, suggesting conjunctival or limbal autografts are associated with very low recurrence rates.[41]

In conditions with more diffuse OSD or limbal stem cell deficiency, KLAL modifications have improved surgical outcomes and ultimate success in the surgical treatment of severe OSD. Croasdale and Holland[37,38] expanded on the KLAL technique of Tsubota by employing two stored corneoscleral rims rather than one. The two rims were each bisected, creating four harvested 180-degree crescents of limbal tissue. Three of the four pieces of cadaveric tissue were transplanted to the recipient eye. This technique allowed for complete coverage of the recipient limbus by donor tissue and delivered one-and-a-half times the

transplanted limbal stem cells than could be derived from a single corneoscleral limbal rim.[36,37]

Another modification to the KLAL procedure was developed for patients with severe conjunctival deficiency in conditions, such as Stevens–Johnson syndrome or ocular cicatricial pemphigoid.[42] The technique has been referred to as the 'Cincinnati procedure' and employs the use of living-related conjunctival and limbal tissue harvested from a sibling or parent. The allograft tissue (lr-CLAL) is applied to the surface deficient eye of the recipient/relative in the superior and inferior four hours after epithelial debridement and a 360-degree conjunctival peritomy. Following this, a cadaveric KLAL is applied to the nasal and temporal limbus of the diseased eye with a technique similar to that described by Croasdale et al.[37] (with the exception of using a single donor corneoscleral rim), making sure to avoid any gap areas in donor tissue at the recipient limbus.[42]

Another significant advance in ocular surface transplantation has been the development of techniques for ex vivo expansion of autologous or living-related stem cells. While the idea of cultured corneal epithelial stem cells was considered as early as 1982,[43] the first clinical reports of cultured autologous limbal stem cell transplantation did not appear until 1996 and 1997.[44,45] Torfi and Schwab first reported success with cultured autologous grafts delivered to the damaged eye and demonstrated improvement in ocular surface function in three of four patients with severe unilateral disease.[44] Similarly, Pellegrini and colleagues described ocular surface restoration in two patients with severe unilateral stem cell deficiency using autologous cultured corneal epithelial stem cells expanded in the laboratory and delivered to the diseased eye as a cultivated corneal epithelial sheet attached to a therapeutic bandage lens.[45] Both groups confirmed that a small 1–2-mm^2 limbal biopsy provides sufficient amounts of cultured corneal epithelial cells to restore the entire corneal–limbal surface after expansion in culture.[44,45] Techniques of ex vivo expansion of both autologous and living-related stem cells continue to evolve, with successful ex vivo expansion of limbal stem cells for grafting.[45–49]

A critical concept that has evolved in ocular stem cell transplantation is the use of adjunct immunosuppression. Immunosuppression has been employed to enhance the outcomes of ocular surface transplantation including the use of both topical as well as oral immunosuppressive agents. Holland and colleagues[50] have stressed the importance of approaching systemic immunosuppression in ocular surface transplantation in a fashion similar to solid organ transplantation. In addition, these authors have demonstrated the safety and efficacy of immunosuppression in ocular surface patients.[50] Studies have demonstrated that ocular surface transplantation in the absence of systemic immunosuppression leads to high failure rates when compared with procedures accompanied by systemic immunosuppression.[38,51,52]

Amniotic membrane transplantation (AMT) has been a useful adjunct to ocular surface transplantation when used in conjunction with limbal stem cell transplant. AMT can provide a scaffold for amplification and delivery of stem cells in ex vivo expansion techniques. While AMT is not used alone in conditions of limbal stem cell deficiency, several studies have shown that it can facilitate epithelial growth and reduce ocular surface inflammation when used in conjunction with other techniques, such as KLAL or ex vivo expansion of stem cells.[53,54]

Just as there have been both advancements in disease classification and a proliferation of new surgical techniques for OSD, immunosuppressive therapy has advanced in parallel. Earlier, adjunct immunosuppressive therapy typically included the use of oral cyclosporine and corticosteroids. Treatment models for immunosuppression have expanded with the development of new systemic anti-inflammatory agents and new classes of immunosuppressive agents, which will be elaborated upon in later chapters. Medication classes, such as immunophilin binders and antimetabolites include agents with decreased systemic side effects. In addition, we have seen the emergence of new drug classes with potent systemic immunosuppressive effects, such as polyclonal and monoclonal antibodies. Topical cyclosporine has been another useful adjunct for postoperative treatment after ocular surface transplantation. Immunosuppressive drugs are now typically combined with topical corticosteroids and topical cyclosporine following limbal stem cell transplantation. This is most effectively accomplished with a multi-disciplinary team approach involving the ocular surface specialist, internal medicine and transplant services for the monitoring of graft success and potential medication-induced local and systemic side effects.[50]

The next advances in ocular surface transplantation will involve the continued development, standardization, and enhancement of ex vivo stem cell expansion techniques for treatment of OSD. A number of materials have been employed as stem cell carriers for ex vivo expansion techniques ranging from collagen and de-epithelialized amniotic membrane to therapeutic soft contact lenses, fibrin gel, oral mucosal cells and silk fibroin.[44–49,55–57] No 'gold standard' has been developed to date. Investigators are exploring additional sources of stem cells, including stem cells from hair follicles, embryonic stem cells, conjunctival epithelial stem cells, dental pulp, umbilical cord lining, and bone marrow-derived mesenchymal stem cells.[58] Despite these advances, a multitude of challenges with ex vivo stem cell expansion persist. These challenges include the development of the ideal carrier for stem cells from the laboratory to the diseased ocular surface, the lack of a definite limbal epithelial stem cell marker to monitor graft quality and the likelihood of a successful expansion and transplantation, and methods of assessment of cultured stem cell therapy in limbal stem cell deficiency without a known marker. Regardless of the challenges, several reports cite improved outcomes for treatment of limbal stem cell deficiency, including a recent meta-analysis performed by Baylis et al.[59] which included the outcomes of cultured limbal epithelial cell therapy published since 1997 (583 patients). The overall success rate of cultured ex vivo expanded stem cell transplantation at the time of the review was 76%.[59] Individual centers have also reported success using cultivated oral mucosal epithelial transplantation to deliver autologous stem cells for the treatment of severe OSD with successfully restored ocular surfaces in patients as long as 35 months after surgery.[56–58] Rama et al.[60] have reported outcomes in 112 patients with corneal damage due to limbal stem cell deficiency who underwent autologous cultivated stem cell transplants using a fibrin carrier, the largest series of patients to date. The study observed permanent restoration of the ocular surface in 77% of patients undergoing autologous cultivated (ex vivo expanded) stem cell transplantation, with the majority of OSD cases resulting from chemical ocular surface burns.[60]

In the following chapters, we plan to cover the broad array of medical and surgical treatment modalities currently available for the management of ocular surface disease. Even at this writing the field is undergoing kaleidoscopic change as our understanding of the pathophysiology of the ocular surface continues to broaden.

References

1. Tu EY, Joslin CE, Sugar J, et al. The relative value of confocal microscopy and superficial corneal scrapings in the diagnosis of Acanthamoeba keratitis. Cornea 2008;27:764–72.
2. Lee WB, Gotay A. Bilateral Acanthamoeba keratitis in synergeyes contact lens wear: clinical and confocal microscopy findings. Eye & Contact Lens 2010;36:164–9.
3. Kieval JZ, Karp CL, Abou Shousha M, et al. Ultra-high resolution optical coherence tomography for differentiation of ocular surface squamous neoplasia and pterygia. Ophthalmology 2012;119:481–6.
4. Pflugfelder S (committee chairman). Management and therapy of dry eye disease: report of the Management and Therapy Subcommittee of the International Dry Eye WorkShop (2007). Ocul Surf 2007;5:163–78.
5. Geerling G, Tauber J, Baudouin C, et al. The international workshop on meibomian gland dysfunction: report of the subcommittee on management and treatment of meibomian gland dysfunction. Invest Ophthalmol Vis Sci 2011;52:2050–64.
6. De Rotth A. Plastic repair of conjunctival defects with fetal membrane. Arch Ophthalmol 1940;23:522–5.
7. Hartman DC. Use of free grafts in correction of recurrent pterygia, pseudopterygia and symblepharon. California Med 1951;75:279–80.
8. Holland EJ, Schwartz GS. The Paton Lecture: ocular surface transplantation: 10 year's experience. Cornea 2004;23:425–31.
9. Albert DM, Miller JW, Azar DT, et al. Albert & Jakobiec's Principles and practice of ophthalmology. Saunders 2008;871–80. Figure 65.4.
10. Thoft RA. Keratoepithelioplasty. Am J Ophthalmol 1984;97:1–6.
11 Lajtha LG. Stem cell concepts. Differentiation 1979;14:23–34.
12. Leblond CP. The life history of cells in renewing systems. Am J Anat 1981;160:114–58.
13. Tseng SCG. Concept and application of limbal stem cells. Eye 1989;3:141–57.
14. Kinoshita S, Adachi W, Sotozono C, et al. Characteristics of the human ocular surface epithelium. Prog Ret Eye Res 2001;20:639–73.
15. Dua HS, Azuara-Blanco A. Limbal stem cells of the corneal epithelium. Surv Ophthalmol 2000;44:415–25.
16. Lehrer MS, Sun TT, Lavker RM. Strategies of epithelial repair: modulation of stem cell and transient amplifying cell proliferation. J Cell Sci 1998;111:2867–75.
17. Thoft RA, Friend J. The X, Y, Z hypothesis of corneal epithelial maintenance. Invest Ophthalmol Vis Sci 1983;24:1442–3.
18. Dua HS, Gomes JA, Singh A. Corneal epithelial wound healing. Br J Ophthalmol 1994;78:401–8.
19. Dua HS, Miri A, Alomar T, et al. The role of the limbal stem cells in corneal epithelial maintenance. Ophthalmology 2009;116:856–63.
20. Friedenwald JS. Growth pressure and metaplasia of conjunctival and corneal epithelium. Doc Ophthalmol 1951;5:184–92.
21. Davanger M, Evensen A. Role of the pericorneal papillary structure in renewal of corneal epithelium. Nature 1971;229:560–1.
22. Goldberg MF, Bron AJ. Limbal palisades of Vogt. Trans Am Ophthalmol Soc 1982;80:155–71.
23. Schermer A, Galvin S, Sun TT. Differentiation-related expression of major 64K corneal keratin in vivo and in culture suggests limbal location of corneal epithelial stem cells. J Cell Biol 1986;103:49–62.

24. Cotsarelis G, Cheng SZ, Dong G, et al. Existence of slow-cycling limbal epithelial basal cells that can be preferentially stimulated to proliferate: implications on epithelial stem cells. Cell 1989;57:201–9.
25. Kasper M, Moll R, Stosiec P, et al. Patterns of cytokeratin and vimentin expression in the human cycle. Histochemistry 1988;89:369–73.
26. Pellegrini G, Golisano O, Paterna P, et al. Location and clonal analysis of stem cells and their differentiated progeny in the human ocular surface. J Cell Biol 1999;145:769–82.
27. Cotsarelis G, Dong G, Sun TT, et al. Differential response of limbal and corneal epithelia to phorbol myristate acetate (TPA). ARVO Abstracts. Invest Ophthalmol Vis Sci 1987;28(suppl.):1.
28. Ebato B, Friend J, Thoft RA. Comparison of limbal and peripheral human corneal epithelium in tissue culture. Invest Ophthalmol Vis Sci 1988;29:1533–7.
29. Lathja LG. Stem cell concepts. Differentiation 1979;14:23–34.
30. Kinoshita S, Friend J, Thoft RA. Biphasic cell proliferation in trans-differentiation of conjunctival to corneal epithelium in rabbits. Invest Ophthalmol Vis Sci 1983;24:1008–14.
31. Kenyon KR, Tseng SCG. Limbal autograft transplantation for ocular surface disorders. Ophthalmology 1989;96:709–23.
32. Tsai RJF, Tseng SCG. Human allograft limbal transplantation for corneal surface reconstruction. Cornea 1994;13:389–400.
33. Tsubota K, Toda I, Saito H, et al. Reconstruction of the corneal epithelium by limbal allograft transplantation for severe ocular surface disorders. Ophthalmology 1995;102:1486–95.
34. Kwitko S, Raminho D, Barcaro S, et al. Allograft conjunctival transplantation for bilateral ocular surface disorders. Ophthalmology 1995;102:1020–5.
35. Kenyon KR, Rapoza PA. Limbal allograft transplantation for ocular surface disorders. Ophthalmology 1995;102:101–2.
36. Holland EJ. Epithelial transplantation for the management of severe ocular surface disease. Trans Am Ophthalmol Soc 1996;19:677–743.
37. Croasdale CR, Schwartz GS, Malling JV, et al. Keratolimbal allograft: recommendations for tissue procurement and preparation by eye banks, and standard surgical technique. Cornea 1999;18:52–8.
38. Holland EJ, Schwartz GS. Changing concepts in the management of severe ocular surface disease over twenty-five years. Cornea 2000;19:688–98.
39. Daya SM, Chan CC, Holland EJ, et al. Cornea Society nomenclature for ocular surface rehabilitative procedures. Cornea 2011;30:1115–9.
40. Kaufman SC, Jacobs DS, Lee WB, et al. Options and adjuvants in surgery for pterygium. Ophthalmology 2013;120:201–8.
41. Hirst LW. Prospective study of primary pterygium surgery using pterygium extended removal followed by extended conjunctival transplantation. Ophthalmology 2008;115:1663–72.
42. Biber JM, Skeens HM, Neff KD, et al. The Cincinnati procedure: technique and outcomes of combined living-related conjunctival limbal allografts and keratolimbal allografts in severe ocular surface failure. Cornea 2011;30:765–71.
43. Friend J, Kinoshita S, Thoft RA, et al. Corneal epithelial cell cultures on stroma carriers. Invest Ophthalmol Vis Sci 1982;23:41–9.
44. Torfi H, Schwab IR, Isseroff R. Transplantation of cultured autologous limbal stem cells for ocular surface disease (abstract). In Vitro 1996;32:47A.
45. Pellegrini G, Traverso CE, Franzi AT, et al. Long-term restoration of damaged corneal surfaces with autologous cultivated corneal epithelium. Lancet 1997;349:990–3.
46. Schwab IR, Reyes M, Isseroff RR. Successful transplantation of bioengineered tissue replacements in patients with ocular surface disease. Cornea 2000;19:421–6.
47. Shimazaki J, Aiba M, Goto E, et al. Transplantation of human limbal epithelium cultivated on amniotic membrane for the treatment of severe ocular surface disorders. Ophthalmology 2002;109:1285–90.
48. Han B, Schwab IR, Madsen TK, et al. A fibrin-based bioengineered ocular surface with human corneal epithelial stem cells. Cornea 2002;21:505–10.
49. Sangwan VS, Matalia HP, Vemuganti GK, et al. Early results of penetrating keratoplasty after cultivated limbal epithelium transplantation. Arch Ophthalmol 2005;123:334–40.
50. Holland EJ, Mogilishetty G, Skeens HM, et al. Systemic immunosuppression in ocular surface stem cell transplantation: results of a 10-year experience. Cornea 2012;31:655–61.
51. Rao SK, Rajagopal R, Sitalakshmi G, et al. Limbal allografting from related live donors for corneal surface reconstruction. Ophthalmology 1999;106:822–8.
52. Daya SM. Living-related conjunctivo-limbal allograft (lr-CLAL) for the treatment of stem cell deficiency: an analysis for long-term outcomes. Ophthalmology 1999;106(suppl.):243.
53. Tsubota K, Satake Y, Ohyama M, et al. Surgical reconstruction of the ocular surface in advanced ocular cicatricial pemphigoid and Stevens–Johnson syndrome. Am J Ophthalmol 1996;122:38–52.
54. Tseng SC, Prabhasawat P, Barton K, et al. Amniotic membrane transplantation with or without limbal allografts for corneal surface reconstruction in patients with limbal stem cell deficiency. Arch Ophthalmol 1998;116:431–41.
55. Harkin DG, George KA, Madden PW, et al. Silk fibroin in ocular tissue reconstruction. Biomaterials 2011;32:2445–58.
56. Nishida K, Yamato M, Hayashida Y, et al. Corneal reconstruction with tissue-engineered cell sheets composed of autologous oral mucosal epithelium. N Engl J Med 2004;351:1187–96.
57. Nakamura T, Inatomi T, Sotozono C, et al. Transplantation of cultivated autologous oral mucosal epithelial cells in patients with severe ocular surface disorders. Br J Ophthalmol 2004;88:1280–4.
58. O'Callaghan AR, Daniels JT. Concise review: limbal epithelial stem cell therapy: controversies and challenges. Stem Cells 2011;29:1923–32.
59. Baylis O, Figueiredo F, Henein C, et al. 13 years of cultured limbal epithelial cell therapy: a review of the outcomes. J Cell Biochem 2011;112:993–1002.
60. Rama P, Matuska S, Paganoni, et al. Limbal stem cell therapy and long-term corneal regeneration. N Engl J Med 2010;363:147–55.

2 Eyelid Anatomy and Function

LILY KOO LIN

Introduction

Maintaining a healthy ocular surface starts with a good understanding of eyelid anatomy and function. The eyelids are vital in promoting the spread of tears, lubricating the corneal surface, and protecting the eye from dust and foreign bodies. A disruption in the eyelid anatomy can prove to be harmful to the integrity of the cornea and ocular surface.

Overview of External Anatomy

The eyelids comprise of an upper and lower eyelid, joined at the medial and lateral canthi. The average aperture of the eyelids measures about 30 mm in horizontal width, and approximately 10 mm in vertical height. The highest peak on the upper eyelid lies slightly nasal, and the lowest contour of the lower eyelid rests slightly lateral. The upper eyelid generally covers 1–3 mm of the upper cornea, and the lower eyelid typically rests at, or near the lower limbus. The upper eyelid crease falls 6–10 mm from the eyelid lash line. The brow is positioned anterior to the superior orbital rim.[1–4]

The eyelid is structurally divided into two anatomical lamellae: the anterior and posterior lamellae. The anterior lamella is comprised of the skin and orbicularis oculi muscle, and the posterior lamella is made up of the tarsal plate and conjunctiva. The gray line is considered the junction of the anterior and posterior lamellae.

EYELID SKIN

The eyelid skin is one of the thinnest of the body, lacking subcutaneous fat, with just loose connective tissue between the eyelid skin and orbicularis oculi. The eyelid skin is less than 1 mm in thickness. The constant dynamic movement of the thin eyelid skin is thought to contribute to age-related eyelid skin laxity.

EYELID MUSCLES: PROTRACTORS

The main protractor of the eyelid, which serves to close the eye, is the orbicularis oculi. It is innervated by the facial nerve, and divided into the pretarsal, preseptal, and orbital portions (Fig. 2.1). The pretarsal and preseptal portions are used in spontaneous blink, and the orbital portion is needed for forced eyelid closure. Facial nerve palsy can lead to lagophthalmos and incomplete blink.

The pretarsal orbicularis deep origins are located on the posterior lacrimal crest, with superficial origins on the anterior limb of the medial canthal tendon. The deep head or Horner's tensor tarsi encircle both canaliculi and are important for lacrimal pump function. The pretarsal orbicularis oculi of the upper and lower lids laterally fuse together to form the lateral canthal tendon.

The preseptal portion originates on the posterior lacrimal crest, as well as the medial portion of the anterior limb of the medial canthal tendon and the lateral portion of the lateral palpebral raphe over the lateral orbital rim.

The orbital portion of the orbicularis oculi arises from the anterior limb of the medial canthal tendon and periosteum.

The corrugators are also protractors, and originate on the superonasal rim and end at head of the brows. Corrugators promote vertical glabellar furrows. The procerus is also a protractor and runs vertically from the frontal bone to the head of the brows and causes horizontal furrows.

EYELID MUSCLES: RETRACTORS

The eyelid muscle retractors serve to open the eye. The retractors of the upper eyelid are the levator palpebrae superioris and Müllers muscles, as well as the frontalis. The lower lid retractors are the capsulopalpebral muscle and the inferior tarsal/palpebral muscle.

Upper Lid Retractor: Levator

The primary retractor of the upper eyelid is the levator muscle. The levator originates on the orbital roof near the apex, in front of the optic foramen and anterior to the superior rectus muscle. The levator muscle portion is 40 mm long, and the levator aponeurosis is 14–20 mm length.

Whitnall's ligament or superior traverse ligament is a condensation of elastic fibers of the anterior sheath of the

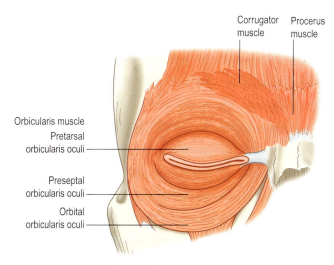

Figure 2.1 The eyelid protractors. (From Nerad JA. Techniques in Ophthalmic Plastic Surgery: A Personal Tutorial. 1st ed. Philadelphia: Elsevier Health Sciences; 2009. Chapter 2, Clinical Anatomy, Fig 2.15 p.37.)

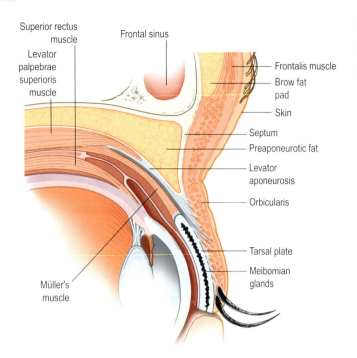

Figure 2.2 Cross-section of the upper eyelid. (From Nerad JA. Techniques in Ophthalmic Plastic Surgery: A Personal Tutorial. 1st ed. Philadelphia: Elsevier Health Sciences; 2009. Chapter 2, Clinical Anatomy, Fig 2.21, p.41.)

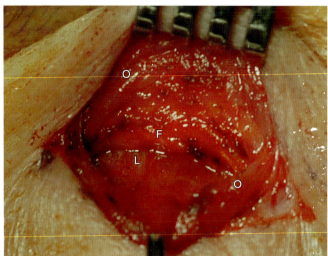

Figure 2.3 The levator aponeurosis: O, orbicularis oculi; F, preaponeurotic fat; L, attenuated levator aponeurosis.

levator muscle. It is located between the transition of the levator aponeurosis and muscle. It provides the suspension support for the upper eyelid and superior orbital tissues. It is thought to transfer the vector of force of the levator muscle from anterior–posterior to superior–inferior. It is analogous to Lockwood's ligament in the lower eyelid. Medially it attaches near the trochlea and superior oblique tendon, and laterally, it runs through the lacrimal gland, and attaches to the inside of the lateral orbital wall, approximately 10 mm above the lateral tubercle.[1–4]

The levator aponeurosis divides into an anterior and posterior portion just above the superior tarsal border. The anterior portion inserts into the pretarsal orbicularis. The most superior portion of these attachments forms the eyelid crease with contraction of the levator complex (Fig. 2.2). The posterior portion inserts onto the anterior surface of the tarsus. The aponeurosis appears as a thick whitish band between Whitnall's ligament and the tarsal plate (Fig. 2.3).

The medial horn of levator aponeurosis inserts onto the posterior lacrimal crest.

The lateral horn divides the orbital and palpebral lobes of the lacrimal gland, then inserts onto the lateral orbital tubercle. The lateral horn is much stronger than the medial horn and this is thought to account for temporal flare in thyroid eye disease.

Upper Lid Retractor: Müller's Muscle

Müller's muscle originates underneath the levator aponeurosis, 12–13 mm above the upper tarsal margin. It is 15–20 mm wide. It is sympathetically innervated, extends inferiorly to insert at the superior tarsal border, and provides 2 mm of elevation. If interrupted, as in Horner's syndrome, it causes a mild ptosis. Müller's muscle is firmly attached to the palpebral conjunctiva. The peripheral

arterial arcade is located between the levator aponeurosis and Müller's muscle above the superior tarsal border and can serve as a useful surgical landmark.[1–4]

Upper Lid Retractor: Frontalis

The frontalis muscle acts to lift the eyebrows and is considered a weak retractor of the upper lids. Elevation of the brow can cause 2 mm of elevation of the upper eyelid. Contraction of the frontalis muscle causes horizontal furrows in the forehead. The absence of frontalis over the tail end of the brow accounts for brow hooding, often seen with age. The frontal nerve, the superior branch of the facial nerve, innervates the frontalis.

Lower Lid Retractors

The lower eyelid retractors serve to depress the eyelid in downgaze, and maintain the upright position of the tarsal plate. The capsulopalpebral fascia in the lower lid is analogous to the levator in the upper lid (Fig. 2.4). It is fibrous tissue that originates from the sheath of the inferior rectus muscle, divides as it encircles the inferior oblique and fuses with the sheath of the inferior oblique. Then the two portions join to form Lockwood's ligament.

The inferior tarsal muscle, also known as the inferior palpebral muscle, is analogous to Müllers muscle in the upper eyelid. It runs between the capsulopalpebral fascia and conjunctiva. It starts at Lockwood's ligament and extends to the inferior conjunctival fornix with insertion onto the inferior tarsal border, where it fuses with the orbital septum. It is also sympathetically innervated. Sympathetic disruption, as in Horner's syndrome, accounts for 'inverse or reverse ptosis' of the lower eyelid. The lower lid retractors are not easily separated and are often collectively referred to as the lower lid retractors.

SEPTUM

The orbital septum lies anterior to fat and serves as an anatomic boundary. The thin fibrous tissue arises from periosteum of the bony rims. The upper eyelid septum fuses with the levator aponeurosis superior to the tarsal plate. The

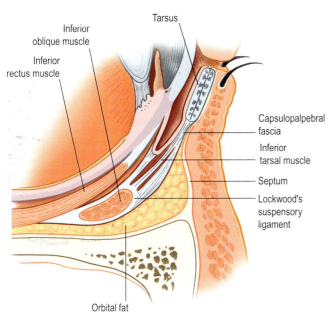

Figure 2.4 Cross-section of the lower eyelid. (From Nerad JA. Techniques in Ophthalmic Plastic Surgery: A Personal Tutorial. 1st ed. Philadelphia: Elsevier Health Sciences; 2009. Chapter 2, Clinical Anatomy, Fig 2.28, p.43.)

lower lid septum fuses with capsulopalpebral fascia, at or below inferior tarsal border.

ORBITAL FAT

The orbital fat serves as a barrier between the orbital structures and eyelid, and can limit the spread of infection and hemorrhage. Orbital fat lies posterior to septum and anterior to aponeurosis in the upper lid. With age-related attenuation of the septum, orbital fat herniation can be seen. The upper eyelid has two fat compartments, the medial fat pad and the larger central fat pad. The central fat pad or pre-aponeurotic fat pad in the upper eyelid is an important surgical landmark. The lower eyelid contains three fat compartments, the medial, central, and lateral.

TARSUS

The tarsal plate is firm, dense connective tissue and measures 1 mm in thickness, and measures 10–12 mm vertically in the upper eyelid, and 4 mm in vertical height in the lower lid. The tarsus contains the meibomian glands. The tarsus is rigidly attached to the periosteum medially and laterally. The marginal arcade is located 2 mm superior to the margin along the upper eyelid tarsus. The peripheral arcade is located superior to the tarsal border, between levator and Müller's muscles. The lower eyelid has one arterial arcade located at the inferior tarsal border.

Meibomian Glands

The meibomian glands originate in the tarsus with 25 glands in the upper lid and 20 in the lower. The meibomian

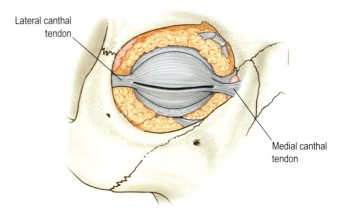

Figure 2.5 The canthal tendons. (From Nerad JA. Techniques in Ophthalmic Plastic Surgery: A Personal Tutorial. 1st ed. Philadelphia: Elsevier Health Sciences; 2009. Chapter 2, Clinical Anatomy, Fig 2.17, p.38.)

glands produce oils, which keep the aqueous of the tear film from evaporating. Both eyelashes and meibomian glands differentiate from the pilosebaceous unit.

During trauma or chronic irritation, a lash follicle may develop from a meibomian gland (acquired distichiasis). An extra row of lashes from the meibomian glands present from birth is congenital distichiasis.

Conjunctiva and the Tear Film

The conjunctiva lines the surface of the eye and the posterior aspect of the eyelids. The bulbar conjunctiva lines the eye, the palpebral portion on the posterior aspect of the eyelids, and the fornix is the reflection. It is most adherent at the limbus, and has redundancy at the fornices. The main function of the conjunctiva is to lubricate the eye. It is made of nonkeratinizing squamous epithelium with mucin-producing goblet cells throughout.

The tear film comprises an inner mucous layer, a middle aqueous layer and a top oil layer. The lacrimal gland and accessory glands produce the aqueous. The lacrimal gland is located superotemporally in the orbit, within the lacrimal gland fossa. The majority of the accessory glands are dispersed along the superior tarsal border and the upper eyelid fornix, and few are located in the inferior fornix. The oil layer is produced by the sebaceous glands, which comprises the meibomian glands and glands of Zeis.

Canthal Tendons

The canthal tendons are extensions of the orbicularis muscle and attach to the periorbita/periosteum over bone (Fig. 2.5).

The medial canthal tendon divides to form attachments onto the anterior and posterior lacrimal crests which surround the lacrimal sac. The attachments overlying the anterior lacrimal crest are strong. The attachments to the posterior lacrimal crest are delicate but are thought to be more critical in maintaining apposition of the eyelid to the globe.

Laterally, the superior and inferior limbs of the lateral canthal tendon attach to the lateral orbital tubercle (Whitnall's tubercle) on the inner aspect of the orbital rim. Eyelid instability or malposition is often attributed to lateral canthal disinsertion or attenuation. The lateral canthal tendon inserts 2 mm higher than the medial canthal tendon.

Eyelid Margin

The eyelid margin measures 2 mm wide. On the most posterior aspect of the eyelid margin lies the mucocutaneous junction, where the palpebral conjunctiva lines the eyelid. More anteriorly are the meibomian gland orifices. The gray line is a section of pretarsal orbicularis (Riolan), located between the meibomian gland orifices and the ciliary follicles. There are approximately 100 eyelash follicles in the upper eyelid, and 50 in the lower.

Lacrimal Drainage System

The gateways of lacrimal drainage are the puncta. The puncta are located medially on the upper and lower eyelids, on lacrimal papilla. The puncta are on the posterior aspect of the eyelid margin, and are medial to the ciliary border. The upper punctum is medial to the lower lid punctum (Fig. 2.6).

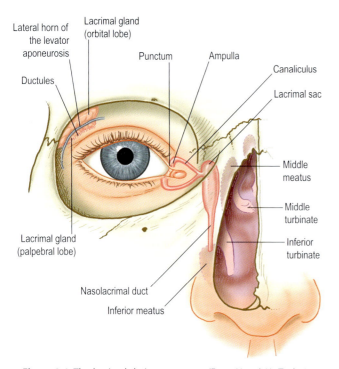

Figure 2.6 The lacrimal drainage system. (From Nerad JA. Techniques in Ophthalmic Plastic Surgery: A Personal Tutorial. 1st ed. Philadelphia: Elsevier Health Sciences; 2009. Chapter 2, Clinical Anatomy, Fig 2.40, p.49.)

The puncta are connected to the canaliculi, which are surrounded by orbicularis. There is a short vertical portion of the canaliculus, which measures 1–2 mm, followed by a horizontal component of approximately 8 mm. In most patients, the upper and lower canaliculi fuse together into the common canaliculus, before entering the lacrimal sac.

The lacrimal sac is protected by the bony lacrimal fossa. The anterior lacrimal crest surrounds the lacrimal fossa anteriorly, with maxillary bone making up the anterior two-thirds of the floor. The posterior aspect is composed of the posterior lacrimal crest.

The medial canthal tendon surrounds the lacrimal sac. In nasolacrimal duct obstruction, the sac can distend with fluid retention, but will not distend superior to the medial canthal tendon.

The collapsed lacrimal sac measures 2 mm in width. It narrows into the nasolacrimal duct and passes within a bony/osseous portion for approximately 15 mm until it exits under the inferior turbinate in the nose.

Vascular Supply

The eyelid benefits from a rich vascular supply that promotes healing and guards against infection. The arterial supply of the eyelids arises from the internal carotid artery and the ophthalmic artery and its branches (supraorbital and lacrimal). The external carotid artery is the arterial source for the face (angular and superficial temporal arteries). The two systems anastomose throughout the upper and lower eyelids and form the marginal arcades. The marginal arcade lies on the surface of the tarsal plate 2–4 mm from the margin. The upper eyelid has a second arcade, the peripheral arcade, which is superior to the border of the tarsus, and lies on the anterior surface of the Müller's muscle.

Lymphatic Drainage

The lateral two-thirds of the upper eyelid and lateral third of the lower lid drain into the preauricular, then deep cervical lymph nodes. The medial third of the upper lid and medial two-thirds of the lower eyelid drain into the submandibular nodes.

Nerves

Sensory innervation of the eyelids is provided by the first and second divisions of the fifth cranial nerve (CN V) which produces the ophthalmic and maxillary nerves.

The ophthalmic (V1) branches include supraorbital, supratrochlear, infratrochlear, nasociliary, and lacrimal. The supraorbital nerve supplies the upper lid, forehead and scalp. The supratrochlear supplies the superior portion of medial canthus, much of the upper lid, conjunctiva, and forehead. The infratrochlear nerve provides sensory innervation to the skin of the inferior medial canthus and lateral nose, conjunctiva, caruncle, and lacrimal sac. The lacrimal nerve supplies the lacrimal gland, the lateral upper lid and conjunctiva.

The infraorbital nerve (V2), supplies the skin and conjunctiva of the lower lid, lower part of nose and upper lip. The zygomaticofacial nerve (V2) supplies the skin of the lateral lower eyelid.

Motor innervations of the eyelids are provided by CN III, CN VII, and sympathetic fibers. CN VII, the facial nerve, innervates the muscles of facial expression: orbicularis oculi, frontalis, procerus, and corrugator supercilii. The levator palpebrae superioris is supplied by CN III while Müller's muscle is sympathetically innervated.

References

1. Nerad JA. Techniques in ophthalmic plastic surgery: a personal tutorial. 1st ed. Philadelphia: Elsevier Health Sciences; 2009.
2. Tyers AG, Collins JRO. Colour atlas of ophthalmic plastic surgery. 2nd ed. Philadelphia: Elsevier Health Sciences; 2001.
3. Kersten RC, Bartley GB, Nerad JA, et al. Basic and clinical science course, section 7: orbit, eyelids, and lacrimal system. San Francisco: American Academy of Ophthalmology; 2001.
4. Levine MR. Manual of oculoplastic surgery. 4th ed. Thorofare: SLACK Incorporated; 2010.

3 The Tear Film: Anatomy, Structure and Function

J. BRIAN FOSTER and W. BARRY LEE

Tear Film Anatomy and Physiology

The healthy ocular surface comprises a functional unit that utilizes a variety of structures, all of which remain intertwined in relation to anatomy, composition, and physiological function. These structures include the tear film, corneal and conjunctival epithelium, meibomian and lacrimal glands, and eyelids. A normally functioning tear film is required to maintain clarity of vision and ocular health. The tear film serves to provide ocular surface comfort, mechanical, environmental, and immune protection, maintain epithelial cellular health, and provide a smooth and very powerful refracting surface for clear vision.

One of the primary functions of the tear film includes providing ocular surface comfort through continuous lubrication. Tears are continually replenished from the inferior tear meniscus by blinking.[1] This counters the forces of gravity and evaporation on the volume of the precorneal tear film and protects corneal and conjunctival epithelial cells from the shear forces exerted by the eyelids during blinking. Tear production is approximately 1.2 microliters per minute, with a total volume of 6 microliters and a turnover rate of 16% per minute.[2] Tear film thickness, as measured by interferometry, is 6.0 μm ± 2.4 μm in normal subjects and is significantly thinner in dry eye patients with measured values as low as 2.0 μm ± 1.5 μm (Fig. 3.1).[3]

The ocular surface is the most environmentally exposed mucosal surface, and the tear film serves to protect against irritants, allergens, environmental extremes of dryness and temperature, potential pathogens and pollutants. Reflex tearing can help flush pathogens and irritants from the ocular surface. Antimicrobial components of the tear film include peroxidase, lactoferrin, lysozyme, and immunoglobulin A, among others. The superficial lipid component of the tear film helps prevent evaporation.[4]

Because the cornea is an avascular structure, the epithelium relies on the tear film to supply glucose, electrolytes, and growth factors, as well as the elimination of waste and free radicals. The tear film is a dilute protein solution that shares similar components to serum, although in different concentrations. Glucose concentration is much lower than in plasma (25 mg/L compared to 85 mg/L), and chlorine and potassium are higher. Other electrolyte components include calcium, magnesium, bicarbonate, nitrate, phosphate, and sulfate. Antioxidants, such as Vitamin C, tyrosine, and glutathione scavenge free radicals to help minimize cellular oxidative damage. The tear film also provides a large number of growth factors, neuropeptides, and protease inhibitors, important in maintaining corneal health and stimulating wound healing (Fig. 3.2, Table 3.1).

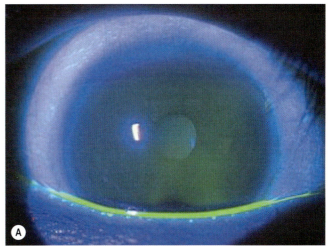

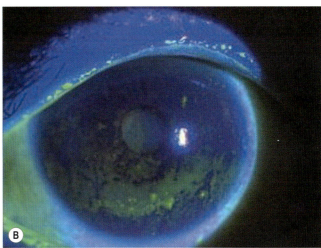

Figure 3.1 Slit lamp photographs with fluorescein staining of a representative dry eye patient and a normal subject. **(A)** Twenty-six-year-old male normal subject. Estimated tear film thickness was 6.4 μm. **(B)** Thirty-six-year-old female dry eye patient with Sjögren syndrome. Estimated tear film thickness was 2.4 μm. (Reprinted with permission from Hosaka E, Kawamorita T, Ogasawara Y, et al. Interferometry in the evaluation of precorneal tear film thickness in dry eye. Am J Ophthalmol 2011;151:18–23.e1.)

The tear film provides a smooth refracting surface over the microvilli of the corneal epithelium. The air–fluid interface of the tear film is a powerful lens that supplies two-thirds of the refracting power of the eye. It is also evident that desiccation and tear film instability can lead to visual degradation and symptoms of fluctuating vision, loss of contrast, and/or discomfort.[5]

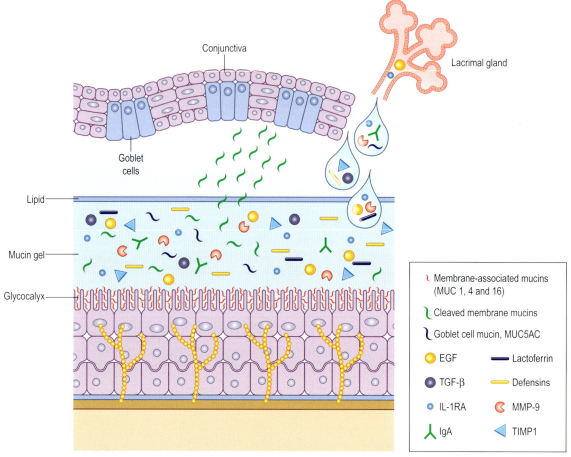

Figure 3.2 Components of the tear film produced by surface epithelium, lacrimal glands and conjunctival goblet cells that lubricate (MUC 1,4,6), protect from inflammation (TGF-β, IL1-receptor antagonist, tissue inhibitor of matrix metalloproteinase-1 (TIMP-1)), infection (IgA, lactoferrin, defensins), and promote healing (epidermal growth factor). (Reprinted with permission from Pflugfelder SC. Tear dysfunction and the cornea: LXVIII Edward Jackson Memorial Lecture. Am J Ophthalmol 2011;152:900–9.e1.)

Table 3.1 Growth factors, neuropeptides, and protease inhibitors in the tear film.

Transforming growth factor (TGF-α,β1,β2)	Mitogenic, inhibits corneal epithelial cell proliferation, pro-fibrotic
Tear hepatocyte growth factor (HGF), keratocyte growth factor	Stimulates corneal epithelial cells, promotes wound healing
Basic fibroblast growth factor (FGFβ, FGF2), Epidermal growth factor	Mitogenic
Substance P	Neuropeptide; stimulates epithelial growth, wound healing
Plasminogen, plasmic, plasminogen activator	Proteases, matrix degradation/wound healing
Matrix metalloproteinases (MMP-2,3,8,9)	Matrix degradation/wound healing
Tryptase, α1-antichymotrypsin, α1-protease inhibitor, α2-macroglobulin	Protease inhibitors

(Adapted with permission from Beuerman R. Tear Film. In: Krachmer JH, Mannis MJ, Holland EJ, editor. Cornea. 2nd ed. Philadelphia, PA: Elsevier Mosby; 2005. p. 45–52.)

Structure and Stability

The ocular surface requires a dynamic yet stable tear film to meet the environmental, immunologic, and optical challenges presented to it. For decades, a discrete three-layer model was accepted, consisting of an anterior lipid layer to provide protection from evaporation; an aqueous component that provided the largest part of tear film volume; and a mucin layer that provided protection and lubrication of the corneal and conjunctival epithelium. A more recently proposed model consists of a mucin/aqueous glycocalyx gel that comprises most of the tear film volume with an external protective lipid layer to resist evaporative forces (Fig. 3.3).[3]

LIPIDS

A heterogeneous mixture of lipids is secreted by the meibomian glands, located posterior to the lash line in the upper and lower eyelids. The low surface tension of the lipid layer enables uniform spread of the tear film and provides an optically smooth refracting surface. The posterior aqueous interface of the lipid layer consists primarily of polar lipids

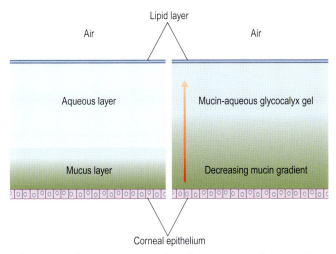

Figure 3.3 Schematic representation of the structure of the tear film. *Left:* Classic: Discrete three layered structure. Contemporary: An aqueous–mucin glycocalyx gel with a mucin gradient has been proposed. (This figure is taken from an article entitled, "McCulley JP, Shine W. A compositional based model for the tear film lipid layer" in the Trans Am Ophthalmol Soc 1997; 95:79–88 and republished with permission of the American Ophthalmological Society.)

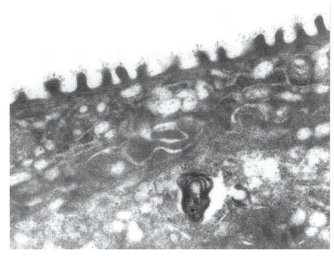

Figure 3.4 Transmission electron micrographs of the surface cell layer of the cornea. Corneal epithelial microvilli with transmembrane mucins that extend into the mucin/aqueous glycocalyx. (Reprinted with permission from Beuerman R. Tear Film. In: Krachmer JH, Mannis MJ, Holland EJ, editor. Cornea. 2nd ed. Philadelphia, PA: Elsevier Mosby; 2005. p. 45–52.)

including ceramides, cerebrosides and phospholipids. Non-polar lipids form the lipid–air interface, including cholesterol esters, triglycerides, and free fatty acids.[6]

AQUEOUS COMPONENT

The aqueous portion of the mucin/aqueous gel contains proteins, electrolytes, oxygen, and glucose (Table 3.1). Electrolyte concentration of this layer is similar to that of serum, resulting in an average osmolarity of 300 mOsm/L. Tear osmolarity correlates highly with dry eye syndrome and will likely be increasingly utilized as a metric for diagnosis and classification of the disorder.[7] Normal osmolarity is essential to maintain cellular volume, enzymatic activity, and cellular homeostasis. Matrix metalloproteinases, particularly MMP-9, serve an important role in wound healing and inflammation, and are substantially up-regulated in dry eye syndrome. Aqueous volume is constantly replenished by the main and accessory lacrimal glands. Most non-reflex tear production is from the glands of Krause and Wolfring, accessory lacrimal glands located in the palpebral conjunctiva of the upper eye lid and the superior conjunctival fornix. The lacrimal glands can provide a substantial volume of aqueous tears when the ocular surface is presented with a noxious stimulus, such as a foreign body, chemical irritant, or epithelial injury. It is unclear what role the lacrimal gland plays in non-reflex tearing, but it appears to be important, as evidenced by the frequency of dry eye syndrome in patients with infiltrative lacrimal gland disease or after surgical removal.

Tear production is neurally driven by a reflex loop that links the ocular surface, central nervous system stimulation, and the glands of the ocular surface. The lacrimal functional unit (LFU) comprises the cornea, conjunctiva, and meibomian glands of the ocular surface, the main and accessory lacrimal glands, and the neural pathways that connect them.[8] Afferent sensory nerves of the cornea and conjunctiva synapse with higher-order sensory neurons, autonomic, and motor efferent nerves in the brainstem. When that stimulus is interrupted by local or general anesthesia, corneal nerve transection after LASIK, or neurotrophic infection, tear production decreases and dryness ensues. Lacrimal and accessory glands, meibomian glands, and conjunctival goblet cells are innervated by autonomic nerve fibers. Motor fibers from the facial nerve innervate the orbicularis oculi muscle and stimulate the blink reflex which distributes tears evenly over the ocular surface.[4]

MUCINS

The mucin component of the glycocalyx gel consists of an organized and heterogeneous group of glycoproteins that promote a firm attachment of the matrix to the corneal epithelium, provide viscosity, and a low surface tension that aids uniform re-wetting of the hydrophobic ocular surface. Corneal and conjunctival epithelium express transmembrane mucins (MUC 1,2,4), which anchor the aqueous/mucin glycocalyx to the cell surface. The lacrimal gland and conjunctival goblet cells secrete mucin into the tear film and these glycoproteins likely play a role in preventing adherence and interaction of microbes, debris, and inflammatory cells with the epithelium.[9] Mucins also provide viscosity that protects the fragile corneal epithelium from the repetitive forces of blinking, and they lower surface tension, which produces the smooth, uniform, optically advantageous properties of the tear film.

The corneal surface is squamous epithelium approximately five cell layers thick. Microvilli on the apical surface have filaments that interact with mucins that expand into the tear film, supporting it and forming a glycocalyx gel (Fig. 3.4). Increased surface area of the microvilli provides a strong anchor that stabilizes the tear film and protects the cornea. The mucin matrix decreases surface tension and facilitates uniform re-wetting of the epithelium and close interaction between the hydrophilic aqueous component and the hydrophobic epithelial cell membranes. Cellular tight junctions on the corneal epithelium form a barrier that provides protection from inflammatory and microbial insults. Corneal epithelial cells live approximately 7 to 10 days and undergo an organized apoptosis and desquamation that is highly regulated by matrix metalloproteinases and other signaling molecules. Complete turnover occurs weekly as deeper basal epithelium moves toward the apex of the cornea.[10]

Tear Dysfunction

Tear dysfunction is a common and potentially debilitating condition that results in a broad spectrum of symptoms with varying degrees of severity. The most common result of tear dysfunction is epithelial disease, which can cause dryness, foreign body sensation, fluctuation in visual quality, decreased contrast, and photophobia. Dysfunction of any component of the lacrimal functional unit can cause tear dysfunction and a resulting epitheliopathy, including conjunctivochalasis, eyelid malposition, and lacrimal or meibomian gland disease. There is general consensus of two main subtypes of dry eye syndrome; evaporative and aqueous dry eye. These are a result of a dysfunction of the meibomian and lacrimal glands. The tests most commonly utilized to assess dry eye severity are the Schirmer test, tear film breakup time (TBUT), fluorescein, rose bengal, lissamine green staining of the ocular surface, and symptom scoring with patient questionnaires, such as the Ocular Surface Disease Index (OSDI).[11]

Osmolarity

One of the principal indicators of tear dysfunction is elevated tear film osmolarity, predominantly due to elevated sodium ion concentration. Elevated osmolarity is considered the central mechanism of ocular surface damage and may be the single best marker for dry eye disease, as reported in the Dry Eye Workshop Report.[12] In rabbit studies, tear osmolarity is directly correlated with tear evaporation and flow rate. Increased osmolarity also correlates with decreased goblet cell density, granulocyte survival, and causes significant morphological changes in tissue culture. In a meta-analysis, Tomlinson et al. report an average tear osmolarity of 302 ± 9.7 in normal subjects (815) and 326.9 ± 22.1 in subjects with keratoconjunctivitis sicca (621). A cut-off value of 316 mOsmol/L appears to provide acceptable sensitivity (69%) and specificity (92%) for the diagnosis of keratoconjunctivitis sicca.[13]

Hyperosmolarity causes significant corneal epithelial stress that may result in increased levels of inflammatory mediators including proinflammatory cytokines and chemokines (Fig. 3.5). These mediators initiate stress-signaling pathways that result in expression of mitogen-activated protein kinase (MAPK) and nuclear-factor B (NFB) in corneal epithelial cells and immune activation and adhesion molecules (HLA-DR and ICAM-1) in conjunctival epithelium. These molecules attract conjunctival inflammatory

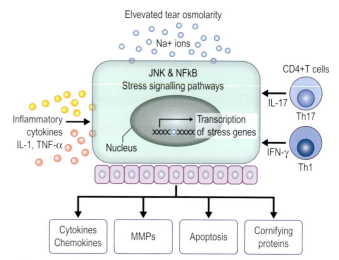

Figure 3.5 Alterations in tear film composition due to tear dysfunction include increased osmolarity and inflammatory cytokines, and CD4+ T cells that activate stress signaling pathways and upregulation of cytokines, chemokines, matrix metalloproteinases, and apoptosis induction. (Reprinted with permission from Pflugfelder SC. Tear dysfunction and the cornea: LXVIII Edward Jackson Memorial Lecture. Am J Ophthalmol. 2011;152:900–9.e1.)

cells and are found in increased frequency in the conjunctiva of dry eye patients, as measured by flow cytometry.[14]

Dry eye patients exhibit increased activity and concentration of matrix metalloproteinases in the tear film, particularly MMP-9. These enzymes play an important role in regulation of epithelial cell desquamation and cleave a variety of substrates in the corneal epithelial basement membrane and tight junction proteins (occludins), that help maintain epithelial barrier function. The sequelae of these activities include corneal surface irregularities, punctate epithelial erosions due to increased epithelial desquamation, apoptosis, and increased fluorescein permeability.[14]

The tear film must respond to a constant barrage of mechanical and chemical irritants, pathogenic invaders, environmental extremes, and be able to mount a healing response quickly. The defensins are a group of naturally occurring peptides present in the tear film that have wound healing and innate antimicrobial properties. Their antimicrobial activity is broad and encompasses viruses (HIV, HSV), fungi, Gram-positive and Gram-negative bacteria. The peptides form a rigid three-dimensional structure that forms voltage-sensitive channels in the plasma membrane of the target organism. Defensins also accelerate wound healing due to their mitogenic effect on fibroblasts and epithelial cells. In addition, these may facilitate a rapid immune response through stimulating monocyte chemotaxis.[15]

A healthy tear film is necessary for clear vision, ocular comfort, and protection from microbial pathogens and environmental insults. Tear film dysfunction is common and carries the potential for significant morbidity.

References

1. Palakuru JR, Wang J, Aquavella JV. Effect of blinking on tear dynamics. Invest Ophthalmol Vis Sci 2007;48:3032–7.
2. Mishima S, Gasset A, Klyce SD, et al. Determination of tear volume and tear flow. Invest Ophthalmol Vis Sci 1966;5:264–9.

3. Hosaka E, Kawamorita T, Ogasawara Y, et al. Interferometry in the evaluation of precorneal tear film thickness in dry eye. Am J Ophthalmol 2011;151:18–23.e1.
4. Stern ME, Beuerman RW, Pflugfelder SC. The normal tear film and ocular surface. In: Pflugfelder SC, Stern ME, Beuerman RW, editors. Dry eye and the ocular surface. New York: Marcel-Dekkar; 2004. p. 11–40.
5. Rolando M, Zierhut M. The ocular surface and tear film and their dysfunction in dry eye disease. Surv Ophthalmology 2001; 45(Suppl 2):S203–10.
6. McCulley JP, Shine W. A compositional based model for the tear film lipid layer. Trans Am Ophthalmol Soc 1997;95:79–88.
7. Lemp MA, Bron AJ, Baudouin C, et al. Tear osmolarity in the diagnosis and management of dry eye disease. Am J Ophthalmol 2011;151:792–8.e1. Epub 2011 Feb 18. PubMed PMID: 21310379.
8. Stern ME, Beuerman RW, Fox RI, et al. The pathology of dry eye: the interaction between the ocular surface and lacrimal glands. Cornea 1998;17:584–9.
9. Gipson IK, Inatomi T. Cellular origin of mucins of the ocular surface tear film. Adv Exp Med Biol 1998;438:221–7.
10. DelMonte DW, Kim T. Anatomy and physiology of the cornea. J Cataract Refract Surg 2011;37:588–98. Review.
11. Korb DR. Survey of preferred tests for diagnosis of the tear film and dry eye. Cornea 2000;19:483–6.
12. International Dry Eye Workshop. The definition and classification of dry eye disease. In: 2007 Report of the International Dry Eye Workshop (DEWS) Ocul Surf 2007;5:75–92.
13. Tomlinson A, Khanal S, Ramaesh K, et al. Tear film osmolarity: determination of a referent for dry eye diagnosis. Invest Ophthalmol Vis Sci 2006;47:4309–15.
14. Luo L, Li DQ, Doshi A, et al. Experimental dry eye stimulates production of inflammatory cytokines and MMP-9 and activates MAPK signaling pathways on the ocular surface. Invest Ophthalmol Vis Sci 2004;45:4293–301.
15. Haynes RJ, Tighe PJ, Dua HS. Antimicrobial defensin peptides of the human ocular surface. Br J Ophthalmol 1999;83:737–41.

4 Conjunctival Anatomy and Physiology

THOMAS M. HARVEY, ANA G. ALZAGA FERNANDEZ, RAVI PATEL, DAVID GOLDMAN, and JESSICA CIRALSKY

Introduction

The conjunctiva is the mucosal surface that extends from the corneoscleral limbus to the eyelid margins and caruncle.[1–4] Often overlooked, conjunctival tissue's complex functions are necessary to maintain ocular surface homeostasis.

Many important functions are performed by the conjunctiva including: (1) protection of the soft tissues of the orbit and the eyelid, (2) provision of the tear film's aqueous and mucous layers, (3) supply of immune tissue, and (4) facilitation of independent globe movement. The conjunctiva can be divided into three distinct regions: bulbar, forniceal, and palpebral. The total surface area of the conjunctiva and cornea in an average adult measures approximately 16 cm² per eye.[2–4]

Anatomy and Histology

BULBAR

The non-keratinized stratified secretory epithelium interfaces with a basement membrane and substantia propria below to create the blanket-like covering of the globe. Bulbar conjunctiva has a preponderance of cuboidal epithelial cells around goblet cells, Langerhans cells, melanocytes, and lymphocytes. In the normal bulbar conjunctiva, epithelial thickness can be more than six cell layers. Apical cell tight junctions, gap junctions, and desmosomes exist to create selective permeability, whereas the epithelial cell microvilli–glycocalyx complex encourages tear film adherence due to hydrophilicity.[1–4]

Mucous-secreting goblet cells constitute 5–10% of the conjunctival epithelial basal cells. The highest density of goblet cells occurs in the inferonasal bulbar conjunctiva and tarsal conjunctiva. Goblet cells are a likely apocrine in nature. Release of secretory granules results from parasympathetic activation.[2,3]

The underlying epithelial basement membrane is primarily composed of type IV collagen. The substantia propria, located beneath the epithelial basement membrane, is a highly vascularized, loose connective tissue. The substantia propria in the limbal conjunctiva is thin and compact.[2–4]

The bulbar conjunctiva is relatively loosely adherent to the underlying Tenon's capsule. The conjunctiva and Tenon's fascia are less mobile within the first few millimeters adjacent to the limbus, where the epithelium transitions to flatter epithelial cell morphology. Radiating infolds

at the limbus are known as the palisades of Vogt. The stem cells of the cornea are located here.[2,3]

The dimensions of the bulbar conjunctiva vary with age, race, eye position, inherent redundancies of tissue and method of measurement. The adult chord length from limbus to fornix averages between approximately 13 and 16 mm superiorly. The inferior fornix is typically between 10 and 12 mm in normals and decreases with age. Cicatrizing conditions can create a foreshortened fornix, thereby decreasing the area of measurable bulbar conjunctiva.[5] Temporally, the bulbar conjunctiva extends for more than 12 mm from the limbus and with a significant portion hidden by the lateral canthus. The nasal bulbar conjunctiva covers the smallest area, limited by the presence of the caruncle and the medial wall of the orbit.[2]

The vascular supply of the bulbar conjunctiva comes principally from anterior ciliary arteries and the peripheral tarsal arcades of the eyelid. The arteries eventually anastomose to create an arteriolar plexus near the limbus to ensure redundancy of oxygenation (Fig. 4.1). The majority of the blood supply for the bulbar conjunctiva near the limbus is derived from the anterior ciliary arteries. The venous drainage is similar: conjunctiva drains into anterior ciliary veins and into many peripheral conjunctival veins that connect to the eyelid's venous plexus, before joining the superior and inferior ophthalmic veins. Bulbar conjunctival veins can become dilated and prominent along with those

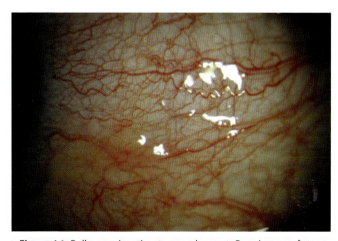

Figure 4.1 Bulbar conjunctiva, temporal aspect. Prominence of conjunctival vasculature is apparent overlying episcleral and scleral vessels. A small pingueculum is present near the limbus. (Photo courtesy of Stuart Watts.)

of the episclera in primary pulmonary hypertension, carotid cavernous fistulas, and other vascular malformations.[2]

The lymphatics of the nasal bulbar conjunctiva drain to the submandibular nodes. Temporal bulbar conjunctival lymphatics drain to preauricular nodes. Bulbar conjunctival lymphatic channels can be seen with injection of dyes at or near the limbus.[2] The darker dye contrasts the lymphatic channel against the white background of sclera (Fig. 4.2).

The ophthalmic branch of the trigeminal nerve contains sensory afferent fibers for the bulbar conjunctiva. Afferent nerves do not synapse until the fifth nerve nucleus. Autonomic efferent nerves supply vessels, accessory lacrimal glands, and the epithelia.[2]

FORNIX

The conjunctiva of the fornix is continuous with the skin and lies between bulbar and palpebral conjunctiva (Fig. 4.3). It contains a nonkeratinized stratified squamous epithelium that is typically three layers thick.[2] The superficial

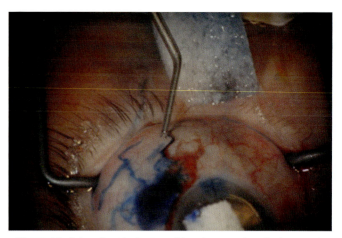

Figure 4.2 Subconjunctival trypan blue dye uses lymphatics to exit from the injection site. The superior conjunctival lymphatics are visible and appear light blue in this photo.

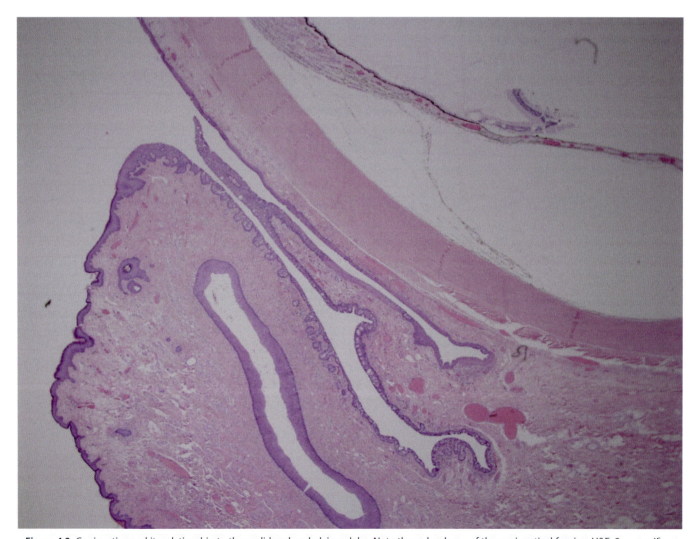

Figure 4.3 Conjunctiva and its relationship to the eyelid and underlying globe. Note the redundancy of the conjunctival fornix – H&E, 2× magnification. (Image courtesy of Daniel M. Albert, M.D., M.S.)

layer is cylindrical, the middle layer is polyhedral, and the deep layer is cuboidal. Within the epithelium, goblet cells, melanocytes and dendritic cells are often encountered.

The substantia propria is thickest in the conjunctival fornix and is anatomically split into two sections: a superficial lymphoid layer and a deeper fibrous layer. The superficial lymphoid layer is microscopically comprised of a loose connective tissue with an admixture of lymphocytes (primarily T lymphocytes), mast cells, plasma cells and neutrophils. The deeper fibrous layer contains the vessels, nerves and glands of Krause. The glands of Krause are accessory lacrimal glands deep within the superior and inferior fornix where they number approximately 42 and 6–8, respectively. These glands collectively form an intricate duct system which opens into the fornices. Like the main lacrimal gland, these glands help produce the aqueous component of the tear film.[2,3]

Two specialized modifications of this conjunctival tissue are present medially: the plica semilunaris and the caruncle. The plica semilunaris (or semilunar fold), a vestigial remnant of the nictitating membrane, is a crescentic fold in the medial fornix. The caruncle, which is medial to the plica semilunaris, is a modified tissue type which contains features of both the conjunctival fornix and of the adjacent cutaneous structures which includes pilosebaceous units and fibroadipose tissue.[2] These structures are around 7 mm from the nasal limbus.

The superior forniceal cul-de-sac is maintained without collapse due to the presence of fine smooth muscle attachments to the levator palpebrae superioris. Unlike the superior fornix, the inferior forniceal cul-de-sac is visible with simple eversion of the lower eyelid. The lateral fornix extends between the lateral canthus and globe and is maintained by fibrous attachments to the lateral rectus tendon. Medially, the fornix is the shallowest and contains the plica semilunaris and caruncle. The medial fornix only exists during adduction due to fibrous attachments to the medial rectus tendon.[2]

Perfusion, innervation, and lymphatic drainage mirror that of the bulbar tissue. The medial fornix has sensory afferents from the maxillary division of the trigeminal nerve. The preponderance of lymphocytes in this region and their role are discussed below.[2]

PALPEBRAL

The marginal mucocutaneous junction marks the transition from eyelid keratinized stratified squamous epithelium to nonkeratinized, stratified squamous epithelium of the palpebral conjunctiva. The palpebral conjunctiva contains cuboidal epithelial cells, similar to the bulbar conjunctiva, and columnar epithelial cells overlying the tarsus. The epithelial cells of the palpebral conjunctiva are smaller compared to the bulbar conjunctiva. The thickness of the epithelium varies from 2–3 cell layers over the upper tarsus to 4–5 over the lower tarsus. Similar to the bulbar and forniceal epithelium, Langerhans cells and goblet cells are present. The substantia propria is thin, compact, and firmly attached over the tarsus.[1–4]

The palpebral conjunctiva lines the inner surfaces of the eyelids. It extends from the mucocutaneous junction of the eyelid margin to the fornices.[2] It is subdivided into marginal, tarsal and orbital conjunctiva.

The marginal conjunctiva measures approximately 2 mm wide. It extends from the mucocutaneous junction to the subtarsal groove, a shallow sulcus that runs parallel to the eyelid margin along the tarsal surface. The transition from nonkeratinized stratified epithelium of the eyelid margin to the cuboidal epithelium of the tarsal conjunctiva occurs at this site.[2]

The tarsal conjunctiva is thin, vascular and firmly adherent to the underlying tarsus, particularly the upper tarsus (Fig. 4.4). This tight adherence provides a smooth tarsal surface, a critical function given its intimate relationship with the cornea. The palpebral conjunctiva contains the accessory lacrimal glands, glands of Wolfring, which are located above or within the tarsus. Epithelial infolds with abundant goblet cells, known as pseudoglands of Henle, are also located here (Fig. 4.5).[2]

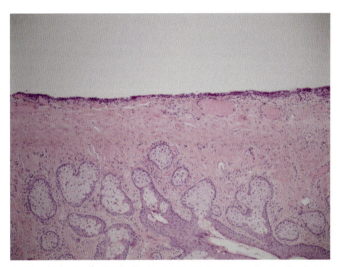

Figure 4.4 Tarsal conjunctiva showing stratified squamous epithelium overlying fibrous stroma. Note the paucity of goblet cells. Meibomian glands can be seen at bottom of picture – H&E, 10× magnification. (Image courtesy of Daniel M. Albert, M.D., M.S.)

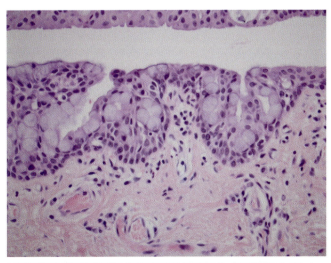

Figure 4.5 Pseudoglands of Henle – H&E, 40× magnification. (Image courtesy of Daniel M. Albert, M.D., M.S.)

Table 4.1   Summary Table of Ocular Surface Mucins

Source	Category	Glycoprotein	Comment
Conjunctival/corneal epithelium	Cell surface-associated	MUC1, MUC4, MUC16	Intimately located at apical cells' microvilli
Conjunctival epithelium	Soluble	(MUC7)	Gene identified; glycoprotein may not be in tear film of normals
Goblet cells	Gel-forming	MUC5AC, MUC2, (MUC19)	MUC19 mRNA is detectable by PCR
Lacrimal glands	Cell surface-associated	MUC1, MUC4, MUC16	Role not well-defined
Lacrimal glands	Gel-forming	MUC5AC, (MUC5B)	Role not well-defined
Lacrimal glands	Soluble	MUC7, (MUC6)	Acini produced

The orbital conjunctiva extends from the posterior edge of the tarsal plate to the fornix. It is loosely attached and forms folds during eyelid opening.

There is a dual blood supply for the palpebral conjunctiva. The main vascular supply arises from the terminal branches of the ophthalmic artery: dorsal, nasal, frontal, supraorbital, and lacrimal arteries. The facial, superficial, temporal, and infraorbital branches of the facial artery provide the supplemental blood supply. Venous drainage occurs through post-tarsal veins of the eyelids, deep facial branches of the anterior facial vein, and the pterygoid plexus.[2]

The lymphatics of the palpebral conjunctiva join the eyelid lymphatics, draining medially to the submandibular lymph nodes and laterally to the preauricular lymph nodes.[2]

Similar to the bulbar and forniceal conjunctiva, the palpebral conjunctiva is mainly innervated by branches of the ophthalmic division of the trigeminal nerve, i.e. the lacrimal, supraorbital, supratrochlear and infraorbital. Additionally, VIP-containing nerve fibers have been shown to innervate accessory lacrimal glands and goblet cells, as well as glands of Moll at the eyelid margin.[2]

Conjunctival Function

TEAR FILM

In addition to the supportive role of accessory lacrimal glands (Krause and Wolfring), arguably the conjunctiva's greatest contribution to the tear film is the production of hydrophilic mucins. Mucins are well-studied products of mucus membranes that are critical for conjunctival health. Mucins are large heavily glycosylated proteins, exhibiting extensive tandem amino acid repeats, and multifunctional utility. Recent assays have helped clarify the mucins' role in: (1) clearance of allergens, pathogens, and debris, (2) lubrication, (3) antimicrobial activity. Their O-glycans have hydrophilic properties to help keep the tear film in contact with the epithelia.[6]

Mucins can be categorized as secreted or cell surface-associated. The secreted mucins are either soluble (located closer to the tear film lipid layer) or gel-forming (located closer to the conjunctival apical cells). Cell surface-associated mucins (also called 'membrane-associated') form the glycocalyx. The gel-forming mucins appear to work together with cell surface-associated mucins to maximally protect the epithelium and limit desiccation. Additionally, shed cell surface-associated mucins contribute to

tear fluid.[3] The various ocular surface mucins are described in Table 4.1.

Secreted mucins have been described as having critical 'cleaning' capabilities, addressing unwanted debris, allergens, and microbes. Combined with efficient tear clearance, lymphatics, inherent immunologic proteins, and secondary immune responses, mucins help the ocular surface to maintain optimal health.[6]

Decreased gel-forming mucin gene expression (e.g. Sjögren's syndrome – MUC5A) and decreased glycosylation of cell surface-associated mucin (e.g. non-Sjögren sicca – MUC16) are two known examples of mucin abnormalities that negatively affect tear film.[4,6]

Conjunctival apical epithelial cell microvilli are integral for proper cell membrane-associated mucin presence.[4] Recent work has shown that conjunctival epithelial microvilli are fewer and smaller (in size) in graft-versus-host disease sicca versus normals and Sjögren's syndrome sicca. Other findings of interest in graft-versus-host disease were abundant CD8+ T cells in the basal epithelium with decreased goblet cell secretory vesicles.

IMMUNOLOGY

The conjunctiva is equipped with several distinct defense mechanisms: anatomical, mechanical, antimicrobial and immunologic. An intact epithelium provides an anatomic defense against pathogen invasion. Eyelid blinking mechanically removes pathogens and foreign substances.[7] Tears contain a variety of antimicrobial proteins, including: lysozyme, immunoglobulins, and lactoferrin. Lysozyme provides protection against Gram-positive organisms through lysis of bacterial cell walls. Immunoglobulins, particularly IgG, neutralize viruses and lyse bacteria.[8] Lactoferrin has bacteriostatic and bactericidal properties (Fig. 4.6).

The conjunctiva's immunologic defense is complex and consists of an innate, adaptive and mucosal component. The innate immune system is a non-specific early host response against pathogens. Pathogens, through pathogen-associated molecular patterns (PAMPs), are recognized by toll-like receptors (TLRs), specific innate immune-recognition receptors. After pathogen recognition by TLRs, an immune response is triggered, leading to inflammation and induction of the adaptive immune system. Recent studies have shown that the conjunctiva expresses β-defensins, important components of the innate immune system, TLR mRNA and proteins.[9]

The adaptive immune system is a delayed host response containing humoral and cellular arms. Immunoglobulins

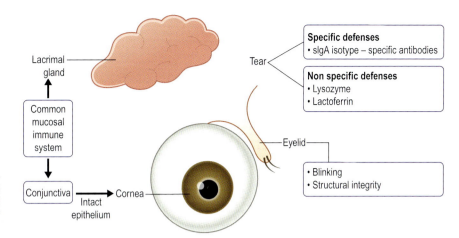

Figure 4.6 The ocular surface has an interconnected defense system to combat pathogens and preserve health. (From McClellan KA. Mucosal Defense of the Outer Eye. Survey of Ophthalmology 1997;42:233–246. Figure 1.)

are the main component of the humoral arm whereas T lymphocytes form the cellular arm. T lymphocytes, cytotoxic and helper T cells, are found in both the conjunctival epithelium and substantia propria; B cells are found rarely in the substantia propria. The adaptive and innate immune systems work together to provide an integrated conjunctival immune system.[8]

There is increasing evidence that the conjunctiva has a specific mucosal immune system, termed conjunctival associated lymphoid tissue (CALT). CALT has previously been described in several different animals; recent studies have shown its existence in humans. CALT is thought to be part of the larger common secretory immune system comprising mucosa-associated lymphoid tissue (MALT) from the gastrointestinal, respiratory and genitourinary tracts.[8,10]

The secretory immune system's main humoral mediator is IgA.[8,10] IgA can provide a protective layer to the mucosa by preventing bacterial binding to mucosal epithelial, binding to antigen to prevent absorption, and neutralizing viruses.[7,8] High endothelial venules, specialized vessels for migration of lymphoid cells between integrated mucosal systems, along with lymphocytes, lymphoid follicles, IgA positive plasma cells and their associated transporter molecule, secretory component (SC), have all been found in the human conjunctiva, further supporting the presence of CALT.[7,9,10]

References

1. Calonge M, Stern ME. In: Pflugfelder SC, Beuerman RW, Stern ME, editors. Dry eye and ocular surface disorders. 1st ed. New York: Marcel Dekker; 2004. p. 89–109.
2. Nelson J, Cameron J. The conjunctiva: anatomy and physiology. In: Krachmer JH, Mannis MJ, Holland EJ, editors. Cornea: fundamentals, diagnosis and management. 3rd ed. Philadelphia: Elsevier-Mosby; 2011;25–31.
3. Tsubota K, Tseng SCG, Nordlund ML. Anatomy and physiology of the ocular surface. In: Holland EJ, Mannis MJ, editors. Ocular surface disease: medical and surgical management. 1st ed. New York: Springer-Verlag; 2002. p. 3–15.
4. Gipson IK, Joyce N, Zieske J. The anatomy and cell biology of the human cornea, limbus, conjunctiva, and adnexa. In: Foster CS, Azar D, Dohlman C, editors. Smolin and Thoft's: The cornea. 4th ed. Philadelphia: Lippincott WIlliams & Wilkins; 2005. p. 3–37.
5. Williams GP, Saw VPJ, Saeed T, et al. Validation of a fornix depth measurer: a putative tool for the assessment of progressive cicatrising conjunctivitis. Br J Ophthalmol 2011;95:842–7.
6. Mantelli F, Argüeso P. Functions of ocular surface mucins in health and disease. Curr Opin Allergy Clin Immunol 2008;8:477–83.
7. McClellan KA. Mucosal defense of the outer eye. Surv Ophthalmol 1997;42:233–46.
8. Foster CS, Streilein J. Basic immunology. In: Foster CS, Azar D, Dohlman C. editors. Smolin and Thoft's: The cornea. 4th ed. Philadelphia: Lippincott Williams & Wilkins; 2005. p. 91–3.
9. Lambiase A, Micera A, Sacchetti M, et al. Toll-like receptors in ocular surface diseases: overview and new findings. Clin Sci 2011;120: 441–50.
10. Knop E, Knop N. The role of eye-associated lymphoid tissue in corneal immune protection. J Anat 2005;206:271–85.

5 *Limbus and Corneal Epithelium*

PEDRAM HAMRAH and AFSUN SAHIN

Introduction

The ocular surface has important functions, including the provision of a smooth external layer required for optical clarity and vision, an unusually efficient mechanical barrier to the entry of microorganisms into the eye, as well as nutrition and metabolic interactions with the underlying stromal tissue. The ocular surface anatomically comprises the cornea, conjunctiva and the corneoscleral junction, called limbus. The cornea and the overlying tear film are responsible for refraction and transmission of light into the eye. However, the limbus and the conjunctiva maintain the clarity and functions of the cornea by providing necessary support. While the anatomical areas of the ocular surface have a continuous multilayered surface epithelial layer in common, significant morphological and functional differences exist between the epithelium of the cornea and the limbus. During the past few decades, our understanding of the limbal morphology and function has dramatically increased and provided us with new key concepts. This chapter reviews the anatomy and cell biology of the limbal and corneal epithelium, providing an insight into some of the recently discovered structural and biological features.

Limbal Epithelium

ANATOMY AND STRUCTURE

The narrow transitional zone between the corneal and bulbar conjunctival epithelium represents the limbal epithelium. However, due to the lack of distinct borders, there are various anatomic definitions of the limbus as defined by anatomists, pathologists, histologists, and surgeons. The most accepted definition delineates the inferior border of the limbus as a line between the outer border of Bowman's layer and Descemet's membrane, and the exterior border as the start of scleral collagen fibers and outside border of the Schlemm's canal, 1.5 to 2 mm outside the inferior border (Fig. 5.1).[1] This region has an important barrier function and prevents conjunctival overgrowth onto the cornea.

Histologically, the non-keratinized stratified limbal epithelium can be differentiated from the conjunctival epithelium, in that it lacks goblet cells. Compared to the corneal epithelium, while the superficial epithelial layers are rather similar, the limbal epithelium contains cell layers, a large number of mature (activated) and immature epithelial dendritic cells, T lymphocytes, highly pigmented melanocytes, and subjacent blood vessels. Moreover, the basal limbal epithelial cells are unique in that they are the least differentiated cells of the ocular surface epithelium.[2] These cells are smaller, less columnar and have more cytoplasmic organelles. A growing body of evidence over the past years

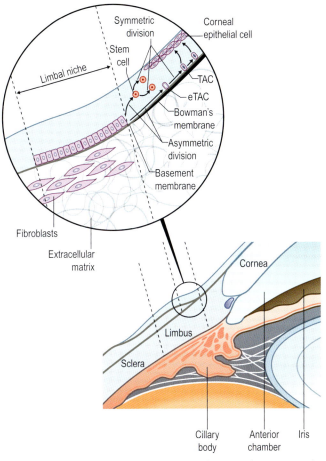

Figure 5.1 The limbus is the transition zone between the cornea and the sclera, which bares the limbal niche and limbal epithelial stem cells (LESCs). The LESCs, which sit on a basement membrane, have a high proliferative capacity. They constantly undergo two types of cell division: a symmetric and asymmetric division in order to maintain ocular surface self-renewal. During symmetric division, either two identical stem cells or alternatively two identical differentiated daughter cells emerge. In contrast, asymmetric division of LESCs results into a stem cell and an early transient amplifying cell (eTAC).

supports the theory that these cells are limbal epithelial stem cells (LESC), giving rise to the more differentiated corneal epithelium.[2]

LIMBAL EPITHELIAL STEM CELLS

Limbal epithelial stem cells reside in the limbal niche,[3] where subepithelial papillae-like structures known as palisades of Vogt are seen clinically.[4] The palisades of Vogt appear as radial linear structures of about 1 mm in length as observed by slit-lamp microscopy and in vivo confocal microscopy.[5] This anatomical landmark provides the

Table 5.1 Known Markers for Basal Limbal and Corneal Epithelial Cells

Marker	Limbal Epithelium (Basal)	Corneal Epithelium (Basal)
KERATINS		
Cytokeratin (CK) 3/CK12	–	+++
CK5/CK14	++	–
CK19	++	–
GAP JUNCTION PROTEINS		
Connexin 43	–	+
Connexin 50	–	–
METABOLIC ENZYMES		
α-enolase	+++	++
Cytochrome oxidase	+++	++
Carbonic anhydrase	+++	++
TRANSPORTERS		
Na+/K+ ATPase	+++	++
ABCG2	+++	–
OTHERS		
p63	+++	±

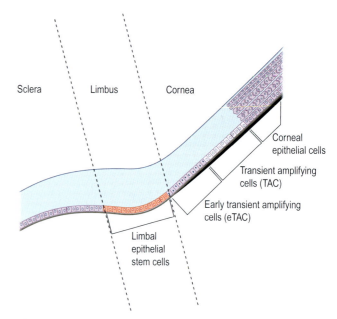

Figure 5.2 Limbal epithelial stem cells, which reside in the limbal niche, give rise to early transient amplifying cells (eTAC). These eTACs further divide and give rise to additional TACs. TACs finally migrate centripetally towards the corneal center, ultimately forming the terminally differentiated corneal epithelial cells.

homeostatic microenvironment that promotes the maintenance of limbal epithelial stem cells (LESCs) in an undifferentiated state. Currently, no single marker can be used to identify LESCs definitively, which lack terminal differentiation markers. However, LESCs can be differentiated from the corneal epithelium by several markers, including p63, vimentin, α9β1 integrin, cytokeratin (CK)19, CK5, CK14, cadherin 342, and the ATP-binding cassette subfamily G member 2 (ABCG2) transporter protein (Table 5.1). Further, LESCs lack CK3 and CK12, which are characteristic for the corneal epithelium. They are heavily pigmented in order to be protected form ultraviolet light damage. LESCs produce several metabolic enzymes and proteins at higher levels than corneal epithelial cells, such as α-enolase, cytochrome oxidase, Na+-K+ ATPase, carbonic anhydrase, and glucose transporter. The functional relevance of these enzymes and proteins are yet to be elucidated.

DIFFERENTIATION OF LIMBAL EPITHELIAL STEM CELLS TO CORNEAL EPITHELIUM

Although LESCs are slowly cycling and divide only occasionally, they have high proliferative and self-renewal capacity.[3] Due to their slow cell cycling, they have a higher retention of DNA precursor analogs. However, in the event of injury, LESCs begin rapid proliferation. In order to retain a constant stem cell pool, LESCs undergo two types of cell division: a symmetric and asymmetric division (Fig. 5.1). During symmetric division, either two identical stem cells or alternatively two identical differentiated daughter cells emerge. In contrast, asymmetric division of LESCs results into a stem cell and an early transient amplifying cell (eTAC).[6] These eTACs further divide and give rise to additional TACs (Fig. 5.2). TACs finally migrate centripetally towards the corneal center, ultimately forming the

terminally differentiated corneal epithelial cells. This terminal differentiation of TACs into corneal epithelial cells is accompanied by specific morphological and biochemical alterations.

LIMBAL NICHE AND LIMBAL EPITHELIAL CRYPTS

The division and differentiation processes of LESCs are strictly regulated by the microenvironment, called the *limbal niche*. The limbal niche is highly vascularized and innervated, and thus, provided by a potential source of nutrients and growth factors for LESCs. In addition, limbal fibroblasts in the underlying stroma secrete acidic and cysteine-rich proteins, thus contributing to LESC adhesion. More recently, the presence of *limbal epithelial crypts* have been demonstrated, extending from the palisades of Vogt.[5,7] All cells within these crypts have been shown to be epithelial in nature as demonstrated by their CK5/14 staining. Further, an ABCG2-positive LESC population has been shown to extend along the basal epithelial cell layer of the limbus.[7]

Corneal Epithelium

The corneal surface is covered by a non-keratinized stratified squamous epithelium and has a thickness of approximately 50 μm. The corneal epithelium is comprised of five to seven layers, consisting of superficial squamous epithelial cells, suprabasal epithelial cells with wing-like extensions, and a monolayer of columnar basal epithelial cells. Basal epithelial cells attach to the epithelial basement membrane, which is adjacent to the Bowman's layer. The characteristics of corneal epithelial cells and their junctional

Table 5.2   Characteristics of Superficial, Suprabasal and Basal Cells of the Corneal Epithelium

	Size of the Layer	Number of Layers	Shape	Mitotic Activity	Junctional Complexes
Superficial cells	50 μm	2–4 layers	Flat, microvilli, microplicae	Absent	Tight junctions, desmosomes
Suprabasal wing-like cells	15 μm	2–3 layers	Wing-like	Absent	Gap junctions, desmosomes
Basal cells	8–10 μm	Monolayer	Cuboidal	Present	Gap junctions, desmosomes, hemidesmosomes

complexes are shown in Table 5.2. Tight junctions (zonula occludens) play an effective barrier role and are present between the superficial cells. Desmosomes, on the other hand, are present in all layers (Fig. 5.3). Further, actin filaments, intermediate filaments, and microtubules, which form the intracellular cytoskeleton, are present in corneal epithelial cells. Cytokeratin 3 and CK12 are expressed on the corneal epithelium but not in the limbal or conjunctival epithelium. There are also immune cells within the corneal epithelium, which have a role in antigen processing. Mature and immature dendritic cells are abundant in the periphery, while immature dendritic cells are present in the central corneal epithelium, where they can now be observed with laser in vivo confocal microscopy.[8] These cells capture antigen, process it, and migrate to draining lymph nodes, where they present antigens to T cells. The numbers of these cells increase dramatically in response to any kind of corneal injury.[8]

The corneal epithelium has unique functions, including the transmission and refraction of light, and a barrier function that prevents the entry of pathogens and other harmful agents into the cornea. The optical properties of the corneal epithelium are facilitated by a wet and smooth surface, as well as the regular epithelial thickness throughout the entire cornea. Furthermore, the relatively low number of intracellular organelles, and the presence and organization of crystallins contribute to these optical properties.

The corneal epithelium covers a highly organized, avascular, and transparent corneal stroma, which requires highly specialized metabolic interactions. The dense and unique neural innervation of the corneal epithelium aids and dictates its specific metabolic functions. A high density of sensory nerve endings supplies the suprabasal cells of the epithelium. This density of nerve endings per unit area is 400 times higher than the epidermal innervation, making the cornea the most innervated tissue in the body. Corneal sensory nerves contain neuropeptides, such as substance P, calcitonin gene-related peptide, and vasoactive intestinal peptide, all of which exert important trophic functions on the corneal epithelium and contribute to the maintenance and self-renewal of epithelial cells on the ocular surface.[9]

As the corneal epithelium is prone to injury, self-renewal is highly critical and imperative. The typical turnover of the epithelium lasts 5 to 7 days. As mitotically active basal epithelial cells proliferate, daughter cells begin their movement, first centripetally and then towards the corneal surface, where they first differentiate into suprabasal cells, wing-like cells, and subsequently into superficial epithelial cells. Fully differentiated squamous cells are then shed from the ocular surface. The X, Y, Z hypothesis of corneal epithelial maintenance (Fig. 5.4) by Thoft and Friend[10] proposed the proliferation of basal cells (X), and the subsequent centripetal migration (Y), was equal to the shedding of superficial epithelial cells (Z). During this balance of proliferation and differentiation, both cell–cell and cell–matrix interactions occur.

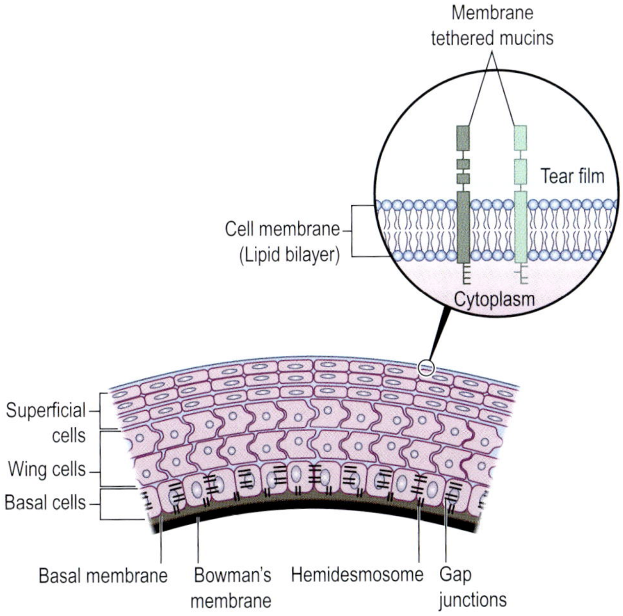

Figure 5.3 The junctional complexes of corneal epithelium are shown. Basal epithelial cells are attached to the basement membrane with hemidesmosomes. Tight junctions (zonula occludens) play an effective barrier role and are present between the superficial cells. Desmosomes, on the other hand, are present in all layers. The superficial epithelial cells have membrane-tethered mucins.

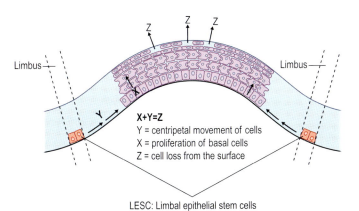

Figure 5.4 The X, Y, Z hypothesis of corneal epithelial maintenance. The proliferation of basal cells (X), and the subsequent centripetal migration (Y), is equal to the shedding of superficial epithelial cells (Z).

SUPERFICIAL EPITHELIAL CELLS

Superficial epithelial cells are present at the outermost layer of corneal epithelium. These differentiated flat and polygonal cells have surface microvilli, which form microplicae. The microplicae increase the cell surface area and improve oxygen and nutrient uptake from the tear film. Further, tight junctions between neighboring cells provide a protective barrier function. Electron microscopic studies have demonstrated two types of superficial epithelial cells: dark cells, and light cells. On the one hand, there are dark cells that are larger with denser microvilli. These cells are older and tend to desquamate. Light cells, on the other hand, are younger, with lighter microvilli. Superficial epithelial cells are terminally differentiated and therefore, do not divide; thus, they contain fewer organelles than other corneal epithelial cells. A unique characteristic of superficial epithelial cells is presence of numerous glycolipid and glycoprotein molecules that are embedded into their cell membranes. These molecules form the glycocalyx particles, which attach to the mucins (MUCs) in the tear film (see Fig. 5.3), and improve tear film stability. Loss of glycocalyx particles causes tear film instability and ocular surface disease. Of the MUCs, three have been identified as major membrane-tethered mucins on the ocular surface (Table 5.3). These include MUCs 1, 4, and 16.

SUPRABASAL WING-LIKE EPITHELIAL CELLS

Suprabasal epithelial cells reside beneath the superficial epithelial layer. Their cell membranes demonstrate lateral interdigitations (wings), with numerous desmosomes and

Table 5.3 The Membrane Mucins that form the Dense Glycocalyx Layer on the Apical Surface of the Corneal Epithelia can Extend up to 500 nm from the Epithelial Surface. Of the Membrane-Tethered Mucins MUCs 1, 3A, 3B, 4, 11, 12, 15, 16, 17, and 20, Three have been Identified as Major Membrane-Tethered Mucins on the Ocular Surface. These Include MUCs 1, 4, and 16.

	Molecular Weight	Functions
MUC-1	120–300 kDa	Anti-adhesion, signaling, pathogen barrier
MUC-4	900 kDa	Signaling, maintenance of tear fluid stability
MUC-16	20 MDa	Association with cytoskeleton, pathogen barrier

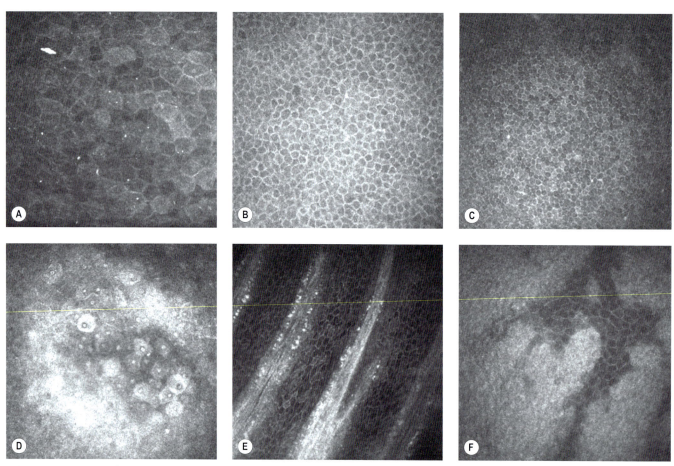

Figure 5.5 In vivo confocal microscopy (IVCM) images of superficial corneal epithelial layer of the cornea (A), wing layer (B), and basal epithelium (C) in a normal subject. Superficial epithelial layer in a dry eye patient demonstrates increased hyper-reflectivity. Note that hyperchromatic nuclei are present (D). IVCM images of inferior palisades. They appear as parallel, elongated structures, separated by 6–10 rows of limbal epithelial cells. Central hyper-reflective fibroconnective tissue is present, surrounded by a combination of a thin layer of minimally reflective epithelium with scattered dense intracellular hyper-reflectivity (E). IVCM images of nasal limbus of a normal eye at the level of superficial squamous cells. It is composed of nests and islands of hypo- and hyper-reflective epithelial cells (F).

gap junctions. There are two to three layers of these cells present in the cornea. They are in a semidifferentiated stage between basal and superficial cells and rarely undergo cell division. Moreover, they migrate superficially to terminally differentiate into superficial squamous epithelial cells.

BASAL EPITHELIAL CELLS

The basal epithelial cells represent a single columnar layer on a basal membrane. They are the only cells within the corneal epithelium with mitotic activity, and have more intracellular organelles compared to other epithelial cells. They have lateral membrane interdigitations that form zonula adherens, desmosomes, and gap junctions. The basal epithelial cells also regulate organization of hemidesmosomes and focal complexes, which maintain attachment to the underlying basement membrane (see Fig. 5.3). They synthesize part of the basal membrane during their life cycle and have anchoring plaques consisting of type I collagen, which span into the corneal stroma. These plaques are important for maintaining the adhesion of the corneal epithelium to the basement membrane. Further, integrins, receptors that mediate attachment between cells and the extracellular matrix are expressed on the corneal epithelium. The integrin subunits $\alpha2$, $\alpha3$, $\alpha5$, $\alpha6$, αv, $\beta1$, $\beta4$, and $\beta5$ have been demonstrated in the human corneal epithelium. Integrins play a critical role in the formation of hemidesmosomes.

BASEMENT MEMBRANE

The basement membrane of corneal epithelium is 0.11 to 0.55 μm in thickness, consisting of the lamina lucida and lamina densa. The basal epithelial cells secrete the necessary constituents for the establishment of the basement membrane. The basement membrane is composed of type IV collagen and laminin. Functionally, it is necessary for the polarization and migration of proliferating epithelial cells. Moreover, it is important for the continuation of a well-organized and stratified corneal epithelium.

Summary

The orchestrated communication between LESCs, the limbal niche, and the corneal epithelium and stroma plays a highly significant role in the maintenance of optical clarity of the cornea, and thus, clear vision. Any insult to the cornea may compromise the LESC functionality. Limbal stem cell deficiency or insufficiency can result from both primary (e.g. aniridia) or secondary etiologies (e.g. chemical burns, Stevens–Johnson syndrome). Progressive disease will lead to persistent epithelial breakdown, superficial corneal vascularization, chronic discomfort, and vision loss. Moreover, the corneal epithelium can be affected by many ocular surface diseases (e.g. dry eye, infectious keratitis). The recent use of in vivo confocal microscopy to study the limbal and corneal epithelium in real time (Fig. 5.5) will undoubtedly advance our knowledge in the pathophysiology of ocular surface diseases. Understanding the precise pathways for differentiation and proliferation of corneal epithelial cells is critical for the development of new effective treatments.

Acknowledgments

The authors acknowledge the contribution of Mr. Peter Mallen for graphic services.

References

1. Gipson IK, Joyce NC. Anatomy and cell biology of the cornea, superficial limbus, and conjunctiva. In: Albert DM, Miller JW, editors. Albert and Jakobiec's principles and practice of ophthalmology. Canada: Saunders Elsevier; 2008. p. 423–40.
2. Dua HS, Azuara-Blanco A. Limbal stem cells of the corneal epithelium. Surv Ophthalmol 2000;44:415–25.
3. Cotsarelis G, Cheng SZ, Dong G, et al. Existence of slow-cycling limbal epithelial basal cells that can be preferentially stimulated to proliferate: implications on epithelial stem cells. Cell 1989;57: 201–9.
4. Davanger M, Evensen A. Role of the pericorneal papillary structure in renewal of corneal epithelium. Nature 1971;229:560–1.
5. Miri A, Al-Aqaba M, Otri AM, et al. In vivo confocal microscopic features of normal limbus. Br J Ophthalmol 2012;96:530–6.
6. Castro-Munozledo F, Gomez-Flores E. Challenges to the study of asymmetric cell division in corneal and limbal epithelia. Exp Eye Res 2011;92:4–9.
7. Dua HS, Shanmuganathan VA, Powell-Richards AO, et al. Limbal epithelial crypts: a novel anatomical structure and a putative limbal stem cell niche. Br J Ophthalmol 2005;89:529–32.
8. Cruzat A, Witkin D, Baniasadi N, et al. Inflammation and the nervous system: the connection in the cornea in patients with infectious keratitis. Invest Ophthalmol Vis Sci 2011;52:5136–43.
9. Müller LJ, Marfurt CF, Kruse F, et al. Corneal nerves: structure, contents and function. Exp Eye Res 2003;76:521–42.
10. Thoft RA, Friend J. The X, Y, Z hypothesis of corneal epithelial maintenance. Invest Ophthalmol Vis Sci 1983;24:1442–3.

6 Classification of Ocular Surface Disease

JOSEPH M. BIBER

Introduction

The ocular surface is one of the most complex and unique tissues in the body. It is also one of the few areas in the body not protected by skin, which is the body's most valuable defense against both desiccation and infection. The ocular surface must remain stable to not only provide protection to the eye, but to maintain the comfort of the eye and provide a refractive surface that allows for good-quality vision. This complex and vulnerable system includes the eyelids and eyelashes, tear film, and the ocular surface, which is made up of the conjunctiva and the corneal epithelium.

The first line of defense is the eyelashes, which collect debris, therefore preventing it from interacting and damaging the surface of the eye. There are roughly 100 lashes in the upper lid and 50 in the lower lid.[1] The layers of the eyelid, from superficial to deep, include the skin, orbicularis muscle, tarsus, and palpebral conjunctiva. The eyelid's primary function is to protect the ocular surface, but they also function in cleansing and lubricating the eye. With each blink, the tear film is continuously spread over the ocular surface, maintaining optical visual clarity of the cornea. The subconscious blink reflex occurs every 6–10 seconds, and it has also been determined that significant restoration of the ocular surface occurs during extended times of closure, such as sleeping.

The conjunctiva is an ectodermally derived mucous membrane that extends from the mucocutaneous junction of the eyelid margins to the corneoscleral limbus.[2] The conjunctival surface reflects onto the palpebral surfaces, creating fornices and folds, which allow for movement of the globe. Nasally, the plica semilunaris is formed by the folding of the conjunctiva. The conjunctival epithelium must be kept continuously moist to avoid desiccation.[3] The conjunctival epithelium is rich in goblet cells, which are mucin-producing cells critical for the tear film. At the corneoscleral junction, the conjunctiva forms radial folds called the palisades of Vogt. The conjunctiva is also the sole source of lymphatic tissue of the eye, and therefore, has an important function in regard to protection against infection.

The tear film is a complex mixture of substances secreted from multiple sources on the ocular surface, including the lacrimal gland, the accessory lacrimal glands, the meibomian glands, and the goblet cells. Historically, the tear film has been broken down into three primary components or layers: the aqueous component, the mucin component, and the oil component. The aqueous component of the tears is secreted by the noninnervated glands of Krause and Wolfring found in the forniceal conjunctiva. The mucin component of tears is produced by goblet cells. The oil component of tears is secreted by the meibomian glands found on the lid margin. Our understanding has evolved and the tear layers are now thought of more as a continuum. Abnormalities in any of these components of the tear film may contribute to instability of the ocular surface.

The final structure of the ocular surface is the cornea, which serves as the transparent window of the eye, allowing light rays to pass into the eye to be processed by the visual system. To accomplish this, the cornea must have a normal contour and be avascular, transparent, and be essentially dehydrated. The corneal epithelium is continuous with the conjunctival epithelium and both are composed of nonkeratinized, stratified, squamous epithelium cells. The corneal epithelium is 50 μm thick and has five or six layers of three different types of cells: superficial cells, wing cells, and basal cells. It is believed that the corneal epithelium is replaced by a population of stem cells found at the anatomical limbus.[4] The corneal epithelium completely sheds and renews itself approximately every 7 days. The corneal epithelium is not a mucus membrane; however, it is susceptible to desiccation if not properly protected by the lids and tear film.

The lacrimal functional unit (LFU) has been described as an encompassing term representing the integrated system that comprises the ocular surface (cornea, conjunctiva, accessory lacrimal and meibomian glands), the main lacrimal glands, the blink mechanism that spreads tears, and the sensory and motor nerves that connect them whose parts act together and not in isolation.[5] Poor function of this unit will often result in dry eye disease.

One of the challenges for clinicians is that disorders of the ocular surface manifest in a number of ways. Regardless of the etiology, conjunctival and corneal inflammation is common and patients will often complain of irritation, redness, burning, itching, blurry vision and photophobia. Unfortunately for patients, diseases of the ocular surface are extremely common and range from asymptomatic to debilitating. In this chapter, we will break down different disorders of the ocular surface by anatomical involvement as well as pathophysiology.

Eyelids and Eyelashes

The critical relationship and dependence of the lid–lash complex to the ocular surface is described above. If the eyelid margin is not apposed to the corneal surface, significant ocular surface inflammation and mechanical trauma can occur. Flaws in the lid–lash complex, which can lead to

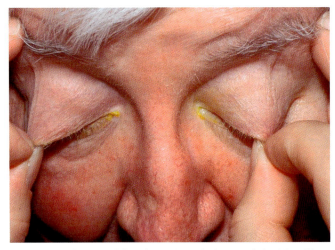

Figure 6.1 Floppy eyelid syndrome. Note the increased elasticity of the upper lids.

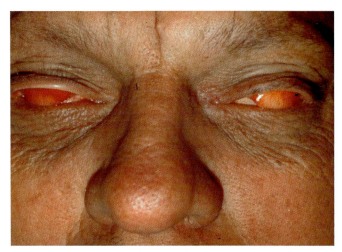

Figure 6.2 Floppy eyelid syndrome. In this patient, the lids are easily everted and maintain that position. Note the increased conjunctival injection of the right superior palpebral conjunctiva.

instability of the ocular surface are myriad, but fall into two basic groups. One group leads to a mechanical rubbing and irritation of the ocular surface and the other is related to poor closure resulting in desiccation of the tissue. Disorders such as trichiasis, distichiasis, epiblepharon, lid imbrication syndrome, and entropion, cause ocular surface problems through the mechanical rubbing of lashes against the conjunctival and corneal surfaces. It is not only the trauma of the lashes rubbing, but also the induced chronic, low-grade inflammation, which further exacerbates the disease process. Most eyelid malpositions involve the lower lid. Trichiasis is distinguished from an entropion or epiblepharon by evaluating the lash orientation when the lid is in its normal position. Trichiasis refers to the condition where the lashes emerge from their normal anterior lamellar origin but are misdirected. Distichiasis is different from trichiasis in that the lashes originate from the more posterior meibomian gland orifices. Both conditions can be congenital or acquired. Another cause of mechanical trauma to the ocular surface creating significant inflammation is floppy eyelid syndrome. In this condition, the rubbery and floppy upper lid is everted during sleep and rubs on the pillow or sheets. This mechanical irritation creates a prominent papillary reaction on the upper palpebral conjunctiva, as well as punctate keratopathy on the cornea. Floppy eyelid is bilateral in 78% of patients, but can be asymmetric. Common external findings include a markedly elongated and lax upper lid and eyelash ptosis of the upper lid (Fig. 6.1). Patients often complain of ocular irritation, mucous discharge, and papillary conjunctivitis[6] (Fig. 6.2). There are also reports of an association between keratoconus and floppy eyelid syndrome. One study reported 18% of their patients with floppy eyelid have clinical keratoconus and possibly up to 71% may have subclinical keratoconus.[7]

Other disorders such as lagophthalmos, eyelid retraction, and ectropion cause damage to the ocular surface by exposure. In these cases, incomplete closure of the lids allows for local increased tear film evaporation and subsequent corneal and conjunctival desiccation. Closure of the eyelids is primarily a function of the upper lid, with the lower lid exhibiting very little upward movement during closure. As a result, many patients tolerate lower lid retraction and scleral show with minimal symptoms, if the upper lid function is normal.[8] Resultant inflammation will cause further insult to the ocular surface. Medical management to stabilize the ocular surface and reduce inflammation is important, but often the critical step is surgically addressing the abnormal lid position.

Lid Margin and Meibomian Glands

Blepharitis and its wide range of clinical symptoms and presentations is one of the most commonly encountered conditions seen in ophthalmology practices. Although blepharitis and lid margin disease has been described throughout the ophthalmic literature for over a hundred years, our understanding and ability to consistently classify and define this challenging, yet common condition has been lacking. In 2010, the International Workshop on Meibomian Gland Dysfunction (MGD) published their findings in hopes of providing a global consensus on the definition, classification, diagnosis, and therapy for MGD.

Blepharitis is a broad term used to describe inflammation of the lid as a whole. Anterior blepharitis is defined as inflammation of the lid margin anterior to the gray line and centered on the lashes. Marginal blepharitis refers to inflammation of the lid margin and includes both anterior and posterior blepharitis. Posterior blepharitis describes inflammation of the posterior lid margin, which may have different causes, including MGD, conjunctival inflammation, and acne rosacea.[9] McCulley et al., in 1982, published six categories for blepharitis, with the first three describing anterior blepharitis and the final three posterior blepharitis and meibomian gland abnormalities. Anterior blepharitis is commonly associated with staphylococcal disease, as well as seborrhea, and presents with inflammation, crusting, and collarettes on the lashes.[10]

Meibomian gland disease is used to describe a broad range of meibomian gland disorders, including neoplasia, congenital disease, and MGD. MGD is defined as a chronic, diffuse abnormality of the meibomian glands, commonly characterized by terminal duct obstruction and/or qualitative/quantitative changes in the glandular secretion. It may result in alteration of the tear film, symptoms of eye irritation, clinically apparent inflammation, and ocular surface disease. Further, MGD is classified into two major categories: low-delivery states and high-delivery states. Low-delivery states are broken down into either hyposecretory (meibomian sicca) or obstructive, with cicatricial and non-cicatricial categories.

Hyposecretory MGD results from decreased meibum secretion without obvious obstruction. Hyposecretory MGD is seen clinically with gland atrophy and dropout. Contact lens wear has been associated with a decrease in the number of functional meibomian glands.[9] Obstructive MGD is a result of obstruction of the duct, resulting in reduced delivery of meibum to the ocular surface. The gland orifice epithelium can become keratinized, creating a low-delivery state. Obstructive MGD is probably the most common form of MGD. Obstructive MGD is further divided into cicatricial and non-cicatricial. The cicatricial form of obstructive MGD results when the duct orifices are dragged posteriorly into the mucosa, as compared to non-cicatricial MGD where the ducts are obstructed but in their normal anatomic position. Causes of cicatricial obstructive MGD include trachoma, ocular cicatricial pemphigoid, erythema multiforme, and atopic eye disease. Non-cicatricial obstructive MGD may be caused by Sjögren's syndrome, seborrheic dermatitis, acne rosacea, atopy, and psoriasis[9] (Fig. 6.3).

High-delivery, hypersecretory MGD is defined by the release of a large volume of lipid at the lid margin that is easily visible on examination with digital pressure on the glands. Seborrheic dermatitis has been reported to be associated with hypersecretory MGD in 100% of cases.[9] Other causes include acne rosacea and atopic disease. In acne, increased sebum excretion on the face is a critical factor in the disease process[9] (Fig. 6.4).

The prevalence of MGD reported in the ophthalmic literature varies widely from as low as 3.5%[11] to almost 70%.[12] One of the challenges of identifying a true prevalence is its wide range of symptoms and clinical findings, creating a broad spectrum that has significant overlap with other ocular surface disorders, specifically dry eye disease. One

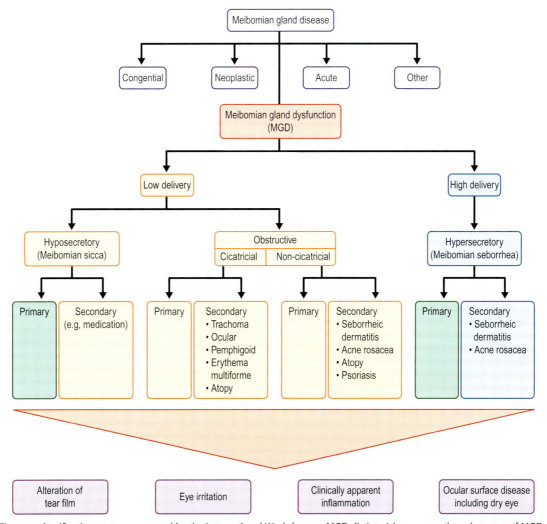

Figure 6.3 The new classification system proposed by the International Workshop on MGD distinguishes among the subgroups of MGD on the basis of the level of secretions and further subdivides those categories by potential consequences and manifestations. One the basis of these proposed classifications, obstructive MGD is the most pervasive. (From Nelson JD, Shimazaki J, Benitez-del-Castillo JM, et al. The International Workshop on Meibomian Gland Dysfunction: Report of the Definition and Classification Subcommittee. IOVS 2011; 52:1930–1937.)

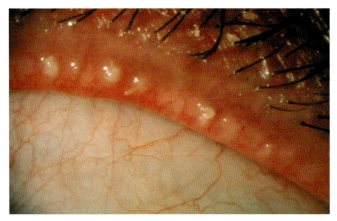

Figure 6.4 Meibomian gland deficiency. Note pouting of the meibum from the orifice. Also note lid margin telangiectasia in a patient with rosacea.

Table 6.1 Clinical Summary of the MGD Staging Used to Guide Treatment

Stage	MGD Grade	Symptoms	Corneal Staining
1	+ (minimally altered expressibility and secretion quality)	None	None
2	++ (mildly altered expressibility and secretion quality)	Minimal to mild	None to limited
3	+++ (moderately altered expressibility and secretion quality)	Moderate	Mild to moderate; mainly peripheral
4	++++ (severely altered expressibility and secretion quality)	Marked	Marked; central in addition
'Plus' disease	Co-existing or accompanying disorders of the ocular surface and/or eyelids		

(From Geerling G, Tauber J, Baudouin C, et al. The International Workshop on Meibomian Gland Dysfunction: Report of the Subcommittee on Management and Treatment of Meibomian Gland Dysfunction. IOVS 2011;52:2050–2064.)

consistent finding has been the increased prevalence in the Asian population. Several studies[12,13] have reported higher than 60% for the Asian population, compared to between 3.5%[11] and 19.9%[14] for Caucasians.

To better guide the clinician with treatment of MGD, the International Workshop devised a staging system for MGD. Four stages were defined based on expressability, secretion quality, symptoms, and corneal staining. Stage 1 refers to patients with minimally altered expressability and secretion quality, no symptoms, and no corneal staining. Stage 2 defines patients with mildly altered expressability and secretion quality, minimal to mild symptoms, and limited corneal staining. Stage 3 is defined as moderately altered expressability and secretion quality, moderate symptoms, and mild to moderate peripheral corneal staining. Stage 4 is defined as severely altered expressability and secretion quality, marked symptoms, and marked central corneal staining. Plus disease is reserved for patients with co-existing disorders of the ocular surface and/or eyelids[15] (Table 6.1). The

classification and staging of lid margin diseases will better aid the clinician, further our understanding of the pathophysiology of this disease process, improve our treatment options and patient outcomes, and guide future research studies in this field.

Tear Film and Dry Eye Syndrome

Dry eye disease (DED), or keratoconjunctivitis sicca (KCS), is one of the most common conditions affecting patients worldwide. Abnormalities of the tear film are characterized by the component that is abnormal or deficient. Dry eye was defined by the International Dry Eye Workshop (DEWS) as a multifactorial disease of the tears and ocular surface that results in symptoms of discomfort, visual disturbance, and tear film instability with potential damage to the ocular surface. It is accompanied by increased osmolarity of the tear film and inflammation of the ocular surface.[16] Historically, and from the DEWS report, DED is divided into two major subtypes: aqueous tear-deficient dry eye (ADDE) and evaporative dry eye (EDE) (Fig. 6.5).

AQUEOUS TEAR-DEFICIENT DRY EYE

Aqueous tear-deficient dry eye (ADDE) refers to dry eye that is due to failure of lacrimal secretion. The failure of lacrimal secretion due to lacrimal acinar destruction or dysfunction results in increased tear osmolarity and starts a cascade of inflammatory mediators to the ocular surface.[16] ADDE is further subdivided into two groups: Sjögren's syndrome dry eye (SSDE) and non-Sjögren's syndrome dry eye. Sjögren's syndrome (SS) is an autoimmune process targeting the lacrimal and salivary glands. It is the second most common autoimmune rheumatologic disease, exceeded only by rheumatoid arthritis. There are two forms of SS: primary SS refers to cases where there is no other associated systemic connective tissue disease; secondary SS consists of the features of primary SS with the features of an overt autoimmune connective tissue disease, such as rheumatoid arthritis, systemic lupus erythematous, polyarteritis nodosa, Wegener's granulomatosis, systemic sclerosis, primary biliary sclerosis, or mixed connective tissue disease. Diagnostic criteria including patient's symptoms, ocular signs, salivary gland involvement, and presence of autoantibodies have been published to aid diagnosis[17] (Table 6.2).

Non-SS dry eye is a form of ADDE due to lacrimal dysfunction, where the systemic autoimmune features characteristics of SSDE have been excluded. Age-related dry eye is the most common form; however, other forms include secondary lacrimal gland deficiencies, obstruction of the lacrimal gland ducts, and reflex hyposecretion.[17] For age-related dry eye, alterations in ductal pathology with increasing age have been postulated as a cause of lacrimal gland dysfunction.[18] Another contributing factor to age-related dry eye is the change in androgen levels with time, which is why postmenopausal women are one of the groups at highest risk of DED. Causes of secondary lacrimal gland deficiency include infiltration of the lacrimal gland in sarcoidosis, lymphoma, AIDS, and graft-versus-host disease (GVHD), lacrimal gland ablation, and lacrimal gland denervation.[17] Cicatricizing conjunctivitis, caused by trachoma, pemphigoid, and

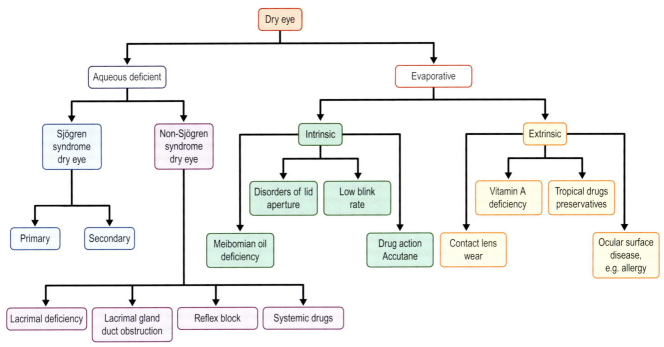

Figure 6.5 Etiologic classification of dry eye disease. The list (*bottom left*) illustrates the environmental risk factors for dry eye disease. The scheme indicates the etiologic classification of dry eye disease into aqueous-deficient or evaporative tear deficiency. (From Krachmer et al., Cornea, 3rd ed., Mosby, Elsevier 2010. Figure 36.1.)

Table 6.2   Revised International Classification Criteria for Ocular Manifestations of Sjögren's Syndrome

I. Ocular symptoms: a positive response to at least one of the following questions:
1. Have you had daily, persistent, troublesome dry eyes for more than 3 months?
2. Do you have a recurrent sensation of sand or gravel in the eyes?
3. Do you use tear substitutes more than three times a day?

II. Oral symptoms: a positive response to at least one of the following questions:
1. Have you had a daily feeling of dry mouth for more than 3 months?
2. Have you had recurrently or persistently swollen salivary glands as an adult?
3. Do you frequently drink liquids to aid in swallowing dry food?

III. Ocular signs: that is, objective evidence of ocular involvement defined as a positive result for at least one of the following two tests:
1. Schirmer I test, performed without anesthesia (≤5 mm in 5 minutes)
2. Rose bengal score or other ocular dye score (≥4 according to van Bijsterveld's scoring system)

IV. Histopathology: in minor salivary glands (obtained through normal-appearing mucosa) focal lymphocytic sialoadenitis, evaluated by an expert histopathologist, with a focus score ≥1, defined as a number of lymphocytic foci (which are adjacent to normal-appearing mucous acini and contain more than 50 lymphocytes) per 4 mm two of glandular tissue

V. Salivary gland involvement: objective evidence of salivary gland involvement defined by a positive result for at least one of the following diagnostic tests:
1. Unstimulated whole salivary flow (≤1.5 mL in 15 minutes)
2. Parotid sialography showing the presence of diffuse sialectasias (punctate, cavitary or destructive pattern), without evidence of obstruction in the major ducts
3. Salivary scintigraphy showing delayed uptake, reduced concentration and/or delayed excretion of tracer

VI. Autoantibodies: presence in the serum of the following autoantibodies:
1. Antibodies to Ro(SSA) or La(SSB) antigens, or both

(From Krachmer et al., Cornea, 3rd ed., Mosby, Elsevier 2010. Table 36.1.)

erythema multiforme, and severe chemical and thermal burns can cause non-SS dry eye due to lacrimal gland duct obstruction. Finally, reflex hyposecretion can lead to non-SS dry eye due to reducing the reflex-induced lacrimal secretion and reducing the blink reflex leading to increasing evaporative loss. This reflex sensory block is common in diabetes mellitus and causes of neurotrophic keratitis, such as herpes simplex virus.[17]

EVAPORATIVE DRY EYE

Evaporative dry eye results from the exposed ocular surface losing water in the presence of normal lacrimal secretory function. Evaporative dry eye is further divided into intrinsic causes and extrinsic. Intrinsic causes include meibomian gland dysfunction, disorders of the lid aperture, and low blink rate. MGD, as discussed above, is the most common cause of evaporative dry eye. Proptosis due to thyroid eye disease, craniosynostosis, and orbital masses increase the area of exposure, resulting in worsening dry eye. Lagophthalmos, especially nocturnal, or incomplete closure after blepharoplasty are other causes of intrinsic evaporative dry eye. A reduced blink rate seen with focused near work or in Parkinson's disease also causes evaporative dry eye.[17]

Extrinsic causes of evaporative dry eye include ocular surface disease, such as allergic conjunctivitis and vitamin A deficiency, contact lens wear, and preservatives in commonly used ophthalmic medicines. Many components of eye drop formulations can induce a toxic response from the ocular surface. Benzalkonium chloride, one of the most common offenders, causes surface epithelial cell damage and punctate epithelial keratitis, which interferes with surface wetability.[17] Glaucoma patients treated for years with preservative-containing drops are at risk for evaporative dry eye. Contact lens use is extremely prevalent in the world today. The primary reasons for contact lens intolerance are dryness and discomfort.[17] About 50% of contact lens wearers report dry eye symptoms.[19] In addition, contact lens wearers are twelve times more likely than emmetropes to report dry eye symptoms and five times more likely than people wearing spectacles.[20]

The classification and defining of dry eye by the DEWS report will continue to enhance our understanding of this complex and common ophthalmic condition. By furthering our understanding and standardizing the terminology, future clinical studies will be able to better identify new modalities of treatments in the hope of providing better care to our patients.

Conjunctiva

The hallmark of disorders of the conjunctiva is inflammation. The conjunctiva has a relatively simple histological structure that limits the response to inflammatory stimuli to five morphologic responses: papillary, follicular, membranous/pseudomembranous, cicatrizing, and granulomatous. Chronicity is also an important criterion for classification of conjunctivitis. Typically, acute conjunctivitis is defined as having a duration of less than 3 weeks.[21] The most obvious sign of conjunctival inflammation is injection, which is typically accompanied by cellular infiltration and chemosis.[21] Conjunctival exudates are often present and can aid the clinician in the diagnosis. The three types of exudates are purulent or hyperacute, mucopurulent or catarrhal, and watery. In addition, identification by the clinician of the most severely affected area of conjunctiva can aid the diagnosis (Fig. 6.6).

Non-specific inflammation may be accompanied by a papillary reaction of the tarsal conjunctiva. Causes of acute papillary conjunctivitis include primarily bacterial causes such as *Neisseria* species and *Staphylococcus* or *Haemophilus*. Chronic papillary changes can be seen in conditions such as superior limbic keratoconjunctivitis, floppy eyelid, masquerade syndromes, mucus-fishing, dry eye disease, and dacryocystitis. If the papillae are greater than 1 mm in diameter they are considered giant papillae. These findings are typically seen in allergic disorders, such as vernal and atopic conjunctivitis, but can also be seen in relation to contact lens wear.[21]

Immune-mediated inflammation may show follicles of the tarsal or limbal conjunctiva. Follicles are yellowish, white, discrete, round, elevated lesions of the conjunctiva, that are more specific than papillary reactions. Acute follicular conjunctivitis is typically associated with viral etiologies, such as adenovirus and herpes simplex, but can also be found in inclusion conjunctivitis secondary to *Chlamydia trachomatis*. Chronic follicular conjunctivitis is most commonly due to *Chlamydia*, as either trachoma or inclusion conjunctivitis. Other causes of chronic follicular changes are *Moraxella*, molluscum contagiosum, and Lyme disease[21] (Fig. 6.7).

In severe cases of conjunctivitis, fibrin membranes that are adherent to the conjunctival surface may develop. True membranes bleed when peeled, which differentiates them from pseudomembranes, and are more indicative of severe inflammation. Historically, bacterial infections from

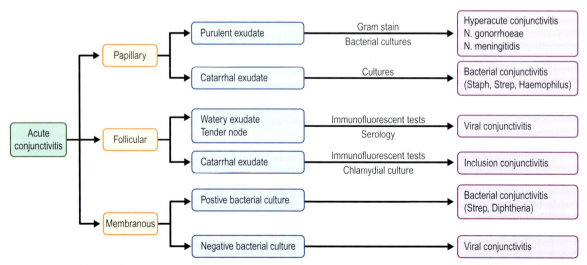

Figure 6.6 An algorithm for diagnosing acute conjunctivitis. (From Krachmer et al., Cornea, 3rd ed., Mosby, Elsevier 2010. Figure 42.1.)

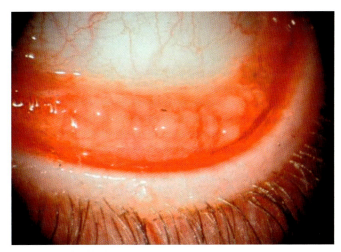

Figure 6.7 Chronic follicular conjunctivitis.

Corynebacterium and beta-hemolytic streptococci were the principal etiologies of acute membranous conjunctivitis; however, viruses such as adenovirus and herpes simplex are more common now.[21] Ligneous conjunctivitis is the only chronic membranous conjunctivitis. Ligneous conjunctivitis is a rare form of conjunctivitis that presents with highly vascularized, friable, whitish membrane on the upper palpebral conjunctiva. Ligneous conjunctivitis has been associated with a plasminogen deficiency and can be treated with systemic and/or topical fresh frozen plasma.[22]

If the conjunctivitis involves only the epithelium and is short-lived, normal conjunctival anatomy and function will return once the inflammation has resolved.[21] The end result of severe and chronic inflammation is irreversible changes, such as goblet cell damage and deficiency. Because goblet cells secrete mucin, which helps the aqueous tears coat the hydrophobic ocular surface, their loss will result in tear film abnormalities. Chronic conjunctival inflammation may lead to changes in the substantia propria of the conjunctiva, resulting in subepithelial fibrosis. With persistent inflammation, scar tissue can change the forniceal architecture and cause foreshortening of the fornix, hallmarks of cicatrizing conjunctivitis. Further progression of the chronic inflammatory process can lead to keratinization of the ocular surface, as well as symblepharon formation, and potentially even ankyloblepharon. Examples of cicatrizing conjunctivitis include Stevens–Johnson syndrome, ocular cicatricial pemphigoid, and chemical burns[21] (Fig. 6.8).

The final morphologic response of the conjunctiva to inflammation is a granuloma. Sarcoid, retained foreign body, and Parinaud's oculoglandular syndrome are often associated with conjunctival granulomas.[21]

Although a distinction exists between actively inflamed conjunctiva and that which is scarred but not inflamed, it must be understood that both situations represent abnormal conjunctiva. Actively inflamed conjunctiva is characterized by injection, chemosis, and the presence of immune mediators. Scarred, noninflamed conjunctiva is characterized by a decrease in mucin and aqueous tears, subepithelial fibrosis, and potentially foreshortening of the fornix and symblepharon. Both situations lead to an unhealthy ocular surface and create significant symptoms for patients.[23]

Corneal Epithelium

The final structure of the ocular surface is the cornea, which serves as the transparent window of the eye allowing light rays to pass into the eye to be processed by the visual system. To accomplish this, the cornea must have a normal contour and be avascular, transparent, and be essentially dehydrated. The corneal epithelium is continuous with the conjunctival epithelium and both are composed of nonkeratinized, stratified, squamous epithelium cells. It is believed that the corneal epithelium is replaced by a population of stem cells found at the anatomical limbus.[4] The corneal epithelium is not a mucous membrane; however, it is susceptible to desiccation if not properly protected by the lids and tear film. As mentioned above, as a continuum of the ocular surface, most of the conditions mentioned in this chapter will have corneal manifestations.

Some conditions not mentioned, that involve the cornea epithelium, include pterygium, corneal adhesion disorders, neurotrophic keratopathy, ocular surface neoplasias, and filamentary keratitis. A pterygium is the triangular-shaped growth consisting of bulbar conjunctival epithelium and hypertrophied subconjunctival connective tissue, which encroaches onto the cornea either nasally or temporally in the palpebral fissure. Corneal epithelial adhesion disorders, such as epithelial basement membrane dystrophy, Meesmann's and Lisch can present with signs and symptoms of recurrent corneal erosion and blurry vision. Reduced corneal sensation renders the corneal surface prone to occult injury and decreases reflex tearing, as well as decreasing wound healing rates with epithelial injury or breakdown. Neurotrophic keratitis is most commonly caused with herpes simplex or herpes zoster infection and can lead to stromal melting and perforation. Filamentary keratitis is a condition in which filaments, adherent complexes of mucus and degenerated corneal epithelial cells, are present on the ocular surface. Filaments are often highly symptomatic and can be found in a number of conditions in which the ocular surface is abnormal, such as post surgery, dry eye disease, and contact lens overwear.

Limbal Stem Cell Deficiency

Problems with the limbal stem cell population result in a decrease in the ability of the corneal epithelium to repopulate itself. Patients often complain of redness, irritation, photophobia, and decreased vision. On examination, early slit lamp findings include loss of the palisades of Vogt, late staining of the epithelium with fluorescein, corneal neovascularization, and development of peripheral pannus. Corneal findings often begin peripherally but may progress to involve the central cornea. Initially, the epithelium becomes irregular and hazy. Punctate epithelial keratopathy may develop, and these may coalesce to form true epithelial defects. Epithelial defects may be persistent, and may lead to stromal scarring, ulceration, and even perforation.[23]

Most cases of stem cell deficiency are acquired; however, congenital causes include aniridia, dominantly inherited keratitis, and ectodermal dysplasia. Acquired cases include chemical/thermal injury, contact lens use, Stevens–Johnson

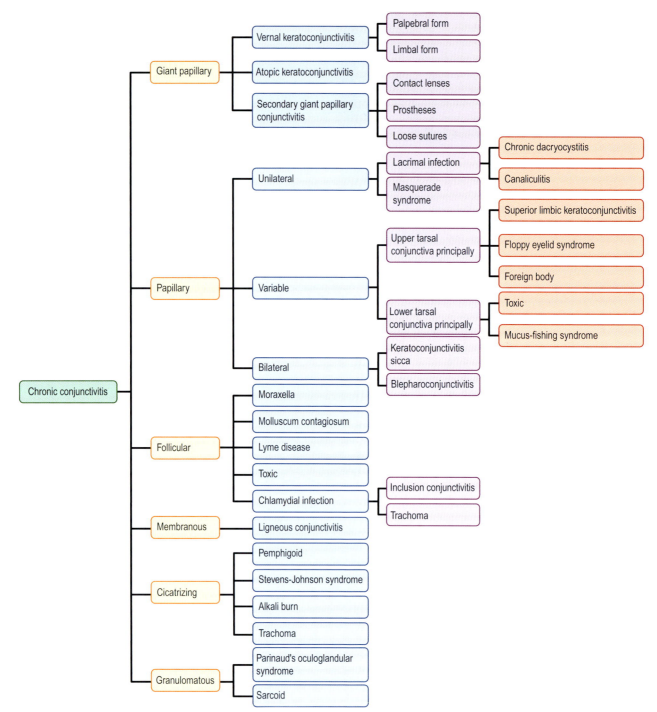

Figure 6.8 An algorithm for diagnosing chronic conjunctivitis. (From Krachmer et al., Cornea, 3rd ed., Mosby, Elsevier 2010. Figure 42.2.)

syndrome, ocular cicatricial pemphigoid, and rheumatoid arthritis.[23]

To aid the clinician and guide treatment approach, staging of severe ocular surface disease has been proposed.[24] First, the patient is categorized based upon the extent of limbal stem cell depletion. Stage I defines patients with involvement of less than half of the limbus, stage II if greater than half of the limbus is deficient. The disease process and clinical findings for stage I are often mild compared to the persistent epithelial defects, vision-hampering conjunctivalization, and even stromal scarring, which

occur more commonly with stage II disease. Next, the patient is categorized based upon the condition of the conjunctiva. If conjunctiva is normal, the patient is staged as 'a.' If the conjunctiva is abnormal from previous inflammation or injury but is currently quiet, the patient is staged as 'b.' If the conjunctiva is actively inflamed, the patient is staged as 'c.' Surgical management as well as prognosis are significantly affected based on the staging of these challenging patients.[24]

Examples of conditions that are classified as stage Ia include iatrogenic limbal stem cell deficiency, contact

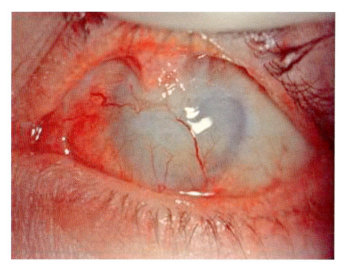

Figure 6.9 Stage IIc limbal stem cell deficiency.

Table 6.3   Staging of Limbal Stem Cell Deficiency

	Stage 'a' Normal Conjunctiva	Stage 'b' Previously Inflamed Conjunctiva	Stage 'c' Inflamed Conjunctiva
Stage I partial Stem cell deficiency	Stage Ia Iatrogenic, CIN, contact lens associated	Stage Ib History of chemical or thermal injury	Stage Ic Mild SJS, OCP, recent chemical injury
Stage II Total/ subtotal cell deficiency	Stage IIa Aniridia, severe contact lens and iatrogenic	Stage IIb History of severe chemical or thermal injury	Stage IIc Severe SJS, OCP, recent chemical or thermal injury

lens-induced keratopathy, and conjunctival intraepithelial neoplasia. Stage Ia disease can progress to IIa with further loss of limbal stem cells. Aniridia, a primary limbal stem cell disorder, is an entity that belongs in the IIa group, as the conjunctiva is often quiet. Patients with a prior history of chemical or thermal injury, with less than 50% limbal deficiency and quiet conjunctiva are labeled as stage Ib. Often, these patients have significant inflammation around the time of their injury (stage Ic or IIc), but the inflammation will quieten down over time, with judicious use of immunosuppressive agents. When planning surgery, it is best to wait for the inflammation to quieten down if possible, thus performing surgery when they are stage Ib rather than Ic. Other examples of stage Ic include conjunctival inflammatory disorders that have not reached the severe stage, such as mild SJS and OCP.[25]

Stage IIb is typically made up of patients with a history of chemical or thermal injury, affecting greater than half of the limbus. These patients are usually staged as IIc around the time of their exposure, and move to the IIb category when the conjunctiva becomes uninflamed. Total limbal stem cell deficiency with active conjunctival inflammation, represents the most severe cases of ocular surface disease. These cases make up stage IIc, and include severe SJS, OCP, and recent chemical injuries (Fig. 6.9). Clinical signs of stage IIc are conjunctival scarring, decreased mucin and aqueous tear production, and ocular surface keratinization. In this setting, stem cell transplantation is difficult due to the poor tear film, active inflammation, and abundance of immune mediators present. For these reasons, stage IIc patients have not only the worst natural disease course, but also the poorest prognosis for surgical rehabilitation[25] (Table 6.3).

Conclusion

In summary, the ocular surface and its many components are a very complex system that is dependant on all parts working together. There is significant overlap in the patient's symptoms as well as clinical findings, which present unique challenges to the clinician. Our understanding of this complex system is continuing to evolve, with that increased knowledge and better treatment regimens will enhance our care. Large studies, such as the DEWS report and International Workshop on Meibomian Gland Dysfunction, have helped define these disease processes and created staging criteria to better assist the clinician. These topics are vast and will be covered individually in later chapters of this book.

References

1. Nerad JA, Chang A. Trichiasis. In: Chen WP, editor. Oculoplastic surgery: the essentials. New York: Thieme; 2001.
2. Nelson J, Cameron J. The conjunctiva. In: Krachmer JH, Mannis MJ, Holland EJ, editor. Cornea. 1st ed. Vol. 1. St. Louis: Mosby; 1997. p. 41–7.
3. Tsubota K, Tseng SCG, Nordlund ML. Anatomy and physiology of the ocular surface. In Holland EJ, Mannis MJ, editors. Ocular surface disease: medical and surgical management. New York: Springer-Verlag; 2002.
4. Cotsarelis G, Cheng S-Z, Dong G, et al. Existence of slow-cycling limbal epithelial basal cells that can be preferentially stimulated to proliferate: implications on epithelial stem cells. Cell 1989;57:201–9.
5. Beuerman RW, Mircheff A, Plugfelder SC, et al. The lacrimal functional unit. In: Plugfelder SC, Beuerman RW, Stern ME, editors. Dry eye and ocular surface disorders. New York: Marcel Dekker; 2004.
6. Schwartz LK, Gelender H, Forster RK. Chronic conjunctivitis associated with floppy eyelids. Arch Ophthalmol 1983;101:1884–8.
7. Culbertson WW, Tseng SCG. Corneal disorders in floppy eyelid syndrome. Cornea 1994;13:33–42.
8. Hall AJ. Some observations on the active opening and closing of the eyes. Br J Ophthalmol 1936;20:257–95.
9. Nelson JD, Shimazaki J, Benitez-del-Castillo JM, et al. The International Workshop on Meibomian Gland Dysfunction: report of the definition and classification subcommittee. IOVS 2011;52:1930–7.
10. McCulley JP, Dougherty JM, Deneau DG. Classification of chronic blepharitis. Ophthalmology 1982;89:1173–80.
11. Schein OD, Munoz B, Tielsch JM, et al. Prevalence of dry eye among the elderly. Am J Ophthalmol 1997;124:723–8.
12. Jie Y, Xu L, Wu YY, et al. Prevalence of dry eye among adult Chinese in the Beijing Eye Study. Eye 2009;23:688–93.
13. Uchino M, Dogru M, Yagi Y, et al. The features of dry eye disease in a Japanese elderly population. Optom Vis Sci 2006;83:797–802.
14. McCarty CA, Bansal AK, Livingston PM, et al. The epidemiology of dry eye in Melbourne, Australia. Ophthalmology 1998;105:1114–9.
15. Nichols KK, Foulks GN, Bron AJ, et al. The International Workshop on Meibomian Gland Dysfunction: Executive Summary. IOVS 2011;52:1922–9.
16. The definition and classification of dry eye disease: report of the Definition and Classification Subcommittee of the International Dry Eye Workshop (2007). Ocular Surf 2007;5:75–92.

17. Vitali C, Bombardieri S, Johnson R, et al. Classification criteria for Sjögren's syndrome: a revised version of the European criteria proposed by the American-European Consensus Group. Ann Rheum Dis 2002;1:554–8.
18. Damato BE, Allan D, Murray SB, et al. Senile atrophy of the human lacrimal gland: the contribution of chronic inflammatory disease. Br J Ophthalmol 1984;68:674–86.
19. Doughty MJ, Fonn D, Richter D, et al. A patient questionnaire approach to estimating the prevalence of dry eye symptoms in patients presenting to optometric practices across Canada. Optom Vis Sci 1997; 74:624–31.
20. Nichols JJ, Ziegler C, Mitchell GL, et al. Self-reported dry eye disease across refractive modalities. Invest Ophthalmol Vis Sci 2005;46: 1911–4.
21. Lindquist TD. Conjunctivitis: an overview and classification. In: Krachmer JH, Mannis MJ, Holland EJ, editors. Cornea. Philadelphia: Mosby Elsevier; 2005. p. 509–20.
22. Neff KD, Holland EJ, Schwartz GS. Ligneous conjunctivitis. In: Krachmer JH, Mannis MJ, Holland EJ, editors. Cornea. Philadelphia: Mosby Elsevier; 2005. p. 629–34.
23. Schwartz GS, Holland EJ. Classification and staging of ocular surface disease. In: Krachmer JH, Mannis MJ, Holland EJ, editors. Cornea. Philadelphia: Mosby Elsevier; 2005. p. 1713–26.
24. Schwartz GS, Gomes JAP, Holland EJ. Preoperative staging of disease severity. In: Holland EJ, Mannis MJ, editors. Ocular surface disease: medical and surgical management. New York: Springer-Verlag; 2002.
25. Holland EJ. Epithelial transplantation for the management of severe ocular surface disease Trans Am Ophthalmol Soc 1996;44:677–743.

PART 2

DISEASES OF THE OCULAR SURFACE

7 Diagnostic Techniques in Ocular Surface Disease

BENNIE H. JENG

Introduction

Ocular surface disease is becoming an increasingly recognized condition that continues to challenge the ophthalmologist to make accurate diagnoses and to institute the correct therapy at the right time. Much of the challenge in making the diagnosis lies in the fact that some of the diagnostic tests that are used, such as the Schirmer test, have notoriously low specificities and sensitivities and are not reproducible from one visit to another within the same patient. Recently, new diagnostic tools that measure tear osmolarity, tear meniscus height, and tear film distribution and thickness have been introduced, and they seemingly promise to help improve our ability to accurately diagnose ocular surface disease. This chapter will discuss the traditional, as well as the newer diagnostic techniques for diagnosing ocular surface disease.

Slit Lamp Examination

The slit lamp examination is a crucial part of the process when evaluating any ophthalmologic patient, and is no different for the individual with ocular surface disease. Careful, systematic examination from the outside to the inside of the eye should be performed each and every time. Care should be taken to specifically evaluate the condition of the meibomian glands (Fig. 7.1) and the entire conjunctival surface, including the palpebral areas, looking for inflammation and scarring. Once this is all performed, without anesthesia and stains, the examination can proceed to the next steps, including Schirmer testing and then ocular surface staining.

Schirmer Testing

The Schirmer test is a simple test that was first described in 1903[1] and it is still commonly performed in the office to assess aqueous tear production. There are three variations of this test, but the most popular is the Schirmer I test which measures both basal and reflex tear production. In this test, a strip of filter paper is placed on the lower eyelid margin without anesthesia, after 5 minutes, the strip is removed,

*Supported in part by an unrestricted grant from Research to Prevent Blindness, Inc and That Man May See, Inc to the Department of Ophthalmology, UCSF. The author has no conflict of interest in any of the techniques or products discussed in this chapter.

and the amount of wetting is measured in millimeters (Fig. 7.2). Although this test is used frequently in the office, it has been found to lack accuracy and reproducibility: the same person's test results taken at the same time each day for several days can fluctuate widely, and the mean Schirmer I test results for normal individuals have been reported to range from 8.1 mm to 33.1 mm.[2] As such, many ophthalmologists do not even use this test anymore, but for those who do, in general, any value below 10 mm is considered abnormal. Many other ophthalmologists consider this test

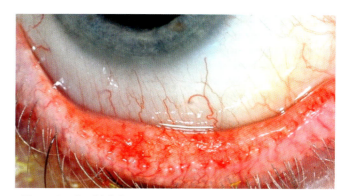

Figure 7.1 Careful slit lamp examination techniques are imperative for diagnosing ocular surface disease. Here, meibomian gland disease is readily seen. (Photo courtesy of Todd P. Margolis, MD, PhD)

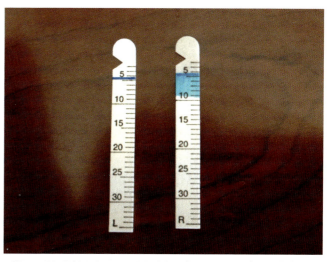

Figure 7.2 Schirmer test strips with millimeter markings. Note blue dye that facilitates measurement of tear wetting.

as a reasonable diagnostic tool only for severe dry eyes, where there is moderate reproducibility,[3] with many practitioners only considering values of less than 5 mm to be significant.

Ocular Surface Staining

Ocular surface stains are used to assess the integrity of the superficial cell layers of the ocular surface, and they are an essential part of the anterior segment examination. Characteristic staining patterns can give clues to the diagnosis: e.g. inferior staining suggests dry eyes or exposure keratopathy. The mainstays of ocular surface stains include: fluorescein, rose bengal, and lissamine green.

Fluorescein sodium is one the most frequently used methods for evaluating corneal staining, and it has been used since the end of the nineteenth century. Fluorescein penetrates poorly into the lipid layer of the corneal epithelium, and therefore, it does not stain normal cornea. Instead, the surface is stained whenever there is disruption of the cell-to-cell junctions.[4] Although fluorescein is a very effective stain for the diseased cornea, it is more difficult to detect fluorescein staining of the conjunctiva because of the poor scleral contrast. However, this staining can be more readily viewed if a yellow (blue-free) filter is used.

Rose bengal stain has also been used for a very long time: in this case for nearly a century. It is a derivative of fluorescein and is used to detect damage on the ocular surface, especially on the conjunctiva (Fig. 7.3). Although originally thought to stain dead or devitalized cells, rose bengal is currently believed to stain any part of the ocular surface that is not adequately protected by the tear film,[4,5] specifically, in areas lacking membrane-associated mucins.[6] Though an excellent diagnostic tool, rose bengal has been shown to be toxic to epithelial cells, and patients often complain about the burning and stinging upon instillation.

Lissamine green is a synthetic organic acid dye that stains in a similar fashion to rose bengal, but without causing stinging and without affecting the viability of the cells. For

this reason, it has gained popularity in its use. However, staining with lissamine green is dose-dependent and an inadequate volume results in weak staining that can be overlooked. A minimal dosage of 10–20 μL is recommended for accurate diagnostic ability (Fig. 7.4).

There are three commonly used methods to grade ocular surface staining: the van Bijsterveld system,[7] the NEI/Industry Workshop guidelines,[8] and the Oxford Scheme.[9] At the present time, there is no evidence that any one method is superior to another for grading the ocular surface staining patterns (Table 7.1).

Tear Break-up Time

The tear break-up time (TBUT) is defined as the time interval between a complete blink and the first appearance of a dry spot in the tear film after fluorescein administration.[10,11] It is believed that this represents an unstable tear film, whereby the mucous layer may rupture, allowing the aqueous to come in contact with exposed epithelium,[12] but the exact mechanism is poorly understood. Like the Schirmer test, the TBUT test has been criticized as being

Table 7.1 Comparison of Three Commonly Used Methods to Grade Ocular Surface Staining

Method	Grading Areas	Scale	Maximum Score
van Bijsterveld	3: nasal bulbar conjunctiva, temporal bulbar conjunctiva, cornea	0–3	9
NEI/Industry Workshop guidelines	5 areas of cornea, 6 areas of conjunctiva	0–3 for cornea 0–3 for conjunctiva	15 for cornea, 18 for conjunctiva
Oxford Scheme	Based on comparison to standard panel	0–5 for entire ocular surface	5

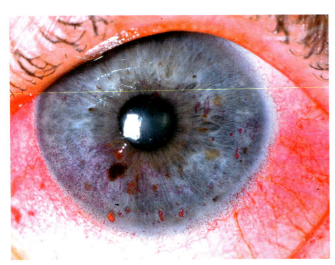

Figure 7.3 Rose bengal staining of the ocular surface. Note the readily visible staining of the conjunctiva. (Photo courtesy of Todd P. Margolis, MD, PhD.)

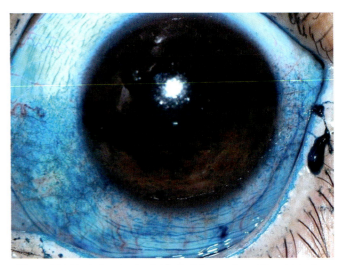

Figure 7.4 Lissamine green staining of the ocular surface. Note the readily visible staining of the conjunctiva, but not the cornea. (Photo courtesy of Todd P. Margolis, MD, PhD.)

unreliable and not reproducible. Many factors may lead to its non-reproducibility, including the volume of fluorescein administered, as well as the presence of preservatives, such as benzalkonium chloride, which may shorten TBUT. Despite this unreliability, it is generally agreed that a TBUT of less than 10 seconds suggests tear film instability, and less than 5 seconds suggests definite dry eye.[13]

Patient Questionnaire

The Ocular Surface Disease Index (OSDI) is a questionnaire that has been validated to discriminate between normal, mild to moderate, and severe dry eye disease as defined by the physician's assessment and a composite disease severity score (Fig. 7.5). The OSDI has also been correlated

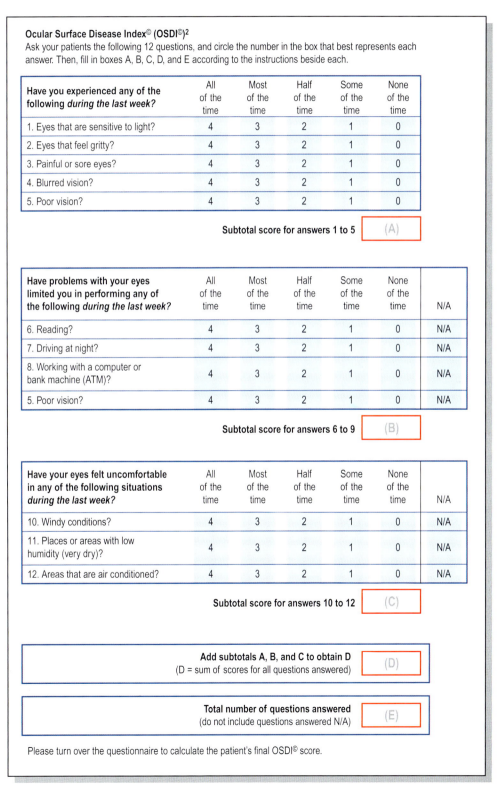

Figure 7.5 Ocular Surface Disease Index questionnaire. (Accessed at: www.dryeyezone.com/documents/osdi.pdf. Copyright © 1995, Allergan.)

Continued on following page

Evaluating the OSDI© Score[1]

The OSDI© is assessed on a scale of 0 to 100, with higher scores representing greater disability. The index demonstrates sensitivity and specificity in distinguishing between normal subjects and patients with dry eye disease. The OSDI© is a valid and reliable instrument for measuring dry eye disease (normal, mild to moderate, and severe) and effect on vision-related function.

Assessing Your Patient's Dry Eye Disease[1,2]

Use your answers D and E from side 1 to compare the sum of scores for all questions answered (D) and the number of questions answered (E) with the chart below.* Find where your patient's score would fall. Match the corresponding shade of red to the key below to determine whether your patient's score indicates normal, mild, moderate, or severe dry eye disease.

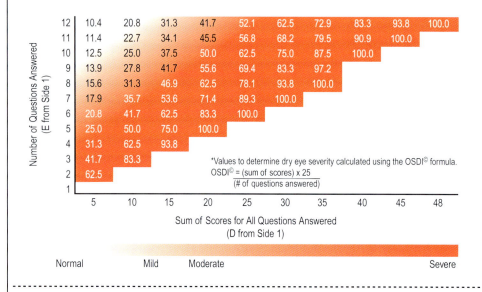

*Values to determine dry eye severity calculated using the OSDI© formula.

$$OSDI^© = \frac{(\text{sum of scores}) \times 25}{(\text{\# of questions answered})}$$

Patient's Name: _____   Date: _____

How long has the patient experienced dry eye disease? _____

Eye Care Professional's Comments: _____

_____

_____

_____

_____

_____

1. Data on file, Allergan, Inc.
2. Schiffman RM, Christianson MD, Jacobsen G, Hirsch JD, Reis BL. Reliability and validity of the Ocular Surface Disease Index. *Arch Ophthalmol.* 2000;118:615-621

Figure 7.5 (Continued)

significantly with the McMonnies Dry Eye Questionnaire, the National Eye Institute Visual Functioning Questionnaire, the physical component summary score of the Short Form-12 Health Status Questionnaire, patient perception of symptoms, and artificial tear usage.[14] It has been demonstrated to have the necessary psychometric properties to be used as an end point in clinical trials, and as such, it could be an important tool for in-office support for the diagnosis of ocular surface disease that is easy to administer.[15]

Impression Cytology

Impression cytology is a powerful tool for the diagnosis of ocular surface disease. This minimally invasive procedure involves applying nitrocellulose filter paper to the area of interest on the ocular surface to remove the superficial 2–3 layers of cells.[16] As first described by Egbert and colleagues,[17] the cells are air dried and stained with periodic acid – Schiff and hematoxylin. This test has been modified several times, and now these cells can then be subject to histological, immunohistochemical, and molecular testing to help diagnose the ocular surface disease. Electron microscopy of the cells can even be done.

Impression cytology can be used routinely to help make the diagnosis of limbal stem cell deficiency, keratoconjunctivitis sicca, atopic eye disease, vernal keratoconjunctivitis, and ocular surface squamous neoplasia. It has also been used to diagnose infections such as *Acanthamoeba* keratitis. Although this technique has been used in recent years to greatly help in the diagnosis of ocular surface disease, it is not a mainstream procedure because it is relatively time consuming for the ophthalmologist, and it requires a willing and trained pathologist to do/assist in the readings.

Confocal Microscopy

In vivo confocal microscopy has evolved into a popular method of imaging the anterior segment at a cellular level because the images obtained are comparable to ex vivo histochemical methods.[18] Not only has this technology been used to evaluate corneal nerves and to aid in the diagnosis of corneal infections, such as *Acanthamoeba* keratitis, but it has also garnered interest for its use in the conjunctiva and the eyelids: studies have demonstrated that confocal microscopy can aid in the diagnosis of dry eye or superior limbic keratoconjunctivitis by its ability to evaluate the conjunctival epithelium for squamous metaplasia.[19] Further, confocal scanning laser microscopy has been found to be an efficient and noninvasive tool for the quantitative assessment of conjunctival inflammation, as well as epithelial cell densities and conjunctival morphologic alterations, such as microcysts in patients with Sjögren's and non-Sjögren's syndrome dry eye disease.[20] The ability to assess for conjunctival inflammation also allows for this technology to help diagnose atopic keratoconjunctivitis. Further, confocal microscopy has also been shown to have high potential in the diagnosis of meibomian gland dysfunction.[21] Although in vivo confocal microscopy technology is still evolving, it has already been demonstrated to have significant value in aiding in the evaluation of patients with ocular surface disease. At the present time, this technology may not be available in a widespread fashion, but its further development in the future will hopefully result in decreasing costs so that it will be available to more practitioners.

Tear Film Interferometry

Additional aqueous tear deficiency assessment includes measuring the thickness of the precorneal tear film. Tear film interferometry can achieve this by using wavelength-dependent fringes: the optical path difference from the reflection at the surface of the tear film and at the interface of the tear film and the cornea results in an interference wave, which is calculated to be the precorneal tear film thickness. Normal precorneal tear thicknesses vary by study from 2.7 to 11.0 µm, but studies that have compared the thicknesses of individuals with dry eyes versus controls demonstrate that the controls have a much thicker tear film.[22–25] Furthermore, this technology can also be used to evaluate specifically for the thickness of the lipid layer of the tear film.[26] Along with a careful evaluation of the meibomian gland status, this technique helps to assess for the mechanism for ocular surface dryness.

The technology of interferometry has also been applied in a kinetic fashion: evaluating the spread of lipids through the tear film with blinking. It has been found that in dry eye disease, due to lipid deficiency from meibomian gland dysfunction, lipids are seen to spread slowly with vertical streaking patterns compared to normal subjects without dry eye who have rapid spreading of the lipids in a horizontal pattern.[27] This technology has significant promise as a powerful diagnostic technique, especially in assessing for changes after institution of therapy, but at the present time it is also not widely available, and it still needs to undergo validation.

Tear Meniscus Measurement

In addition to precorneal tear film thickness, the measurement of tear meniscus dimensions has also been shown to be of great value in the assessment of the patient with ocular surface disease.[28] In the past, the meniscus variables, such as height, width, cross-sectional area, and meniscus curvature, have all been reported to be useful in the diagnosis of dry eye, but with limitations in the measurement techniques, due to their invasive nature causing stimulation of the reflex tearing. Recently, however, the Visante Anterior Segment Optical Coherence Tomography (OCT; Carl Zeiss Meditec, International, Dublin, CA, USA), has been shown to produce accurate measurements of tear height in a noninvasion fashion with acceptable sensitivity, specificity, and reproducibility when compared with slit lamp tear meniscus height measurements, tear function vital staining scores, and Schirmer testing[29] (Fig. 7.6). The Spectral OCT (also known as Fourier domain, high-speed, or three-dimensional OCT) has also been shown to be well correlated with Schirmer testing, TBUT, and subjective symptoms. The advantage of the Spectral OCT is that it has improved sensitivity and a short acquisition time, which

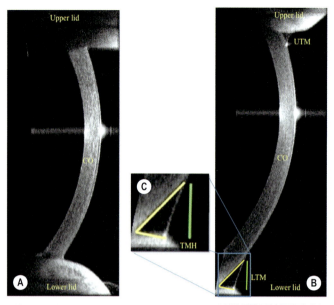

Figure 7.6 Visante optical coherence tomography images. (**A**) Dry eye patient. (**B**) Healthy subject. A vertical 10 mm long scan across the corneal apex obtained immediately after a blink. Upper tear meniscus (UTM) and cornea (CO) are marked on the image. (**C**) Yellow lines delineate the corneal surface and lower lid margin. The green perpendicular line indicates the tear meniscus height (TMH) processed in the digital image software. Note the difference between the upper and lower TMH between the dry eye subject and healthy control. (Reproduced with permission from Ibrahim OMA, Dogru M, Takano Y, et al. Application of Visante Optical Coherence Tomography tear meniscus height measurement in the diagnosis of dry eye disease. Ophthalmology 2010; 117:1923–9.)

improves the quality of the two-dimensional images and thereby enables accurate three-dimensional modeling. The high acquisition speed also allows for the evaluation of tear meniscus changes in real time.[30] As with the other previously described technologies, OCT imaging of the tear meniscus has proven to be a powerful diagnostic tool, but at the present time it is not widely available to all practitioners.

Esthesiometry

Because corneal epithelial disturbances are frequently due to decreased corneal sensation, esthesiometry is an important adjunctive technique for diagnosing ocular surface disease. The classic technique for performing esthesiometry is with the Cochet – Bonnet esthesiometer,[31] which consists of a fine nylon filament, the length of which can be adjusted to apply different intensities of stimuli. While seemingly an objective measurement, this test is fraught with limitations including difficulties with alignment, placement, and replication of the force applied with the nylon filament. In addition, use of this test causes disruption of the epithelial surface by the filament. Rather than use this instrument, some practitioners simply use a cotton swab with the cotton pulled into a wisp, and then used with a subjective semi-quantitative grading scale. Recently, a non-contact air jet esthesiometer has been introduced and tested.[32] This instrument, the CRCERT – Belmonte esthesiometer, allows for better stimulus reproducibility and better control over

stimulus characteristics. Since this technique relies on having the patient in their baseline sensitivity state, this technique must be employed prior to anesthetic instillation in the eye.

Osmolarity

The Dry Eye Workshop Report introduced the concept that an increase in tear osmolarity is a hallmark of dry eye disease, and it is now thought to be the central mechanism in the cause of ocular surface damage in dry eyes.[33] From this report, tear osmolarity has been reported to be the single best objective marker for dry eye disease. Unfortunately, at that time, measurements were limited to laboratory instruments which required very large volumes of tears. Recently, with the introduction of the TearLab Test (TearLab Corp, San Diego, CA, USA), the clinician can easily collect and measure osmolarity in a 50 μL tear sample with minimal disturbance to the tear film.[34] This microfluidic technology produces a reading within seconds before evaporation can influence the concentration of solutes in the tear sample.

In a prospective, observational case series to determine the clinical usefulness of tear osmolarity compared to commonly used objective tests to diagnose dry eye, tear osmolarity was found to be the best single metric to diagnose and classify dry eye disease. In this study, it was found that a cutoff of more than 308 mOsms/L achieved a 90.7% rate of a correct diagnosis of severe dry eye patients, and had a true negative rate of 81.3%.[35]

Rapid Testing For Inflammatory Markers

Matrix metalloproteinase 9 (MMP-9) plays a critical role in wound healing and inflammation, and is primarily responsible for the pathologic alterations to the ocular surface in various conditions.[36] MMP-9 has been demonstrated to be significantly elevated in the tears of patients with blepharitis, allergic eye disease, dry eye disease, and conjunctivochalasis.[37,38] The ability to test for MMP-9 in the tear film may prove to be an important tool to help in the diagnosis of ocular surface disease. Recently, a commercially available point-of-care test, RPS InflammaDry Detector (RPS, Inc, Sarasota, FL, USA) offers an easy-to-administer and rapid turn-around test (10 minutes) for measuring MMP-9 levels in the tear film.

Ocular Surface Scraping

Despite the plethora of novel ideas and tests for evaluating ocular surface disease, sometimes it is necessary to revert to the tried and true method of taking a sample and evaluating it under light microscopy. Conjunctival scrapings (or swabbings) can be performed to obtain a specimen for cytologic examination (Fig. 7.7). The specimens that are collected may reveal cells or microorganisms under light microscopy that may be helpful in the diagnostic process. Although the use of these techniques requires either the

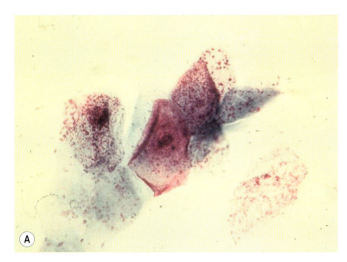

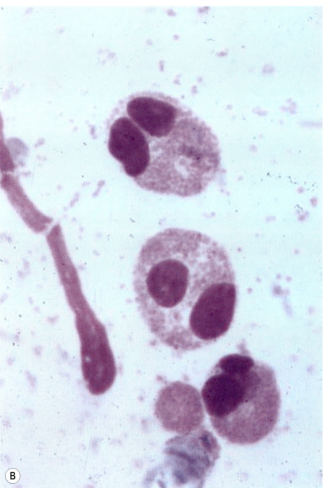

Figure 7.7 Ocular surface scrapping demonstrating (**A**) keratinized epithelial cells (note keratin granules) that could be seen in dry eyes, superior limbic keratoconjunctivitis, or exposure keratopathy; (**B**) eosinophil (note bi-lobed nuclei and eosinophilic granules) that could be seen in vernal keratoconjunctivitis, atopic keratoconjunctivitis, or other allergic processes. (Photos courtesy of Vicky Cevallos, MT.)

ophthalmologist or a microbiologist to evaluate the specimen, it is a technique that can be used widely compared to the expensive new technology that has been described above.

Conclusion

The diagnostic process for ocular surface disease is frequently complex, and patients require accurate and prompt diagnoses, such that targeted and appropriate therapies can be instituted quickly to relieve the patients of their symptoms. Although many patients with ocular surface disease have conditions that are annoying and bothersome to them, with a low likelihood of serious complications, ocular surface disease can seriously adversely affect quality of life. In addition, complications, such as corneal perforation from extreme dry eyes can occur. As traditional diagnostic techniques have been shown to not always be useful, with this in mind, it behooves us to continuously strive to develop diagnostic techniques that can help better diagnose, and treat our patients. The newer diagnostic techniques described above, present an exciting and promising array of modalities that may change the way we take care of our patients.

References

1. Schirmer O. Studien zur physiologie und pathologie der tranenabsonderung und tranenabfuhr. Graefes Arch Clin Exp Ophthalmol 1903; 56:197–291.
2. Savini G, Prabhawasat P, Kojima T, et al. The challenge of dry eye diagnosis. Clin Ophthalmol 2008;2:31–55.
3. Tsubota K, Xu KP, Fujihara T, et al. Decreased reflex tearing is associated with lymphocytic infiltration in lacrimal glands. J Rheumatol 1996;23:313–29.
4. Feenstra RP, Tseng SC. Comparison of fluorescein and rose bengal staining. Ophthalmology 1992;99:605–17.
5. Feenstra RP, Tseng SC. What is actually stained by rose bengal? Arch Ophthalmol 1992;110:984–93.
6. Argüeso P, Tisdale A, Spurr-Micharud S, et al. Mucin characteristics of human corneal-limbal epithelial cells that exclude the rose bengal anionic dye. Invest Ophthalmol Vis Sci 2006;47: 113–9.
7. van Bijsterveld OP. Diagnostic tests in the sicca syndrome. Arch Ophthalmol 1969;82:10–4.
8. Lemp MA. Report of the National Eye Institute/Industry Workshop on clinical trials in dry eyes. CLAO J 1995;21:221–32.
9. Bron AJ, Evans VE, Smith JA. Grading of corneal and conjunctival staining in the context of other dry eye tests. Cornea 2003;22: 640–50.
10. Norn MS. Desiccation of the precorneal tear film. I. Corneal wetting-time. Acta Ophthalmol (Copenh) 1969;47:865–80.
11. Lemp MA. Breakup of the tear film. Int Ophthalmol Clin 1973; 13:97–102.
12. Sharma A, Ruckenstein E. Mechanism of tear film rupture and its implications for contact lens tolerance. Am J Optom Physiol Opt 1985;62:246–53.
13. Shimazaki J. Definition and criteria of dry eye. Ganka 1995; 37:765–70.
14. Schiffman RM, Chirstianson MD, Jacobsen G, et al. Reliability and validity of the Ocular Surface Disease Index. Arch Ophthalmol 2000;118:615–21.
15. Ozcura F, Aydin S, Helvaci MR. Ocular surface disease index for the diagnosis of dry eye syndrome. Ocular Immunol Inflamm 2007; 15:389–93.
16. Singh R, Joseph A, Umapathy T, et al. Impression cytology of the ocular surface. Br J Ophthalmol 2005;89:1655–9.
17. Egbert PR, Lauber S, Maurice DM. A simple conjunctival biopsy. Am J Ophthalmol 1977;84:798–801.

18. Crazat A, Pavan-Langston D, Hamrah P. In vivo confocal microscopy of corneal nerves: analysis and clinical correlation. Semin Ophthalmol 2010;25:171–7.

19. Kojima T, Matsumoto Y, Ibrahim OMA, et al. In vivo evaluation of superior limbic keratoconjunctivitis using laser scanning confocal microscopy and conjunctival impression cytology. Invest Ophthalmol Vis Sci 2010;51:3986–92.

20. Wakamatsu TH, Sato EA, Matsumoto Y, et al. Conjunctival in vivo confocal scanning laser microscopy in patients with Sjögren syndrome. Invest Ophthalmol Vis Sci 2010;51:144–50.

21. Ibrahim OMA, Matsumoto Y, Dogru M, et al. The efficacy, sensitivity, and specificity of in vivo laser confocal microscopy in the diagnosis of meibomian gland dysfunction. Ophthalmology 2010;117:665–72.

22. Danjo Y, Nakamura M, Hamano T. Measurement of the precorneal tear film thickness with a non-contact optical interferometry film thickness measurement system. Jpn J Ophthalmol 1994;38:260–6.

23. King-Smith PE, Fink BA, Fogt N, et al. The thickness of the human precorneal tear film: evidence from reflection spectra. Invest Ophthalmol Vis Sci 2001;41:3348–59.

24. King-Smith PE, Fink BA, Hill RM, et al. The thickness of the tear film. Curr Eye Res 2004;29:357–68.

25. Hosaka E, Kawamorita T, Ogasawara Y, et al. Interferometry in the evaluation of precorneal tear film thickness in dry eye. Am J Ophthalmol 2011;151:18–23.

26. Goto E, Dogru M, Kojima T, et al. Computer-synthesis of an interference color chart of human tear lipid layer by a colorimetric approach. Invest Ophthalmol Vis Sci 2003;44:4693–7.

27. Goto E, Tseng SC. Kinetic analysis of tear interference images in aqueous tear deficiency dry eye before and after punctual occlusion. Invest Ophthalmol Vis Sci 2003;44:1897–905.

28. Mainstone JC, Bruce AS, Golding TR. Tear meniscus measurement in the diagnosis of dry eye. Curr Eye Res 1996;15:653–61.

29. Ibrahim OMA, Dogru M, Takano Y, et al. Application of Visante Optical Coherence Tomography tear meniscus height measurement in the diagnosis of dry eye disease. Ophthalmology 2010;117:1923–9.

30. Czajkowski G, Kaluzny BJ, Laudencka A, et al. Tear meniscus measurement by spectral optical coherence tomography. Optom Vis Sci 2012;89:1–7.

31. Cochet P, Bonnet R. L'Esthesie corneenne. Sa mesure clinique. Ses variations physiologiques et pathologieques. La Clinique Ophtalomologique 1960;4:3–27.

32. Golebiowshi B, Papas E, Stapleton F. Assessing the sensory function of the ocular surface: implications of use of a non-contact air jet aesthesiometer versus the Cochet–Bonnet aesthesiometer. Exp Eye Res 2011;92:408–13.

33. International Dry Eye Workshop. The definition and classification of dry eye disease. In: 2007 Report of the International Dry Eye Workshop (DEWS). Ocul Surf 2007;5:75–92.

34. Sullivan BD, Whitmer D, Nichols KK. An objective approach to severity in dry eye disease. Invest Ophthalmol Vis Sci 2010;51:6125–30.

35. Lemp MA, Bron AJ, Baudouin C, et al. Tear osmolarity in the diagnosis and management of dry eye disease. Am J Ophthalmol 2011;151:792–8.

36. Sambursky R, O'Brien TP. MMP-9 and the perioperative management of LASIK surgery. Curr Opin Ophthalmol 2011;22:294–303.

37. Acera A, Rocha G, Vecino E, et al. Inflammatory markers in the tears of patients with ocular surface disease. Ophthalmic Res 2008;40:315–21.

38. Chotikavanich S, de Paiva CS, Li de Q, et al. Production and activity of matrix metalloproteinase-9 on the ocular surface increase in dysfunctional tear syndrome. Invest Ophthalmol Vis Sci 2009;50:3203–9.

8 Blepharitis: Classification

LISA M. NIJM

Historical Classification of Blepharitis

Blepharitis represents one of the most common anterior segment disorders encountered in ophthalmology. Data from the National Disease and Therapeutics Index reported 590 000 patient visits in 1982 due to blepharitis.[1] More recent studies have shown that ophthalmologists and optometrists observe blepharitis in 37–47% of their patients.[2,3] Indeed, epidemiologic data from one study in Britain indicated that blepharitis and conjunctivitis account for 71% of ocular cases of inflammation that presented to the emergency room.[4]

Despite the prevalence of blepharitis in both presentation and contribution to ocular conditions, the etiology of blepharitis remains largely unknown. Available evidence suggests that the etiology is most likely multifactorial and this has led to a fair amount of variation in classification of the disease (Table 8.1). Historically, Elsching first described the condition in 1908[5] and Thygeson classified blepharitis into different types in 1946.[6] Thygeson initially described the entity as a 'chronic inflammation of the lid border' and further divided it into two general categories: squamous and ulcerative. He went on to describe findings associated with seborrheic blepharitis, staphylococcal blepharitis and a combination of the two clinical entities. Thygeson established the association of blepharitis with abnormal *Staphylococcus* colonization and attributed infection of the meibomian glands to be the primary cause of blepharitis.[6]

Interestingly, over three decades passed before McCulley et al. first reported blepharitis caused by non-infectious means. Studies conducted by McCulley and others revealed that the disease of blepharitis encompassed much more than infection of the meibomian glands.[7] In fact, one study,

comparing 26 control patients to 26 patients with chronic blepharitis, demonstrated that all of the blepharitis patients possessed a generalized sebaceous gland dysfunction, which included the meibomian glands.[8] Further, investigators of these initial studies noted that stagnation of the meibomian glands seemed to cause a defect in the tear lipid layer, resulting in a superficial punctate keratopathy consistent with tear film deficiency states.[7] Further investigations led to the notion that the disease of blepharitis encompassed several factors in addition to *Staphylococcus aureus* that were not of an infectious nature.

Subsequently, McCulley and colleagues designed a more elaborate classification system based on the intense study of changes induced in the lid, lashes, hair follicles, meibomian glands, conjunctiva and cornea in blepharitis patients.[7] They divided blepharitis into six distinct categories: (1) staphylococcal blepharitis, (2) seborrheic blepharitis, (3) mixed seborrheic and staphylococcal, (4) seborrheic with meibomian seborrhea, (5) seborrheic blepharitis with secondary meibomianitis, and (6) primary meibomianitis.[4] The authors noted the distinct clinical features of each entity that separated them into different categories. For instance, those patients with staphylococcal blepharitis tended to have relatively more inflammation of the anterior portion of the lid, but for a shorter duration, compared to the other categories. Further more, unlike patients with primary or secondary meibomitis, these patients were culture positive for either *S. aureus or S. epidermidis* (compared to controls). Strikingly, those patients with seborrheic blepharitis, of any type demonstrated a 95% incidence of associated seborrheic dermatitis, while staphylococcal patients had relatively no dermatologic findings.[7] This detailed classification and study greatly expanded on the early observations of Thygeson and emphasized the complex nature of the disease.

Table 8.1 Summary of Major Proposals for Classification of Chronic Blepharitis

Primary Study Author(s)	Year Published	Proposed Classification System
Thygeson	1946	Ulcerative and squamous.
McCulley	1982	Classification of blepharitis into 6 categories: (1) staphylococcal blepharitis, (2) seborrheic blepharitis, (3) mixed seborrheic with staphylococcal, (4) seborrheic with meibomian seborrhea, (5) seborrheic blepharitis with secondary meibomianitis, and (6) primary meibomianitis.
Huber-Spitzy	1991	Classification into 3 groups based on clinical features: (1) blepharitis sicca, (2) blepharitis seborrheica and (3) blepharitis ulcerosa.
AAO Preferred Practice Patterns	2003	Blepharitis divided into two main categories based on anatomic delineation of lid margin: (1) anterior and (2) posterior blepharitis, then further subcategorized by presentation (anterior blepharitis referring to staphylococcal and seborrheic, posterior blepharitis referring to meibomian gland dysfunction).
Mathers	2004	Using cluster analysis, categorized blepharitis into one of 9 groups based on meibomian gland dropout, lipid volume, Schirmer test value, evaporation, and lipid viscosity.
Shapiro and Abelson	2006	Standardized photograph grading scale for blepharitis and meibomitis based on anatomical classifications.

In 1991, Huber-Spitzy proposed a simplified classification compared to McCulley, consisting of only three groups based on clinical features: (1) blepharitis sicca, (2) blepharitis seborrheica and (3) blepharitis ulcerosa.[9] The authors described blepharitis sicca as a local eczematous disease, consisting of only superficial inflammation with dry scaling of the lid margin.[9] On the other hand, blepharitis seborrheica was characterized as having marked inflammation with large 'greasy scales' and excessive sebaceous gland secretions. Finally, the most severe form, blepharitis ulcerosa, was diagnosed only when the follicles of the lashes were encrusted with thickly matted, hardened crusts which frequently resulted in bleeding on forceps removal.[9]

Further research detailing the coexistence of blepharitis with dry eye, led Mathers and colleagues to create a multifaceted classification system for blepharitis, ocular surface disease and dry eye, based on cluster analysis of several different variables.[10] In 2004, the investigators presented data suggesting that by assessing meibomian gland dropout, lipid volume, Schirmer test value, evaporation, and lipid viscosity, patients could be placed in one of nine distinct diagnostic groups.[9] These groups were identified as: (1) obstructive MGD with rosacea and dry eye, (2) obstructive MGD and dry eye, (3) seborrheic MGD, (4) seborrheic MGD with dry eye, (5) seborrheic, obstructive MGD with dry eye, (6) low evaporation and dry eye, (7) high evaporation and high schirmer's test, (8) low Schirmer's, high evaporation and dry eye, and (9) normal Schirmer's high evaporation and dry eye.

In 2003, the American Academy of Ophthalmology advocated the anatomic model of classification that many ophthalmologists were using to divide blepharitis into two main categories, based on anatomic delineation of lid margin: anterior and posterior blepharitis.[11] The AAO preferred practice pattern then further subcategorized blepharitis by its presentation, i.e., anterior blepharitis, encompassing both staphylococcal and seborrheic blepharitis and posterior blepharitis, referring mainly to meibomian gland dysfunction.[11]

More recently, Shapiro and Abelson devised a photographic standardized scale for blepharitis and meibomitis based on anatomical classifications.[12] These anatomical classifications include assessing the lash follicles, dermis, eyelid, vascularity, mucocutaneous junction, meibomian gland orifices and tarsal conjunctiva. Digital images were reviewed by a panel of clinicians and were arranged from least severe to most severe; representative images were then selected to generate a scale of 0 to 3 or 0 to 4 (normal to severe) and subsequently used for several FDA studies.[13,14]

Though many detailed classification systems have been proposed, there is no single universally accepted system of classification. Practically, most clinicians continue to classify blepharitis by anatomic location and subcategorize by disease components. Therefore, for purposes of discussion, this chapter will discuss the classification of blepharitis in terms of anterior and posterior lid margin disease and the conditions associated with each entity.

Anterior Blepharitis

Common symptoms of blepharitis include burning, itching, a gritty or foreign body sensation, crusting and redness or irritation of the lid margins. However, there is significant overlap of these symptoms in all forms of blepharitis, and therefore, clinical features must be utilized to distinguish between different etiologies of blepharitis (Table 8.2). Of note, the symptoms of blepharitis are traditionally bilateral and any unilateral presentation, marked asymmetry or resistance to therapy, should alert the clinician to the presence of other diseases masquerading as blepharitis, such as sebaceous cell carcinoma (Fig. 8.1).[15]

The two most common subcategories of anterior blepharitis are staphylococcal blepharitis and seborrheic blepharitis (though it is important to note that some patients have mixed disease with features of both conditions).

STAPHYLOCOCCAL BLEPHARITIS

Staphylococcal blepharitis is typically characterized by scaling, crusting, and erythema of the lid margin.[16] This form of anterior blepharitis tends to occur more often in females and at a slightly younger age than seborrheic blepharitis (mean age 42, compared with 51 years old).[7]

Clinical Features

Collarettes are typically found in staphylococcal infection. Staphylococcal debris and white blood cells congeal to form hard, brittle fibrinous scales at the base of the lash. As the

Table 8.2 Clinical Features of the Most Common Forms of Blepharitis

	Anterior Blepharitis – Staphylococcal	Anterior Blepharitis – Seborrheic	Posterior Blepharitis – Meibomian Gland Dysfunction
Eyelash	Frequent loss/thinning, breakage or misdirection	Rare eyelash loss or misdirection	May have misdirection in long standing disease
Eyelid	Collarettes extending along lashes; may also contain sleeves if demodex folliculorum present	Greasy scales on lid margins	Foamy, thick meibum, meibomian gland dropout, pouting meibomian glands, inspissated glands
Tear film deficiency	Frequent	Frequent	Frequent
Conjunctiva	Mild to mod injection, chronic papillary conjunctivitis	Mild injection	Mild to mod injection, Associated with GPC
Cornea	Punctate epithelial keratitis, marginal infiltrates, phlyctenules	Corneal erosions	Corneal pannus, ulceration, corneal edema, scarring, neovascularization, corneal thinning, punctuate keratitis
Chalazia/hordoleum	Rare	Rare	May have frequent
Dermatologic disease	Atopic dermatitis	Seborrheic dermatitis	Rosacea

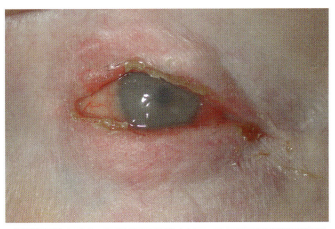

Figure 8.1 Sebaceous cell carcinoma of the eyelid can masquerade as blepharitis and should be suspected in any case of unilateral blepharitis, marked asymmetry between eyes or blepharitis unresponsive to traditional therapy. (Courtesy of Dr. Mark Mannis.)

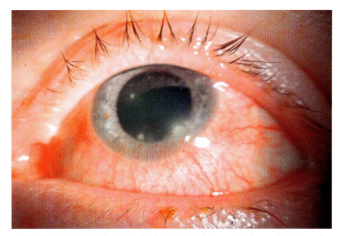

Figure 8.3 Marginal corneal infiltrates associated with staphylococcal blepharitis. (Courtesy of Dr. Mark Mannis.)

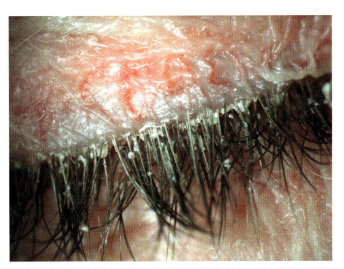

Figure 8.2 Scaling, crusting and collarette formation at the base of the cilia in a patient with staphylococcal blepharitis.

lash grows, these scales encircle the lash and form what is known as collarettes (Fig. 8.2).[11] In addition, sleeves may be found along the lash shaft, which are representative of *Demodex follicularum*. The parasite mite is found in both normal patients and those with blepharitis; as such, its role in blepharitis is unclear.[11] In addition, dilated blood vessels at the base of the lashes produce erythema and chronic inflammation of the anterior lid, which may lead to changes, such as notching and thickening of the lid, loss or thinning of lashes, and misdirected lashes.[17]

The lids in staphylococcal blepharitis tend to be more inflamed than other forms of blepharitis and in some cases, external hordeolum or chalazia may occur from acute inflammation of the surrounding meibomian glands.[5] In addition, the conjunctiva in staphylococcal blepharitis may appear mild to moderately hyperemic and may demonstrate a chronic papillary conjunctivitis, thought to occur from release of the bacterial toxins.[4] Further more, this form of anterior blepharitis may also be associated with punctate epithelial keratitis, marginal infiltrates or ulcerations and phlyctenular keratitis (Fig. 8.3).[7]

Infectious Etiology

Classically, staphylococcal blepharitis is considered to be the form of blepharitis associated with bacterial colonization of the anterior lid margin. The most common organisms isolated from patients with chronic blepharitis include *S. epidermidis*, *Propionibacterium acnes*, *Corynebacterium* and *S. aureus*.[7,18] Some studies have shown that though *S. epidermidis* is isolated in high concentrations from both normal patients and those with blepharitis, *S. aureus* seems to be isolated in greater frequency in patients with a clinical diagnosis of staphylococcal blepharitis.[7] However, other studies suggest that rather than having higher concentration of one bacterial isolate, blepharitis patients have a more heavily colonized lid surface than normal controls.[16] Additionally, there has been speculation that staphylococcal toxins may be responsible for the symptoms of blepharoconjunctivitis. Yet, a study by Seal et al. demonstrated that *S. aureus* colonized 6% of normal lids without producing blepharitis, even though all isolates produced alpha toxin.[18]

SEBORRHEIC BLEPHARITIS

On the other hand, seborrheic blepharitis has been associated with an overproduction of sebum, leading to greasy scaling of the anterior eyelid. Seborrheic blepharitis tends to occur in an older age group, compared to staphylococcal blepharitis and does not appear to have a gender predilection.[19] Overall, there is less inflammation than staphylococcal blepharitis, unless there is a staphylococcal superinfection.[7] McCulley et al. reported that in seborrheic blepharitis, the meibomian glands had dilated ductules with normal secretions.[7] Approximately one-third of patients with seborrheic blepharitis had keratoconjunctivitis sicca[4] and corneal erosions have been reported in up to 15% of cases.[20]

ASSOCIATED CONDITIONS

For the most part, staphylococcal blepharitis does not have any definitive associated systemic conditions. Both anterior and posterior blepharitis are associated with rosacea, but rosacea is more often found in posterior disease. Some

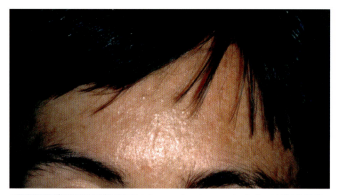

Figure 8.4 Seborrheic dermatitis with characteristic hypersecretion of oil on the skin and seborrheic hypertrophy. (Courtesy of Dr. Mark Mannis.)

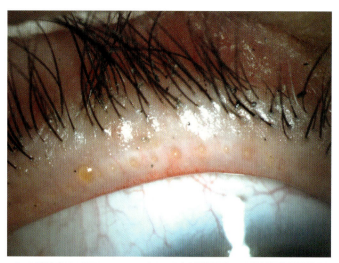

Figure 8.5 Inspissated meibomian gland present in posterior blepharitis. Note the turbid secretions present in adjacent meibomian glands.

patients with chronic atopy have increased susceptibility to the development of chronic staphylococcal infections and appear to be predisposed to developing staphylococcal blepharitis as well.[17]

On the contrary, as McCulley et al.[7] noted, a great preponderance of seborrheic blepharitis patients also have seborrheic dermatitis. Seborrheic dermatitis is a common, chronic condition characterized by symmetric erythematous inflammation, with scaling that is often greasy in areas of the skin with a high concentration of sebaceous glands.[21] Most patients with seborrheic blepharitis and dermatitis present with similar yellow, greasy scaling on the eyelids, eyebrows, and scalp (Fig. 8.4). Other commonly affected areas include the ears, sides of the nose, chest, axilla, and inguinal area.[20]

All categories of blepharitis appear to be associated with some degree of aqueous tear deficiency or keratoconjunctivitis sicca.[22,23]

Posterior Blepharitis

MEIBOMIAN GLAND DYSFUNCTION

Contrary to patients with anterior blepharitis, patients with meibomian gland disease have inflammation associated with the posterior lid margin. In meibomian gland dysfunction (MGD), the glands tend to be minimally inflamed, but the meibomian orifices are dilated with stagnant secretions. Clinically, posterior blepharitis patients seem to have more pronounced symptoms with fewer distinct clinical signs, in comparison to anterior blepharitis patients. The subcommittee for diagnosis and classification of MGD, at the International workshop on meibomian gland dysfunction, noted that MGD encompasses myriad signs including meibomian gland dropout, altered composition of meibum, and changes in lid morphology.[24]

Meibomian Gland Dropout

Though meibomian gland dropout increases with age in normal patients, it has been postulated that this occurs at an increased rate in patients with severe MGD, leading to an evaporative dry eye state with its associated symptoms.[20] Several techniques have been described to quantify meibomian gland dropout, including meiboscopy, meibography,

and confocal microscopy.[20] Meiboscopy involves a clinical examination with transilluminated biomicroscopy of the glands,[25] while meibography captures images of the glands using near-infrared light and camera.[26] Confocal microscopy has also been described to assess meibomian gland structure and changes in MGD.[27,28] Ibrahim et al. proposed parameters for confocal microbioscopic analysis of meibomian gland function and dropout, including meibomian gland acinar longest diameter, shortest diameter, and inflammatory cell density.[29]

Altered Biochemical Composition of Meibum

In obstructed meibomian gland disease, studies have shown the lipid secretions to be altered, leading to thickening of the secretions, plugging of the glands and pouting of the meibomian orifices.[30] The secretions of meibomian glands in posterior blepharitis range from a cloudy, turbid fluid, to a granular substance to inspissated glands with a 'toothpaste-like consistency' that may be extruded as a plug or curled thread.[19] In addition, there may be 'meibomian foam,' a frothy accumulation, which is postulated to be attributed to the presence of soaps in the tear film.[31] Dougherty and McCulley et al. reported in several studies the alterations of specific polar and nonpolar lipid secretions of meibomian glands, compared to normal controls and even within different classifications of blepharitis, as the rationale behind the varying symptomatology and classification of blepharitis.[31,32] For instance, the investigators have proposed that the increase in oleic acid found in the meibum of patients with posterior blepharitis may be responsible for complaints of increased burning sensation in this subset of patients.[33] Further more, they showed a significant difference in the fatty wax and sterol ester fraction of meibum, which represents a large portion of the total lipid secretion from the meibomian glands in patients with chronic blepharitis.[33]

Changes in Lid Morphology

Pouting of the meibomian glands serves as an early, pathognomonic sign of morphological changes in the lid that occur in MGD (Fig. 8.5).[25] The meibomian orifice becomes

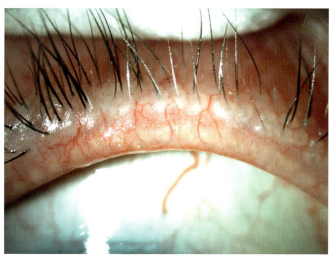

Figure 8.6 Lid telangiectasia in a patient with blepharitis and ocular rosacea.

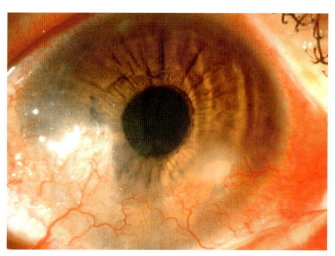

Figure 8.7 Corneal pannus, neovascularization and scarring secondary to uncontrolled ocular rosacea. (Courtesy of Dr. Mark Mannis.)

elevated above the surface of the lid, secondary to obstruction of the terminal ducts and extrusion of the abnormal meibum described earlier. These changes are compounded by retroplacement of the meibomian orifices behind the mucocutaneous junction over time.[31] The orifices may become ovally elongated and result in duct exposure in severe cases.[31] Additional lid changes in MGD include rounding, notching, dimpling, telangiectasia, increased vascularity of the posterior lid margin, and epithelial ridging between gland orifices.[25] With chronic inflammation, hyperemia, lid thickening, and irregularity of lid contour may occur. As a result, secondary changes in the anterior lid margin may occur, such as loss of eyelashes, crusting of the lid margin, and hyperkeratinization of the mucocutaneous junction from squamous metaplasia.[34]

ASSOCIATED CONDITIONS

A large number of patients with posterior blepharitis also present with rosacea.[35] Rosacea is a chronic skin condition characterized by persistent pustules, papules, erythema, telangiectasia, and sebaceous gland hypertrophy.[17] Typically, dilated, telangiectatic blood vessels are found on the nose, cheeks and forehead. Ocular rosacea may be present with or without chronic skin changes and is typically associated with obstructed meibomian glands and telangiectatic vessels (Fig. 8.6). Sequelae of ocular rosacea include corneal pannus, dendritic keratopathy, corneal edema, scarring, neovascularization, thinning, lipid deposition, phlyctenules, ulceration, and perforation (Fig. 8.7).[34] These potentially grave complications of ocular rosacea, highlight the importance of recognition and treatment of this disease in association with posterior blepharitis.

Chalazia are also more common in patients with posterior blepharitis. On pathology, the lesion appears as a localized, chronic granulomatous reaction to extravasated meibomian gland secretions from a plugged gland (Fig. 8.8).[16] Therefore, it would follow that chalazia tend to occur more often in uncontrolled posterior blepharitis with plugging of the meibomian glands. Clinicians must be aware of

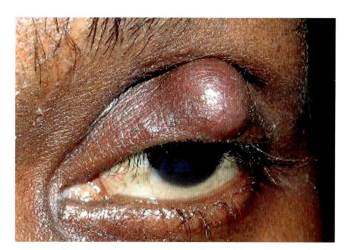

Figure 8.8 A chalazion, commonly associated with meibomian gland dysfunction, presents as a large, localized firm nodule. (Courtesy of Dr. Mark Mannis.)

the rare but ominous masquerade conditions that may mimic chalazia, such as sebaceous cell carcinoma and Merkle cell carcinoma.

Patients with giant papillary conjunctivitis secondary to contact lens use, may also have a greater incidence of posterior blepharitis.[35]

Conclusion

Blepharitis represents one of the most common ocular conditions where true pathogenesis remains largely unknown. The multiple classification systems that have emerged allow for some distinctions to be made, but also underscores our need to investigate this multifaceted disease to a greater depth. Focused research and continued improvements in techniques for evaluating blepharitis, will lead to a deeper understanding of the disease process and improved therapy.

References

1. National Disease and Therapeutics Index (NDTI), IMS America, Dec 1982.
2. Hom MM, Martinson JR, Knapp LL, et al. Prevalence of meibomian gland dysfunction. Optom Vis Sci 1990;67:710–2.
3. Lemp MA, Nichols KK. Blepharitis in the United States 2009: a survey based perspective on prevalence and treatment. Ocul Surf 2009; 7(Suppl. 2):S1–S14.
4. Edwards RS. Ophthalmic emergencies in a district general hospital casualty department. Br J Ophthalmol 1987;71:938–42.
5. Mathers WD, Shields WJ, Sachdev MS, et al. Meibomian gland dysfunction in chronic blepharitis. Cornea 1991;10:277–85.
6. Thygeson P. Etiology and treatment of blepharitis. Arch Ophthalmol 1946;36:445–77.
7. McCulley JP, Dougherty JM, Deneau DG. Classification of chronic blepharitis. Ophthalmology 1982;89:1173–80.
8. McCulley JP, Sciallis GF. Meibomian keratoconjunctivitis. Am J Ophthalmol 1977;84:788–93.
9. Huber-Spitzy V, Baumgartner I, Böhler-Sommeregger K, et al. Blepharitis – a diagnostic and therapeutic challenge. A report on 407 consecutive cases. Graefes Arch Clin Exp Ophthalmol 1991;229:224–7.
10. Mathers WD, Choi D. Cluster analysis of patients with ocular surface disease, blepharitis, and dry eye. Arch Ophthalmol 2004;122: 1700–4.
11. American Academy of Ophthalmology Cornea/External Disease Panel. Preferred Practice Pattern Guidelines. San Francisco, CA: Blepharitis—Limited Revision, AAO; 2011.
12. Torkildsen GL, Cockrum P, Meier E, et al. Evaluation of clinical efficacy and safety of tobramycin/dexamethasone ophthalmic suspension 0.3%/0.05% compared to azithromycin ophthalmic solution 1% in the treatment of moderate to severe acute blepharitis/blepharoconjunctivitis. Curr Med Res Opin 2011;27:171–8.
13. Comparative study of AzaSite plus compared to AzaSite alone and dexamethasone alone to treat subjects with blepharoconjunctivitis. http://clinicaltrials.gov/ct2/show/NCT00754949. 2012.
14. A single-center, double-masked, randomized, vehicle controlled study to evaluate the safety and efficacy of testosterone 0.03% ophthalmic solution compared to vehicle for the treatment of meibomian gland dysfunction. http://clinicaltrials.gov/ct2/show/NCT00755183?term=single-center+testosterone&rank=1. 2012.
15. Akpek EK, Polcharoen W, Chan R, et al. Ocular surface neoplasia masquerading as chronic blepharoconjunctivitis. Cornea 1999; 18:282–8.
16. Raskin EM, Speaker MG, Laibson PR. Blepharitis. Infect Dis Clin North Am 1992;6:777–87.
17. Ghanem VC, Mehra N, Wong S, et al. The prevalence of ocular signs in acne rosacea: comparing patients from ophthalmology and dermatology clinics. Cornea 2003;22:230–3.
18. Seal D, Ficker L, Ramakrishnan M, et al. Role of staphylococcal toxin production in blepharitis. Ophthalmology 1990;97:1684–8.
19. Bron AJ, Benjamin L, Snibson GR. Meibomian gland disease. Classification and grading of lid changes. Eye 1991;5(Pt 4):395–411.
20. Peralejo B, Beltrani V, Bielory L. Dermatologic and allergic conditions of the eyelid. Immunol Allergy Clin North Am 2008;28:137–68, vii.
21. Bernardes TF, Bonfioli AA. Blepharitis. Semin Ophthalmol 2010; 25:79–83.
22. Shine WE, McCulley JP. Keratoconjunctivitis sicca associated with meibomian secretion polar lipid abnormality. Arch Ophthalmol 1998;116:849–52.
23. Bron AJ, Tiffany JM. The contribution of meibomian disease to dry eye. Ocul Surf 2004;2:149–65.
24. Tomlinson A, Bron AJ, Korb DR, et al. The international workshop on meibomian gland dysfunction: report of the diagnosis subcommittee. Invest Ophthalmol Vis Sci 2011;52:2006–49.
25. Robin JB, Jester JV, Nobe J, et al. In vivo transillumination biomicroscopy and photography of meibomian gland dysfunction: a clinical study. Ophthalmology 1985;92:1423–6.
26. Nichols JJ, Berntsen DA, Mitchell GL, et al. An assessment of grading scales for meibography images. Cornea 2005;24:382–8.
27. Matsumoto Y, Sato EA, Ibrahim OM, et al. The application of in vivo laser confocal microscopy to the diagnosis and evaluation of meibomian gland dysfunction. Mol Vis 2008;14:1263–71.
28. Wang Y, Le Q, Zhao F, et al. Application of in vivo laser scanning confocal microscopy for evaluation of ocular surface diseases: lessons learned from pterygium, meibomian gland disease, and chemical burns. Cornea 2011;30:525–8.
29. Ibrahim OM, Matsumoto Y, Dogru M, et al. The efficacy, sensitivity, and specificity of in vivo laser confocal microscopy in the diagnosis of meibomian gland dysfunction. Ophthalmology 2010;117:665–72.
30. Jackson WB. Blepharitis: current strategies for diagnosis and management. Can J Ophthalmol 2008;43:170–9.
31. Dougherty JM, Osgood JK, McCulley JP. The role of wax and sterol ester fatty acids in chronic blepharitis. Invest Ophthalmol Vis Sci 1991;32:1932–7.
32. McCulley JP, Shine WE. Eyelid disorders: the meibomian gland, blepharitis, and contact lenses. Eye Contact Lens 2003;29(Suppl. 1): S93–5.
33. Smith RE, Flowers Jr CW. Chronic blepharitis: a review. CLAO J 1995;21:200–7.
34. Lee WB, Darlington JK, Mannis MJ, et al. Dendritic keratopathy in ocular rosacea. Cornea 2005;24:632–3.
35. Martin NF, Rubinfeld RS, Malley JD, et al. Giant papillary conjunctivitis and meibomian gland dysfunction blepharitis. CLAO J 1992; 18:165–9.

9 Anterior Blepharitis: Treatment Strategies

JAY C. BRADLEY

Introduction

Blepharitis is one of the most common ocular disorders seen by eye care specialists and is found in almost 47% of ophthalmic patients. Approximately 30 million Americans may be affected.[1] Blepharitis is common in middle-aged patients, and its incidence increases with age. Blepharitis may be under-reported as the primary reason for an office visit, since the patient may present for a dry eye assessment, surgical evaluation or routine examination.[2] Although common, blepharitis is often overlooked, misdiagnosed or inadequately treated. The lack of diagnosis may be due to poor understanding of the condition and the absence of a widely accepted definition and classification scheme, as well as the lack of a clinically straightforward algorithm to aid in the diagnosis and treatment of blepharitis. Recently, diagnostic and treatment algorithms for practitioners have been developed. A simplified clinically relevant terminology based on anatomic location is key to improve diagnosis and management.[3]

Anterior blepharitis refers to acute or chronic inflammation and its associated signs and symptoms involving the anterior portion of the eyelid (eyelashes and follicles) (Fig. 9.1).[1] In one study, anterior blepharitis was found to account for 12% of all eyecare patients seeking treatment for generalized ocular discomfort or irritation.[4] Unlike posterior blepharitis, which primarily involves the meibomian glands, anterior blepharitis appears to be more common in younger (mean age of 42) and female (80%) patients. A variety of conditions (including age, allergy, immune system problems, hormonal changes, bacteria, rosacea and dermatitis) may contribute to its development.[1,5]

Anterior blepharitis typically involves an excessive colonization of normal lid bacteria (*Staphylococcus aureus*, *Staphylococcus epidermidis*, *Corynebacterium*, or others) and inflammation.[1,3,6-7] Infection occurs at the origins of the eyelashes and involves the follicles and surrounding tissues.[5] Bacteria elaborate virulence factors including toxins, enzymes, and waste products that enter the tear film and contribute to ocular surface inflammation and irritation.[5,8] Lipolytic exoenzymes produced by the lid bacteria hydrolyze wax and sterol esters release irritating free fatty acids.[3] These breakdown products can contribute to the disruption of tear film integrity.[5,8]

Clinical Presentation and Diagnosis

Diagnosis of anterior blepharitis is typically based on signs, symptoms, history, and external/lid examination. Typically bilateral, anterior blepharitis is both chronic and intermittent and can significantly impact quality of life.[1] In its acute phase, patients often present with bright red, puffy, irritated eyes that itch or burn.[3] Additional signs include lid and lash debris, watery eyes, and intermittent effects on vision.

Staphylococcal-related anterior blepharitis affects predominantly young to middle-aged women, and keratoconjunctivitis sicca (dry eye) can present in up to 50% of these patients[6,8] Eyelash loss or breakage and misdirection, collarettes or scurf on the eyelids and lashes, and fine eyelid ulcerations along the lash margin can also be seen (Fig. 9.2).[8] In severe cases, staphylococcal hypersensitivity syndrome may cause ocular surface inflammation, corneal

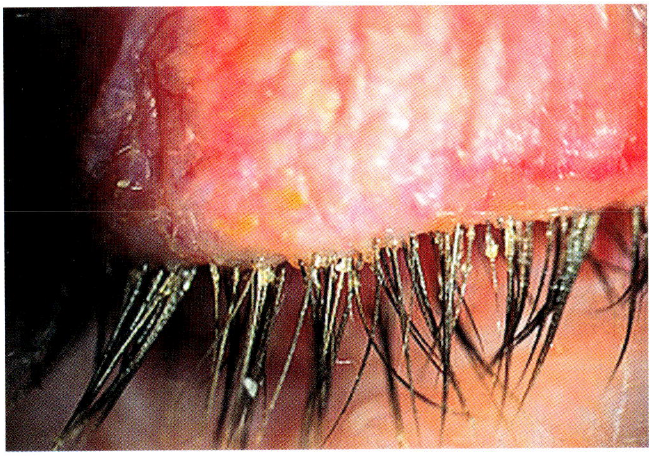

Figure 9.1 Anterior blepharitis with lid erythema, scurf and collarettes.

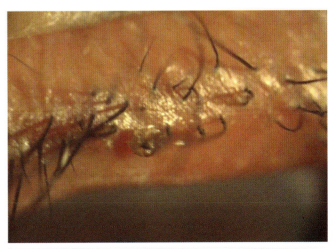

Figure 9.2 Eyelash loss, breakage and misdirection with collarettes.

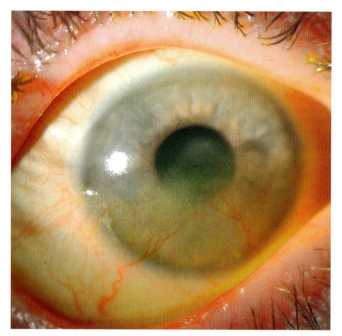

Figure 9.3 Staphylococcal hypersensitivity syndrome with anterior blepharitis, corneal neovascularization and dry eye.

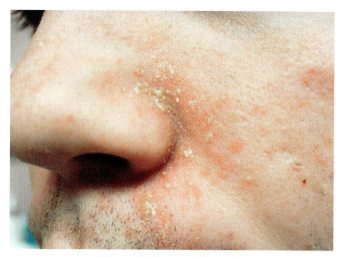

Figure 9.4 Seborrheic dermatitis.

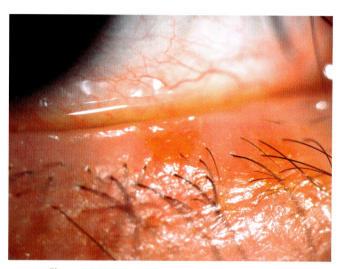

Figure 9.5 Herpes simplex-related anterior blepharitis.

neovascularization and scarring, and decreased vision (Fig. 9.3).

Seborrhea-related disease generally affects older patients and is indiscriminate of gender.[6,9] Aqueous tear deficiency can be seen in 25% to 40% of these patients.[8] Seborrheic dermatitis is a skin condition associated with flaking and scaling, involving the eyebrows and eyelids (Fig. 9.4). The cause of this skin condition is not well understood. Seborrhea sometimes appears in patients with weakened immune systems. Fungi or certain types of yeast that feed on lipids in the skin may also contribute to seborrheic dermatitis with accompanying blepharitis.

A thorough history and comprehensive eye examination is critical to confirming a diagnosis. Patient history can help, as the presence of underlying skin conditions such as seborrheic dermatitis or atopic eczema may point to the diagnosis of seborrheic disease.[8] Clinicians should look for signs of both infection and inflammation.

The differential diagnosis can be confounded by similar conditions with other etiologies, and includes infectious, inflammatory, and seborrheic etiologies.[10] Infectious etiologies include staphylococcal and other bacteria, herpes simplex virus (Fig. 9.5), *Demodex* (Figs 9.6 and 9.7) and *Phthrisis pubis* (Fig. 9.8). Rosacea-related anterior blepharitis is primarily inflammatory but is often associated with bacterial overgrowth as well. Rosacea-related disease, if untreated or inadequately treated, may lead to severe corneal neovascularization and scarring with resultant poor vision (Fig. 9.9). Anterior blepharitis is also found in patients with seborrhea.

With *Demodex* blepharitis, microscopic mites (*Demodex folliculorum*) and their waste materials cause clogging of eyelash follicles and associated inflammation (Figs 9.6 and 9.7). *Demodex brevis* can also affect the oil glands of the skin and eyelids causing secondary blepharitis. While presence

of these tiny mites is common, the development of *Demodex* blepharitis may be due to unusual allergic or immune system responses.

In addition, patients may experience signs or symptoms involving both the anterior and posterior eyelids, since anterior blepharitis is often found concomitantly with meibomian gland disease.[3] Chalazion formation and bacterial conjunctivitis may be seen in these patients, due to posterior lid involvement and bacterial overgrowth. In addition, the proximity of the eyelids to ocular structures can lead to other disorders (such as dry eye) due to inflammatory mediator release and/or tear film instability.[11]

Presentation should be categorized by the presence or absence of key signs and symptoms. Symptoms include stickiness, crusting, burning of the eyelids upon awakening and eyelid irritation, both acute and chronic. Principle signs include erythema, edema and eyelid and lash debris (collarettes and scurf) (Figs 9.10 and 9.11).

Eyelid and lash examinations are generally sufficient to aid in the differential diagnosis of anterior blepharitis. Slit lamp biomicroscopy is necessary for evaluating the tear

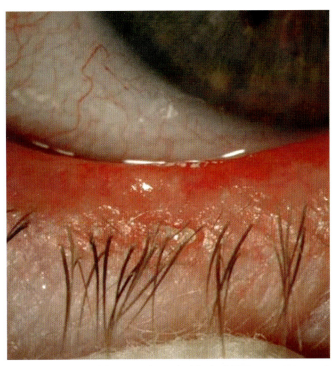

Figure 9.6 *Demodex* blepharitis.

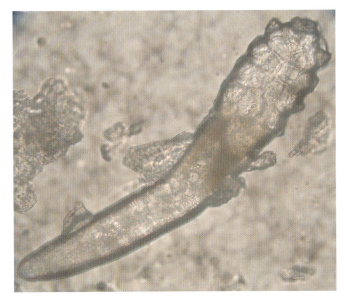

Figure 9.7 *Demodex* microscopic image (400× magnification).

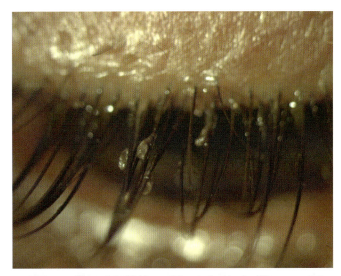

Figure 9.8 *Phthirus pubis* anterior blepharitis.

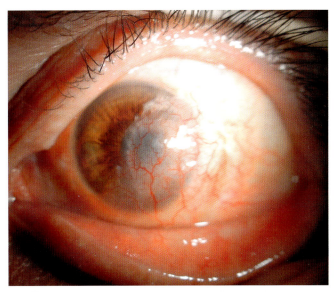

Figure 9.9 Rosacea-related anterior blepharitis with severe corneal scarring and neovascularization.

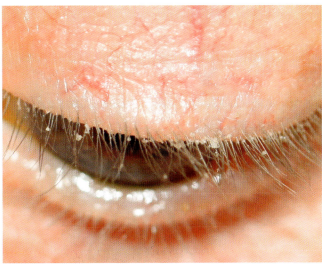

Figure 9.10 Anterior blepharitis with scurf.

film, anterior eyelid margin, tarsal conjunctiva, bulbar conjunctiva and the cornea. The external examination should include attention to the anterior portion of the eyelid margins and eyelid skin. Culture and biopsy may facilitate the differential diagnosis of anterior blepharitis but should be reserved for special circumstances (such as resistance to therapy, atypical asymmetric presentation or unifocal recurrent chalazia).

Classification of patients based upon disease severity is a critical element which guides treatment decisions. Anterior blepharitis can be divided into asymptomatic and

Table 9.1   Anterior Blepharitis Severity Classification Table

	Asymptomatic	Mild	Moderate	Severe
Symptoms	None	Occasional morning eyelid sticking or burning/lid irritation	Frequent morning eyelid sticking or burning/lid irritation	Persistent eyelid sticking, burning, or lid irritation that interferes with normal activities
Eyelash debris	None to rare	Scattered	Half of eyelashes with debris (scurf/collarettes)	Most of eyelashes with debris (scurf/collarettes)
Erythema	Redness at eyelash bases, no eczematous appearance	Redness at eyelash bases, pink appearance	Redness at eyelash bases, light red appearance (or presence of eczema)	Redness at eyelash bases, dark red appearance
Lid edema	None	Just noticeable	0.5 to 1 mm	>1 mm

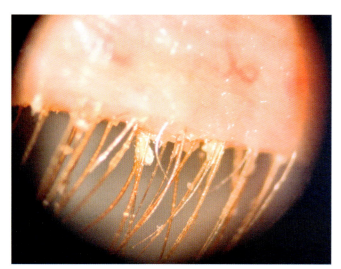

Figure 9.11 Anterior blepharitis with collarettes.

symptomatic disease. Patients presenting with symptomatic blepharitis may be further subdivided into mild, moderate or severe categories based upon signs and symptoms present and degree of severity (Table 9.1).

Treatment

An algorithm for patient management based upon disease severity has been proposed. While treatment goals can vary based on the clinical picture, they should focus upon and include providing symptomatic relief, managing inflammation, treating the underlying etiology, and minimizing recurrence. In patients presenting acutely, treatment should aim to provide symptomatic relief and improve quality of life by decreasing bacterial burden and inflammation of the eyelid. In patients with chronic disease, minimizing acute flare-ups and damage to ocular structures secondary to chronic inflammation are the primary objectives.

Chronic untreated or inadequately treated disease can result in ectropion, thickened lid margins, dilated and visible capillaries, trichiasis, and entropion. The cornea may exhibit significant erosion and secondary infectious keratitis. In severe cases, corneal scarring and neovascularization, corneal thinning or perforation, and decreased or loss of vision can occur. Due to these potential untoward

effects, early and appropriate treatment of anterior blepharitis is crucial.

In patients with anterior blepharitis undergoing ocular surgery (such as cataract or laser in situ keratomileusis), a 'quiet eye' without evidence of infection or inflammation is desired, in order to optimize results and prevent the development of postoperative infection.[2] Therapy should induce remission by impacting these etiologies in the event of an acute exacerbation, followed by some type of maintenance strategy to prevent recurrence. The use of topical antibiotic therapy preoperatively and betadine skin prep on the day of surgery is crucial to decrease the risk of postoperative infection.

The multifactorial nature of anterior blepharitis and the high frequency of mixed anterior/posterior disease, often require combination therapies for optimal patient management. In cases with significant associated posterior disease or tear dysfunction, therapies targeting these pathologies are needed for successful management. Omega-3 nutritional supplements (such as flaxseed oil, fish oil, and other commercially available products) are beneficial and should be utilized in these patients.

Patient education, warm compresses, and lid hygiene should be initiated early and are critical to successful treatment. Patients should be taught to cleanse the eyelid margin and the base of the eyelashes. Warm compresses help liquefy debris for easier removal with scrubs. Initially, warm compresses and scrubs may be needed frequently and for several minutes each time. Once controlled, frequency and duration can be significantly reduced, often to once daily for a few minutes. Finally, medicated scrubs may be used to reduce bacterial colonization, remove lid and lash debris and bacterial toxins and restore ocular health. All three elements (education, warm compresses and lid hygiene) are key to any plan for the treatment of anterior blepharitis.

Contact lens wear in patients with anterior blepharitis can be problematic due to increased propensity for the formation of lens deposits and intolerance, due to borderline tear film. Daily contact lens wear, rigid gas-permeable wear or contact lens discontinuation may be beneficial if problems arise. During flares, use of make-up should be minimized or discontinued since it may interfere with eyelid hygiene and prevent flare treatment or prolong the course of disease.

Pharmacologic therapy for anterior disease should focus on symptomatic relief, inflammation control, and treatment of the underlying etiology. Ideally, treatment should provide rapid symptom resolution, patient-friendly administration, inflammation reduction and bacterial overgrowth eradication.

Since anterior blepharitis is commonly associated with dry eye and ocular surface irritation, frequent artificial tear use can aid in symptomatic relief, during and between flares. Some commercially available artificial tears contain a lipid component and may be helpful in selected patient with concomitant meibomian gland disease.

Topical antibiotic therapy is necessary in the management of moderate to severe disease, especially when bacterial overgrowth is observed. Historically, bacitracin and aminoglycosides (gentamicin and tobramycin) comprised the most commonly used topical antibiotics for the treatment of blepharitis. Administration was generally limited to acute anterior blepharitis flares, to minimize the opportunity for development of resistance and minimize associated ocular surface toxicity. Antibiotic ointments can also be utilized to increase the contact time with the eyelid surface and aid in symptomatic relief from ocular surface irritation.[11]

Recently, macrolide antibiotics (such as erythromycin and azithromycin) have been advocated since they possess both anti-inflammatory and anti-infective properties. Topical azithromycin has exceptional affinity for tissue and a long half-life, making it an attractive treatment option for eyelid disease.[12] Erythromycin is also available as an ophthalmic ointment but does not penetrate tissue well.

Longer courses of topical antibiotic drops or ointments have been advocated in severe or recurrent disease. Topical azithromycin can be used twice daily, initially to rapidly decrease bacterial load and quiet symptoms, and then once daily to prevent recurrence and improve lid inflammation. To increase its effectiveness, topical azithromycin should be applied immediately after performing warm compresses and scrubs. The optimal duration of this therapy has not been determined. Long-term antibiotic ointment, such as erythromycin or bacitracin at bedtime may also be an effective treatment option to quieten flares and prevent recurrences.

In staphylococcal or rosacea-related anterior blepharitis, long-term oral tetracycline therapy may be beneficial. Minocycline and doxycycline are most commonly used, due to their efficacy and favorable side effect profile. Therapy is generally started at an antimicrobial dosage to decrease bacterial load and then tapered to an anti-inflammatory (via anti-matrix metalloproteinase inhibition) dosage once stable. Sustained-release formulations are available and can be useful in patients experiencing medication-related side effects.

Topical corticosteroids target the inflammatory component of blepharitis. They are generally reserved for moderate to severe inflammation and complicated presentations.[8] The selection of steroid used should take into account the potency needed for adequate therapeutic response while balancing the risk of side effects.

Simultaneous steroid and antibiotic use as induction therapy can be beneficial in patients with moderate to severe disease. This treatment should be used judiciously since long-term corticosteroid use can increase the risk of elevated intraocular pressure, exacerbate the infectious process leading to superinfection, and stimulate cataract development.[13] For safety reasons, the lowest effective steroid dose should be used and patients should be monitored closely for safety and efficacy. In patients with moderate or severe disease, the use of fixed-dose combination products may facilitate patient administration and increase convenience. For patients in need of chronic anti-inflammatory therapy to prevent recurrences, low-dose topical steroid (such as fluorometholone or loteprednol) or topical cyclosporine 0.05% may be considered to prevent disease recurrence, while minimizing the risk of long-term side effects.

Treatment of seborrheic anterior blepharitis includes regular cleansing with eyelid scrubs and gentle nondetergent antidandruff shampoos. These therapies can provide significant relief and improve the appearance of the eyelids. In patients with severe seborrheic dermatitis, a dermatologic consultation may be considered.

Treatment of other less common causes of anterior blepharitis targets the underlying etiology. For herpes simplex virus-related blepharitis, topical and/or oral antiviral therapy along with ocular surface lubrication and cool compresses control symptoms and shorten the duration of the active disease. For fungi and yeast overgrowth associated with seborrhea, treatment of the underlying disease and lid hygiene are generally curative. For *Demodex*-associated anterior blepharitis, eyelid scrubs combined with tea tree oil have been advocated. Sulfur oil and antiparasitic gels (metronidazole) have also been recommended. Topical steroid use may be beneficial in controlling inflammation seen in association with *Demodex*-related disease.[14] In cases of *Phthiriasis pubis*-related anterior blepharitis, therapy includes careful removal of the lice and nits (louse eggs) and local application of pediculocide. Patient and sexual contacts need treatment of the infection source to prevent disease recurrence.

Conclusion

Blepharitis is a common ocular condition. Anterior blepharitis involves presenting signs and symptoms reflecting infection and inflammation. Clinical classification is based on severity of signs and symptoms. This condition can negatively affect vision and quality of life for millions of patients and increase the risk of postoperative complications in ocular surgery patients.

Treatment of anterior blepharitis should be individualized, based upon severity and whether the presentation represents chronic disease or an acute flare-up. Patient education, warm compresses, and lid hygiene are vital to treatment at all severity levels. Drug therapy should target infection, inflammation, and symptom resolution. Clinicians should be vigilant when using topical antibiotics and steroids to manage symptoms and pathology and to ensure safety.

References

1. Donnenfeld ED, Mah FS, McDonald MD, et al. New considerations in the treatment of anterior and posterior blepharitis. Refr Eyecare 2008;12:1–15.
2. Lemp MA, Nichols KK. Blepharitis in the United States 2009: a survey-based perspective on prevalence and treatment. Ocul Surf 2009;7(Suppl. 2):S1–S14.

3. Foulks GN, Lemp MA. Blepharitis: a review for clinicians. Refr Eyecare 2009;13:1–10.
4. Venturino G, Bricola G, Bagnis A, et al. Chronic blepharitis: treatment patterns and prevalence. Invest Ophthalmol Vis Sci 2003;44:E-Abstract 774.
5. Dougherty JM, McCulley JP. Bacterial lipases and chronic blepharitis. Invest Ophthalmol Vis Sci 1986;27:486–91.
6. McCulley JP, Dougherty JM, Deneau DG. Classification of chronic blepharitis. Ophthalmology 1982;89:1173–80.
7. Groden LR, Murphy B, Rodnite J, et al. Lid flora in blepharitis. Cornea 1991;10:50–3.
8. Jackson WB. Blepharitis: current strategies for diagnosis and management. Can J Ophthalmol 2008;43:170–9.
9. McCulley JP, Dougherty JM. Blepharitis associated with acne rosacea and seborrheic dermatitis. Int Ophthalmol Clin 1985;25:159–72.
10. Bernardes TF, Bonfioli AA. Blepharitis. Semin Ophthalmol 2010; 25:79–83.
11. Abelson M, Shapiro A, Tobey C. Breaking down blepharitis. Rev Ophthalmol 2011;74–8.
12. Giamarellos-Bourboulis EJ. Macrolides beyond the conventional antimicrobials: a class of potent immunomodulators. Int J Antimicrob Agents 2008;31:12–20.
13. David DS, Berkowitz JS. Ocular effects of topical and systemic corticosteroids. Lancet 1969;294:149–51.
14. Kheirkhah A, Casas V, Li W, et al. Corneal manifestations of ocular Demodex infestation. Am J Ophthalmol 2007;143:743–9.

10 *Meibomian Gland Disease: Treatment*

GARY N. FOULKS

Introduction

Meibomian gland disease is one of the most commonly encountered clinical problems and can occur as focal or diffuse involvement of the meibomian glands. Meibomian glands are anatomically located in the tarsal plate of both upper and lower eyelids, as holocrine sebaceous glands that open directly on the eyelid margin and discharge their entire contents onto the lid margin. A full description of the anatomy and physiology of the glands is provided in the Report of the Meibomian Gland Workshop published in 2011.[1] The meibomian gland is a type of sebaceous gland and it is susceptible to disease entities that affect all sebaceous glands, such as seborrhea and rosacea.[1] Since obstruction of the gland orifice and alteration of the meibomian secretion are the predominant pathophysiological causes of disease, management of the clinical problem centers around relief of obstruction and modification of the abnormal secretion, as well as control of inflammation when it occurs as part of the disease process.

Classification of Meibomian Gland Disease

The etiology of meibomian gland disease can be congenital or acquired. A classification system proposed by the International Workshop on Meibomian Gland Dysfunction is depicted in Figure 10.1.[2] Congenital absence of the meibomian gland occurs and is particularly severe in association with anhidrotic ectodermal dysplasia.[3]

Acquired disease occurs as both focal (internal hordeolum or chalazion) or diffuse (meibomian gland dysfunction: MGD) involvement. Although obstruction of the glandular orifice is the likely first event, the clinical appearance is very different, as the internal hordeolum (Fig. 10.2) is the result of an acute bacterial infectious inflammation, while chalazion (Fig. 10.3) is the result of a chronic localized lipogranulomatous inflammation, and meibomian gland dysfunction (MGD) (Figs 10.4 and 10.5) is primarily obstructive with variable inflammatory reaction and typically no active infectious component, although lid margin flora may influence metabolism of the meibum secretion.[4] Thus, the management of the various clinical manifestations of meibomian gland disease differs in both the pathophysiological target and recommended therapy.

Pathophysiological Targets and Goals of Therapy

Since internal hordeolum is acute suppurative inflammation of the meibomian gland, antibiotic therapy of the infectious component and anti-inflammatory therapy to control the acute inflammation are both appropriate treatments. Relief of obstruction of the gland is also important. The infecting organism is most often *Staphylococcus* but other bacteria can be present.[5] No good comparative clinical trials have been published to compare effectiveness of treatment options for internal hordeolum,[6] but the use of topical antibiotic drops or ointments includes topical erythromycin, bacitracin, tobramycin, or fluoroquinolones. In adults with severe or recurrent disease, oral doxycycline can be prescribed as systemic therapy. Application of warm compresses periodically during the day helps to reduce inflammation and encourages the infection to localize to a point which may spontaneously erupt to relieve the obstruction. Occasionally, surgical lancing of the pointing hordeolum speeds resolution. Anti-inflammatory therapy with topical corticosteroid can be helpful when inflammation is severe.

Since chalazion is a chronic focal reaction of the tissue to altered lipid components of meibum occurring in an obstructed gland, the primary therapy is first anti-inflammatory. Warm compresses and massage of the eyelid are a usual first step but this alone is often not curative.[7] Antiinflammatory therapy with topical corticosteroid drops can reduce inflammation but the chronic granulomatous nature of the inflammatory response may not completely resolve with topical therapy. Intralesional steroid injection has been advocated to reduce inflammation.[7–9] In recalcitrant cases, evacuation of the chalazion by surgical incision and curettage is necessary.[10] Randomized controlled clinical trials have been published that compare efficacy and safety of treatment options and show that treatment with intralesional steroid is as effective as incision and curettage (84 % versus 87%, respectively) in contrast to the conservative management with hot compresses, that resulted in only a 46% resolution.[8,9]

Repeatedly recurrent or unusually irregular lid lesions mimicking chalazion can be more difficult to diagnose and can certainly be more dangerous, as they are neoplasms of the meibomian gland. It is, therefore, wise to submit curettage specimens for histopathological evaluation in

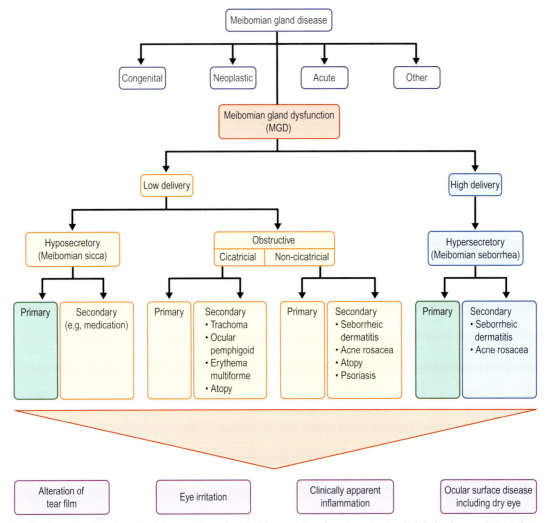

Figure 10.1 Classification of meibomian gland disease. (Reproduced with permission from Investigative Ophthalmology and Vision Science: Nelson JD, Shimazaki J, Benitez-del-Castillo JM, et al. The international workshop on meibomian gland dysfunction: report of the definition and classification subcommittee. Invest Ophthalmol Vis Sci 2011;52:1930–7.)

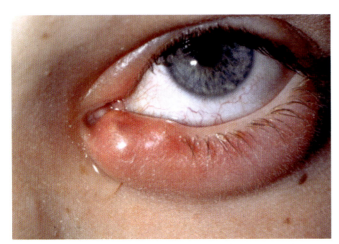

Figure 10.2 Internal hordeolum. Note the acute focal swelling and erythema of the lower eyelid with obstruction of meibomian gland orifice behind lash line.

recurrent or unusual circumstances. Sebaceous cell carcinoma is the most worrisome lesion to be identified, but intratarsal keratinous cysts are also an uncommon etiology of a lesion mimicking chalazion.[11,12]

Meibomian gland dysfunction is probably the most common affliction of the meibomian glands and the pathophysiology is amply described in the MGD Report of 2011.[1] Obstruction of the meibomian gland orifice by keratinized epithelium or thickened abnormal secretion is the primary initiating pathological event.[1,13] Therefore, relief of obstruction is a central goal of therapy. The obstruction of the meibomian gland orifice can be visualized in many cases of MGD but as Blackie, Korb and others have emphasized, nonobvious obstruction is frequent and expression of the eyelid glands as part of the physical examination is essential to diagnosis (Fig. 10.6).[14] Including expression of the meibomian glands as part of the routine evaluation of the eyelids during an eye examination, is a pivotal recommendation of the MGD Report. Mechanical options for treatment typically begin with application of warm compresses, two or more times daily, followed by firm massage of the eyelids.[15] A variety of techniques have been advocated but

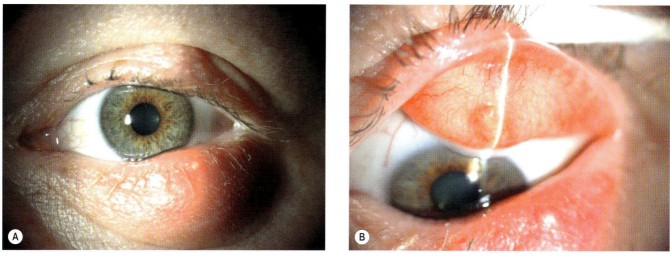

Figure 10.3 (**A**) Chalazion: external view. Note the focal swelling in the upper eyelid without significant erythema. (Note also the external hordeolum with acute inflammation in the lower eyelid). (**B**) Chalazion inner palepebral view.

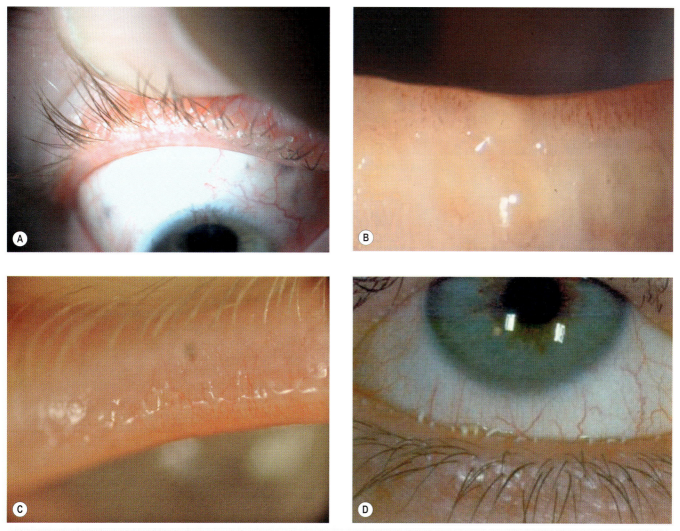

Figure 10.4 (**A**) MGD with epithelial obstruction of meibomian gland orifice. (**B**) MGD with meibomian gland secretion turbidity. (Reproduced with permission of Elsevier. From Foulks GN, Bron AJ. Meibomian Gland Dysfunction. A Clinical Scheme for Description, Diagnosis, Classification, and Grading. The Ocular Surface 2003;1:107–26.) (**C**) MGD with meibomian gland secretion that is turbid with clumps. (**D**) MGD with meibomian gland secretion that is paste consistency.

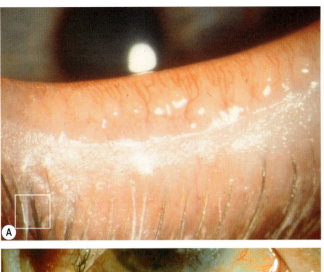
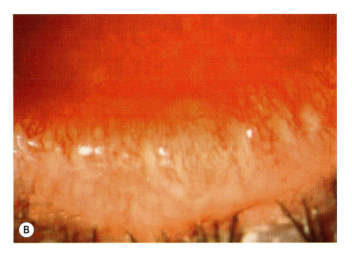
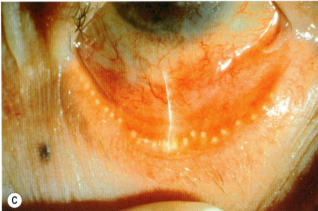

Figure 10.5 (**A**) Chronic MGD change of telangiectasia of eyelid margin. (**B**) Chronic MGD with cicatricial obstruction of meibomian gland orifice. (Reproduced with permission of Elsevier. From Foulks GN, Bron AJ. Meibomian Gland Dysfunction. A Clinical Scheme for Description, Diagnosis, Classification, and Grading. The Ocular Surface 2003;1:107–26.) (**C**) Chronic MGD with posterior traction of meibomian gland orifice due to cicatricial change. (Reproduced with permission of Elsevier. From Foulks GN, Bron AJ. Meibomian Gland Dysfunction. A Clinical Scheme for Description, Diagnosis, Classification and Grading. The Ocular Surface 2003;1:107–26.)

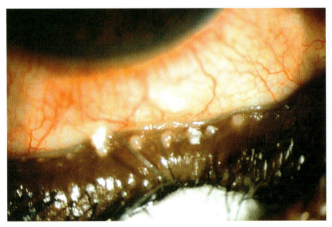

Figure 10.6 Expression of the meibomian glands by cotton-tipped swab pressed on lower eyelid. (Reproduced with permission of Elsevier from Foulks GN, Bron AJ. Meibomian Gland Dysfunction. A Clinical Scheme for Description, Diagnosis, Classification and Grading. The Ocular Surface 2003;1:107–26.)

one effective, simple approach is well described.[15] Other techniques are described in the MGD Report.[16] Warming of the eyelid has been accomplished by application of a washcloth soaked in hot water, but more elaborate methods have also been described. Heating a washcloth or a potato in a microwave oven has been advocated to provide a lasting heat, but overheating can occur and lead to burns of the facial skin.[17] Reports from the Japanese literature describe heating of the eyelids with an infrared lamp, applied as a controlled mask.[18] The application of warm, moist air or steam has also been evaluated.[19] A novel approach to application of controlled temperature concurrent with mechanical expression of the eyelids is the Lipiflow™ system, which utilizes pulsed compression of the eyelids during continuous monitored thermal control (Fig. 10.7).[20]

Meibum is a complex mixture of various polar and nonpolar lipids containing cholesteryl esters (CEs), triacylglycerol, free cholesterol, free fatty acids (FFAs), phospholipids, wax esters (WEs), and diesters.[21–24] Reported alterations of the behavior and composition of meibum in MGD are summarized in Table 10.1. Changes in the composition and behavior of the meibomian gland secretion (meibum), occurring both with age and due to meibomian gland dysfunction, have been documented by a variety of

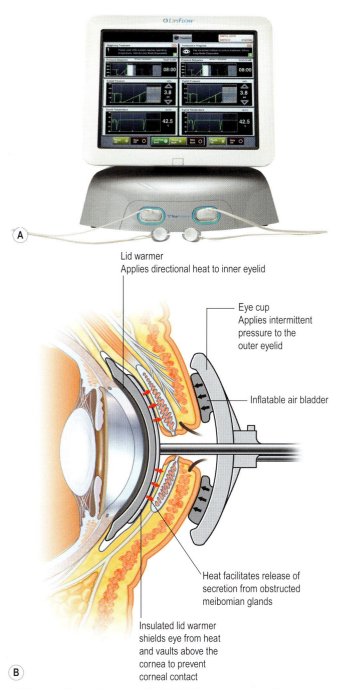

Table 10.1 Behavior and Composition Changes in Meibum with MGD

Behavior	
Increased phase transition temperature	Borchman, et al. (FTIR)[25]
Increased ordering of lipid	Foulks, et al. (FTIR)[26]
Increased viscosity	Borchman, et al. (FTIR)[25]
Composition	
Reduced cholesterol	Mathers, Lane[27]
Reduced triglycerides	Mathers, Lane[27]
Reduced polar lipids (PE, SM)	Shine, et al.[28]
Increased lipid peroxides	Augustin, et al.[29]
Increased free fatty acids	Shine, et al.[30]
Increased branched chain fatty acids	Joffre, et al.[31]
Increased triglyceride saturation	Joffre, et al.[31]
Change in diglyceride content	Dougherty, et al.[32]
Increased phospholipid unsaturation	Shine, et al.[33]
Increased protein content	Borchman, et al.[34]
Change in saturation of carbohydrate chains	Borchman, et al.[10]
Decrease oleic acid content	Shine, et al.[35]
Decreased cholesteryl esters	Shrestha, et al.[36]
Decrease in terpenoid content	Borchman, et al.[37]

FTIR, Fourier transform infrared spectroscopy; PE, phosphoethanolamine; SM, sphingomyelin.

Lid warmer
Applies directional heat to inner eyelid

Eye cup
Applies intermittent pressure to the outer eyelid

Inflatable air bladder

Heat facilitates release of secretion from obstructed meibomian glands

Insulated lid warmer shields eye from heat and vaults above the cornea to prevent corneal contact

Figure 10.7 (A) Illustration of the Lipiflow™ System that provides monitored temperature warming and intermittent pulsation of the eyelids. (Courtesy of Tear Sciences, Inc; Morrisville, North Carolina.) **(B)** Cross-sectional view of Lipiflow™ System when applied to eyelid. (www.tearscience.com/physician/in-officeprocedure/lipid-science (accessed Jan., 2013))

spectroscopic techniques.[38,39] These studies reveal that abnormal behavior of the secretion is due to increased viscosity, resulting from an elevated phase transition temperature that correlates with a higher degree of ordering of the lipid molecules (Fig. 10.8).[40] These abnormal properties of the altered meibum can be reversed with several pharmacological therapies (Fig. 10.9).[4,41–43] Tetracycline-class drugs (tetracycline, doxycycline, and minocycline) have been shown to alter the abnormal meibum, presumably by interfering with lipase enzymes that degrade the normal lipids into smaller diglycerides.[4] Doxycycline has been shown to produce a number of other changes in lipid composition and the presence of caratenoids in the meibum.[39] Azithromycin applied topically to the eye and eyelid over a month of therapy is a very effective agent to restore lipid behavior towards normal (Fig. 10.9).[41–43] The effect is probably due to a combination of antilipase activity and anti-inflammatory activity as well.[45]

Finally, control of inflammation is an important part of the therapy of MGD. Although topical corticosteroids are probably the most effective and most rapid method for controlling inflammation, the duration of such therapy is limited by the side effects of elevated intraocular pressure and cataract formation. Topical therapy with cyclosporine avoids those complications with improvement of MGD but the duration of therapy required is longer than steroids.[46] Supplementation of the diet with omega-3 essential fatty acids may also provide some anti-inflammatory benefit, although there are few controlled clinical trials that verify such a benefit, and measurement of meibum does not demonstrate specific effect on the production or composition of the secretion.[47,48] The recommended doses of omega-3 essential fatty acids vary but it is probably wise to follow the guidelines of the American Heart Association which advise limiting omega-3 supplements to 2 to 4 grams per day, unless under physician observation.[49]

Management of MGD

The management strategies for MGD have been well defined and referenced in the 2011 Report of the TFOS Meibomian

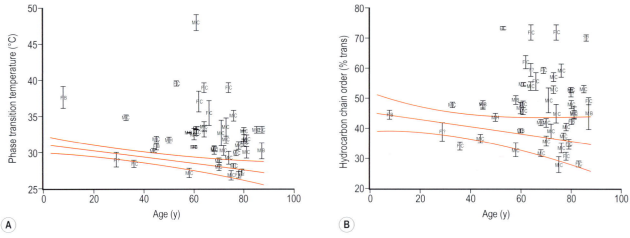

Figure 10.8 Spectroscopic analysis of meibum in MGD. The data is obtained by Fourier Transform Infrared (FTIR) spectroscopy and illustrates the change in lipid ordering (**B**) as it correlates with phase transition temperature (**A**) of meibum. The linear plot and 95% confidence limits are shown for values of normal meibum with respect to age. (Reproduced with permission of Investigative Ophthalmology and Vision Science from Borchman D, Foulks GN, Yappert MC, et al. Human Meibum Lipid Conformation and Thermodynamic Changes with Meibomian Gland Dysfunction. Invest Ophthalmol Vis Sci 2011;52:3805–17.)

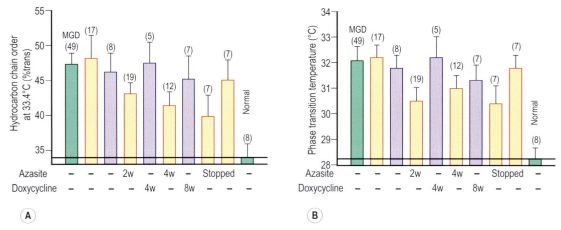

Figure 10.9 Change in meibum behavior with therapy: topical azasite versus oral doxycycline. Note that phase transition temperature returns towards normal with azithromycin therapy and with a more rapid response than to doxycycline. (Reproduced with permission of Lippincott Williams Wilkins from Foulks, Borchman, Yappert, Kakar. Topical Azithromycin and Oral Doxycycline Therapy of Meibomian Gland Dysfunction: A Comparative Clinical and Spectroscopic Pilot Study. Cornea 2013;32:44-53.)

Gland Workshop with therapy based upon clinical staging of the disease process and the concurrent effect on the tear film and ocular surface.[16] In brief, the clinical staging of the meibomian gland dysfunction evaluates the degree of obstruction of the gland orifices, due both to the number of glands obstructed and the amount of pressure needed to release expressate from the gland.[50,51] Grading of the character of the meibum is typically done in four categories: clear, turbid, turbid with clumps, and paste (see Fig. 10.4).[43,44] The amount of lid swelling and erythema of the lid margin determines the grading of degree of inflammation.[50,51] Other lid margin changes indicate the chronicity of the MGD, as cicatricial dragging of the orifices posteriorly onto the conjunctiva, telangiectasia of the lid margin, notching of the eyelid at the site of scarred orifices, and loss of eyelashes occur over time and do not resolve with therapy (see Fig. 10.5).[50,51]

The Meibomian Gland Workshop recommends grading the meibum quality by assessing each of eight glands of the central third of the lower lid on a scale of 0 to 3 for each gland:

0, clear
1, cloudy
2, cloudy with debris (granular)
3, thick, like toothpaste (total score range, 0–24).

Expressibility is assessed on a scale of 0 to 3 in five glands in the lower or upper lid, according to the number of glands expressible:

0, all glands
1, three to four glands
2, one to two glands
3, no glands.

Staining scores are obtained by summing the scores of the exposed cornea and conjunctiva:

Oxford staining score range, 1–15[52]
DEWS staining score range, 0–33.[53]

Once the severity level of MGD is determined, an appropriate level of therapy can be selected from the treatment algorithm (Table 10.2).[16] Asymptomatic but evident MGD (stage 1) should prompt education of the patient as to the nature and potential progression of disease and the value of prophylactic lid hygiene and massage. Mildly symptomatic disease with increasing evidence of MGD (stage 2) should be treated. If it is determined that the patient's diet is deficient in omega-3 essential fatty acids, oral supplementation can also be considered.[47,48] The clinical trials evaluating the effectiveness of omega-3 essential fatty acid

Table 10.2 Treatment Algorithm for MGD

Stage	Clinical Description	Treatment
1	No *symptoms* of ocular discomfort	*Inform* patient about MGD, the potential impact of diet, the effect of work/home environments on tear evaporation, and the possible drying effect of certain systemic medications.
	Clinical signs of MGD based on gland expression: Minimally altered secretions: grade 2–4 Expressibility: 1 No ocular surface *staining*	*Consider* eyelid hygiene including warming and expression of glands.
2	Minimal to mild *symptoms* of ocular discomfort	*Advise* patient on improving ambient humidity; optimizing workstations and increasing dietary omega-3 fatty acid intake.
	Minimal to mild MGD *clinical signs*: Scattered lid margin features Mildly altered secretions: grade 4–8 Expressibility: 1	*Institute* eyelid hygiene with eyelid warming once or twice daily, followed by firm massage and expression of MG secretions.
	None to limited ocular surface *staining*: DEWS grade 0–7; Oxford grade 0–3	*All the above, plus:* Artificial lubricants (for frequent use, nonpreserved) Topical azithromycin Topical emollient lubricant or liposomal spray Consider oral tetracycline derivatives
3	Moderate *symptoms* of ocular discomfort with limitations of activities	*All the above, plus* oral tetracycline derivatives
	Moderate MGD *clinical signs*: ⇑ lid margin features: plugging, vascularity Moderately altered secretions: grade 8–13 Expressibility: 2	Lubricant ointment at bedtime Anti-inflammatory therapy for dry eye as indicated
	Mild to moderate ocular surface staining conjunctival and peripheral corneal *staining*, DEWS grade 8–23; Oxford grade 4–10	All of the above plus anti-inflammatory therapy
4	Marked *symptoms* of ocular discomfort with definite limitation of activities	All of the above plus combination anti-inflammatory therapy: topical cyclosporine bid and pulse corticosteroids
	Severe MGD *clinical signs*: ⇑ lid margin features: dropout, displacement Severely altered secretions: grade 13 Expressibility: 3	
	Increased ocular surface staining conjunctival and corneal *staining*, including central DEWS grade 24–33; Oxford grade 11–15	
	⇑ signs of inflammation: moderate conjunctival hyperemia, phlyctenules	
'Plus' disease	Specific conditions occurring at any stage and requiring treatment 1. Exacerbated inflammatory ocular surface disease 2. Mucosal keratinization 3. Phlyctenular keratitis 4. Trichiasis (e.g. in cicatricial conjunctivitis, ocular cicatricial pemphigoid) 5. Chalazion 6. Anterior blepharitis 7. Demodex-related anterior blepharitis with cylindrical dandruff	May be causal or secondary to MGD or may occur incidentally 1. Pulsed soft steroid as indicated 2. Bandage lens/scleral contact lens 3. Steroid therapy 4. Epilation, cryotherapy 5. Intralesional steroid or excision 6. Topical antibiotic or antibiotic/steroid 7. Tea tree oil scrubs

(Adapted and modified from the treatment algorithm of the International Workshop on Meibomian Gland Dysfunction. Geerling G, Tauber J, Baudouin C, et al. The international workshop on meibomian gland dysfunction: report of the subcommittee on management and treatment of meibomian gland dysfunction. Invest Ophthalmol Vis Sci 2011 Mar 30;52:2050–64.)

supplementation are few, but the anecdotal evidence is encouraging that there is benefit. The optimal dosage has not been determined for MGD therapy but it is reasonable to follow the American Heart Association guidelines that recommend 2000 to 4000 milligrams per day but no more than 4000 milligrams per day without physician supervision.[49] Use of essential fatty acid supplements in patients taking oral anticoagulants is not advisable, as they may alter coagulation of the blood.

If the staging of disease determines stage 2 severity, the use of topical 1% azithromycin solution applied nightly in addition to lid massage after application of warm compress is indicated. It is best to apply a drop of the azithromycin solution into the conjunctival sac and then rub the excess fluid on the eyelid, into the base of the eyelashes. Consideration of oral doxycycline at this stage is also reasonable but if the severity is stage 3, the doxycycline regimen is certainly indicated and anti-inflammatory therapy may also be added as topical corticosteroid drops in the short term with concurrent or subsequent topical cyclosporine therapy for longer-term treatment.

Concurrent with the evaluation of meibomian gland function, evaluation of the ocular surface/tear film effects of MGD needs to be done by evaluation of tear film stability (tear break up time (TBUT)) and ocular surface staining.[51,53] Therapy to stabilize the tear film is generally directed at restoring the lipid layer of the tear film by use of topical lipid-enhanced lubricants used two to four times daily.[54,55] A more recent option to restore the lipid layer stabilizing effect to the tear film is liposomal spray.[56] If inflammation of the ocular surface is also present, the use of topical steroid drops or cyclosporine is indicated.

The category of 'Plus' disease identifies associated problems that can occur as a result of MGD or in association with MGD. Treatments specific for each associated problem are recommended and are listed in Table 10.2.

There are a number of possible options for relieving obstruction of the meibomian glands that have not yet been fully evaluated in randomized clinical trials but which have been reported to provide relief of symptoms by reducing meibomian gland orifice obstructions. The Lipiflow™ System provides pulsed thermal compression of the eyelids. Cannulation of the gland orifices with a specially designed small-bore needle has been reported to relieve symptoms in 75% of patients with MGD.[57] Further evaluation of these options in controlled clinical trials is warranted.

The use of topical androgen has also been advocated as there is a growing body of evidence that androgen controls meibomian gland secretion and that reduction of androgen, due to advancing age, menopause in women, or the use of antiandrogen drugs in men undergoing prostate cancer therapy leads to meibomian gland deficiency.[58] No randomized clinical trials have yet proved that topical administration of androgen reverses MGD.

Therapeutic Summary (Refer to Table 10.2)

Having identified the pathophysiologic targets of the various manifestations of meibomian gland disease, a treatment algorithm is clearly defined.

1. Focal disease

1. Internal hordeolum with acute inflammation
   a. Apply hot compresses (to localize and reduce inflammation)
   b. Apply topical antibiotic (erythromycin ointment t.i.d., azithromycin b.i.d, or topical fluoroquinolone t.i.d.)
   c. If pointing purulent focus, consider lancing at point of lesion.
   d. If severe swelling consider:
      1) Oral doxycycline (100 mg p.o. b.i.d.) or minocycline
      2) Topical steroid: prednisolone acetate 1% or lotoprednol etrabonate t.i.d.
2. Chalazion
   a. Apply hot compress (to reduce inflammation)
   b. Apply topical antibiotic/steroid combination b.i.d.
   c. If no response to topical anti-inflammatory, consider intralesional steroid injection or incision and curettage
3. Unusual or recurrent 'chalazion'
   a. If incision and curettage performed, submit specimen for histopathology
   b. Consider eyelid biopsy and/or referral to ophthalmic oncologist

2. Diffuse disease (meibomian gland dysfunction (MGD))

1. Evaluate and stage level of severity according to MGD Workshop Report
   a. Express glands to determine degree of obstruction and character of meibum
   b. Evaluate tear film stability and ocular surface damage by use of topical fluorescein or lissamine green
2. Stage 1:
   a. Educate patient about presence of MGD and possible progression
   b. Educate patient about effects of environment and activity on tear evaporation and drying effects of systemic medications
   c. Evaluate dietary intake of omega-3 essential fatty acids and encourage including fish in diet
   d. Consider eyelid hygiene including warming and expression of glands
3. Stage 2:
   a. Increase dietary omega 3 intake, including supplements
   b. Institute eyelid hygiene with lid warming and firm eyelid expression of MG secretions
   c. Consider topical azithromycin daily therapy for at least one month
   d. Add lipid-containing artificial tear stabilizing drop b.i.d.
   e. Consider topical liposomal spray or emollient lubricant
   f. Consider oral tetracycline derivatives
4. Stage 3:
   a. All of the above therapy inclusive of oral doxycycline therapy
   b. Anti-inflammatory topical therapy as indicated: corticosteroids and/or cyclosporine

5. Stage 4:
   a. All of the above therapy and combination anti-inflammatory therapy: topical cyclosporine and pulse corticosteroid
6. Plus disease:
   a. Exacerbated inflammatory ocular surface disease: pulsed soft steroid as indicated
   b. Mucosal keratinization: bandage contact lens/scleral contact lens
   c. Phlyctenular keratitis: steroid therapy
   d. Trichiasis (e.g. in cicatricial conjunctivitis, ocular cicatricial pemphigoid): epilation, cryotherapy, radiofrequency ablation
   e. Chalazion: intralesional steroid or excision
   f. Anterior blepharitis: topical antibiotic or antibiotic/steroid
   g. *Demodex*-related anterior blepharitis, with cylindrical dandruff: tea tree oil scrubs or topical metronidazole lotion

3. Diffuse disease with associated dermatologic condition

1. Rosacea: topical metronidazole cream to facial skin
2. Anhidrotic ectodermal dysplasia: dermatologic consultation

Acknowledgement

The author thanks Douglas Borchman, PhD, Professor of Ophthalmology and Professor of Biochemistry at the University of Louisville School of Medicine for valuable advice regarding lipid chemistry of the meibomian gland secretion.

References

1. Knop E, Knop N, Millar T, et al. The international workshop on meibomian gland dysfunction: report of the subcommittee on anatomy, physiology, and pathophysiology of the meibomian gland. Invest Ophthalmol Vis Sci 2011;52:1938–78.
2. Nelson JD, Shimazaki J, Benitez-del-Castillo JM, et al. The international workshop on meibomian gland dysfunction: report of the definition and classification subcommittee. Invest Ophthalmol Vis Sci 2011;52:1930–7.
3. Allali J, Roche O, Monnet D, et al. Anhidrotic ectodermal dysplasia: congenital ameibomia. J Fr Ophtalmol 2007;30:525–8.
4. Dougherty JM, McCulley JP, Silvany RE, et al. The role of tetracycline in chronic blepharitis-Inhibition of lipase production in staphylococci. Invest Ophthalmol Vis Sci 1991;32:2970–5.
5. Ramesh S, Ramakrishnan R, Bharathi MJ, et al. Prevalence of bacterial pathogens causing ocular infections in South India. Ind J Pathol Microbiol 2010;53:281–6.
6. Lindsley K, Nichols JJ, Dickersin K. Interventions for acute internal hordeolum. Cochrane Database Syst Rev 2010;8(9):CD007742. Review.
7. Chung CF, Lai JS, Li PS. Subcutaneous extralesional triamcinolone acetonide injection versus conservative management in the treatment of chalazion. Hong Kong Med J 2006;12:278–81.
8. Goawalla A, Lee V. A prospective randomized treatment study comparing three treatment options for chalazia: triamcinolone acetonide injections, incision and curettage and treatment with hot compresses. Clin Experiment Ophthalmol 2007;35:706–12.
9. Ben Simon GJ, Rosen N, Rosner M, et al. Intralesional triamcinolone acetonide injection versus incision and curettage for primary chalazia: a prospective randomized study. Am J Ophthalmol 2011;151:714–8.
10. Duarte AF, Moreira E, Nogueira A, et al. Chalazion surgery: advantages of a subconjunctival approach. J Cosmet Laser Ther 2009;11:154–6.
11. Shields JA, Demirci H, Marr BP, et al. Sebaceous carcinoma of the eyelids: personal experience with 60 cases. Ophthalmology 2004;111:2151–7. Review.
12. Jakobiec FA, Mehta M, Iwamoto M, et al. Intratarsal keratinous cysts of the Meibomian gland: distinctive clinicopathologic and immunohistochemical features in 6 cases. Am J Ophthalmol 2010;149:82–94.
13. Green-Church KB, Butovich I, Willcox M, et al. The international workshop on meibomian gland dysfunction: report of the subcommittee on tear film lipids and lipid-protein interactions in health and disease. Invest Ophthalmol Vis Sci 2011;52:1979–93.
14. Blackie CA, Korb DR, Knop E, et al. Nonobvious obstructve meibomian gland dysfunction. Cornea 2010;29:1333–45.
15. Paranjpe DR, Foulks GN. Therapy of meibomian gland disease. Ophthalmol Clin NA 2003;16:37–42.
16. Geerling G, Tauber J, Baudouin C, et al. The international workshop on meibomian gland dysfunction: report of the subcommittee on management and treatment of meibomian gland dysfunction. Invest Ophthalmol Vis Sci 2011;52:2050–64.
17. Jones YJ, Georgesuc D, McCann JD, et al. Microwave warm compress burns. Ophthal Plast Reconstr Surg 2010;26:219.
18. Mori A, Oguchi Y, Goto E, et al. Efficacy and safety of infrared warming of the eyelids. Cornea 1999;18:188–93.
19. Matsumoto Y, Dogru M, Goto E, et al. Efficacy of a new warm moist air device on tear functions of patients with simple meibomian gland dysfunction. Cornea 2006;25:644–50.
20. Lane SS, Dubiner HB, Epstein RJ, et al. a new system, the lipiflow, for the treatment of meibomian gland dysfunction (mgd). Cornea 2012;31:396–404.
21. Butovich IA. The Meibomian puzzle: combining pieces together. Prog Retin Eye Res 2009;28:483–98.
22. Butovich IA, Uchiyama E, Di Pascuale MA, et al. Liquid chromatography-mass spectrometric analysis of lipids present in human meibomian gland secretions. Lipids 2007;42:765–76.
23. Chen J, Green-Church KB, Nichols KK. Shotgun lipidomic analysis of human meibomian gland secretions with electrospray ionization tandem mass spectrometry. Invest Ophthalmol Vis Sci 2010;51:6220–31.
24. Green-Church KB, Butovich I, Willcox M, et al. The International Workshop on Meibomian Gland Dysfunction: Report of the Subcommittee on Tear Film Lipids and Lipid–Protein Interactions in Health and Disease. Invest Ophthal Vis Sci 2011;52:1979–93.
25. Borchman D, Foulks GN, Yappert MC, et al. Human meibum lipid conformation and thermodynamic changes with meibomian gland dysfunction. Invest Ophthalmol Vis Sci 2011;52:3805–17.
26. Foulks GN, Borchman D, Yappert M, et al. Topical azithromycin therapy for meibomian gland dysfunction: clinical response and lipid alterations. Cornea 2010;29:781–8.
27. Mathers WD, Lane JA. Meibomian gland lipids, evaporation, and tear film stability. Adv Exp Med Biol 1998;438:349–60.
28. Shine WE, McCulley JP. Keratoconjunctivitis sicca associated with meibomian secretion polar lipid abnormality. Arch Ophthalmol 1998;116:849–52.
29. Augustin AJ, Spitznas M, Kaviani N, et al. Oxidative reactions in the tear fluid of patients suffering from dry eyes. Graefes Arch Clin Exp Ophthalmol 1995;233:694–8.
30. Shine WE, McCulley JP. Meibomian gland triglyceride fatty acid differences in chronic blepharitis patients. Cornea 1996;15:340–6.
31. Joffre C, Souchier M, Gregoire S, et al. Differences in meibomian fatty acid composition in patients with meibomian gland dysfunction and aqueous-deficient dry eye. Br J Ophthalmol 2008;92:116–9.
32. Dougherty JM, McCulley JP. Analysis of the free fatty acid component of meibomian secretions in chronic blepharitis. Invest Ophthalmol Vis Sci 1986;27:52–6.
33. Shine WE, McCulley JP. Meibomianitis: polar lipid abnormalities. Cornea 2004;23:781–3.
34. Borchman D, Yappert MC, Foulks GN. Changes in human meibum lipid with meibomian gland dysfunction using principal component analysis. Exp Eye Res 2010;91:246–56.
35. Shine WE, McCulley JP. Association of meibum oleic acid with meibomian seborrhea. Cornea 2000;19:72–4.
36. Shrestha RK, Borchman D, Foulks GN, et al. Analysis of the composition of lipid in human meibum from normal infants, children, adolescents, adults and adults with meibomian gland dysfunction using 1H-NMR spectroscopy. Invest Ophthalmol Vis Sci 2011;52:7350–8.

37. Borchman D, Foulks GN, Yappert MC, et al. differences in human meibum lipid composition with meibomian gland dysfunction using nmr and principal component analysis. Invest Ophthalmol Vis Sci 2012;53:337–47.

38. Borchman D, Foulks GN, Yappert MC, et al. Spectroscopic evaluation of human tear lipids. Chemistry and Physics of Lipids 2007;147:87–102.

39. Wojtowicz, JC, Butovich I, McCulley JP. Historical brief on human meibum lipids composition. The Ocular Surface 2009;7:145–53.

40. Borchman D, Foulks GN, Yappert MC, et al. Human meibum lipid conformation and thermodynamic changes with meibomian gland dysfunction. Invest Ophthalmol Vis Sci 2011;52:3805–17.

41. Foulks GN, Borchman D, Yappert MC, et al. Topical azithromycin and oral doxycycline therapy of meibomian gland dysfunction: a comparative and spectroscopic pilot study. Cornea 2013;32:44–53.

42. Luchs J. Azithromycin in DuraSite for the treatment of blepharitis. Clin Ophthalmol 2010;4:681–8.

43. Utine CA. Update and critical appraisal of the use of topical azithromycin ophthalmic 1% (AzaSite) solution in the treatment of ocular infections. Clin Ophthalmol 2011;5:801–9.

44. Borchman D, Foulks GN, Yappert MC, et al. Differences in human meibum lipid composition with meibomian gland dysfunction using NMR and principal component analysis. Invest Ophthalmol Vis Sci 2012;53:337–47.

45. Sadrai Z, Hajrasouliha AR, Chauhan S, et al. Effect of topical azithromycin on corneal innate immune responses. Invest Ophthalmol Vis Sci 2011;52:2525–31.

46. Perry HD, Doshi-Carnevale S, Donnenfeld ED, et al. Efficacy of commercially available topical cyclosporine A 0.05% in the treatment of meibomian gland dysfunction. Cornea 2006;25:171–5.

47. Macsai MS. The role of omega-3 dietary supplementation in blepharitis and meibomian gland dysfunction (an AOS thesis). Trans Am Ophthalmol Soc 2008;106:336–56.

48. Wojtowicz JC, Butovich I, Uchiyama E, et al. Pilot, prospective, randomized, double-masked, placebo-controlled clinical trial of an omega-3 supplement for dry eye. Cornea 2011;30:308–14. Erratum in: Cornea. 2011;30:1521.

49. American Heart Association Recommendations for Fish in Diet. Available at http://www.heart.org/HEARTORG/GettingHealthy/NutritionCenter/Fish-101_UCM_305986_Article.jsp (last accessed 18 Jan 2013).

50. Foulks GN, Bron AJ. Meibomian Gland dysfunction. a clinical scheme for description, diagnosis, classification, and grading. The Ocular Surface 2003;1:107–26.

51. MGD Workshop diagnosis and grading, Tomlinson A, Bron AJ, Korb DR, et al. The international workshop on meibomian gland dysfunction: report of the diagnosis subcommittee. Invest Ophthalmol Vis Sci 2011;52:2006–49.

52. Bron AJ, Evans VE, Smith JA. Grading of corneal and conjunctival staining in the context of other dry eye tests. Cornea 2003;22:640–50.

53. The 2007 Report of the International Dry Eye Workshop (DEWS). Ocular Surface 2007;5:107–52.

54. Foulks GN. The correlation between the tear film lipid layer and dry eye disease. Surv Ophthalmol 2007;52:369–74.

55. Benelli U. Systane lubricant eye drops in the management of ocular dryness. Clin Ophthalmol 2011;5:783–90.

56. Craig JP. Purslow C. Murphy PJ, et al. Effect of a liposomal spray on the pre-ocular tear film. Cont Lens Anterior Eye 2010;33:83–7

57. Maskin SL. Intraductal meibomian gland probing relieves symptoms of obstructive meibomian gland dysfunction. Cornea 2010;29:1145–52.

58. Sullivan DA, Sullivan BD, Evans JE, et al. Androgen deficiency, meibomian gland dysfunction, and evaporative dry eye. Ann NY Acad Sci 2002;966:211–22.

11 *Dry Eye Disease: Epidemiology and Pathophysiology*

MICHAEL A. LEMP

Introduction

Epidemiology is that branch of medical study which concerns itself with the frequency, distribution, determinants and assessments associated with disease. In this chapter we shall cover major studies and results, concentrating on the most recent ones, which affect clinical understanding of dry eye disease (DED). For a comprehensive review of this field, including an assessment of symptom questionnaires, the reader is referred to the 2007 Report of the International Dry Eye Workshop (DEWS), chapter on the epidemiology of dry eye disease.[1] As noted in the above referenced publication, there has been a significant increase in both interest in and studies of the prevalence and incidence of DED, particularly since the 1990s. At the first Tear Film and Ocular Surface Society international meeting in 1992, a call for a 'consensus conference' was made. This resulted in the National Eye Institute/Industry workshop report, which determined that there was a paucity of data concerning prevalence and incidence of DED. New methodologies in the field of epidemiology and statistical analysis have been employed to expand our knowledge in this regard.

Clinicians have long recognized that complaints relating to DED are common in clinical practice. In an attempt to apply scientifically valid methodologies to this enquiry, an agreed definition is essential. The DEWS report, building on an earlier text, defined DED as '*a multifactorial disease of tears and ocular surface that results in symptoms of discomfort, visual disturbance and tear instability with potential damage to the ocular surface. It is accompanied by increased osmolarity of the tear film and inflammation of the ocular surface*'.[2] Armed with this widely agreed definition, many studies have been published. These studies address different population groups throughout the world. They agree that DED is a very common condition, increasing in frequency with advancing age. The estimates of prevalence (proportion of a population with the disease at a given time), range from about 5% to over 30%. These differences may be related to different population characteristics but primarily to differences in the characterization of subjects with disease.

There are many tests in clinical use for identifying DED. However, these tests correlate poorly with each other and, depending on which tests were used, study results can vary widely. It is also recognized that the symptoms of ocular irritation, which are characteristic of DED, do not correlate well with signs. Finally, each of the tests, including symptom questionnaires, gives variable results over time. This variability, which is thought to be a consequence of the instability of the tear film, a hallmark of DED not seen in normal subjects, is a challenge not only to diagnosis but also for determining effects of treatments in clinical trials. This will be discussed further. Similar constraints exist for determining incidence figures (new cases of disease over a period of time).

Some of the most recent prevalence estimates, including not only chronic DED but also episodic cases in response to environmental stress, range as high as 20% of the population. Recent interest in determining prevalence figures are, in part, driven by the recognition that DED, in addition to causing ocular irritation and damage to the ocular surface, can have a significant impact on vision between blinks, as well as an adverse effect on visual outcomes following cataract and refractive surgery.

There are a limited number of studies concerning the natural history of DED. However, there are several multiyears studies of treated DED, which suggest that while the untreated disease progresses, not all subjects develop severe disease but rather that a certain severity point is reached around which signs and symptoms fluctuate. This may be true of most cases of DED, but certain subsets of the disease, i.e. those associated with systemic autoimmune disease, such as Sjögren's syndrome, graft-versus-host disease and other systemic diseases, tend to progress more rapidly to a more severe state. In these situations there is more clinically obvious inflammation. As disease progresses, more of the disease markers become abnormal, making diagnosis more obvious.

Nomenclature

Various names have been attached to dry eye. These include keratoconjunctivitis sicca (KCS), dry eye syndrome, and dysfunctional tear syndrome (DTS). KCS is a traditional name implying dryness and inflammation of the ocular surface. Its use began to wane with the recognition that all cases of the condition do not demonstrate a lack of tears and with recognition of the role of inflammation in the pathogenesis of the disease process. Dry eye or dry eye syndrome became the predominant terms in use throughout the English-speaking world and even in non-English-speaking countries, in which the term is widely recognized. With publication of the Delphi report in 2006,[3] a new term, *dysfunctional tear syndrome*, was proposed. The issue was put to a vote at the Tear Film and Ocular Surface Society meeting prior to publication of the DEWS report. A majority of the expert participants preferred the term 'dry eye' or 'dry eye disease,' citing its wide recognition, not only by clinicians and researchers but also by patients.[4] The latter term emphasizes the increasingly well-characterized

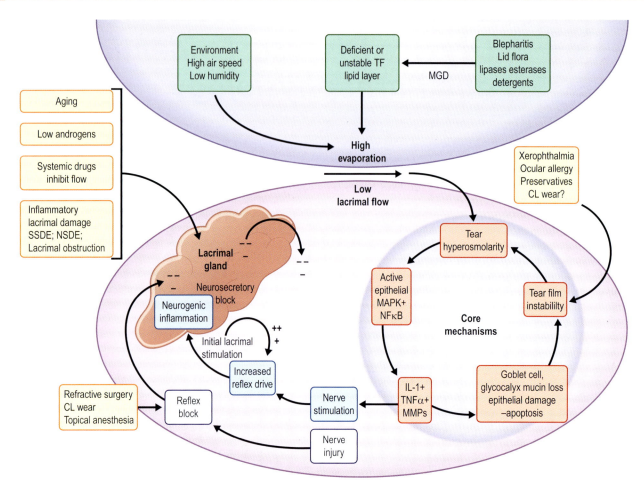

Figure 11.1 Mechanisms of dry eye. The core mechanisms of dry eye are driven by tear hyperosmolarity and tear film instability. The cycle of events is shown on the right of the figure. Tear hyperosmolarity causes damage to the ocular surface epithelium by activating a cascade of inflammatory events at the ocular surface and a release of inflammatory mediators into the tears. Epithelial damage involves cell death by apoptosis, a loss of goblet cells and disturbance of the mucin expression. Individual etiologies often cause dry eye by several interacting mechanisms. ((Text attenuated) Originally published in Report of the International Dry Eye Workshop (DEWS). The Ocular Surface 2007;5:85. Reproduced with permission of Elsevier, the publisher.)

pathophysiological processes of a discrete disease. Both DED and DTS are currently in use.

Risk Factors for Dry Eye Disease

There are a number of risk factors for the development of DED (Fig. 11.1). Reference 1 lists these factors and stratifies them based on levels of evidence. The most obvious factors associated with DED are increasing age, female gender and hormonal changes. Connective tissue disease is associated with more severe forms of DED, e.g. Sjögren's syndrome and graft-versus-host disease. Dry eye disease occurs with greater frequency in women, particularly in the menopausal and postmenopausal years. The preponderance of evidence has demonstrated that androgen insufficiency is a principal risk factor for both lacrimal gland involvement and meibomian gland dysfunction (MGD). The female:male ratio decreases with advancing age as large segments of males with MGD become affected. The distribution of subtypes of DED, based on glands primarily affected is discussed in the section on pathophysiology later.

Impact on Visual Function

A recent recognition is the impact that DED has on visual function. A hallmark of DED is tear film instability.[2] This is manifest in a rapid tear breakup time, during the inter-blink interval. This effect is not apparent in standard high-contrast visual acuity testing, in which the subject can blink and transiently re-form the tear film. However, within several seconds in dry eye patients, the tear film breaks up causing a significant loss of resolving power and a drop in acuity. A Japanese study has documented that inter-blink visual acuities of 20/60 and greater are common.[5,6] Patients rarely recognize the connection between their visual problem and dry eye, usually complaining of decreased reading time, or ocular fatigue. This is probably caused by repeated blinking in an unconscious effort to clear vision. Other parameters of visual loss in DED, such as contrast sensitivity and Shack Hartmann aberrometry measurements may be also affected.[7,8] These features of DED lead to the substantial degradation of quality of life measures in the disease. In one study, the equivalent burden of having moderate to severe dry eye was similar to that of moderate to severe angina.[9]

Perhaps the most significant recent clinical consequence of the visual changes has been reported in patients undergoing refractive surgery and cataract surgery with the implantation of high-resolution intraocular lenses. An unstable tear film interferes with the optical image sufficiently, such that the level of acuity expected is not achieved. Although large studies have yet to be published, recognition and identification of patients with DED preoperatively and medical management of the condition may improve visual outcomes.

Role of Symptoms in DED

The literature states that dry eye is a symptom-driven disease.[1] This implies that symptoms are a requisite component of the diagnosis. While symptoms certainly play a major role in the disease, recent studies have noted two seemingly paradoxical observations, i.e. that many patients with early/mild disease have symptoms greater than any objective findings, and that in a subset of patients with severe disease there is a paucity of symptoms. The latter is thought to be due to a decrease in sensory perception associated with inflammation; the former has been linked to a hyperalgesia, associated with early nerve ending response to injury. In a recent presentation of an observational study, only 60–70% of patients with DED were reported to have symptoms (as measured by the Ocular Surface Disease Index).[10] The remaining 30–40% do not present with measurable symptoms. Reliance on symptoms alone for diagnosis would therefore, seem unwise.

Pathophysiology of Dry Eye Disease

Although there are numerous risk factors for the development of dry eye disease, the final common expression of the pathophysiology includes tear film hyperosmolarity and instability. The concept of a functional lacrimal unit has been developed in which the secretory glands (lacrimal, meibomian and mucin-producing surface cells), the entire ocular surface, and the lids are linked by a neural network, which responds to external stimuli to maintain a stable tear film and underlying ocular surface, necessary for subserving clear vision.[11] This unit has recently been enlarged to include the nasolacrimal duct, which has receptors that respond to volume changes.

A key concept to understanding the development of DED is the breakdown in this unit leading to an unstable, concentrated (hyperosmolar) tear film. In Table 11.1, this concept is illustrated in a graphic, which the entry points or risk factors in the periphery lead to the core central mechanisms.[2] As these mechanisms (e.g. lacrimal hyposecretion and/or meibomian gland dysfunction) come into play, there is a mutually reinforcing cycle of dysfunction leading to inflammation in the ocular surface and lacrimal glands. This vicious cycle concept has been developed by Baudouin[12] and is illustrated in Figure 11.1.

Table 11.1   Risk Factors for Dry Eye Disease

Mostly Consistent[1]	Suggestive[2]	Unclear[3]
Older age	Asian race	Cigarette smoking
Female sex	Medications	Hispanic ethnicity
Postmenopausal estrogen therapy	Tricyclic antidepressants	
Omega-3 and Omega-6 fatty acids	Selective serotonin reuptake inhibitors	Anticholinergics
Medications	Diuretics	Anxiolytics
Antihistamines	Beta-blockers	Antipsychotics
Connective tissue disease	Diabetes mellitus	Alcohol
LASIK and refractive excimer laser surgery	HIV/ HTLVI infection	Menopause
Radiation therapy	Systemic chemotherapy	Botulinum toxin injection
Hematopoietic stem cell transplantation	Large incision ECCE and penetrating keratoplasty	
	Isotretinoin	Acne
Vitamin A deficiency	Low humidity environments	Gout
Hepatitis C infection	Sarcoidosis	Oral contraceptives
Androgen deficiency	Ovarian dysfunction	Pregnancy

1 Mostly consistent evidence implies the existence of at least one adequately powered and otherwise well-conducted study published in a peer-reviewed journal, along with the existence of a plausible biological rationale and corroborating basic research or clinical data.
2 Suggestive evidence implies the existence of either: (1) inconclusive information from peer-reviewed publications or (2) inconclusive or limited information to support the association, but either not published or published somewhere other than in a peer-reviewed journal.
3 Unclear evidence implies either directly conflicting information in peer-reviewed publications or inconclusive information but with some basis for a biological rationale.
(This table was published in Report of the International Dry Eye Workshop (DEWS) The Ocular Surface 2007;5:99. Reproduced with permission from Elsevier, the publisher.)

Principal Causative Factors

Tear hyperosmolarity is considered the central mechanism in DED, leading to inflammation at the ocular surface with resulting tissue damage and symptoms.[2] The hyperosmolar state is the result of either an insufficient secretion of fluid from the lacrimal glands (low aqueous flow) and/or excessive evaporation of the tear film. Normal tear osmolarity averages around 295 mOsmol/L which is isotonic with blood. Tear osmolarity over the ocular surface is greater than that in other tear compartments (e.g. the menisci), because of the larger surface area of the interpalpebral space, allowing for evaporative water loss between blinks. Indirect evidence of this comes from studies exposing the ocular surface in humans to increasing concentrations of solutions until ocular irritation occurs.[13] It is also probable that, were it possible to sample tears from the preocular surface, the values would change over the ocular surface as the lid moves over the surface. There is a transfer of fluid from this preocular surface compartment to the tear menisci at their nasal extent with each complete blink. The menisci serve as a compartment of mixed tears and in normal subjects, is remarkably stable. As disease develops, the osmolarity in the tear menisci rises. While not the same as that over the ocular surface, there is a relationship that permits use of menisci to evaluate and monitor activity on the surface.

Hyperosmolarity affects the ocular surface in multiple ways. Hyperosmolarity initiates a cascade of inflammatory events mediated by at least two separate pathways, leading to the recruitment and activation of inflammatory cells on the ocular surface and the production of inflammatory cytokines and chemokines (see below). Associated with these changes is an increase in surface cell death (apoptosis), changes in mucin production and a loss of lubrication between the lid and the ocular surface.[2]

The lacrimal functional unit is capable of responding to these changes by increasing aqueous tear production in an attempt to lower the osmolarity. This may result in a transiently lower tear osmolarity but in aqueous tear deficient dry eye (ADDE). The lacrimal glands lack the secretory capacity to maintain this effort. In evaporative dry eye (EDE), most commonly caused by meibomian gland dysfunction (MGD), the excessive evaporative tear loss is associated with a thin or defective tear lipid layer which stimulates reflex tearing.[14] Prolonged overstimulation of the lacrimal gland results in a *neurogenic inflammation* in the lacrimal gland, characterized by increased autoantigen expression, T-cell targeting and release of inflammatory cytokines into the tear film. These lead to compromise of the gland and a mixed or hybrid form of the disease. Other compensatory mechanisms may include increased blinking and squinting. Tear osmolarity has a linear relationship with increasing severity of dry eye[10] and is the best most reliable metric for the diagnosis of DED.[15]

TEAR FILM INSTABILITY

The other hallmark of DED is tear film instability. In normal healthy subjects the lacrimal functional unit is remarkably stable in response to environmental stress. This is seen in tests of tear stability, such as the *tear break-up time* test (TBUT). With the onset of disease, an early feature is a breakdown in the homeostatic control of a stable tear film between blinks. This instability and tear hyperosmolarity are closely linked, but the primary event is unclear. Early studies suggested that a TBUT of less than 10 seconds was indicative of DED. Newer techniques to refine reproducibility and precision of the test include capture of the break-up process on video and the use of programmed videokeratography to decrease operator variability. Normative values between 5 and 7 seconds have been suggested.

The tear film should provide for a complete tear layer throughout the blink interval. When break-up of the tear film occurs prior to the next blink, there is a discontinuity that degrades the visual image and produces irritation. The ratio of the TBUT to the *inter-blink interval* has been called the *ocular protection index*.[16] Values less than 1 are considered pathological.

Disturbances in the mucin cover of the cornea are responsible for rapid break-up. Tear break-up can occur over areas of corneal irregularity and are more rapid and extensive. Damage to the mucin layer or glycocalyx have been reported with the use of preservative-containing eye drops, particularly those containing benzalkonium chloride, which is a constituent of many glaucoma medications. Up to three-quarters of patients with long-term use of topical glaucoma medications exhibit symptoms and signs of DED, and the frequency increases with the number of medications used.[17] Contact lens wear has also been associated with tear instability.

THE ROLE OF INFLAMMATION

A major shift in our understanding of DED occurred with the recognition that inflammation plays a pivotal part in the pathogenesis of the disease. This is an important concept that has gained wide acceptance and is driving pharmaceutical development for more effective treatments. What follows is a summary of the evidence supporting the role of inflammation. For a more detailed discussion of this complex subject, readers are referred to the *Cullen Symposium on Corneal and Ocular Surface Inflammation* (Baylor College of Medicine, Houston, TX, January, 2005, The Ocular Surface, Vol. 3, Supplement). Patients with moderate to severe disease, usually show clinical evidence of inflammatory changes to the ocular surface and lids. In mild cases, these clinical signs are frequently absent.

Laboratory Studies

Both in vitro studies and animal models of dry eye disease have been utilized to study DED. Initial studies in canines demonstrated that topical treatment with cyclosporine A could effectively treat dry eye.[18] The use of human conjunctival cell lines has demonstrated that inflammatory cytokines can up-regulate markers of inflammation, such as HLA-DR and ICAM-1. Studies utilizing mouse models, which usually involve initiation of disease by environmental stress, with or without systemic scopolamine injections, show inflammation of the conjunctiva and T-cell activation, which are seen in human DED.[19] Figure 11.2 from Reference 19 illustrates the mechanisms thought to be involved in acute and chronic immune-associated inflammation in DED.

Human Studies

Histopathological studies, measurement of inflammatory cytokines, chemokines and immunomodulatory molecules in tears, and tests for expression of cell surface antigens, all support the role of inflammation in human dry eye. Inflammation leads to tissue damage and is an intimate part of the vicious cycle of mutually reinforcing events in DED.[2] All of these markers of inflammation, which are seen in moderate to severe disease, are present to a lesser extent in mild to moderate cases. Many of the studies of inflammation in DED have employed patients suffering from Sjögren's syndrome, graft-versus-host disease and other systemic conditions associated with autoimmune disease. In these cases, inflammation may play a primary role with autoimmune attack of the lacrimal gland as an early feature. In cases of dry eye associated with hormonal and aging changes, inflammation may play a more downstream role as a consequence of tear hyperosmolarity.

As mentioned above, the presence of tear hyperosmolarity has been shown to elicit a cascade of inflammatory events which involves both MAP kinases and NFκB

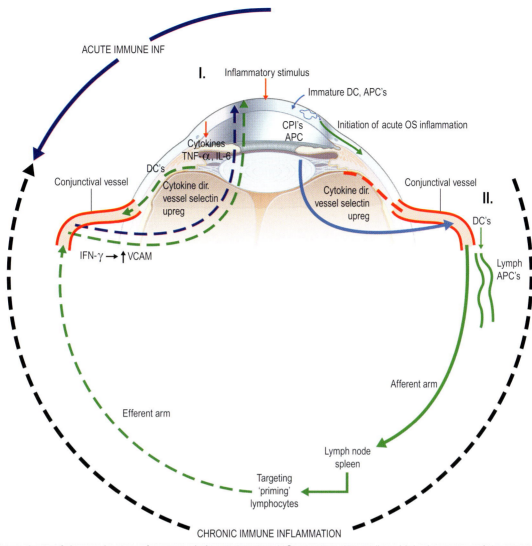

Figure 11.2 Hypothesis of the mechanism of acute and chronic immune inflammation. (Originally published in Report of the International Dry Eye Workshop (DEWS). The Ocular Surface 2007;5:185. Reproduced with permission of Elsevier, the publisher.)

signaling pathways from the ocular surface cells activating several pathways, leading to breakdown in the ocular surface and the presence of inflammatory cytokines, chemokines and tissue modulating markers in the tear film. Markers identified include IL, IL-1α,IL-17, TNF-α, and MMP-9. Inflammatory markers such as these and others are under study for their diagnostic possibilities.

ROLE OF ANDROGENS IN DED

There is an extensive literature on the role of androgen deficiency in the pathogenesis of DED. Both low levels of systemic androgen and high levels of estrogen are risk factors for the development of DED. Biologically active androgens support the secretory activities of the lacrimal and meibomian glands. In addition, there are a number of associations between DED and other diseases characterized by decreased androgen activity, including complete androgen insensitivity syndrome, premature ovarian failure, and patients undergoing treatment with antiandrogen

compounds for prostate cancer. A comprehensive review of this subject is published.[20]

Distribution of Subtypes of Dry Eye Disease

As noted earlier, DED based on the glandular structures primarily involved has been divided into two mechanistic subtypes, i.e. aqueous tear deficient dry eye (ADDE) and evaporative dry eye (EDE). Although there are a number of conditions leading to the latter, the predominant factor is meibomian gland dysfunction (MGD). Aqueous deficiency has commonly been treated as synonymous with DED, with MGD occupying a position as a co-morbid condition. In recent years, there has been increased interest in the role of MGD in the pathogenesis of DED and its integral role in the lacrimal functional unit. Figure 11.3 from (Reference 2) depicts a comprehensive description of the mechanistic division of the different components of the ocular surface.

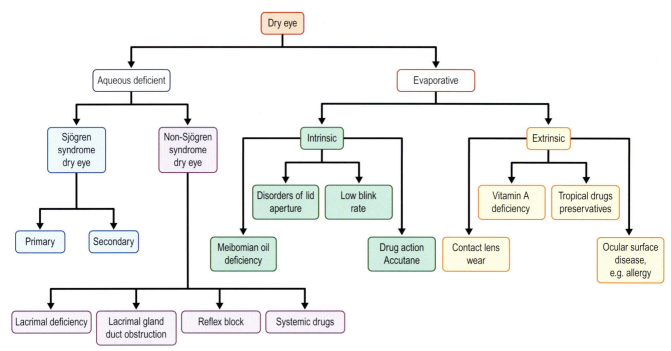

Figure 11.3 Major etiological causes of dry eye. (Originally published in Report of the International Dry Eye Workshop (DEWS). The Ocular Surface 2007; 5:185. Reproduced with permission of Elsevier, the publisher.)

Studies in Asia, Europe, and more recently in the US, have documented the high prevalence of MGD, particularly in populations over the age of 50. MGD has become a major focus of research, and a comprehensive monograph on this subject was published in 2011. Early reports of the high prevalence of MGD in Asian populations led to the impression that MGD was more common in Asians.[21] However, recent studies in Europe and the US have reported similarly high prevalences.[22,23] In the most recent report of 224 subjects, MGD alone far outweighs ADDE alone, 79 to 24, with 57 subjects showing evidence of a combined form of DED.[24] With increasing severity, there is a marked increase in the combined form of the disease, as initial compensatory mechanisms fail, compromising the other structures of the lacrimal functional unit. Most cases of Sjögren-associated DED are a mixed form of the disease. The recently published report of the MGD workshop thoroughly treats this topic.[25] A large population-based study in Spain has reported that more subjects with clear objective signs of MGD are asymptomatic than those with symptoms.[26]

Conclusion

Recent developments over the last decade have provided important data that are changing perceptions of dry eye disease and its pathogenesis. This is leading to a new understanding of the processes involved in the development of disease, which in turn, can explain some of the poorly understood characteristics of the disease. Central to understanding DED is that the disease process involves a loss of the homeostatic control of the lacrimal functional unit. This unit, which comprises the lacrimal glands, cornea, conjunctiva, lids with the meibomian glands, and the nasolacrimal outflow channels, is linked by a neural network. The unit can react to changes in environmental conditions by altering the function of each of its components, as dictated by signaling changes in response to changing environmental needs. An increase in wind, for example, can accelerate evaporative water loss from the pre-ocular surface tear film, stimulating an increase in secretion by the lacrimal gland and/or an increased blink rate which can increase the thickness of the lipid layer of the tear film. As DED begins to develop, whether it starts with a decrease in aqueous tear production in the lacrimal glands or changes in the meibomian glands, there is a loss of control of this finely regulated system designed to maintain a stable tear film. This leads to alterations in vision, symptoms of irritation in most subjects, and an inability to react to changing environmental demands to maintain a stable tear film.

The key factors in this disease are twin hallmarks of the disease, i.e. tear film instability and an elevated tear osmolarity. These two facets are closely linked and are responsible for many of the observed changes in DED. Of the many tests that have been used to diagnose the condition, most exhibit variability over time and between eyes. In addition, the individual tests do not correlate well with each other, nor do they correlate well with patient-reported symptoms. In several recently published studies these observations were analyzed. The most commonly used objective tests are quite variable over a 3 month period of observation in dry eye patients. In addition, patient symptoms as measured by the Ocular Surface Disease Index (OSDI) are variable and do not correlate well with objective signs. Indeed, recent findings point out that many patients with DED do not report symptoms, undermining the notion that DED is defined as a symptomatic disease. The variability seen is thought to be due to tear film instability.[27] The lack of correlation between signs of disease (i.e., Schirmer test, tear break-up times, corneal and conjunctival staining, lid margin scoring) suggests that each test provides important but independent information, that may become positive at different stages of the disease. For example, fewer than 50% of patients with mild to moderate disease demonstrate any corneal staining. Another characteristic of patients with mild to moderate disease is conflict between various signs of disease. This has led to the development of composite index of disease severity, incorporating all of the commonly performed tests.[10] The contribution of each test at different stages of disease can then be evaluated. Of all the tests used, only tear osmolarity demonstrates a linear relationship to increasing severity of DED.

As our knowledge base continues to enlarge, we will undoubtedly garner further insights that will allow the development of better treatments for the management of this highly prevalent disease.

References

1. No authors listed. The epidemiology of dry eye disease. Report of the epidemiology subcommittee of the International Dry Eye Workshop. Ocular Surf 2007;5:93–107.
2. No authors listed. The definition and classification of dry eye disease. Report of the definition and classification subcommittee of the international dry eye workshop. Ocular Surf 2007;5:75–92.
3. Behrens A, Doyle JJ, Stern M, et al. Dysfunctional tear syndrome syndrome: a Delphi approach to treatment recommendations. Cornea 2006;25:900–7.
4. Baum J, Foulks G, Lemp MA. What's in a name? Cornea 2006; 25:871–2.
5. Kaido M, Dogru M, Ishida R, et al. Concept of functional visual acuity and its application. Cornea 2007;26(9 Suppl. 1):S29–35.
6. Goto E, Yagi Y, Matsumoto Y, et al. Impaired functional visual acuity of dry eye patients. Amer J Ophthalmol 2002;133:181–6.
7. Montes-Mico R, Caliz A, Alio JL. Wavefront analysis of higher order aberrations in dry eye patients. J Refract Surg 2004;20:243–7.
8. Thibos LN, Hong X. Clinical applications of the Shack Hartmann aberrometer. Optom Vis Sci 1999;76:817–25.
9. Schiffman RM, Walt JG, Jacobsen G, et al. Utility assessment among patients with dry eye disease. Ophthalmology 2003;110:1412–9.
10. Sullivan BD, Whitmer D, Nichols KK, et al. An objective approach to dry eye disease severity. Invest Ophthalmol Vis Sci Dec 2010; 51:6125–30.
11. Beuerman RW, Mircheff A, Pflugfelder SC, et al. The lacrimal functional unit. In: Pflugfelder SC, Beuerman RW, Stern ME, editors. Dry eye and ocular surface disorders. New York: Marcel Dekker; 2004.
12. Baudouin C. The vicious cycle in dry eye syndrome: a mechanistic approach. J Fr Ophtalmol 2007;30:239–46.
13. Liu H, Begley C, Chen M, et al. A link between tear instability and hyperosmolarity in dry eye. Invest Ophthalmol Vis Sci 2009; 50:3671–369.
14. Bron AJ, Yokoi N, Gafney E, et al. Predicted phenotypes of dry eye: proposed consequences of its natural history. Ocul Surf Apr 2009; 7:78–92.
15. Lemp MA, Bron AJ, Baudouin C, et al. Tear osmolarity in the diagnosis and management of dry eye disease. Am J Ophthalmol 2011; 151:792–798.
16. Ousler GW, Hagberg KW, Schindelar M, et al. The ocular protection index. Cornea 2008;27:509–13.
17. Leung EW, Medeiros FA, Weinreb RN. Prevalence of ocular surface disease in glaucoma patients. J Glaucoma 2008;17:50–5.
18. Kaswan R. Characteristics of a canine model of KCS: effective treatment with topical cyclosporine. Adv Exp Med Biol 1994;350: 583–94.
19. No authors listed. Research in dry eye: Report of the Research Subcommittee of the International Dry Eye Workshop. Ocular Surf 2007;5:179–93.
20. Sullivan DA. Tearful relationships? Sex, hormones, the lacrimal gland and aqueous-deficient dry eye. Ocul Surf 2004;2:92–123.
21. Uchino M, Dogru M, Yagi Y et al. The features of dry eye disease in a Japanese elderly population. Optom Vis Sci 2006;83(11): 797–802.
22. Lemp MA, Nichols KK. Blepharitis in the United States 2009: a survey-based perspective on prevalence and treatment. Ocul Surf 2009;7(Suppl. 2):S1–S14.
23. Viso E, Gude F, Rodriguez-Ares MT. The association of meibomian gland dysfunction and other common ocular disease with dry eye: a population-based study in Spain. Cornea 2011;30:1–6.
24. Lemp MA, Crews LA, Bron AJ, et al. Distribution of aqueous deficient and evaporative dry eye in a clinic-based patient cohort: a retrospective study. Cornea 2012;31:472–8.
25. Schaumberg DA, Nichols JJ, Papas EB, et al. The international workshop on meibomian gland dysfunction: report of the subcommittee on the epidemiology of and associated risk factors for MGD. Invest Ophthalmol Vis Sci 2011;52:1994–2005.
26. Viso E, Rodríguez-Ares MT, Abelenda D, et al. Prevalence of asymptomatic and symptomatic meibomian gland dysfunction in the general population of Spain. Invest Ophthalmol Vis Sci 2012;53: 2601–2606.
27. Sullivan BD, Crews LA, Sönmez B, et al. Clinical utility of objective tests for dry eye disease: variability over time and implications for clinical trials and disease management. Cornea 2012;31:1000–8.

12 *Treatment of Dry Eye Disease*

STEPHEN C. PFLUGFELDER and GREGORY R. NETTUNE

Introduction

Dry eye develops when disease or dysfunction of one or more components of the integrated lacrimal functional unit is no longer able to maintain a stable tear film.[1] Dry eye is a common condition with a reported prevalence ranging from 2% to 14.4%.[2–6] Patients with dry eye typically complain of eye irritation, such as foreign body sensation, burning, and dryness, as well as visual symptoms, including photophobia and fluctuating vision. Dry eye causes pathological changes to the ocular surface epithelium with disruption of corneal epithelial barrier function and loss of mucus-secreting goblet cells. Dry eye may decrease quality of life, and in the most severe cases, dry eye disease can cause functional and occupational disability. The impact of dry eye on quality of life was rated to be equivalent to unstable angina using utility assessments.[7]

Therapy of dry eye is aimed at improving irritation symptoms, visual quality and sight-threatening corneal epithelial disease. This chapter reviews current evidence and consensus-based treatment recommendations for dry eye, that are based on previously published recommendations of the International Dry Eye Workshop (DEWS) and Meibomian Gland Workshop.[8,9]

Diagnostic Classification of Dry Eye

Optimal management of dry eye or tear dysfunction requires performance of a minimal number of diagnostic tests to: identify character, frequency and severity of patient complaints; confirm presence of an unstable tear film; identify aqueous tear deficiency; detect meibomian gland disease; identify conditions altering tear clearance and/or distribution (conjunctivochalasis, lid or punctal ectropion, punctal stenosis, pterygium, pingueculum, Salzmann's nodular degeneration) and detect location and extent of ocular surface epithelial disease. Results of these tests, combined with clinical impressions, can be used to grade disease severity. The Dry Eye Workshop proposed four levels of severity (Table 12.1);[8] however, disease severity may be better characterized on a continuous spectrum.

Aqueous deficiency requires therapies to minimize or eliminate environmental factors, lubricate and hydrate the ocular surface, protect against osmotic stress and stimulate tear production. Replacement of tear constituents with autologous serum or plasma and protection of the ocular surface with therapeutic contact lens, such as PROSE are necessary in more severe cases (levels 3 and 4). Ocular surface inflammation is a pathological feature shared by

Table 12.1 Severity Grading Scheme for Dry Eye

Dry Eye Severity Level	1	2	3	4
Discomfort, severity & frequency*	Mild and/or episodic Occurs under environ stress	Moderate episodic or chronic Stress or no stress	Severe frequent or constant without stress	Severe and/or disabling and constant
Visual symptoms	None or episodic Mild blurring	Annoying and/or activity limiting, episodic	Annoying, chronic and/or constant limiting activity Mild to moderate photophobia	Constant and/or possibly disabling Moderate to severe disabling photophobia
Conjunctival injection	None to mild	None to mild	+/–	+/++
Conjunctival staining	None to mild	Variable	Moderate to severe	Severe, unless cornified
Corneal staining (severity/location)	None to mild	Variable and inferior	Marked, including central	Severe diffuse, unless cornified
Corneal/Tear signs	None to mild	Mild debris, ↓ meniscus	Filamentary keratitis, mucus clumping, ↑ tear debris	Filamentary keratitis, mucus clumping, ↑ tear debris, epithelial defect
Lid/meibomian glands	Variable	Variable	Frequent MGD	Trichiasis, MGD, irregularity, keratinization, symblepharon
TBUT (sec)	Variable	≤8	≤5	Immediate
Schirmer score (mm/5 min)	Variable	≤10	≤5	≤2

*Discomfort symptoms may be minimal or absent in levels 3 and 4 due to nerve degeneration.
eviron: environmental; MGD: meibomian gland disease.
Modified from scheme proposed by Dry Eye Workshop (Pflugfelder S (committee chairman) Management and therapy of dry eye disease: report of the Management and Therapy Subcommittee of the International Dry Eye WorkShop (2007). Ocul Surf 2007;5:163–78.)

aqueous deficient and aqueous sufficient dry eye conditions and many currently utilized therapies, inhibit production of inflammatory cytokines and proteases. A severity-based treatment algorithm for treatment of dry eye is presented in Figure 12.1. Therapies can be added or removed based on objective and subjective response.

ENVIRONMENTAL MODIFICATION

Systemic and environmental factors contributing to dry eye should be modified or eliminated. Systemic medications with anticholinergic side effects (e.g. antihistamines, antidepressants, and antispasmodics) should be eliminated if possible. Exposure to desiccating environmental stresses (e.g. low humidity and air conditioning drafts) that cause irritation symptoms or increase tear evaporation, should be minimized or eliminated. The height of video display terminals should be adjusted to sit at slightly below eye level to decrease the interpalpebral aperture and exposure. Room humidifiers may be beneficial in dry climates and high altitudes. Moisture chamber eyeglasses can reduce tear evaporation and maintain high humidity around the eye. Nocturnal lagophthalmos can be treated with swim goggles, taping the eyelids closed, or performing a lateral tarsorrhaphy. Patients should be encouraged to eat a balanced diet, rich in n-3 polyunsaturated fatty acids from fish and low in saturated n-6 fatty acids.[10] Smoking has been identified to destabilize the tear film and should be stopped.[11]

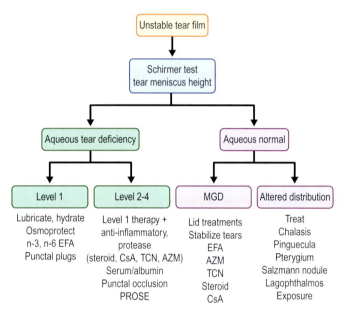

Figure 12.1 Treatment algorithm. In patients presenting with an unstable tear film, a Schirmer test or tear meniscus measurement should be performed to determine whether the patient has aqueous deficient or aqueous normal tear dysfunction. Treatment in the aqueous tear deficient group is based on clinical severity. Therapy should be tailored to the underlying problem (meibomian gland disease or altered distribution) in the aqueous normal group. Treatment is based on recommendations of the Dry Eye Workshop and Meibomian Gland Workshop. (From: Pflugfelder S. (committee chairman). Management and therapy of dry eye disease: report of the Management and Therapy Subcommittee of the International Dry Eye WorkShop (2007). Ocul Surf 2007;5:163–78. Geerling G, Tauber J, Baudouin C, et al. The international workshop on meibomian gland dysfunction: report of the subcommittee on management and treatment of meibomian gland dysfunction. Invest Ophthalmol Vis Sci 2011;52:2050–64.)

Artificial Tears

Artificial tears are considered a first-line therapy for dry eye. They increase tear volume, minimize desiccation and lubricate the ocular surface. They often provide temporary relief of irritation symptoms in many dry eye conditions. There are a variety of commercially available artificial tears, that contain various agents (Table 12.2) that increase their viscosity, lubricity, retention time and adhesion to the ocular surface. Certain artificial tear formulations contain electrolytes or ions, such as potassium and bicarbonate ions, that are found in normal tears. Tears with a lipid component, such as castor oil (*Refresh Optive™ ADVANCED, Systane® Balance*, and *Soothe® XP*) may retard tear evaporation and prevent intrusion of irritating skin lipids.

Artificial tears lubricate the ocular surface, reduce tear osmolarity and protect the ocular surface from desiccation. They often provide temporary improvement in eye irritation and blurred vision symptoms, visual contrast sensitivity, tear break-up time, corneal surface regularity and ocular surface dye staining. They have not been found to reverse conjunctival squamous metaplasia.[12–19]

Tears can be used on an as-needed basis by most dry eye patients. In patients with severe keratitis sicca, corneal anesthesia, blink paralysis or lagophthalmos should be instructed to use artificial tears on a regular basis (every 1–2 hours) and to increase the frequency of instillation

Table 12.2 Composition of Artificial Tears

Viscosity Enhancing Agent	Concentration	Found in Commercial Brands
Cellulose derivatives [carboxymethylcellulose (CMC), hydroxypropylmethylcellulose (HPMC)]	0.2–1%	*Refresh Tears, TheraTears® (CMC); Bion® Tears, Tears Naturale®, Visine®, GenTeal®, Artelac® (HPMC)*
CMC + glycerin	0.5-0-9	*Refresh Optive™*
Polyols [polyethylene glycol (PEG), propylene glycol, glycerin]	0.25–1%	*Systane®, Systane Ultra®, Soothe® Lubricant preservative free, Advanced Eye Relief®, Oasis®*
Polyvinyl alcohol (PVA)	1–1.4%	*HypoTears®, Akwa Tears®, Tears Again®, Tears Naturale® PM, Freshkote*
Hyaluronic Acid	0.1–0.18%	*Blink Tears®, Hyalistil™ Oasis®, Vismed®*
Oil-based emulsions (mineral and castor oil)		*Solutions: Refresh Optive™ ADVANCED, Systane® Balance, Soothe® XP Emollient, Ointments: AKWA Tears, LACRI-LUBE®, Systane Nighttime Ointment®,Tears Naturale® PM, REFRESH PM®*

when reading or when they are exposed to dry or drafty environments, until a more definitive treatment can be instituted. No distinct advantage in ocular surface protection has been found with any particular brand of artificial tears, the decision on which tear to use can be based on patient preference and the presence or type of a preservative. It is well recognized that the preservative benzalkonium chloride (BAC) can cause severe corneal and ocular surface toxicity. Patients with aqueous tear deficiency are particularly susceptible to the toxic effects of BAC because of their reduced tear volume and tear clearance. This risk is further worsened by punctal occlusion.

Benzalkonium chloride is known to disrupt tight junctions and accelerate desquamation of the apical epithelial layer of the cornea in a dose-dependent fashion.[20] BAC has detrimental effects on cell membrane integrity and viability. BAC was found to promote apoptosis at lower concentrations and necrosis at higher concentrations following treatment of a conjunctival epithelial cell line.[21] It has also been found to stimulate production of inflammatory cytokines (IL-1 and TNF-α) by cultured ocular surface epithelial cells.[22]

Fortunately, there are currently very few artificial tears on the market that are preserved with BAC. Unit dose, preservative-free, artificial tears, eliminate the risks of epithelial preservative toxicity. They should be considered for treatment of patients who instill them more than four times. There are several multidose artificial tears that contain less toxic preservatives, such as Purite® or sodium perborate that are an alternative to more costly unit dose preservative-free tears.

Gels (Genteal™, Novartis, East Hanover, NJ; Tears Again® NIGHT & DAY™ Gel, Ocusoft, Richmond, TX) composed of polyacrylic acid are more viscous and have longer retention times than artificial tear solutions. Petroleum – mineral oil-based ointments are usually reserved for nocturnal use or in treatment of lagophthalmos or blink paralysis because they blur vision and feel sticky.

Punctal Occlusion

Punctal occlusion should be considered for patients with aqueous tear deficiency and low tear volume. Punctal occlusion is a simple and practical method for conserving endogenously produced tears or instilled artificial tears, increasing tear volume and decreasing tear osmolarity. Punctal occlusion has been reported to decrease ocular irritation symptoms, to improve ocular surface dye staining, and to decrease dependence on artificial tears.[23–27] It should be used with caution in patients with normal aqueous tear production (Schirmer 1 scores >10 mm) and poor tear clearance or in patients with overt lid or ocular surface inflammation, such as meibomian gland disease or ocular rosacea. In these cases, ocular surface inflammation should be controlled prior to punctal occlusion.

Dissolvable intracanalicular plugs (lasting 7–10 days for collagen and up to 3 months for synthetic polymers) can be placed into the canaliculis on a trial basis, to determine the efficacy and tolerability of punctal occlusion prior to placement of semipermanent plugs or permanent occlusion. Reversible punctal occlusion can be accomplished with a variety of 'semipermanent' dumbbell-shaped silicone plugs that are inserted into the punctal orifice. These plugs are available in a variety of sizes ranging in diameter from 0.4 to 0.8 mm and a gauge can be used to determine the size of the punctum prior to insertion. Silicone plugs are typically retained for weeks to years and have a reported extrusion rate of approximately 7% at 1 month, increasing to 37% at 6 months.[28] They can be easily removed with forceps. They are generally well tolerated, but occasionally patients will experience discomfort from the head of the plug rubbing against the medial bulbar conjunctiva. There is also a small risk of pyogranuloma formation at the punctal opening and migration of the plug into the lacrimal canaliculus, that may require surgical removal of the displaced plug.

Permanent punctal occlusion is most commonly performed with a disposable thermocautery or with a radiofrequency needle. These procedures can be performed rapidly in the examination room, after topical anesthesia and/or local infiltration of the lid with anesthetic. Punctal occlusion can also be performed with the argon laser, but the results of this technique are variable. One advantage of the laser technique is that laser spots can surround the puncta, causing stenosis, but not permanent closure. Therefore, the amount of stenosis can be titrated based on the patient's tear function. Temporary or semipermanent plugs should be considered before permanent punctal occlusion, to determine if the patient will experience bothersome epiphora symptoms.

Anti-inflammatory Therapy

Basic and clinical research indicates that anti-inflammatory therapies significantly improve signs and symptoms of dry eye. Anti-inflammatory therapy should be considered for patients who continue to experience irritation symptoms or have corneal signs, despite the use of artificial tears. It should be instituted prior to punctual occlusion in patients with clinically apparent ocular surface inflammation (lid or conjunctival injection, corneal vascularization or infiltrates). There are several anti-inflammatory therapies with demonstrated efficacy for treatment of dry eye. These agents target one or more components of the inflammatory response to dry eye.

CYCLOSPORINE A

Cyclosporine is a fungal-derived peptide that prevents activation and nuclear translocation of cytoplasmic transcription factors that are required for T-cell activation and inflammatory cytokine production. Cyclosporine also inhibits mitochondrial mediated pathways of apoptosis.

Cyclosporine emulsion (Restasis™, Allergan) is the only FDA approved anti-inflammatory therapy of dry eye. Administered twice a day, topical cyclosporine stimulates aqueous tear production by suppressing ocular surface and glandular inflammation and inhibiting apoptosis (programmed cell death) of the tear-producing epithelial cells in the lacrimal glands and ocular surface. In FDA clinical trials, cyclosporine emulsion was found to be effective in decreasing corneal fluorescein staining, improving blurred vision symptoms and decreasing artificial tear use in patients with moderate to severe keratoconjunctivitis sicca. Clinical improvement may be observed within several weeks and continues up to 6 months. Preliminary clinical experience suggests that cyclosporine may be effective in patients with less severe disease. Cyclosporine emulsion is a nontoxic medication that can be continued indefinitely, although once daily dosing may be sufficient after 1 year[29] and discontinuing routine use may lead to worsening symptoms.[30] Topical cyclosporine has also been found to increase density of mucus-filled goblet cells in the conjunctiva.[31,32] Some dry eye patients benefit from more frequent dosing than the standard twice daily regimen.[33]

TACROLIMUS

Tacrolimus is a calcineurin inhibitor with a similar mechanism of action to cyclosporine, reduction in T-cell activation. Although tacrolimus is not approved for the treatment of dry eye in the United States, a recent small study suggests that it may benefit patients with dry eye.[34] Further studies are needed to address safety and efficacy.

CORTICOSTEROIDS

Corticosteroids are potent immunosuppressors, and when administered topically they inhibit multiple pathways of the inflammatory response. Topical corticosteroids also decrease ocular surface inflammation and have been reported to improve corneal epithelial disease in dry eye. They are most appropriately used for pulse therapy, such as 2–4 times per day for up to 4 weeks, to minimize their well-known side effects.[35,36] Clinical improvement is usually observed within a week and the therapeutic effect may be sustained for weeks or months after a pulse.[35] To minimize the potential to raise intraocular pressure, agents such as fluorometholone and loteprednol etabonate or low-dose dexamethasone (0.01%) should be considered.[36,37] Topical steroids can be combined with other anti-inflammatory therapies, such as cyclosporine, to provide more rapid relief of symptoms and greater improvement of ocular surface disease.

TETRACYCLINES

In addition to their antibiotic activity, tetracyclines are recognized to have numerous anti-inflammatory properties. They inhibit the production of inflammatory cytokines, decrease nitric oxide production and inhibit matrix metalloproteinase production.[38] The semisynthetic tetracycline doxycycline has been recognized to improve irritation symptoms, increase tear film stability and decrease the severity of ocular surface disease in meibomian gland dysfunction and ocular rosacea.[8] Doxycycline has also been reported to be effective for treating recurrent corneal epithelial erosions.[39]

Oral tetracycline therapy should be considered in patients with ocular rosacea, severe corneal epithelial disease, corneal vascularization, marginal infiltrates, non-healing corneal epithelial defects and corneal ulceration associated with tear film deficiency. In a randomized clinical trial of doxycycline for treatment of meibomian gland dysfunction, a dose of 20 mg orally twice a day, for 1 month was found to be as effective as 200 mg orally twice a day.[40] The trend

has been to treat patients with lower doses (20–50 mg orally twice a day) to minimize gastrointestinal upset and candidiasis, for 4 weeks and stop or taper to once a day if improvement in signs and symptoms is observed.

AZITHROMYCIN

Azithromycin is an azalide, macrolide antibiotic with broad-spectrum antibacterial activity and an antimicrobial mechanism of action that involves binding to the 50S subunit of the bacterial ribosome. Like the tetracycline, antibiotics, azithromycin may also have anti-inflammatory properties[41] beneficial to treating the ocular surface.[42] Azithromycin is available as a topical ophthalmic preparation (Azithromycin 1% solution) approved for the treatment of bacterial conjunctivitis. Azithromycin applied to the lids may have an antibacterial effect on common agents of anterior blepharitis, including *Staphylococcus*. A number of studies have shown improvement in signs and symptoms of meibomian gland dysfunction-related dry eye in patients using topical azithromycin solution.[43–46] Topical azithromycin ophthalmic solution on the lid margin may be a practical alternative in patients unwilling or unable to take oral doxycycline.

ESSENTIAL FATTY ACIDS

Diet has been implicated as a cause for dry eye. In the Woman's Health Study, the group with the highest dietary consumption of omega-3 (n-3) polyunsaturated fatty acids (PUFA) carried a significantly lower risk of dry eye than the group with the lowest consumption. Furthermore, a high dietary omega-6 (n-6) to n-3 ratio was associated with a twofold higher risk of developing dry eye.[10] This benefit was attributed to the anti-inflammatory properties of n-3 PUFAs that are found in certain cold water fish (salmon, cod, mackerel). The n-3 PUFA eicosapentaenoic acid (EPA) found in fish oil has been found to decrease production of arachidonic acid-derived eicosanoids, to decrease the production of proinflammatory cytokines and reactive oxygen species and inhibit lymphocyte proliferation.[47,48] The n-6 PUFA γ-linolenic acid (GLA) also has anti-inflammatory activity.[48] Supplementation with EPA has been found to potentiate the anti-inflammatory activity of GLA by decreasing synthesis of arachidonic acid. Formulations containing one or both of these PUFAs have been observed to be effective in treating chronic inflammatory diseases, such as rheumatoid arthritis.[49] Clinical trials of nutritional supplements containing linoleic acid and/or GLA alone or combined with fish oil[50–53] for treatment of dry eye have reported improvement in symptoms and/or signs.

SECRETOGOGUES

The oral secretogogues pilocarpine and cevilemine stimulate aqueous tear production. They should be considered in conditions, such as Sjögren's syndrome and neurotrophic disease, where the ability to reflex tear is lost. Oral pilocarpine (Salagen, MGI Pharma, Minneapolis) is a muscarinic cholinergic parasympathomimetic agonist that stimulates exocrine glands. Subjective improvement in dry eye symptoms has been reported[54–56] and one study also noted improvement in conjunctival staining.[55] Pilocarpine is typically prescribed at a dose of 5 mg q.i.d. The most common side effects from this medication are excessive sweating and gastrointestinal cramping, occurring in approximately 40% of patients.[56]

Cevimeline (Evoxac; Daiichi, Montvale, NJ) is another oral cholinergic agonist that has been found to improve ocular irritation symptoms[57] and aqueous tear production.[57–59] This agent appears to have fewer adverse systemic side effects than oral pilocarpine, although it may also cause mild to moderate gastrointestinal symptoms and sweating.[59] It is typically prescribed at a dose of 30 mg p.o. t.i.d.

SERUM/PLASMA

Autologous serum, which is known to contain albumin and various growth and anti-inflammatory factors, can be used to treat Sjögren's syndrome-associated keratoconjunctivitis sicca[60,61] and to promote healing of persistent corneal epithelial defects.[62–65] Autologous plasma has also been reported to heal neurotrophic keratopathy in dry eye.[66] Because of the difficulty and expense in preparing serum drops and the potential for microbial contamination, they should be reserved for patients with severe disease who are unresponsive to other therapies. Furthermore, studies have reported varying degrees of efficacy with serum ophthalmic preparations, possibly due to different concentrations and preparation regimens. Close cooperation with a blood bank or formulation pharmacy with an established protocol for serum/plasma may improve outcomes and minimize complications.

CONTACT LENSES

Patients with severe corneal epithelial disease (e.g. filamentary keratitis and non-healing corneal epithelial defects) and those with lid margin keratinization, irregularity or trichiasis (as typically seen with Stevens Johnson syndrome) may benefit from therapeutic contact lenses. Hydrogel and silicone hydrogel soft lenses provide some protection from microtrauma, from irregular lids and trichiasis, but they are often poorly tolerated in severe aqueous tear deficiency. A better option for this subset of patients is the prosthetic replacement of the ocular surface ecosystem (PROSE™), a specially designed scleral-bearing contact lens with a fluid-filled reservoir over the cornea. PROSE has proven to be an excellent option for improving irritation symptoms and visual acuity.[67–69] The fluid-filled reservoir hydrates the cornea and shields it from blink trauma, noxious environmental stimuli and inflammatory mediators in the tears. The body-temperature saline reservoir also prevents corneal cooling and nerve firing that occurs during the inter-blink intervals. Patients may experience almost immediate relief in photophobia and irritation symptoms after placing the device on the cornea. The PROSE is an excellent substitute for tarsorrhaphy; however, this surgical procedure should be considered in patients where PROSE is not an option. Other options for treatment of filamentary keratitis include topical corticosteroids, topical acetylcysteine and onabotulinumtoxin A injection into the orbicularis muscle to decrease lid frictional force on the corneal surface.[70]

References

1. Stern ME, Beuerman RW, Fox RI, et al. The pathology of dry eye: The interaction between ocular surface and lacrimal glands. Cornea 1998;17:584–9.
2. Moss SE, Klein R, Klein BE. Prevalence of and risk factors for dry eye syndrome. Arch Ophthalmol 2000;118:1264–8.
3. Moss SE, Klein R, Klein BE. Incidence of dry eye in an older population. Arch Ophthalmol 2004;122:369–73.
4. Schaumberg DA, Sullivan DA, Buring JE, et al. Prevalence of dry eye syndrome among US women. Am J Ophthalmol 2003;136:318–26.
5. Schaumberg DA, Dana R, Buring JE, et al. Prevalence of dry eye syndrome among US men: estimates from the Physicians' Health Studies. Arch Ophthalmol 2009;127:763.
6. Shimmura S, Shimazaki J, Tsubota K. Results of a population-based questionnaire on the symptoms and lifestyles associated with dry eye. Cornea 1999;18:408–11.
7. Schiffman RM, Walt JG, Jacobsen G, et al. Utility assessment among patients with dry eye disease. Ophthalmology 2003;110:1412–9.
8. Pflugfelder S (committee chairman). Management and therapy of dry eye disease: report of the Management and Therapy Subcommittee of the International Dry Eye WorkShop (2007). Ocul Surf 2007;5: 163–78.
9. Geerling G, Tauber J, Baudouin C, et al. The international workshop on meibomian gland dysfunction: report of the subcommittee on management and treatment of meibomian gland dysfunction. Invest Ophthalmol Vis Sci 2011;52:2050–64.
10. Miljanović B, Trivedi KA, Dana MR, et al. Relation between dietary n-3 and n-6 fatty acids and clinically diagnosed dry eye syndrome in women. Am J Clin Nutr 2005;82:887–93.
11. Altinors DD, Akça S, Akova YA, et al. Smoking associated with damage to the lipid layer of the ocular surface. Am J Ophthalmol 2006; 141(6):1016–21.
12. Nelson JD, Farris RL. Sodium hyaluronate and polyvinyl alcohol artificial tear preparations: a comparison in patients with keratoconjunctivitis sicca. Arch Ophthalmol 1988;106:484–7.
13. Lemp MA. Artificial tear solutions. Int Ophthalmol Clin 1973; 13:221–9.
14. Toda I, Shinozaki N, Tsubota K. Hydroxypropyl methylcellulose for the treatment of severe dry eye associated with Sjögren's syndrome. Cornea 1996;15:120–8.
15. Huang FC, Tseng SH, Shih MH, et al. Effect of artificial tears on corneal surface regularity, contrast sensitivity and glare disability in dry eyes. Ophthalmology 2002;109:1934–40.
16. Iskeleli G, Kizilkaya M, Arslan OS, et al. The effect of artificial tears on corneal surface regularity in patients with Sjögren syndrome. Ophthalmologica 2002;216:118–22.
17. Liu Z, Pflugfelder SC. Corneal surface regularity and the effect of artificial tears in aqueous tear deficiency. Ophthalmology 1999; 106:939–43.
18. Donshik PC, Nelson JD, Abelson M, et al. Effectiveness of BION tears, Cellufresh, Aquasite, and Refresh Plus for moderate to severe dry eye. Adv Exp Med Biol 1998;438:753–60.
19. Calonge M. The treatment of dry eye. Surv Ophthalmol 2001; 45(suppl. 2):S227–39.
20. Pauly A, Meloni M, Brignole-Baudouin F, et al. Multiple endpoint analysis of the 3D-reconstituted corneal epithelium after treatment with benzalkonium chloride: early detection of toxic damage. Invest Ophthalmol Vis Sci 2009;50:1644–52.
21. De Saint Jean M, Brignole F, Bringuier AF, et al. Effects of benzalkonium chloride on growth and survival of Chang conjunctival cells. Invest Ophthalmol Vis Sci 1999;40:619–30.
22. Epstein SP, Chen D, Asbell PA. Evaluation of biomarkers of inflammation in response to benzalkonium chloride on corneal and conjunctival epithelial cells. J Ocul Pharmacol Ther 2009;25:415–24.
23. Freeman JM. The punctum plug: evaluation of a new treatment for the dry eye. Trans Am Acad Ophthalmol Otolaryngol 1975;79: 874–9.
24. Tuberville AW, Frederick WR, Wood TO. Punctal occlusion in tear deficiency syndromes. Ophthalmology 1982;89:1170–2.
25. Willis RM, Folberg R, Krachmer JH, et al. The treatment of aqueous deficient dry eye with removable punctual plugs. A clinical and impression-cytological study. Ophthalmology 1987;94:514–8.
26. Gilbard JP, Rossi SR, Azar DT, et al. Effect of punctal occlusion by Freeman silicone plug insertion on tear osmolarity in dry eye disorders. CLAO J 1989;15:216–8.

27. Baxter SA, Laibson PR. Punctal plugs in the management of dry eyes. Ocul Surf 2004;2:255–65.
28. Balaram M, Schaumberg DA, Dana MR. Efficacy and tolerability outcomes after punctal occlusion with silicone plugs in dry eye syndrome. Am J Ophthalmol 2001;131:30–6.
29. Su MY, Perry HD, Barsam A, et al. The effect of decreasing the dosage of cyclosporine A 0.05% on dry eye disease after 1 year of twice-daily therapy. Cornea 2011;30:1098–104.
30. Rao SN. Reversibility of dry eye deceleration after topical cyclosporine 0.05% withdrawal. J Ocul Pharmacol Ther 2011;27:603–9.
31. Pflugfelder SC, De Paiva CS, Villarreal AL, et al. Effects of sequential artificial tear and cyclosporine emulsion therapy on conjunctival goblet cell density and transforming growth factor-beta 2 production. Cornea 2008;27:64–9.
32 Kunert KS, Tisdale AS, Gipson IK. Goblet cell numbers and epithelial proliferation in the conjunctiva of patients with dry eye syndrome treated with cyclosporine. Arch Ophthalmol 2002;120:330–7.
33. Dastjerdi MH, Hamrah P, Dana R. High-frequency topical cyclosporine 0.05% in the treatment of severe dry eye refractory to twice-daily regimen. Cornea 2009;28:1091–6.
34. Moscovici BK, Holzchuh R, Chiacchio BB, et al. Clinical treatment of dry eye using 0.03% Tacrolimus eye drops. Cornea 2012;31:945–9.
35. Marsh P, Pflugfelder SC. Topical non-preserved methylprednisolone therapy of keratoconjunctivitis sicca in Sjögren syndrome. Ophthalmology 1999;106:811–6.
36. Pflugfelder SC, Maskin SL, Anderson B, et al. A randomized, double-masked, placebo-controlled, multicenter comparison of loteprednol etabonate ophthalmic suspension, 0.5%, and placebo for treatment of keratoconjunctivitis sicca in patients with delayed tear clearance. Am J Ophthalmol 2004;138:444–57.
37. Jonisch J, Steiner A, Udell IJ. Preservative-free low-dose dexamethasone for the treatment of chronic ocular surface disease refractory to standard therapy. Cornea 2010;29:723–6.
38. Pflugfelder SC. Anti-inflammatory therapy for dry eye. Am J Ophthalmol 2004;137:337–42.
39. Dursun D, Kim MC, Solomon A, et al. Treatment of recalcitrant recurrent corneal epithelial erosions with inhibitors of matrix metalloproteinases-9, doxycycline and corticosteroids. Am J Ophthalmol 2001;132:8–13.
40. Yoo SE, Lee DC, Chang MH. The effect of low-dose doxycycline therapy in chronic meibomian gland dysfunction. Korean J Ophthalmol 2005;19:258–63.
41. Ianaro A, Ialenti A, Maffia P, et al. Anti-inflammatory activity of macrolide antibiotics. J Pharmacol Exp Ther 2000;292:156–63.
42. Igami TZ, Holzchuh R, Osaki TH et al. Oral azithromycin for treatment of posterior blepharitis. Cornea 2011;30:1145–9.
43. Foulks GN, Borchman D, Yappert M, et al. Topical azithromycin therapy for meibomian gland dysfunction: clinical response and lipid alterations. Cornea 2010;29:781–8.
44. Luchs J. Efficacy of topical azithromycin ophthalmic solution 1% in the treatment of posterior blepharitis. Adv Ther 2008;25:858–87.
45. Haque RM, Torkildsen GL, Brubaker K, et al. Multicenter, open-label study evaluating the efficacy of azithromycin ophthalmic solution 1% on the signs and symptoms of subjects with blepharitis. Cornea 2010;29:871–7.
46. Opitz DL, Tyler KF. Efficacy of azithromycin 1% ophthalmic solution for treatment of ocular surface disease from posterior blepharitis. Clin Exp Optom 2011;94:200–6.
47. Zurier RB, Rossetti RG, Seiler CM, et al. Human peripheral blood T lymphocyte proliferation after activation of the T cell receptor: effects of unsaturated fatty acids. Prost Leuk Essent Fatty Acids 1999;60:371–5.
48. DeMarco DM, Santoli D, Zurier RB. Effects of fatty acids on proliferation and activation of human synovial compartment lymphocytes. J Leuk Biol 1994;56:612–5.
49. Calder PC, Zurier RB. Polyunsaturated fatty acids and rheumatoid arthritis. Curr Opin Clin Nutr Metab Care 2001;4:115–21.
50. Aragona P, Bucolo C, Spinella R, et al. Systemic omega-6 essential fatty acid treatment and PGE1 tear content in Sjogren's syndrome patients. Invest Ophthalmol Vis Sci 2005;46:4474–9.
51. Barabino S, Rolando M, Camicione P, et al. Efficacy of systemic linoleic and gamma-linolenic acid therapy in dry-eye syndrome with inflammatory component. Cornea 2003;22:97–101.
52. Kokke KH, Morris JA, Lawrenson JG. Oral omega-6 essential fatty acid treatment in contract lens association dry eye. Cont Lens Anterior Eye 2008;31:141–6.
53. Creuzot C, Passemard M, Viau S, et al. Improvement of dry eye symptoms with polyunsaturated fatty acids. J Fr Ophtalmol 2006;29:868–73.
54. Tsifetaki N, Kitsos G, Paschides CA, et al. Oral pilocarpine for the treatment of ocular symptoms in patients with Sjögren's syndrome: a randomised 12 week controlled study. Ann Rheum Dis 2003;62:1204–7.
55. Papas AS, Sherrer YS, Charney M, et al. Successful treatment of dry mouth and dry eye symptoms in Sjögren's syndrome patients with oral pilocarpine: a randomized, placebo-controlled, dose-adjustment study. J Clin Rheumatol 2004;10:169–77.
56. Vivino FB, Al-Hashimi I, Khan Z, et al. Pilocarpine tablets for the treatment of dry mouth and dry eye symptoms in patients with Sjögren syndrome: a randomized, placebo-controlled, fixed-dose, multicenter trial. P92-01 Study Group. Arch Intern Med 1999;159:174–81.
57. Fife RS, Chase WF, Dore RK, et al. Cevimeline for the treatment of xerostomia in patients with Sjögren syndrome: a randomized trial. Arch Intern Med 2002;162:1293–300.
58. Petrone D, Condemi JJ, Fife R, et al. A double-blind, randomized, placebo-controlled study of cevimeline in Sjögren's syndrome patients with xerostomia and keratoconjunctivitis sicca. Arthritis Rheum 2002;46:748–54.
59. Ono M, Takamura E, Shinozaki K, et al. Therapeutic effect of cevimeline on dry eye in patients with Sjögren's syndrome: a randomized, double-blind clinical study. Am J Ophthalmol 2004;138:6–17.
60. Fox RI, Chan R, Michelson JB, et al. Beneficial effects of artificial tears made with autologous serum in patients with keratoconjunctivitis sicca. Arthritis Rheum 1984;27:459–61.
61. Yoon KC, Heo H, Im SK, et al. Comparison of autologous serum and umbilical cord serum eye drops for dry eye syndrome. Am J Ophthalmol 2007;144:86–92.
62. Schrader S, Wedel T, Moll R, et al. Combination of serum eye drops with hydrogel bandage contact lenses in the treatment of persistent epithelial defects. Graefes Arch Clin Exp Ophthalmol 2006;244:1345–9.
63. Jeng BH, Dupps WJ, Jr. Autologous serum 50% eyedrops in the treatment of persistent corneal epithelial defects. Cornea 2009;28:1104–8.
64. Del Castillo JM, de la Casa JM, Sardina RC. Treatment of recurrent corneal erosions using autologous serum. Cornea 2002;21:781–3.
65. Young AL, Cheng AC, Ng HK, et al. The use of autologous serum tears in persistent epithelial defect. Eye 2004;18:609–14.
66. Rao KV, Leveque C, Pflugfelder SC. Corneal nerve regeneration in neurotrophic keratopathy following autologous plasma therapy. Br J Ophthalmol 2010;51:844–9.
67. Romero-Rangel T, Stavrou P, Cotter J, et al. Gas-permeable scleral contact lens therapy in ocular surface disease. Am J Ophthalmol 2000;130:25–32.
68. Rosenthal P, Croteau A. Fluid-ventilated, gas-permeable scleral contact lens is an effective option for managing severe ocular surface disease and many corneal disorders that would otherwise require penetrating keratoplasty. Eye Contact Lens 2005;31:130–4.
69. Gumus K, Gire A, Pflugfelder SC. The impact of the Boston ocular surface prosthesis on wavefront higher-order aberrations. Am J Ophthalmol 2011;151:682–90.
70. Gumus K, Lee S, Yen MT, et al. Botulinum toxin injection for the management of refractory filamentary keratitis. Arch Ophthalmol 2012;130:446–50.

13 Seasonal and Perennial Allergic Conjunctivitis

DENISE DE FREITAS

Introduction

Seasonal allergic conjunctivitis (SAC) and perennial allergic conjunctivitis (PAC) are the common and mild acute forms of ocular allergy, usually accompanied by seasonal allergic rhinitis,[1] with SAC comprising 25% to 50% of the total cases of allergic conjunctivitis.[2] Several authors have emphasized that ocular allergies, especially SAC, are underdiagnosed, thus underestimating their true prevalence.[3] Although SAC and PAC are relatively mild conditions, rarely causing permanent visual impairment, their effects on the quality of life can be profound, with significant morbidity.[4]

The seasonal incidence of SAC is closely related to the cycles of released plant-derived airborne allergens, or aeroallergens. The allergens that produce SAC vary from one geographic area to another, but tree, grass, and ragweed pollens are the most common encountered allergens. PAC is more likely to occur year-round, although about 79% of patients may still have seasonal exacerbations. Some have theorized that warming trends, accompanying long-term climate change, may cause greater exposure times to seasonal allergens, with subsequent effects on allergic eye disease prevalence.[5]

The majority of PAC and SAC affect both young and middle-aged people of both sexes.[6]

Pathophysiology

Both SAC and PAC are type I (immediate) immunoglobulin E (IgE)-mediated hypersensitivity reactions, due to environmental airborne allergens, divided into two phases, with the mast cell (MC) playing a central role. A reaction occurs when a sensitized individual is exposed to a specific antigen. IgE has a strong affinity for MCs, predominantly MCTC phenotype, triggering its degranulation. The number of MCs present within the conjunctiva stroma may be increased up to 60% in patients with SAC compared to normal patients.[7]

The reaction involves a very complex series of immunological events, coordinated by various mediators, initiated by the allergen. An allergen such as pollen reacts with specific IgE antibodies bound to a sensitized MC, triggering cross-linkage of the IgE molecules and an influx of calcium ions into the MC. This causes the MC to degranulate and release preformed inflammatory mediators, such as histamine, which causes the signs and symptoms associated with the early-phase response in sensitized individuals. There are two components of MC activation. The first is the release of preformed mediators, including histamine. The second is the synthesis of arachidonic acid and the subsequent metabolic cascade, resulting in the production of prostaglandins and leukotrienes. The released histamine binds H_1 and H_2 receptors on the target tissue cell surfaces. Binding to the H_1 receptor results in the primary allergic symptoms of itching, burning, and stinging sensation and tearing, while binding to the H_2 receptor releases leukotrienes and prostaglandins, stimulating mucus production and also increasing vascular permeability.[7] This early-phase response is immediate and lasts clinically for 20–30 minutes.

MC degranulation also initiates a series of cellular and extracellular events, which lead to the late-phase response, including production of prostaglandins, thromboxanes and leukotrienes derived from arachidonic acid.[8] MCs also release cytokines and chemotactic factors which induce the production of IgE from B cells, enhance production of Th_2 lymphocytes, attract eosinophils and activate vascular endothelial corneal and conjunctival cells to release chemokines and adhesion molecules. The chemokines and adhesion molecules mediate the infiltration of eosinophils, basophils, neutrophils and Th_2 lymphocytes to the site of inflammation, coupled with the newly formed mediators and sustained MC activation, resulting in the late-phase response. This may occur 3–12 hours after the initial reaction, and symptoms can continue up to 24 hours.[9]

After the MCs are activated, cytokines are released. These cytokines attract eosinophils, lymphocytes, and neutrophils. Eosinophil infiltration of the conjunctiva is present in about 43% of patients with SAC, and about 25–84% of patients with PAC. Degranulating eosinophils release toxic proteins, including eosinophil major basic protein and eosinophil cationic protein. These proteins have cytotoxic effects and further enhance MC degranulation. These products of eosinophils are toxic to the corneal epithelium and, if present chronically, may result in ulceration. The late-phase response is characterized by an influx of multiple inflammatory cells, including eosinophils, basophils, neutrophils, and macrophages, along with CD4+ and CD8+ cells. Conjunctival epithelial cells may also prolong the allergic inflammatory response by releasing chemotactic mediators. The year-round symptoms associated with PAC are the result of chronic MC activation and Th_2 lymphocyte infiltration.[10,11]

In summary, acute allergy is caused by IgE-mediated MC degranulation, whereas chronic allergies are also associated with continuous activation of MC but with predominance of mediators, such as eosinophils and Th_2-generated cytokines.[12]

Clinical Findings of SAC and PAC

Signs and symptoms of SAC and PAC are essentially the same and typically develop on a gradual basis but can also develop suddenly following contact with the offending allergen. The difference relies on specific allergens to which patients are sensitive and the chronicity of exposure. SAC and PAC remain self-limited without ocular surface damage, while atopic and vernal keratoconjunctivitis can compromise the cornea, causing ulcers and scarring and can ultimately lead to vision loss. SAC and PAC are usually bilateral, although they may be asymmetrical. If the allergic insult occurs with a particular allergen entering only one eye, ocular changes may exceptionally be unilateral. The symptoms and signs are recurrent, occurring rapidly following the exposure to seasonal allergens.

Individuals with SAC typically have symptoms of acute allergic conjunctivitis for a defined period of time, usually of short duration, that is, when the predominant airborne allergen is present. Typically, persons with SAC are symptom-free during the winter months in cooler climates because of the decreased airborne transmission of some allergens, such as pollen. Molds, house dust, and animal dander may also participate in the disease process. The severity of symptoms varies depending on the type of allergen, its concentration, and time of exposure.[4] Dry eye facilitates allergen contact with the ocular surface since the capability of the tears to 'wash away' the allergen is usually compromised.[13] The most significant symptom in SAC is itching. Patients usually complain of intense itching of the eyes, sometimes along with a burning sensation and tearing.[14] Discharge is usually serous, clear and watery, but with a ropy characteristic.

Signs in SAC include lid edema, conjunctival hyperemia and injection, and chemosis. Chemosis may be apparent in the bulbar and lower tarsal conjunctiva, giving to it a 'milky' or pale pink appearance. Some patients refer to a dramatic unilateral bulging of the conjunctiva, frequently described as the acute formation of a 'bubble' in the eye, mainly when patients rub their eyes. In reality, the conjunctiva balloons, due to intense and acute infiltration of cells and fluids, causing the chemosis (Fig. 13.1). The conjunctival chemosis can be very intense and may even cause unstable tear film and consequently corneal dellen (Fig. 13.2). These conditions tend to disappear with the resolution of the chemosis. Rarely, SAC and PAC affect the cornea, but the presence of punctate keratitis or dellen might lead to symptoms of pain, photophobia and blurred vision. SAC and PAC usually result in few to no sequelae.[15]

PAC is less common than SAC and, as patients are chronically exposed to allergen, symptoms and signs occur year-round. The most common triggers are mold spores, animal dander, and dust mites usually found in the household. Patients may also be sensitive to seasonal allergen with a superimposed offender to their symptoms. Symptoms and signs in PAC are similar to those in SAC but are usually milder and with longer duration. Because of the prolonged exposure, the conjunctiva may become boggy, chronically red, and irritated. Papillary hypertrophy along the tarsal conjunctival surface (Fig. 13.3) may occur with chronic exposure to allergens in PAC. The discharge is whitish but thick, and even stringy.[4]

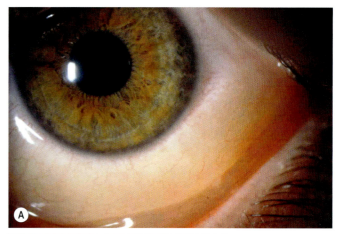
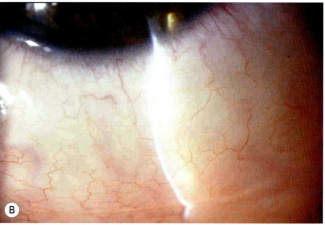

Figure 13.1 Conjunctiva bulging due to intense and acute infiltration of cells and fluids causing the chemosis in a patient with seasonal allergic conjunctivitis (SAC).

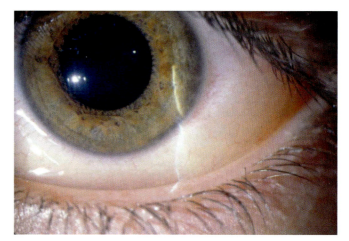

Figure 13.2 Intense conjunctival chemosis causing unstable tear film and corneal dellen in a patient in acute phase of seasonal allergic conjunctivitis (SAC).

Diagnosis of SAC and PAC

The diagnosis of SAC and PAC is generally based on clinical history and careful biomicroscopic examination.[16] Important features of the history include a personal or family history of atopic disease, such as allergic rhinitis, bronchial

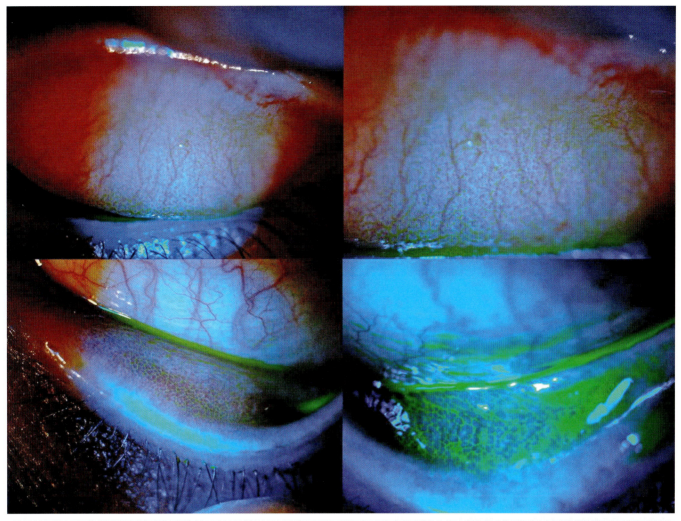

Figure 13.3 Mild papillary reaction in the upper and lower tarsal conjunctivas in a patient with perennial allergic conjunctivitis (PAC).

asthma, and/or atopic dermatitis. As cited earlier, patients with PAC are more likely to also have perennial rhinitis.[1]

Perhaps the most important symptom is itching. Without itching, the diagnosis of allergic conjunctivitis is suspect. With the intense itching, the diagnosis of SAC and PAC is very likely, but one should also consider dry eye, toxic conjunctivitis, contact dermatitis, blepharitis, and other forms of allergic conjunctivitis in the differential diagnosis.[17] In these other disorders, itching is usually mild and occasional. It is worthwhile to pinpoint the location of itching. For example, patients who complain of ocular itching may be describing symptoms related to the skin of their eyelids. Careful questioning can distinguish itching of the conjunctiva from itching of the eyelid skin. Moreover, patients with dry eye tend to have mild itching located in the nasal inner part of the bulbar conjunctiva, due to allergen accumulation in the area of tear drainage.[13]

Superficial conjunctival scrapings may help to establish the diagnosis by revealing characteristic eosinophils (Fig. 13.4), which are not normally present on the conjunctiva. However, eosinophils are observed in the most severe cases, but are generally present in the deep layers of the substantia propria of the conjunctiva. For this reason,

the absence of eosinophils on conjunctival scraping does not rule out the diagnosis of allergic conjunctivitis.[18] Even the presence of one eosinophil or eosinophilic granules is consistent with a diagnosis of allergy. About 25% of patients with diagnosed SAC have eosinophils on cytological examination.[8]

The diagnosis can also be made by performing the conjunctival provocation tests, which consist of instilling offending pollen into the conjunctival sac, producing the typical symptoms of SAC. Conjunctival provocation tests are rarely necessary for the diagnosis of SAC and PAC, and it has rather proven to be a reliable method to evaluate ocular therapeutics.[19,20] There is also a possible involvement of nasal allergy in some patients with allergic conjunctivitis, such as SAC and PAC, and therefore, there may be value to a nasal challenge with allergen combined with registration of the ocular features.[1]

The standard clinical test for the diagnosis of type I hypersensitivity reaction is the intradermal skin test. Cutaneous tests, such as the scratch or prick, and more rarely, the intracutaneous injections, may be utilized to determine the antigens causing the hypersensitivity. The prick test is the preferred method because it is more sensitive, less

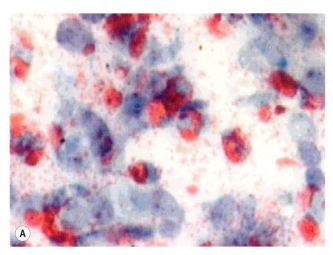
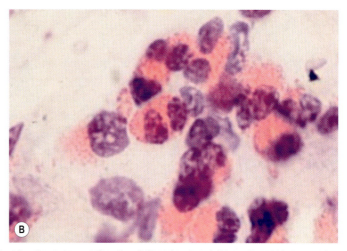

Figure 13.4 Conjunctival scrapings in low (**A**) and high (**B**) magnification showing the presence of eosinophils and eosinophil granules consistent with the diagnosis of allergy.

variable, and more comfortable to patients than the intra-cutaneous test.[21]

The radioallergosorbent test (RAST), a blood test, may also help to define the allergens. Elevated IgE levels in serum (RAST, ELISA) and in tear fluid are present in almost all patients with SAC and PAC.[22]

Treatment of SAC and PAC

Treatment of SAC and PAC includes reducing the amount of allergen exposure.[17] One important goal of treatment is to prevent transformation of SAC to a chronic inflammatory process.

Because SAC usually involves allergens, such as tree, grass, and ragweed pollens, patients should avoid outside activities until late afternoon or after a heavy rain, when pollen levels are lower. SAC tends to be worse in warm, dry weather and to lessen with rain and cool temperatures. Patients should also keep windows in their home and car closed to lessen exposure to pollen. Hair and clothes should be washed after being outdoors. Patients should also be aware that pollen can also be transported indoors on people and pets. Wearing glasses or goggles can also serve as a barrier to allergens.[17]

As already mentioned, allergens in PAC are usually mold spores, animal dander, dust mites, and are predominantly found in the household. Therefore, carpets must be cleaned, changed or removed, as well as children's stuffed animals, soft toys, and curtains. The mattress top and sides must also be cleaned and enclosed in plastic bags or other dust mite proof cover. Sheets, pillows and blankets should be washed in hot water (130°F or 54°C). Pillows and the base of the bed must be vacuumed regularly. Pets should be kept out of the bedroom, and the bathroom should be kept clean and dry to inhibit mold growth. While it is better to stop dust mites at the source, reducing the dust levels in the air could be an adequate strategy. Air purifiers that use HEPA filtration are more effective and safer. Most filters remove 50–70% of material. HEPA filters will remove up to 99% of the material; not just dust mite feces, but also all types of other

allergens, such as animal dander, dust, pollen, cockroach feces, etc.[23]

Supportive treatment of both conditions includes cold compresses to decrease inflammation, avoidance of eye rubbing and the use of preservative-free artificial tears to wash or dilute allergens and inflammatory mediators away from the ocular surface. Artificial tear solutions should be kept in the refrigerator, since the use of cold drops produces vasoconstriction ameliorating symptoms and signs. There are several pharmacologic agents for the treatment of SAC and PAC, and their use will depend on the disease severity (Table 13.1).[3]

Topical vasoconstrictors, alone or in combination with antihistamines, may provide short-term relief, mainly in SAC. The antihistamine is effective for the acute onset and reduces pruritus, while the decongestant reduces chemosis, eyelid edema, and redness via vasoconstriction. Examples of vasoconstrictors are naphazoline[24] and oxymetazoline.[25] However, vasoconstrictors may cause rebound conjunctival injection and inflammation, and they are ineffective in severe ocular allergy.

Antihistamine eye drops are prescribed for the relief of acute symptoms and signs of SAC and PAC by blocking the histamine receptors in the conjunctiva. These medications do not affect other proinflammatory mediators, such as prostaglandins and leukotrienes, which remain uninhibited. A number of topical antihistamines are available, including azelastine,[26] emedastine,[27] epinastine,[28] and levocabastine.[29] Systemic antihistamines may also relieve symptoms and signs of eye allergy. Second-generation H_1 antihistamines, such as cetirizine and loratadine, are much more selective for peripheral H_1 receptors, as opposed to the central nervous system H_1 receptors, cholinergic receptors, and some H_2 receptors that cause cardiac arrhythmia. This selectivity significantly reduces the occurrence of adverse drug reactions, such as drowsiness, dry eye[30] and dry mouth.[31]

Topical mast cell stabilizers decrease the degranulation of conjunctival MCs, preventing the release of histamine and other chemotactic factors.[32] However, the drug does not relieve existing symptoms and has no role in the treatment

Table 13.1 Treatment options for SAC and PAC

Agent	Mechanisms of Action	Drugs
Topical vasoconstrictor	Vasoconstriction reducing chemosis and edema	Naphazoline, oxymetazoline
Antihistamines	Histamine receptors blockage	Azelastine, emedastine, epinastine, levocabastine
Mast cell stabilizers	Decrease degranulation of conjunctival mast cells preventing release of histamine	Cromolyn sodium, lodoxamide
Dual acting agents	Histamine receptor antagonist and mast cell stabilizer	Alcaftadine, bepotastine, olopatadine, nedocromil, ketotifen
Non-steroidal anti-inflammatory drugs	Inhibition of prostaglandin and thromboxane production	Ketorolac tromethamine
Corticosteroids	Inhibition of phospholipase and arachidonic acid formation	Loteprednol, fluorometholone, prednisone acetate, dexamethasone
Immunomodulators	Inhibition of eosinophilic infiltration in conjunctiva (cyclosporine) or inhibition of T-cell action (tacrolimus)	Cyclosporine, tacrolimus

of the acute phase of SAC; mast cell stabilizers should be used on a prophylactic basis, mainly in cases of PAC. They need to be used long term (treatment effect usually requires continued use over 5 to 7 days) or in conjunction with other classes of medications, such as antihistaminics. Examples of MC stabilizers are cromolyn sodium[33] and lodoxamide.[34]

Dual-acting agents exert multiple pharmacological effects, such as histamine receptor antagonist action, stabilization of MC degranulation and, subsequently, suppression of activation and infiltration of eosinophils. Examples are alcaftadine,[31] bepotastine,[35] olopatadine,[36] nedocromil,[37] and ketotifen.[38]

Nonsteroidal anti-inflammatory drugs (NSAIDs) act on the cyclooxygenase metabolic pathway and inhibit production of prostaglandins and thromboxanes. They have no role in blocking mediators formed by the lipoxygenase pathway, such as leukotrienes.[39] Example of an NSAID that is approved for allergic indications is ketorolac tromethamine.[40,41]

Corticosteroid eye drops are very effective in treating SAC and PAC, but the numerous adverse effects, such as secondary infection, elevated intraocular pressure, and formation of cataract, make their use judicious and selective.[42] Corticosteroids act at the first step of the arachidonic acid pathway by inhibiting phospholipase and arachidonic acid formation. Therefore, the anti-inflammatory and immunosuppressive effects of corticosteroids are broad and nonspecific. Corticosteroids exist in various forms and concentrations. Steroids, such as loteprednol and fluorometholone, have less potency in the eye but fewer ocular adverse effects.[43] In contrast, prednisolone acetate and dexamethasone are more potent but have a higher incidence of adverse effects. Topical steroids must be prescribed only for a short period of time and for severe cases that do not respond to other options of therapy. Pulse dosing of topical steroids may be employed, followed by maintenance with an MC stabilizer.[23] There is some evidence supporting the ability of intranasal corticosteroids, used by patients with seasonal allergic rhinitis, to reduce allergic conjunctivitis symptoms.[44] Fluticasone aqueous nasal spray has been effective in relieving nasal symptoms in adolescents and adults with seasonal allergic rhinitis.[45] Patients using corticosteroids should be closely monitored.

Immunomodulatory agents, such as cyclosporine (0.05% to 2% drops)[46] and tacrolimus (0.03% ointment)[47] have demonstrated efficacy in the treatment of ocular allergy. Cyclosporine A is an immunosuppressant that acts by inhibiting eosinophilic infiltration by interfering with the type IV allergic reactions in the conjunctiva. Tacrolimus acts mainly by inhibiting the action of T cells. Both agents are associated with fewer side effects and are preferred over chronic use of corticosteroids in the treatment of allergic conjunctivitis. Immunomodulatory agents are reserved for more severe forms of allergic conjunctivitis, such as vernal and atopic keratoconjunctivitis and have limited indications in cases of SAC and PAC.

Allergen-specific immunotherapy is an effective treatment used to induce immunologic tolerance when the allergen is well known. The primary objectives of allergen-specific immunotherapy are to decrease the symptoms triggered by allergens and to prevent recurrence of the disease in the long term.[3] It is indicated in patients who have evidence of specific IgE antibodies to clinically relevant allergens. Skin prick testing is the preferred method of testing for specific IgE antibodies and identification of allergen for the immunotherapy. Candidates for immunotherapy include those who: (1) have symptoms that are not well controlled by pharmacological therapy or avoidance measures, (2) require high doses of medication, multiple medications, or both to maintain control of their disease, (3) experience adverse effects of medications, or (4) wish to avoid the long-term use of pharmacological therapy.[48]

It is important to note that in the treatment of acute or chronic forms of allergic eye diseases, patient compliance may not be ideal, given the false impression of poor efficacy of treatment.[49]

References

1. Pelikan Z. Seasonal and perennial allergic conjunctivitis: the possible role of nasal allergy. Clin Experiment Ophthalmol 2009;37:448–57.
2. Bielory L. Ocular allergy. Mt Sinai J Med 2011;78:740–58.
3. Bilkhu PS, Wolffsohn JS, Naroo SA. Non-pharmacological and pharmacological management of seasonal and perennial allergic conjunctivitis. Cont Lens Anterior Eye 2012;35:9–16.
4. Friedlaender MH. Ocular allergy. Curr Opin Allergy Clin Immunol 2011;11:477–82.
5. Ziska L, Knowlton K, Rogers C, et al. Recent warming by latitude associated with increased length of ragweed pollen season in central North America. Proc Natl Acad Sci USA 2011;108:4248–51.
6. Rosario N, Bielory L. Epidemiology of allergic conjunctivitis. Curr Opin Allergy Clin Immunol 2011;11:471–6.

7. Offiah I, Calder VL. Immune mechanisms in allergic eye diseases: what is new? Curr Opin Allergy Clin Immunol 2009;9:477–81.

8. Kari O, Haahtela T, Laine P, et al. Cellular characteristics of non-allergic eosinophilic conjunctivitis. Acta Ophthalmol 2010;88:245–50.

9. Katelaris CH, Bielory L. Evidence-based study design in ocular allergy trials. Curr Opin Allergy Clin Immunol 2008;8:484–8.

10. Choi SH, Bielory L. Late-phase reaction in ocular allergy. Curr Opin Allergy Clin Immunol 2008;8:438–44.

11. Leonardi A, Fregona IA, Plebani M, et al. Th1- and Th2-type cytokines in chronic ocular allergy. Graefes Arch Clin Exp Ophthalmol 2006;244:1240–5.

12. Leonardi A, Curnow SJ, Zhan H, et al. Multiple cytokines in human tear specimens in seasonal and chronic allergic eye disease and in conjunctival fibroblast cultures. Clin Exp Allergy 2006;36:777–84.

13. Hom MM, Nguyen AL, Bielory L. Allergic conjunctivitis and dry eye syndrome. Ann Allergy Asthma Immunol 2012;108:163–6.

14. Kosina-Hagyo K, Veres A, Fodor E, et al. Tear film function in patients with seasonal allergic conjunctivitis outside the pollen season. Int Arch Allergy Immunol 2012;157:81–8.

15. Trocme SD, Sra KK. Spectrum of ocular allergy. Curr Opin Allergy Clin Immunol 2002;2:423–7.

16. Mantelli F, Lambiase A, Bonini S. A simple and rapid diagnostic algorithm for the detection of ocular allergic diseases. Curr Opin Allergy Clin Immunol 2009;9:471–6.

17. Bielory BP, O'Brien TP, Bielory L. Management of seasonal allergic conjunctivitis: guide to therapy. Acta Ophthalmol 2012;90:399–407.

18. Wiszniewska M, Pas-Wyroslak A, Palczynski C, et al. Eosinophilia in conjunctival tear fluid among patients with pollen allergy. Ann Allergy Asthma Immunol 2011;107:281–2.

19. Nivenius E, Van der Ploeg I, Gafvelin G, et al. Conjunctival provocation with airborne allergen in patients with atopic keratoconjunctivitis. Clin Exp Allergy 2012;42:58–65.

20. Mourao EM, Rosario NA. Adverse reactions to the allergen conjunctival provocation test. Ann Allergy Asthma Immunol 2011;107:373–4.

21. Radcliffe MJ, Lewith GT, Prescott P, et al. Do skin prick and conjunctival provocation tests predict symptom severity in seasonal allergic rhinoconjunctivitis? Clin Exp Allergy 2006;36:1488–93.

22. Leonardi A, Fregona IA, Gismondi M, et al. Correlation between conjunctival provocation test (CPT) and systemic allergometric tests in allergic conjunctivitis. Eye (Lond) 1990;4(Pt 5):760–4.

23. Bielory L. Ocular allergy treatment. Immunol Allergy Clin North Am 2008;28:189–224, vii.

24. Dockhorn RJ, Duckett TG. Comparison of Naphcon-A and its components (naphazoline and pheniramine) in a provocative model of allergic conjunctivitis. Curr Eye Res 1994;13:319–24.

25. Duzman E, Warman A, Warman R. Efficacy and safety of topical oxymetazoline in treating allergic and environmental conjunctivitis. Ann Ophthalmol 1986;18:28–31.

26. Canonica GW, Ciprandi G, Petzold U, et al. Topical azelastine in perennial allergic conjunctivitis. Curr Med Res Opin 2003;19:321–9.

27. Borazan M, Karalezli A, Akova YA, et al. Efficacy of olopatadine HCl 0.1%, ketotifen fumarate 0.025%, epinastine HCl 0.05%, emedastine 0.05% and fluorometholone acetate 0.1% ophthalmic solutions for seasonal allergic conjunctivitis: a placebo-controlled environmental trial. Acta Ophthalmol 2009;87:549–54.

28. Pradhan S, Abhishek K, Mah F. Epinastine: topical ophthalmic second generation antihistamine without significant systemic side effects. Expert Opin Drug Metab Toxicol 2009;5:1135–40.

29. Takamura E, Nomura K, Fujishima H, et al. Efficacy of levocabastine hydrochloride ophthalmic suspension in the conjunctival allergen challenge test in Japanese subjects with seasonal allergic conjunctivitis. Allergol Int 2006;55:157–65.

30. Torkildsen GL, Ousler GW 3rd, Gomes P. Ocular comfort and drying effects of three topical antihistamine/mast cell stabilizers in adults with allergic conjunctivitis: a randomized, double-masked crossover study. Clin Ther 2008;30:1264–71.

31. Bohets H, McGowan C, Mannens G, et al. Clinical pharmacology of alcaftadine, a novel antihistamine for the prevention of allergic conjunctivitis. J Ocul Pharmacol Ther 2011;27:187–95.

32. Lambiase A, Micera A, Bonini S. Multiple action agents and the eye: do they really stabilize mast cells? Curr Opin Allergy Clin Immunol 2009;9:454–65.

33. James IG, Campbell LM, Harrison JM, et al. Comparison of the efficacy and tolerability of topically administered azelastine, sodium cromoglycate and placebo in the treatment of seasonal allergic conjunctivitis and rhino-conjunctivitis. Curr Med Res Opin 2003;19:313–20.

34. Das D, Khan M, Gul A, et al. Safety and efficacy of lodoxamide in vernal keratoconjunctivitis. J Pak Med Assoc 2011;61:239–41.

35. Williams JI, Kennedy KS, Gow JA, et al. Bepotastine Besilate Ophthalmic Solutions Study Group. Prolonged effectiveness of bepotastine besilate ophthalmic solution for the treatment of ocular symptoms of allergic conjunctivitis. J Ocul Pharmacol Ther 2011;27:385–93.

36. Shimura M, Yasuda K, Miyazawa A, et al. Pre-seasonal treatment with topical olopatadine suppresses the clinical symptoms of seasonal allergic conjunctivitis. Am J Ophthalmol 2011;151:697–702, e2.

37. Alexander M, Patel P, Allegro S, et al. Supplementation of fexofenadine therapy with nedocromil sodium 2% ophthalmic solution to treat ocular symptoms of seasonal allergic conjunctivitis. Clin Experiment Ophthalmol 2003;31:206–12.

38. Torkildsen GL, Abelson MB, Gomes PJ. Bioequivalence of two formulations of ketotifen fumarate ophthalmic solution: a single-center, randomized, double-masked conjunctival allergen challenge investigation in allergic conjunctivitis. Clin Ther 2008;30:1272–82.

39. Swamy BN, Chilov M, McClellan K, et al. Topical non-steroidal anti-inflammatory drugs in allergic conjunctivitis: meta-analysis of randomized trial data. Ophthalmic Epidemiol 2007;14:311–9.

40. Yaylali V, Demirlenk I, Tatlipinar S, et al. Comparative study of 0.1% olopatadine hydrochloride and 0.5% ketorolac tromethamine in the treatment of seasonal allergic conjunctivitis. Acta Ophthalmol Scand 2003;81:378–82.

41. Schechter BA. Ketorolac tromethamine 0.4% as a treatment for allergic conjunctivitis. Expert Opin Drug Metab Toxicol 2008;4:507–11.

42. Bielory BP, Perez VL, Bielory L. Treatment of seasonal allergic conjunctivitis with ophthalmic corticosteroids: in search of the perfect ocular corticosteroids in the treatment of allergic conjunctivitis. Curr Opin Allergy Clin Immunol 2010;10:469–77.

43. Ilyas H, Slonim CB, Braswell GR, et al. Long-term safety of loteprednol etabonate 0.2% in the treatment of seasonal and perennial allergic conjunctivitis. Eye Contact Lens 2004;30:10–3.

44. Bielory L. Ocular symptom reduction in patients with seasonal allergic rhinitis treated with the intranasal corticosteroid mometasone furoate. Ann Allergy Asthma Immunol 2008;100:272–9.

45. LaForce CF, Dockhorn RJ, Findlay SR, et al. Fluticasone propionate: an effective alternative treatment for seasonal allergic rhinitis in adults and adolescents. J Fam Pract 1994;38:145–52.

46. Utine CA, Stern M, Akpek EK. Clinical review: topical ophthalmic use of cyclosporine A. Ocul Immunol Inflamm 2010;18:352–61.

47. Garcia DP, Alperte JI, Cristóbal JA, et al. Topical tacrolimus ointment for treatment of intractable atopic keratoconjunctivitis: a case report and review of the literature. Cornea 2011;30:462–5.

48. Moote W, Kim H. Allergen-specific immunotherapy. Allergy Asthma Clin Immunol 2011;7(Suppl. 1):S5.

49. Mishra GP, Tamboli V, Jwala J, et al. Recent patents and emerging therapeutics in the treatment of allergic conjunctivitis. Recent Pat Inflamm Allergy Drug Discov 2011;5:26–36.

14 Vernal Keratoconjunctivitis

KENNETH C. MATHYS and W. BARRY LEE

Vernal Keratoconjunctivitis

Vernal Keratoconjunctivitis (VKC) is an allergic ocular surface disease that affects primarily the conjunctiva and cornea and is characterized by chronic ocular surface inflammation. The chronicity of VKC can lead to debilitating ocular surface disease, with myriad potential complications, that may permanently affect vision. The name 'vernal' itself implies spring and youth, reflecting two common characteristics of VKC. It primarily affects children, although it may rarely occur in adults. In addition, the disease course is often seasonal with exacerbations in the warmer months (typically the spring), but in some patients it can become a chronic condition and occur throughout the year.[1] Males are affected more than females; however, one series reports a female preponderance in cases.[2] The diagnosis of VKC is clinical and is based on typical signs and symptoms. The classic signs include conjunctival hyperemia, tarsal papillae, limbal papillae, and ropy mucous discharge. Symptoms of VKC are itching, photophobia, and tearing. There may also be pain if the cornea is involved. The disorder is found with varying frequency in all geographic areas, but has a higher incidence in warmer climates. VKC has been described in the ophthalmic literature for over 150 years. The condition has been referred to in the literature by many names, including spring catarrh, phlyctaena palladia, circumcorneal hypertrophy and conjunctivitis verrucosa, but the current nomenclature of vernal keratoconjunctivitis is now almost universally used.[3]

The precise etiology and pathogenesis of VKC are still unknown. There have been many clinical and laboratory studies performed in recent years in an attempt to answer these questions. While it is established that VKC is an IgE- and Th2-mediated allergic condition, it is clear that the simplified concept of a type I allergic hypersensitivity reaction does not fully describe the complex immune process involved in VKC.[4–6]

VKC may affect the superior palpebral conjunctiva, the bulbar conjunctiva, or both, with patients exhibiting two forms of disease: palpebral vernal and limbal vernal. The inferior palpebral conjunctiva is less often involved with VKC. In the palpebral form, the superior tarsal conjunctiva is the primary location of pathology, making ptosis a common associated finding of palpebral VKC. Papillae of various sizes develop on the superior tarsal conjunctiva (Fig. 14.1). As the disease progresses, the papillae may coalesce into larger lesions referred to as 'cobblestone' or 'paving-stone' papillae (Fig. 14.2). Deep furrows are seen in between the papillae. These large papillae may cause mechanical damage to the cornea. The discharge is thick and ropy and characteristically has a dirty white or cream color. Microscopic examination of the discharge shows large numbers of eosinophils, mononuclear, and polymor-

phonuclear inflammatory cells.[1] Scarring of the conjunctiva is not seen in VKC.

In the limbal form, there is a broadening and opacification of the limbus. This can produce a semitransparent, thickened appearance of the limbus. These signs are often seen first in the superior limbus, but can spread 360 degrees. Discrete yellow or gray nodules may appear in the thickened limbus. In severe cases, these nodules can become confluent. White, punctate lesions known as Horner–Trantas dots may develop in the hypertrophied limbus (Fig. 14.3).

Either form of VKC can affect the cornea, with the earliest corneal manifestation typically found as a superficial punctate keratitis, referred to as keratitis of Tobgy.[1] It can progress to multiple, discrete, dull gray points of epithelial

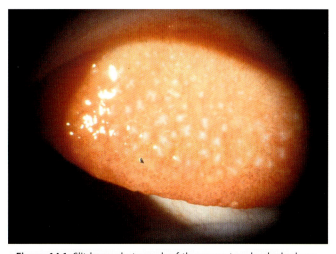

Figure 14.1 Slit lamp photograph of the upper tarsal palpebral conjunctiva, demonstrating a diffuse papillary reaction.

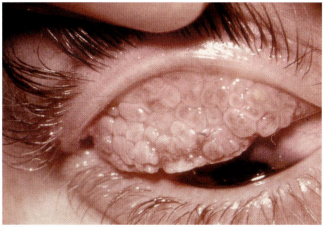

Figure 14.2 Giant papillae of the upper tarsal palpebral conjunctiva. The classic cobblestone appearance of VKC.

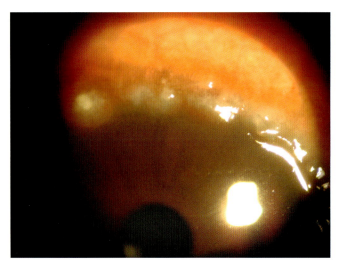

Figure 14.3 Slit lamp photograph of Horner–Trantas, dots characteristic of limbal vernal keratoconjunctivitis.

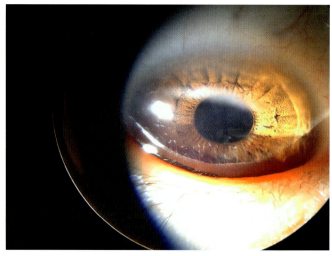

Figure 14.5 Slit lamp photograph of pseudogerontoxon, in the superior midperipheral cornea.

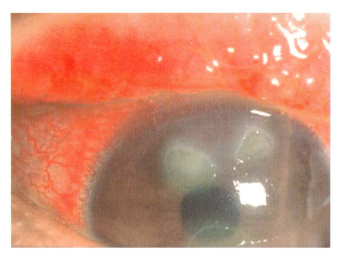

Figure 14.4 Slit lamp photograph of two vernal shield ulcers in association with injection and papillary changes of the superior tarsal conjunctiva.

irregularity and degeneration, which stain with fluorescein or rose bengal. These spots may become confluent and coalesce into a corneal erosion or ulcer, referred to as a vernal shield ulcer (Fig. 14.4). The ulcer is typically indolent, characteristically oval in shape, and most commonly found in the upper half of the cornea. The ulcer is often shallow with white edges. A grayish opacification of Bowman's membrane may develop which will eventually harden into a gray plaque in the base of the ulcer. Often, plaque removal is needed to promote healing of the ulcer. After an ulcer is healed, corneal neovascularization and scarring are often seen.[1,7] Another potential complication of the shield ulcer is secondary bacterial or fungal infection by colonized pathogens.[8]

Another corneal manifestation of VKC is pseudogerontoxon, which resembles a segment of arcus senilis or gerontoxon, and is seen in many individuals with limbal VKC. The lesion is typically found a few millimeters anterior to the limbus in the midperipheral cornea and is often arcuate in pattern. It may be unifocal or multifocal (Fig. 14.5). It is an

important clinical finding because pseudogerontoxon is often the only clinical evidence of previous allergic eye disease.[9]

Demographics

Vernal keratoconjunctivitis is predominantly a disease of children and adolescents. Two large case series from central Italy, where there is a relatively high incidence of VKC, have reported the mean age at diagnosis as between 6.8 ± 5 years and 11 ± 5 years.[10,11] Only 4% of newly diagnosed patients were older than 20 at the time of initial diagnosis.[10] There are more males with VKC than females. Multiple case series have reported a male to female ratio of approximately $3:1$.[10,11] Interestingly, the higher number of males affected seems to only be present in children and adolescents. When looking at adults with VKC over the age of 20 years, the male to female ratio is $1:1$.[11] Estrogen and progesterone receptors are present in the epithelium and subepithelium of patients with VKC, while not normally present in healthy epithelium. The role these hormonal receptors play in VKC is not known.[12]

Prevalence

The prevalence of vernal keratoconjunctivitis varies by geographic region. The disease is most prevalent in warm climates. In geographic regions with temperate seasonal change, a relapsing pattern of VKC is often seen, with flare-ups occurring in the spring and summer months, and remission of symptoms in the cooler winter months. In climates that remain hot all year round, a perennial form of VKC is commonly seen. This is not an absolute finding, and individual patients with either relapsing or perennial VKC are seen in any climate. The estimated overall prevalence of VKC is $3.2/10\,000$ across all of western Europe. A higher prevalence is seen in Italy ($27.8/10\,000$) where the climate is warmer, while a lower prevalence of VKC is seen in Norway ($1.9/10\,000$) where the climate is cooler.[13]

Co-Morbid Conditions

Since VKC is an allergic condition, other allergic co-morbid conditions may be associated. A family history of atopic disease is seen in 48% of patients with VKC.[11] Among patients with VKC, 15–64% also have asthma, 30–49% also have allergic rhinitis, and 16–24% also have eczema.[10,11] Not all patients with VKC have co-morbid conditions. VKC is the only clinical issue in 59% of patients.[11] Allergen skin prick testing for common allergens is positive in 44–58% of VKC patients. Specific serum IgE levels are positive in 57% of VKC patients,[10] and are increased in VKC patients compared to serum IgE levels in normal controls.[11] Other than allergic conditions, keratoconus is the disease most commonly associated with VKC. Prevalence of clinical keratoconus in VKC patients is 2–9%. In a large cohort of patients with VKC, 27% were identified as having keratoconus based on videokeratography maps.[14] Eye rubbing, which is common among patients with VKC, due to chronic eye itching, has been proposed as an explanation for the high rate of keratoconus in this cohort.[15] Iatrogenic cataracts from steroid use, as well as steroid-induced glaucoma complications, have been reported. Bacterial keratitis and shield ulcers are seen in 10% of patients with VKC and these are typically the most severe cases. Fungal keratitis is rare, but has been reported in VKC.[16]

Genetics

To date, no specific genotype has been demonstrated to have a relationship with vernal keratoconjunctivitis. Current research is investigating this question. The presence of eosinophilia, increased expression of cytokines, and other cellular mediators, including increased CD4 lymphocyte cells in the epithelium and subepithelium of affected patients suggests VKC may be associated with up-regulation of the cytokine gene cluster on chromosome 5q. This gene regulates production of IL-3, -4, -5, granulocyte/macrophage-colony-stimulating factor (GM-CSF), type 2 T-helper cells, growth of mast cells and eosinophils and production of IgE, all of which are seen in the pathology of VKC.[17]

Clinical Features

The classic and most constant clinical symptoms of vernal keratoconjunctivitis are itching, redness, photophobia, and tearing; these are all seen in >90% of patients with VKC.[11] The tarsal form of the disease is the most common, with superior tarsal papillae seen in 44–83% of patients. Limbal papillae are seen in 8–11%, and a mixed clinical picture is found in 9–46% of patients with VKC. Giant cobblestone papillae occur in 16% of patients.[10,11,14] Ninety-eight percent of cases are bilateral.[11] Other common signs include Horner–Trantas dots in 15% of reported cases and mucous discharge in 53% of reported cases.[11] Treatment of VKC is guided by the severity of symptoms. The response to treatment is variable. In one case series, with long-term follow up of greater than 3 years, 27% of patients had a complete resolution, 35.4% showed improvement but mild to moderate persistence of symptoms, and 32% had no change in signs or symptoms as a response to therapy. Severe worsening involving visual loss is rare and is seen in cases with ulcerative keratitis. 6% of patients had a loss of two or more lines of best corrected vision due to corneal scarring and neovascularization.[11] A clinical grading system has been developed to help standardize communication regarding clinical features and severity (Table 14.1).

Pathophysiology

Many immunohistochemical and molecular biological studies have demonstrated that there are a multitude of cellular signaling pathways involved in the allergic response in vernal keratoconjunctivitis. The mechanisms governing the coordination and recruitment of inflammatory cells in the conjunctiva of patients with VKC is complex and not fully understood. As with other allergic conditions, patients with VKC display signs of a type 1 hypersensitivity reaction. In this acute allergic reaction, allergens bind to IgE on mast cells and basophils, stimulating degranulation and release of cytokines and histamine. Levels of IgE may be elevated in the serum and tears of patients with VKC when compared to normal controls.[18,19] Concentration of histamine in tears has been shown to be higher in patients with VKC

Table 14.1 Clinical Grading of Vernal Keratoconjunctivitis

VKC Grading	Symptoms	Conjunctival Hyperemia	Conjunctival Secretion	Papillary Reaction	Trantas Dots	Corneal Involvement
Grade 0 quiescent	None	None/mild	None	Mild to moderate	None	None
Grade 1 mild	Mild and occasional	Mild	None/mild	Mild to moderate	None	None
Grade 2A moderate	Moderate and intermittent	Mild	Mild	Mild to severe	None	None
Grade 2B moderate	Moderate and persistent	Mild to moderate	Mild to moderate	Mild to severe	None	Superficial punctate keratitis
Grade 3 severe	Moderate to Severe and persistent	Moderate to severe	Severe	Severe injection and edema	Few	Superficial punctate keratitis
Grade 4 critical	Severe and persistent	Moderate to severe	Severe	Severe injection and edema	Numerous	Corneal erosion or ulceration
Grade 5 evolution	None or mild	None or mild	None	Fibrosis and scarring	None	None

Adapted from Bonini S, Sacchetti M, Mantelli F, et al. Clinical grading of vernal keratoconjunctivitis. Curr Opin Allergy Clin Immunol 2007;7:436–41.

compared to controls. This may be due to reduced inactivation of histamine by histaminase and increased local production by basal and mast cells.[20] The theory of a type 1 hypersensitivity reaction alone cannot explain the pathology of VKC. Fifty percent of patients with VKC had negative skin tests to common allergens.[11] In addition, tear samples of VKC patients, as well as conjunctival biopsies, demonstrate many cytokines and immune cells.[4] Figure 14.6 demonstrates a schematic diagram of the allergic cascade responsible for VKC.

Activated helper T cells, mast cells, basophils, eosinophils, macrophages, plasma cells, and fibroblasts are found in the conjunctiva of patients with VKC. The immune cells are often organized as small lymphoid follicles without a germinal center. Th2 lymphocytes and their cytokines IL-3, IL-4, and IL-5 are found at elevated levels in tears of VKC patients.[21] Research has shown that Th2 cells are important in the pathophysiology of VKC, while Th1 lymphocytes and the cytokines produced by these cells, IL-2, interferon gamma, and tumor necrosis factor beta (TNF-β), are not found at elevated levels in VKC patients.[22] Thus, it is believed that Th2 cells are important in mediating the inflammatory response in VKC.

Chemokines are involved in leukocyte recruitment and chemotaxis in the inflammatory response. Chemokines bind to G-protein coupled receptors and signal via secondary messengers to alter cell behavior. Monocyte chemotactic protein (MCP), regulated upon activation, normal T cells expressed and secreted (RANTES), exotaxin, and macrophage inhibitory protein (MIP), may have an important role in regulating the allergic response in VKC.[23]

Mast cell-released proteases, tryptase, and chymase are elevated in tears of patients with VKC.[24] Matrix metalloproteinases (MMPs) are extracellular enzymes that are active in promotion of inflammation and degradation of the extracellular matrix. MMP-1, -3, -9, and -13 have been found in high concentration of conjunctival biopsies of VKC patients.[25] Transforming growth factor (TGF) β1, β2 and their intracellular downstream effector proteins, Sma- and Mad- related protein (Smad) -2, -3 are increased in the stroma of VKC patients, compared to normal controls.[26] Both nerve growth factor (NGF) and substance P, which is modulated by NGF, are found at increased plasma levels in VKC patients, compared to controls.[27] Immunohistochemical study of the collagen in the conjunctival epithelium and stroma of patients with VKC shows increased amounts of type I and III collagen, as well as a thickened basement membrane, consisting of type IV collagen.[28,29]

Corneal confocal microscopy has been used to examine morphologic changes of the cornea in vivo in patients with VKC. Increased numbers of activated keratocytes and inflammatory cells are seen in the anterior stroma of VKC patients, compared to normal controls. Also, increased epithelial cell diameter and reflectivity is seen in the superficial epithelium of the cornea.[30] The combined effect of these cellular mediators is promotion of inflammation, stimulation of fibroblast growth and proliferation, and increased collagen production in the conjunctival and corneal stroma.[31] When chronic, these changes lead to tissue remodeling and scarring.

Differential Diagnosis

The diagnosis of vernal keratoconjunctivitis is based on the clinical findings. As indicated previously, the typical symptoms of chronic itching, redness, and photophobia, found with clinical signs of large superior tarsal papilla, limbal papilla, or ropy mucous discharge in a young boy are very characteristic of VKC. Milder cases may pose more of a diagnostic dilemma. Other ocular conditions that could be confused with VKC include atopic keratoconjunctivitis, giant papillary conjunctivitis, and trachoma in endemic areas. If needed, conjunctival cytology, tear film analysis, and conjunctival cultures can be used to help establish the diagnosis.

Treatment

There are varying clinical presentations of vernal keratoconjunctivitis, ranging from mild itching and redness to vision threatening corneal scarring. Due to this wide variation in presentation, there is not a specific treatment for VKC that is appropriate for all patients. Moreover, since exacerbations are common among individuals with VKC, treating physicians must monitor and adjust therapy and treatment plans as needed. Options for treatment of VKC encompass environmental, medical, and surgical therapies.

As VKC is a form of allergic conjunctivitis, most treatment options are focused on interruption of the inflammatory immune response. As with other allergic conditions, removal of known allergens from contact with a patient can improve symptoms. Skin testing can be performed to

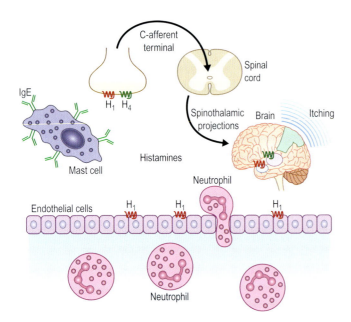

Figure 14.6 A schematic diagram depicting the pathophysiology of the allergic cascade responsible for VKC. The diagram shows the local reaction of IgE, histamine, and mast cells and their interaction with local histamine 1 (H_1) and histamine 2 (H_2) receptors and how they create the signal of itching generated from the brain after a local interaction with antigen in tissue. (From From Thurmond RL, Gelfand EW, Dunford PJ. The role of histamine H1 and H2 receptors in allergic inflammation: the search for new antihistamines. Nat Rev Drug Discov 2008;7(1):41–53.)

determine a patient's specific allergen sensitivities. For patients with seasonal flares associated with warmer humid climates, relocation to a cooler dry climate could be beneficial. There are obvious economic and geographic restrictions to the feasibility of these measures. Application of cool compresses to the closed eyelids will offer symptomatic relief for patients, but will not treat the underlying condition. Preservative-free artificial tears, used judiciously at room temperature or chilled in a refrigerator, will help to soothe the ocular surface and clear allergic antigens and mucous from the ocular surface.

There are many options for pharmacologic therapy for VKC. Topical vasoconstrictors, such as naphazoline and tetrahydrozoline are available over the counter and commonly used. Through vasoconstriction, they decrease conjunctival redness temporarily; however, rebound hyperemia with prolonged use limits their utility. Antiallergy eye drops, such as antihistamines and mast cell stabilizers, are the primary agents used to treat the chronic symptoms of itching, redness and irritation associated with mild to moderate VKC. Histamine released by mast cells found in submucosal tissue, is an important mediator in a type I allergic hypersensitivity reaction. Levocabastine 0.05%, a selective histamine (H_1) receptor antagonist, has been proven effective for treating ocular allergic symptoms of VKC.[32,33] Extensive research has documented the efficacy of mast cell stabilizers in treatment of VKC.[34–37] Mast cell stabilizers, including cromolyn sodium 4%, nedocromil sodium 2%, and lodoxamide 0.1%, work by inhibiting mast cell degranulation, suppressing the inflammatory cascade resulting from release of inflammatory mediators, including histamine from mast cells.

Newer topical agents combine the anti-inflammatory effect of a H_1 receptor antagonist and a mast cell stabilizer. These medications, including olopatadine 0.2%, epinastine, 0.05%, ketotifen 0.025%, and alcaftadine 0.25%, have been studied extensively for use in treatment of allergic conjunctivitis and vernal keratoconjunctivitis.[38] They are suitable for treatment of mild chronic symptoms of VKC, due to the low side effect profile and ease of use, with daily or twice-daily dosing. Oral H_1 receptor antagonists may also be used to control these symptoms.

Additionally, topical acetylcysteine can be beneficial for treatment and reduction of the thick mucus discharge seen with VKC. Acetylcysteine breaks disulfide bonds, thereby dissolving mucus, and it is effective as a mucolytic agent in this disease. It is formulated from commercially available Mucomyst, diluted to a 5% or 10% solution with artificial tears, and is applied four times a day.

Preservative-free topical nonsteroidal anti-inflammatory drops, ketorolac 0.5% and diclofenac 0.1% have been used effectively to treat VKC. Forty percent of patients treated with diclofenac for 120 days showed clinical improvement of symptoms.[39] Ketorolac 0.5% was shown to reduce the signs and symptoms of VKC more rapidly than topical cyclosporine 0.5%.[40]

Stronger anti-inflammatory medication is often required to treat a flare of vernal keratoconjunctivitis. Topical corticosteroid eye drops, including fluorometholone 0.1%, loteprednol 0.5%, prednisolone acetate 1%, and dexamethasone phosphate 0.1% are the primary treatment modality for flares of VKC. Fluorometholone 0.1% was shown to be more effective than nedocromil sodium for treating

symptoms of severe VKC.[41] Due to complications associated with prolonged use, topical corticosteroids should be administered in pulsed dosing with symptom flares and tapered off when symptoms are controlled. Complications of prolonged topical steroid use includes cataract and steroid-induced glaucoma, which have been reported in 2% of patients with VKC.[11] In addition, a solution (e.g. prednisolone sodium phosphate) may be preferred to a suspension (e.g. prednisolone acetate) in VKC, due to the adverse mechanical effects of the suspension particles in combination with large papillae. When topical corticosteroid drops are not effective or when a longer duration of the theraputic effect is desired, supratarsal injection of dexamethasone sodium phosphate (2 mg) or triamcinolone acetonide (20 mg) has been shown to improve symptoms.[42,43] Similar to corticosteroid drop use, supratarsal corticosteroid injection can cause an increase of intraocular pressure; therefore, it is imperative to monitor the intraocular pressure of patients following treatment.

Cyclosporine A has been studied as another therapeutic option for moderate to severe cases of vernal keratoconjunctivitis. Cyclosporine produces an anti-inflammatory effect by selectively suppressing the production of interleukin 2 by T lymphocytes. Multiple randomized, placebo controlled trials have demonstrated the effectiveness of cyclosporine A 1–2% at decreasing signs and symptoms of VKC, including itching, tearing, photophobia, conjunctival hyperemia, Trantas dots, and punctate keratitis.[44–47] Treatment benefit was noted as early as 2 weeks after treatment onset. Cyclosporine has been used for up to 4 months continuously without significant side effects, other than burning upon administration of the drops. Cyclosporine was not detected in the serum of patients using the drops.[47,48] Compared to dexamethasone 0.1%, cyclosporine A 2% was equally effective in reducing signs and symptoms of VKC when used for 1 month.[46] Symptoms often recur after cessation of the medication. For patients with moderate to severe VKC experiencing side effects of topical steroids, such as elevated IOP, cyclosporine may be an effective alternative treatment. Cyclosporine A 2% is not commercially available and must be made by a compounding pharmacy. Tacrolimus ointment (0.03%) is another antiinflammatory agent that has been shown effective against VKC by inhibiting the inflammatory actions of T cells.

Mitomycin-C (MMC) 0.01% has been used successfully to treat exacerbations of severe vernal keratoconjunctivitis.[49,50] It is an antibiotic drug which also acts as a nonselective inhibitor of cell proliferation. To limit toxic effects of the medication to the ocular surface, MMC is used for short intervals, up to 2 weeks and then stopped. The most common side effect is corneal punctate keratitis. Due to its inhibitory effect on wound healing, MMC should not be used in patients with corneal epithelial defects or shield ulcers. The authors have no experience with this technique and advocate caution with use of topical MMC.

Since no medical treatment has been universally effective at treating vernal keratoconjunctivitis, development of novel therapies continue. Intravenous immunoglobulin infusion, topical probiotic *Lactobacillus acidophilus* drops and oral montelukast sodium, have all been shown effective in treating VKC in small case series.[51–53] Further study is needed of these and other new treatment options.

References

1. Duke-Elder S. Vernal keratoconjunctivitis. In: Duke-Elder S, editor. System of ophthalmology, Vol. III, Diseases of the outer eye. London: Henry Kimpton; 1965. p. 476–93.
2. Tuft SJ, Dart JK, Kemeny M. Limbal vernal keratoconjunctivitis: Clinical characteristics and immunoglobulin E expression compared with palpebral vernal. Eye 1989;3:420–7.
3. Barney NP. Vernal and atopic keratoconjunctivitis. In: Krachmer JH, Mannis MJ, Holland EJ, editors. Cornea. 2nd ed. Philadelphia: Elsevier Mosby; 2005. p. 667–70.
4. Kumar S. Vernal keratoconjunctivitis: a major review. Acta Ophthalmol 2009;87:133–47.
5. Leonardi A, Secchi AG. Vernal keratoconjunctivitis. Int Ophthalmol Clin 2003;43:41–58.
6. Bonini S, Coassin M, Aronni S, et al. Vernal keratoconjunctivitis. Eye 2004;18:345–51.
7. Cameron JA. Shield ulcers and plaques of the cornea in vernal keratoconjunctivitis. Ophthalmology 1995;102:985–93.
8. Gedik S, Akova YA, Gür S. Secondary bacterial keratitis associated with shield ulcer caused by vernal conjunctivitis. Cornea 2006; 25:974–6.
9. Jeng BH, Whitcher JP, Margolis TP. Pseudogerontoxon. Clin Exp Ophthalmol 2004;32:433–4.
10. Leonardi A, Busca F, Motterle L, et al. Case series of 406 vernal keratoconjunctivitis patients: a demographic and epidemiological study. Acta Ophthalmol Scand 2006;84:406–10.
11. Bonini S, Bonini S, Lambiase A, et al. Vernal keratoconjunctivitis revisited: a case series of 195 patients with long-term follow-up. Ophthalmology 2000;107:1157–63.
12. Bonini S, Lambiase A, Schiavone M, et al. Estrogen and progesterone receptors in vernal keratoconjunctivitis. Ophthalmology 1995;102: 1374–9.
13. Bremond-Gignac D, Donadieu J, Leonardi A, et al. Prevalence of vernal keratoconjunctivitis: a rare disease? Br J Ophthalmol 2008; 92:1097–102.
14. Totan Y, Hepşen IF, Cekiç O, et al. Incidence of keratoconus in subjects with vernal keratoconjunctivitis: a videokeratographic study. Ophthalmology 2001;108:824–7.
15. Cameron JA, Al-Rajhi AA, Badr IA. Corneal ectasia in vernal keratoconjunctivitis. Ophthalmology 1989;96:1615–23.
16. Sridhar MS, Gopinathan U, Rao GN. Fungal keratitis associated with vernal keratoconjunctivitis. Cornea 2003;22:80–1.
17. Bonini S, Bonini S, Lambiase A, et al. Vernal keratoconjunctivitis: a model of 5q cytokine gene cluster disease. Int Arch Allergy Immunol 1995;107:95–8.
18. Samra Z, Zavaro A, Barishak Y, et al. Vernal keratoconjunctivitis: the significance of immunoglobulin E levels in tears and serum. Int Arch Allergy Appl Immunol 1984;74:158–64.
19. Fujishima H, Saito I, Takeuchi T, et al. Immunological characteristics of patients with vernal keratoconjunctivitis. Jpn J Ophthalmol 2002; 46:244–8.
20. Ableson MB, Leonardi AA, Smait LM, et al. Histaminease activity in patients with vernal keratoconjunctivitis. Ophthalmology 1995;102: 1958–63.
21. Metz DP, Hingorani M, Calder VL, et al. T-cell cytokines in chronic allergic eye disease. J Allergy Clin Immunol 1997;100:817–24.
22. Leonardi A, Borghesan F, Faggian D, et al. Tear and serum soluable leukocyte activation markers in conjunctival allergic disease. Am J Ophthalmol 2000;129:151–8.
23. Abu El-Asarar AM, Struyf S, Van Damme J, et al. Role of chemokines in vernal keratoconjunctivitis. Int Ophthalmol Clin 2003;43:33–9.
24. Ebihara N, Funaki T, Takai S, et al. Tear chymase in vernal keratoconjunctivitis. Curr Eye Res 2004;28:417–20.
25. Leonardi A, Brun P, Di Stefano A, et al. Matrix metalloproteases in vernal keratoconjunctivitis, nasal polyps and allergic asthma. Clin Exp Allergy 2007;37:872–9.
26. Leonardi A, Di Stephano A, Motterle L, et al. Transforming growth factor-B/Smad signalling pathway and conjunctival remodeling in vernal keratoconjunctivitis. Clin Exp Allergy 2011;41:52–60.
27. Lambiase A, Bonini S, Micera A, et al. Increased plasma levels of substance P in vernal keratoconjunctivitis. Invest Ophthalmol Vis Sci 1997;38:2161–4.
28. Abu El-Asar AM, Geboes K, al-Kharashi SA, et al. An immunohistochemical study of collagens in trachoma and vernal keratoconjunctivitis. Eye 1998;12:1001–6.
29. Leonardi A, Abatangelo G, Cortivo R, et al. Collagen types I and III in giant papillae of vernal keratoconjunctivitis. Br J Ophthalmol 1995; 79:482–5.
30. Leonardi A, Lazzarini D, Bortolotti M, et al. Corneal confocal microscopy in patients with vernal keratoconjunctivitis. Ophthalmology 2012;119:509–15.
31. Bonini S, Lambiase A, Sgrulletta R, et al. Allergic chronic inflammation of the ocular surface in vernal keratoconjunctivitis. Curr Opin Allergy Clin Immunol 2003;3:381–7.
32. Bonini S, Pierdomenico R. Levocabastine eye drops in vernal keratoconjunctivitis. Eur J Ophthalmol 1995;5:283–4.
33. Verin P, Allewaert R, Joyaux JC, et al. Comparison of lodoxamide 0.1% ophthalmic solution and levocabastine 0.05% ophthalmic suspension in vernal keratoconjunctivitis. Eur J Ophthalmol 2001;11:120–5.
34. Foster SC. Evaluation of topical cromolyn sodium in the treatment of vernal keratoconjunctivitis. Ophthalmology 1988;95:194–201.
35. Kazdan JJ, Crawford JS, Langer H, et al. Sodium cromoglycate (intal) in the treatment of vernal keratoconjunctivitis and allergic conjunctivitis. Can J Ophthalmol 1976;11:300–3.
36. Foster CS, Duncan J. Randomized clinical trial of topically administered cromolyn sodium for vernal keratoconjunctivitis. Am J Ophthalmol 1980;90:175–81.
37. Hennawi M. A double blind placebo controlled group comparative study of ophthalmic sodium cromoglycate and nedocromil sodium in the treatment of vernal keratoconjunctivitis. Br J Ophthalmol 1994; 78:365–9.
38. Corum I, Yeniad B, Bilgin LK, et al. Efficiency of olopatadine hydrochloride 0.1% in the treatment of vernal keratoconjunctivitis and goblet cell density. J Ocul Pharmacol Ther 2005;21:400–5.
39. D'Angelo G, Lambiase A, Cortes M, et al. Preservative free diclofenac sodium 0.1% for vernal keratoconjunctivitis. Graefes Arch Clin Exp Ophthalmol 2003;241:192–5.
40. Kosrirukvongs P, Luengchaichawange C. Topical cyclosporine 0.5 per cent and preservative-free ketorolac tromethamine 0.5 per cent in vernal keratoconjunctivitis. J Med Assoc Thai 2004;87:190–7.
41. Tabbara KF, Al-Kharashi SA. Efficacy of nedocromil 2% versus fluorometholone 0.1%: a randomised, double masked trial comparing the effects on severe vernal keratoconjunctivitis. Br J Ophthalmol 1999; 83:180–4.
42. Sani JS, Gupta A, Pandey SK, et al. Efficacy of supratarsal dexamethasone versus triamcinolone injection in recalcitrant vernal keratoconjunctivitis. Acta Ophthalmol Scand 1999;77:515–8.
43. Holslaw DS, Whitcher JP, Wong IG, et al. Supratarsal injection of corticosteroid in the treatment of refractory vernal keratoconjunctivitis. Am J of Ophthalmol 1996;121:243–9.
44. Bleik JH, Tabbara KF. Topical cyclosporine in vernal keratoconjunctivitis. Ophthalmology 1991;98:1679–84.
45. Gupta V, Sahu PK. Topical cyclosporine A in the management of vernal keratoconjunctivitis. Eye 2001;15:39–41.
46. De Smedt S, Nkurikiye J, Fonteyne Y, et al. Topical cyclosporine in the treatment of vernal keratoconjunctivitis in Rwanda, Central Africa: a prospective, randomised, double-masked, controlled clinical trial. Br J Ophthalmol 2012;96:323–8. doi:10.1136/bjophthalmol-2011-300415.
47. Spadavecchia L, Fanelli P, Tesse R, et al. Efficacy of 1.25% and 1% topical cyclosporine in the treatment of severe vernal keratoconjunctivitis in childhood. Pediatr Allergy Immunol 2006;17:527–32.
48. Mendicute J, Aranzasti C, Eder F, et al. Topical cyclosporine A 2% in the treatment of vernal keratoconjunctivitis. Eye 1997;11:75–8.
49. Akpek EK, Hasiripi H, Christen WG, et al. A randomized trial of low-dose, topical mitomycin-C in the treatment of severe vernal keratoconjunctivitis. Ophthalmology 2000;107:263–9.
50. Jain AK, Sukhija J. Low dose mitomycin-C in severe vernal keratoconjunctivitis: a randomized prospective double blind study. Indian J Ophthalmol 2006;54:111–6.
51. Derriman L, Nguyen DQ, Ramanan AV, et al. Intravenous immunoglobulin (IVIg) in the management of severe refractory vernal keratoconjunctivitis. Br J Ophthalmol 2010;94:667–9.
52. Iovieno A, Lambiase A, Sacchetti M, et al. Preliminary evidence of the efficacy of probiotic eye-drop treatment in patients with vernal keratoconjunctivitis. Graefes Arch Clin Exp Ophthalmol 2008;246: 435–41.
53. Lambiase A, Bonini S, Rasi G, et al. Montelukast, a leukotriene receptor antagonist, in vernal keratoconjunctivitis associated with asthma. Arch Ophthalmol 2003;121:615–20.

15 *Atopic Keratoconjunctivitis*

PRITI BATTA and ELMER Y. TU

Introduction

Within the spectrum of allergic eye diseases, atopic kerato-conjunctivitis (AKC), along with perennial allergic conjunctivitis (PAC) (Ch. 13), vernal keratoconjunctivitis (VKC) (Ch. 14) and, to a certain extent, giant papillary conjunctivitis (GPC) (Ch. 16), is categorized as a form of chronic allergic conjunctivitis (CAC). Along with the milder, more acute seasonal allergic conjunctivitis (SAC) (Ch. 13), these conditions characteristically involve an IgE-mediated type I hypersensitivity response, manifested by papillary conjunctivitis, with itching as a universal early symptom. However, the more chronic AKC, along with VKC, is distinguished from seasonal and perennial allergic conjunctivitis, by the complex recruitment of other immunologic mechanisms, including a prominent T-cell-mediated type IV hypersensitivity response, as well as a variety of other inflammatory cell types and cytokines. The potential for corneal involvement and opacification increases significantly with the CACs because of the severity and sustained nature of their inflammation. The highest incidence of visual loss is therefore, found in the most chronic of these disorders, AKC.

Definition and Associated Risk Factors

Atopic keratoconjunctivitis (AKC) was first described in 1952 by Hogan, who described five cases of atopic eczema associated with bilateral keratoconjunctivitis.[1] He recognized an association between the skin and eye findings, coining the term 'atopic keratoconjunctivitis.' His patients were notable for chronic conjunctival hyperemia and thickening, corneal epitheliopathy, and later corneal scarring and neovascularization. Based on his observations, he outlined several criteria to aid in diagnosing this unique condition: the presence or history of eczematous dermatitis, a family history of atopic disease, associated allergies (asthma, hay fever), eosinophilia, and a characteristic keratoconjunctivitis associated with exacerbations of the dermatitis.

Few studies have established the incidence of AKC. However, atopic dermatitis (AD), its most frequent extra-ocular association, has been estimated to affect between 5% and 20% of the general population, making it the most common chronic inflammatory condition of the skin. The incidence of AD is greatest in the pediatric population Twenty-five to forty-two percent of AD patients are found to have ocular involvement.[2,3] AKC may occur at any time after the onset of the associated dermatitis or other atopic condition, and is not necessarily correlated with exacerbations of these conditions.[4] The initial presentation of ocular symptoms in AKC most commonly occurs in the second to third decade of life, with some patients presenting earlier or

later. Visually significant complications most frequently occur in the fourth to fifth decades, with more men affected than women. The condition then remains chronic for years, usually requiring lifelong treatment. Studies suggest that an earlier onset of AKC, for example in childhood, carries the greatest risk for tear film abnormalities and greater ocular surface damage.[5] A survey of CAC in a referral practice found that AKC and VKC were equally observed (39% each), while 13% were diagnosed with PAC.[6] However, the chronicity and visual complications of AKC would be expected to skew this population, causing AKC to be over-represented in referral practice, when compared to the general population.

As suggested by Hogan, the strong association between AKC and eczematous dermatitis cannot be overemphasized, with at least 95% of AKC cases presenting in patients with some history of this chronic skin condition.[7] Other atopic conditions associated with AKC include asthma and allergic rhinitis, each seen in 65–87% of AKC patients.[8] Although a handful of case reports have described AKC without other atopic disease, later investigation will usually reveal some form of systemic atopy. Patients will also frequently describe a family history of atopy. Recently, Guglielmetti et al. have suggested that Hogan's definition be modified to include the clinical features described below, combined with the presence of any atopic condition (e.g. atopic dermatitis, periocular eczema, asthma), occurring at any time point during the atopy, independent of its severity, and exhibiting corneal involvement at some point in the course of disease.[4]

Clinical Presentation

The initial symptoms of AKC include non-specific tearing and irritation. Similar to other allergic eye conditions, chronically itchy, red eyes are usually a prominent feature. Patients will complain of a stringy mucoid discharge, sometimes leading to difficulty opening the eyelids upon awakening. Patients rarely complain of pain, but often have discomfort and photophobia. Initially, blurred vision may be intermittent when due to tear film and ocular surface issues, but may become chronic if due to later corneal scarring. Unlike SAC and PAC, symptoms of AKC are usually present year-round, though a significant number of patients may note seasonal exacerbations.

EYELIDS

The periorbital skin and eyelids display a scaling, flaky dermatitis consistent with eczema (Fig. 15.1). There may be periorbital hyperpigmentation, which may lighten in response to control of the inflammation. In long-standing AKC, de Hertoghe sign, or absence of the lateral brow, is

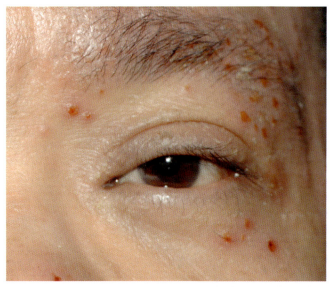

Figure 15.1 Atopic eczema. Note flaking dermatitis, excoriated skin lesions and thickening and erythema of skin overlying medial brow.

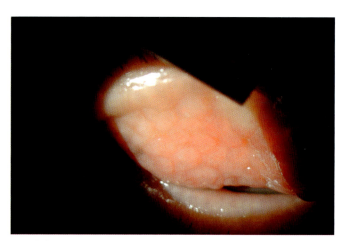

Figure 15.3 Giant papillae on superior palpebral conjunctiva. This patient recently underwent superior intratarsal corticosteroid injection for treatment of atopic symptoms. Note resultant flattening of papillae.

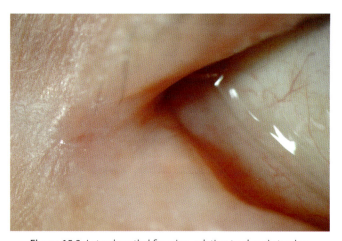

Figure 15.2 Lateral canthal fissuring, relating to chronic tearing.

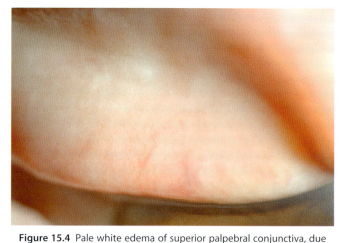

Figure 15.4 Pale white edema of superior palpebral conjunctiva, due to diffuse inflammatory infiltrate. Note obscuration of underlying blood vessels.

occasionally seen and may also be related to chronic eye rubbing. Vertical corrugations near the medial canthus of the upper and lower eyelid may also result. The eyelid margins may be thickened, edematous, and hyperemic. Eyelid edema may lead to Dennie–Morgan lines, single or double creases in the lower eyelid. The eyelid skin is often fissured, and lateral canthal ulceration related to chronic tearing may be present (Fig. 15.2). Lid malposition (usually ectropion), ptosis, lagophthalmos and madarosis may all result from chronic eyelid edema and inflammation. The chronic edema can lead to permanent lid swelling, a hallmark of long-standing atopic eye disease. Keratinization of the eyelid margins is sometimes observed, along with associated meibomianitis and obliteration of meibomian glands.

CONJUNCTIVA

The palpebral conjunctiva reveals papillary hypertrophy, more prominent on the lower tarsus. There may be giant papillae as in VKC (Fig. 15.3). Diffuse sheet-like infiltration of the conjunctiva may lead to pale white edema and obscuration of blood vessels (Fig. 15.4). Conjunctival scarring may occur, often in a reticular or septal pattern (Fig. 15.5). Subepithelial fibrosis can, in severe cases, lead to symblephara, inferior forniceal foreshortening, and cicatricial ectropion. The bulbar conjunctiva typically displays diffuse chemosis and injection. The limbus may become infiltrated and edematous, and gelatinous limbal hyperplasia, consisting of confluent macropapillae, is sometimes seen. Trantas dots, tiny white lesions consisting of necrotic epithelial cells and eosinophils, may be observed, similar to those in VKC (Fig. 15.6).

CORNEA

Corneal disease may be complicated by the late development of corneal hypesthesia in patients with AKC, resulting in a paradoxic reduction in surface symptoms, including itching. Punctate epithelial keratopathy is the most common corneal finding. Filamentary keratitis may occur,

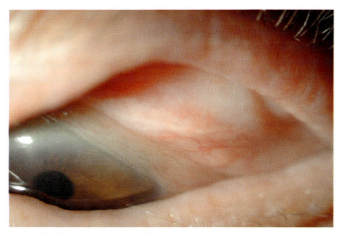

Figure 15.5 Reticular scarring of superior palpebral conjunctiva. Note chemosis of bulbar conjunctiva, overriding superior cornea.

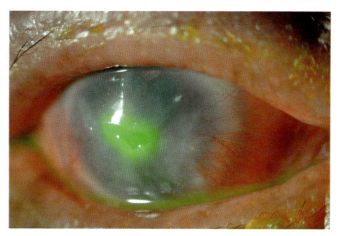

Figure 15.7 Persistent epithelial defect. Note diffuse corneal scarring and extensive corneal neovascularization.

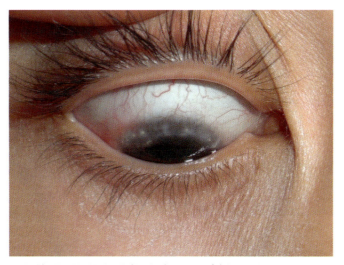

Figure 15.6 Trantas dots and pannus of the superior cornea.

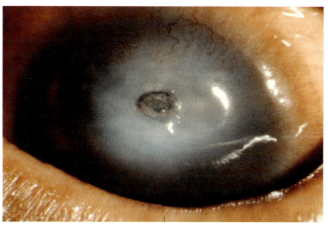

Figure 15.8 Central corneal scar in patient with prior shield ulcer.

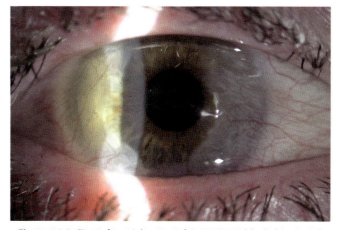

Figure 15.9 Circumferential pannus formation and limbal stem cell deficiency, associated with atopic keratoconjunctivitis.

sometimes with very thick mucoid filamentary strands and possibly related to tear film instability, due to goblet cell abnormalities and deficient mucin secretion, also commonly featured in AKC. Persistent epithelial defects frequently occur in the setting of a dry and inflamed ocular surface and may eventually lead to macroerosions (Fig. 15.7). These pose a particular problem in the atopic patient and can progress to frank bacterial ulcers. Atopic shield ulcers with 'vernal' plaque formation may also develop. Histologically, these adherent mucus plaques contain epithelial debris, eosinophils, and inflammatory cells, and probably result from a combination of mechanical irritation from giant papillae, as well as toxic epithelial changes secondary to inflammation. Persistence of these plaques may eventually cause stromal thinning and perforation (Fig. 15.8). The chronic inflammation and mechanical insult from palpebral scarring may eventually result in partial or total limbal stem cell deficiency (Fig. 15.9). Chronic inflammation and superimposed infection may lead to corneal scarring, neovascularization, and lipid deposition. Severe pannus often develops, typically affecting the superior one-third of the cornea. Vision may decline due to obscuration of the visual axis, irregular astigmatism, and/or ocular surface

compromise. A pseudogerontoxon may be seen in the peripheral cornea, which resembles a short, circumferential segment of arcus senilis. This localized area of lipid deposition, related to abnormal vascular permeability at the limbus, may be the only evidence of previous atopic disease in a quiet eye.[9]

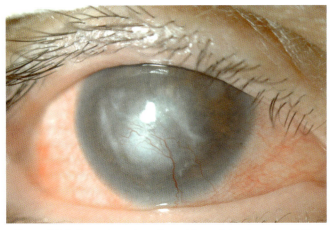

Figure 15.10 Herpetic scar in patient with atopic keratoconjunctivitis.

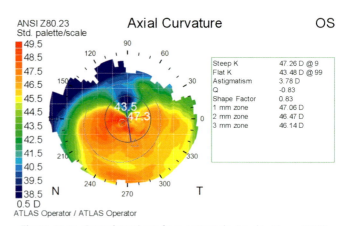

Figure 15.11 Contralateral eye from patient depicted in Figure 15.10, showing keratoconus on corneal topography.

OTHER COMPLICATIONS

Eyelid inflammation is common in AKC, often related to staphylococcal blepharitis. In fact, patients with atopic dermatitis are found to have high rates of bacterial skin colonization, specifically with staphylococcal species. AKC patients are at higher risk of corneal superinfections because of an unstable ocular surface, the local bacterial colonization of the eyelids, and a dysfunctional innate immune system.[10] Herpes simplex keratitis, frequently bilateral, is another well-known complication of AKC, and is presumably related to abnormalities in the atopic host's immune defenses (Fig. 15.10). Herpetic epithelial lesions may be recurrent, especially when topical or systemic immunosuppressants are required to control the atopic state.[11] Management is especially difficult because epithelial AKC lesions may be difficult to distinguish from HSV keratitis.

Rapidly progressive cataracts frequently develop in AKC patients, classically described as anterior subcapsular opacities, usually stellate or shield-like in appearance. The pathogenesis for atopic cataract is unclear, though some have suggested that high levels of IgE may be correlated with development of cataract in these patients.[12] The chronic use of topical steroids also predisposes to posterior subcapsular cataracts in AKC patients. Other forms of cataract may form independent of corticosteroid use, especially in patients with severe systemic atopic disease.

A higher incidence of keratoconus and pellucid marginal degeneration has been reported in AKC patients, likely related in part to chronic eye rubbing (Fig. 15.11).[3,13] Interestingly, a slightly higher rate of retinal detachment has also been noted in AKC patients. This may also be related to chronic eye rubbing, inducing degenerative vitreous changes.[14]

Power and colleagues reported on the frequency of different clinical features in AKC, based on long-term follow-up (average, 7 years) of a cohort of 20 AKC patients.[8] In their series, all 20 patients had eczema, and half had a family member affected with atopy. All patients had conjunctival hyperemia, and 65% had papillary reaction. Roughly half displayed some form of conjunctival scarring, including subepithelial fibrosis, forniceal foreshortening and symblepharon formation. All patients had superficial punctate keratitis. Fourteen of the 20 patients had severe corneal complications, including persistent epithelial defect (seen in half of the patients), corneal ulceration, or bacterial keratitis. Three patients developed herpetic keratitis. Two had keratoconus. Seven patients (nine eyes) required penetrating keratoplasty, some for corneal perforation.

Immunology and Pathogenesis

All ocular allergic disorders are characterized by a hypersensitivity response, defined as an excessive reaction of the normal immune system, usually by exposure to an inciting antigen. Type I hypersensitivity, or IgE-mediated immediate hypersensitivity, predominates in PAC and SAC, but is also involved in other CACs, including AKC. By its nature, common inciting antigens are more easily identified in SAC because of the acute inflammatory response, and is evidenced by the exposure and seasonal pattern seen in SAC. Serum IgE levels are chronically elevated in AKC patients, as seen in individuals with other forms of atopy, but their levels are not necessarily correlated to severity of disease. Notably, serum IgE levels in AKC patients are higher than in patients with allergic conjunctivitis, probably reflecting a more chronic atopic state.[15] IgE levels in tear samples are also increased in AKC, and correlate with serum IgE levels.[15] However, AKC additionally involves a chronic inflammation of the ocular surface, a type IV delayed hypersensitivity response, where an immediate antigen is not easily identified.

A genetic predisposition combined with antigen sensitization is suspected in AKC and in its associated disease, atopic dermatitis. AKC may, however, represent either a common manifestation end point for a number of abnormal gene processes, or a single gene defect with variable phenotypic expression, modified by other gene polymorphisms and the environment. Tabbara et al. described the acquisition of new VKC and AKC after bone marrow transplantation, suggesting that the origin of atopy might lie in an abnormality of the pluripotential marrow stem cells.[16] Furthermore, a recently recognized Th2 cytokine, which may be involved in mast cell activation, IL-33, has been found to be up-regulated in giant papillae in AKC.[17] IL-33 is a ligand for ST2L, the gene for which an association with atopic dermatitis has been suggested. More recent studies suggest that an epithelial barrier defect may be responsible rather than a defect in immunoregulatory function. A strong association of a defect in the Filaggrin gene (FLG) with atopic dermatitis, asthma, eczema and ichthyosis vulgaris, has been described and confirmed in multiple pedigrees of families with AD. The filaggrin protein is not only an abundant and essential component of epithelial barrier function; its breakdown products are responsible for epithelial homeostasis, forming the skin's natural moisturizing factor (NMF).[18] Despite its association with asthma, filaggrin is not found in the bronchioles, suggesting that FLG mutations lead to a defective barrier which may allow earlier and stronger systemic antigen sensitization. A similar mechanism may contribute to AKC, where external eyelid administration of immunosuppressant creams has been found to reduce ocular surface signs and symptoms. Reductions of NMF has also been shown to raise the pH of keratinized epithelium which promotes the growth and colonization of *Staphylococcus aureus*, commonly found in atopic dermatitis, which contribute to the activation of innate immunity.

HISTOLOGIC STUDIES

However, most of the immunologic characterizations of AKC, to date, have involved the characterization of the pathways up-regulated in this inflammatory state, without specific regard to its genesis. In contrast to seasonal and perennial conjunctivitis, in which mast cells are primarily implicated, histologic examination and immunohistochemical studies of conjunctival specimens reveal increased numbers of mast cells, eosinophils, T lymphocytes, and neutrophils in AKC patients, relative to normal controls.[19–23] Mast cells and eosinophils have not only been detected in conjunctival epithelium, a pathologic finding, but are also present in increased numbers in the substantia propria. A surplus of Langerhans cells, macrophages and B cells in the substantia propria is also seen.[19] Indeed, while topical mast cell stabilizers are often effective in managing the signs and symptoms of allergic conjunctivitis, they are rarely adequate in controlling AKC.

T LYMPHOCYTES

T-lymphocyte infiltration is apparent in both the conjunctival epithelium and substantia propria in AKC. T-helper (Th) cells predominate in all allergic eye diseases. Of the major T-cell subtypes, the Th1 subtype is involved in cellular immunity, whereas the Th2 subtype is involved in humoral immune responses, including those mediated by IgE, and is therefore, strongly implicated in allergic eye disease. Th2 cells characteristically secrete several interleukins (IL), including IL-4, IL-5, IL-6, and IL-13; notably, IL-4 stimulates IgE production from B cells, while IL-5 is involved in eosinophil recruitment.

The cytokines involved in the recruitment and activation of inflammatory cells in AKC have been studied extensively, with particular attention to T-cell cytokines. In most studies, Th2 cytokines are prominent, with increased levels of IL-4, IL-5, IL-6, and IL-13 detected in both conjunctival and tear samples from AKC patients.[23–25] Tear levels of IL-5 have been suggested as a marker for severity of AKC, and IL-4

levels may be correlated with exacerbations in dermatologic atopy.[25] Elevated levels of IL-4-producing T cells were also observed in peripheral blood samples of AKC patients.[23] However, other studies suggest, a preferential up-regulation of Th1 cytokines, such as interferon-γ (IFN-γ), in AKC.[20]

EOSINOPHILS

Activated eosinophils are instrumental in recruiting additional inflammatory cells to the ocular surface. They release chemoattractants, such as IL-8, which attracts neutrophils to the conjunctiva; IL-8 is found to be highly expressed by eosinophils in AKC.[26] They secrete IL-4, attracting Th2 cells, as well as the chemoattractants RANTES and MCP-1.[24] Eosinophils are also major players in the development of sight-threatening corneal complications in AKC. Upon degranulation, they secrete leukotrienes, promoting allergic inflammation, as well as toxic proteins, including major basic protein (MBP) and eosinophilic cationic protein (ECP). MBP and ECP are known to induce damage to the corneal epithelium, causing superficial punctate keratopathy as well as frank corneal ulceration.[27] In vitro, these proteins have been observed to reduce corneal epithelial cell viability and cause morphologic changes.[28] Pathologic studies of corneal buttons from AKC patients show evidence of eosinophils and eosinophil byproducts in shield ulcers; notably, this applied to the area of the ulcer as well as surrounding 'healthy' stroma.[29]

CONJUNCTIVAL EPITHELIAL CELLS AND FIBROBLASTS

In addition to traditional inflammatory cells, other cell types express pro-inflammatory mediators in AKC. Recently, the active role played by conjunctival epithelial cells and fibroblasts has been recognized. The expression of surface adhesion molecules and the release of cytokines by epithelial cells enhance recruitment of eosinophils; notably, the surface adhesion molecule ICAM-1, which binds eosinophils, is strongly expressed by conjunctival epithelial cells in AKC.[30] Expression of Toll-like receptor 3 has also been detected on the surface of conjunctival epithelial cells, and may be involved in recruitment of eosinophils.[31] Conjunctival fibroblasts, when activated by Th cytokines, such as IL-4, TNF-α, or IL-13, produce the chemokines eotaxin-1 and eotaxin-2. These promote local accumulation of eosinophils and enhance eosinophil degranulation.[32] Interestingly, eotaxin can also be produced by activated corneal keratocytes (corneal fibroblasts), attracting eosinophils into the cornea and causing degranulation of epitheliotoxic proteins. Conjunctival fibroblasts were found to constitutively express IL-6, IL-8, MCP-1, and RANTES, all of which enhance inflammatory cell accumulation in the conjunctiva.[24] Recently, it has been suggested that thymic stromal lymphopoietin (TLSP), which recruits Th2 cells and may be involved in allergic inflammation, can be expressed on conjunctival epithelial cells.[33]

SECONDARY STRUCTURAL CHANGES

Extensive inflammation in AKC leads to chronic ocular surface alterations. Both goblet cell loss, based on impression cytology,[34] as well as goblet cell hyperplasia, based on conjunctival biopsy,[8] have been reported. Tear film instability, with increased tear break-up time but normal tear production, has also been described. Goblet cell production of mucins is altered, with decreased levels of the primary tear mucin MUC5AC, and increased levels of MUC 1, 2 and 4.[35] Of note, MUC5AC production was most dramatically reduced in patients with significant epithelial disease or shield ulcers. These patients also had increased numbers of conjunctival eosinophils and neutrophils, compared to AKC patients without significant epithelial disease, consistent with the role these cells play in corneal epithelial damage.[34] It is likely that goblet cell proliferation and mucin production are affected by inflammatory cytokines present in the conjunctiva in AKC patients. Corneal sensitivity is also reduced in AKC, and this may be related to abnormal corneal nerve architecture, noted in AKC patients on confocal microscopy. AKC patients had thicker corneal nerves with deflection and bifurcation anomalies, as well as increased tortuosity.[36] Squamous metaplasia has also been described in AKC.[34]

Differentiation from Vernal Keratoconjunctivitis

Atopic keratoconjunctivitis (AKC) and VKC are similar conditions, both in their presentation and their pathogenesis. Both are chronic, potentially blinding conditions, present in individuals predisposed by an atopic background, and involving both type I and type IV hypersensitivity responses. Clinically, they are similar, with conjunctival inflammation, epithelial defects, shield ulcers, and corneal scarring as major features of both. Eosinophils and T lymphocytes are found to infiltrate the conjunctiva in both conditions.

Distinguishing the two entities can therefore, be difficult, but is important given the worse visual prognosis for AKC. AKC presents at an older age than VKC; VKC typically presents in childhood, while the peak incidence of AKC is between the ages of 30 and 50 years. VKC usually 'burns out' by late puberty, whereas AKC remains chronic for years, often persisting into old age, when it may spontaneously resolve. However, by then, vision and quality of life are often compromised due to years of conjunctival and corneal inflammation, leading to ocular surface scarring, as well as cicatricial lid abnormalities.

Increased eyelid and periorbital skin involvement is another feature differentiating AKC from VKC, the latter generally sparing the skin. The eyelid margins are also not significantly affected in VKC, and cicatricial changes, forniceal foreshortening, and symblephara are not usually seen. The papillary reaction in each condition is also distinct. AKC usually presents with micropapillae on the palpebral conjunctiva. While giant papillae are sometimes seen in AKC, this is a definitive hallmark of VKC. Additionally, the lower tarsus is preferentially involved in AKC, in contrast to VKC, in which papillae are much more prominent on the upper tarsus. Corneal findings are similar in both diseases, albeit with more scarring and neovascularization seen in AKC. Limbal gelatinous hyperplasia can be seen in either condition, though Trantas dots are more frequently associated with VKC.

While the immunopathogenesis of AKC and VKC is very similar, a few differences have been reported. Tear levels of IL-4 have been found to be significantly higher in AKC patients, compared to those with VKC; it has been suggested that this may reflect a higher systemic level of Th-mediated inflammation in AKC patients, related to atopic dermatitis, rather than local ocular inflammation.[25] A study of cytokine expression in conjunctival-derived T-cell lines from AKC and VKC patients found greater expression of Th1 cytokines in AKC, compared to VKC, in which Th2 cytokines were more predominantly expressed.[20] However, another study found that the Th1 cytokine IFN-γ was more highly expressed in VKC tear levels, compared to AKC.[24] Additional studies are needed to better characterize differences in the immune pathology between AKC and VKC.

Management

Because of the chronic nature of AKC, the balance of treatment efficacy and risk is often difficult. However, disease-related complications, such as corneal scarring, limbal destruction, and structural lid changes are often less amenable to therapy than medication-related complications, such as steroid-induced glaucoma and cataract. The benefits of immunosuppressants, both systemic and local, must further be balanced against the significant risk of infection, both bacterial and viral. The goal of therapy should therefore, be complete control of the ocular surface inflammation with the safest medications and lowest dosing needed to achieve this. A multidisciplinary approach is best for the patient, and these patients should be co-managed with internists, allergists, and dermatologists to ensure adequate control of all the ocular, skin, and systemic manifestations of atopy. Advanced AKC may necessitate systemic immunosuppression, in order to prevent sight-threatening complications, and this requires the input of an internist to manage dosing and monitor for side effects. Control of environmental allergens is of little risk and may be helpful in controlling symptoms. Allergy testing may be helpful in this regard, but antigen avoidance is usually an adjunctive therapy.

Because AKC involves the eyelids, in addition to the ocular surface, basic eyelid hygiene is essential. Eyelid scrubs should be part of the AKC patient's daily routine in order to control blepharitis and the risk of staphylococcal keratitis. Antibiotic ointment may also be applied to the eyelid margins. Warm compresses will improve tear film stability in patients with meibomian gland dysfunction related to eyelid margin inflammation. However, if severe itching or an exacerbation of periocular atopic dermatitis is present, cool compresses will be more likely to provide symptomatic relief. Emollients and mild steroid ointments applied to the eyelid skin help control periocular eczema. Tacrolimus 0.03% ointment (Protopic), a steroid-sparing immunosuppressive agent, has also been shown to be effective in treating atopic dermatitis of the eyelids.

Initial management of conjunctival inflammation may involve topical mast cell stabilizers and antihistamines. The mast cell stabilizers include sodium cromoglycate, nedocromil and lodoxamide, which may be effective as maintenance therapy in mild cases of AKC. The selective H1-blocking antihistamines, such as levocabastine and emedastine, have limited effectiveness alone. Agents, such as olapatadine and ketotifen have both mast cell-stabilizing and antihistamine properties, and are more frequently employed for allergic eye diseases. Although these agents have little direct effect on the T-cell-mediated inflammation, they may reduce overall induction of inflammation and, importantly, reduce mechanical eye rubbing, associated with the development of keratoconus and possibly AKC-associated cataract.

More severe inflammation in AKC usually requires topical corticosteroid therapy. Initially, prednisolone acetate 1% or difluprednate 0.05% may be used, with gradual tapering to milder steroids, such as loteprednol or fluorometholone as signs and symptoms improve. Since the inflammation in AKC is on the ocular surface, corticosteroids with significant intraocular penetration should be avoided when possible. However, even with judicious use of these medications, steroid-related side effects, such as cataract and elevated intraocular pressure are often inevitable for AKC patients. Superior intratarsal injection of corticosteroids is effective in refractory cases, though this treatment option may also be limited by side effects.

More recently, effective control of AKC has been described with steroid-sparing immunosuppressive drugs, such as cyclosporine, a calcineurin inhibitor that reduces production of the cytokine IL-2, thereby reducing Th production. Immunohistochemical analysis of superior tarsal conjunctival biopsies in AKC patients treated with 2% topical cyclosporine A, revealed a reduction in the number of Th cells, B cells and macrophages after treatment, confirming the immunomodulatory effect of topical cyclosporine.[37] A randomized, placebo-controlled trial found that topical cyclosporine A 2% in maize oil, was effective in treating signs and symptoms of AKC.[38] However, side effects included intense stinging and prolonged blurred vision, which led some patients in the study to use the drops less frequently. A more recent randomized, controlled trial found that topical cyclosporine A 0.05% (Restasis) was also beneficial in treating AKC, and was tolerated much better, with fewer side effects.[39] Tacrolimus, mentioned earlier, is also a calcineurin inhibitor, and inhibits T-cell production with greater potency than cyclosporine. An eye drop form is currently only available for use in Japan, but some reports describe improvement in AKC with tacrolimus ointment available as compounded formulation, either applied directly to the eye[40] or to the eyelids, with presumed spillover onto the ocular surface.

Systemic immune suppression is sometimes necessary in refractory cases of AKC; agents reported to be beneficial include prednisone, cyclosporine, tacrolimus, mycophenolate, and azathioprine. Low-dose systemic tacrolimus has been found to be effective in controlling AKC symptoms, with only minor side effects reported.

Corneal epitheliopathy, erosions, and ulcerations in AKC should initially be managed as they would be in non-atopic individuals, albeit with appropriate titration of immunosuppressive therapy. Superficial punctate keratopathy requires aggressive lubrication, with preservative-free artificial tears and lubricating ointments, with the goal of increasing comfort and avoiding frank epithelial defects, which are typically more difficult to manage in atopes. If epithelial erosion does occur, topical antibiotic prophylaxis should be added to prevent bacterial superinfection and

infectious keratitis, a complication of epithelial defects in AKC. All new epithelial defects should be cultured prior to initiation of broad-spectrum antibiotics. Therapeutic measures, such as bandage contact lens placement and tarsorrhaphy should be utilized when needed, in order to facilitate healing of the defect. Shield ulcer plaques, consisting of epithelial and inflammatory debris at the base of an ulcer, are often resistant to treatment with topical anti-inflammatory therapy. Some have recommended surgical debridement of the plaque in such cases; in one report describing three patients, this led to complete re-epithelialization in all patients within a few weeks.[41] Occasionally, it may be hard to distinguish a shield ulcer plaque from herpetic keratitis, and the latter should be kept in mind when faced with a plaque-like ulcerative lesion in an AKC patient.

Despite aggressive management, corneal scarring and occasionally perforation may occur in severe cases, necessitating penetrating keratoplasty. Results of penetrating keratoplasty are often poor in AKC patients, due to atopic inflammation and a compromised ocular surface. In a report of nine AKC patients who underwent penetrating keratoplasty, four of the nine patients required more than one graft. All patients were preoperatively treated with oral antihistamines, topical mast cell stabilizers, and topical corticosteroid for at least 5 days. Postoperatively, two patients were treated with topical cyclosporine A 2% and another with systemic cyclosporine in order to enhance graft survival. The authors note that final visual acuity results were quite favorable, but obtaining such results required aggressive control of inflammation and surface disease.[42] Many advocate starting systemic immunosuppression with agents, such as prednisone or cyclosporine, beginning a few weeks prior to planned corneal transplant surgery, in order to limit risk of graft rejection. In patients with corneal epithelial or stromal irregularity but with good control of their AKC, scleral contact lenses may afford good vision and increased comfort without the need for surgery. Patients who develop limbal stem cell deficiency may require ocular surface stem cell transplantation for visual rehabilitation.

Other surgical measures may be considered in the management of AKC. Papillary resection with or without mitomycin-C application has been described as a method to reduce ocular surface inflammation. Clinical improvement was noted after resection, and decreased conjunctival inflammation was observed on cytologic analysis.[43] In advanced AKC, extensive scarring of the ocular surface and eyelid margins may necessitate eyelid surgery. This includes lid margin tightening and rotational procedures for lid malposition, as well as symblephara lysis and forniceal reconstruction for severe conjunctival scarring. Many patients will require cataract surgery at a relatively young age due to atopic and steroid-induced cataract development. A few patients may need glaucoma filtering surgery or valve placement if steroid-induced glaucoma develops.

Conclusion

Atopic keratoconjunctivitis is characterized by chronic periocular eczema, conjunctival inflammation, corneal epitheliopathy and ulceration, and eventually vision-threatening corneal scarring as a primary consequence or secondary to bacterial or herpetic keratitis. It is similar to vernal conjunctivitis, but unlike VKC, it usually presents in adulthood and may persist for decades, resulting in significant morbidity. Patients almost universally have atopic dermatitis. The pathophysiology is complex, involving mast cells, lymphocytes, eosinophils, and conjunctival epithelial cells. T-helper lymphocytes and activated eosinophils play particularly important roles. Management is often difficult and requires multiple treatment arms, including topical mast cell stabilizers, corticosteroids, and steroid-sparing immunosuppressive agents, such as topical cyclosporine. In more severe cases, systemic immunosuppression may be required. Penetrating keratoplasty may be considered, for either visual rehabilitation or tectonic purposes; however, outcomes are often poor due to inflammation and surface disease, and systemic immunosuppression is recommended to optimize outcomes.

References

1. Hogan MJ. Atopic keratoconjunctivitis. Trans Am Ophthalmol Soc 1952;50:265–81.
2. Garrity JA, Liesegang TJ. Ocular complications of atopic dermatitis. Can J Ophthalmol 1984;19:21–4.
3. Tuft SJ, Kemeny DM, Dart JK, et al. Clinical features of atopic keratoconjunctivitis. Ophthalmology 1991;98:150–8.
4. Guglielmetti S, Dart JK, Calder V. Atopic keratoconjunctivitis and atopic dermatitis. Curr Opin Allergy Clin Immunol 2010;10:478–85.
5. Onguchi T, Dogru M, Okada N, et al. The impact of the onset time of atopic keratoconjunctivitis on the tear function and ocular surface findings. Am J Ophthalmol 2006;141:569–71.
6. Marback PM, de Freitas D, Paranhos Junior A, et al. [Epidemiological and clinical features of allergic conjunctivitis in a reference center]. Arq Bras Oftalmol 2007;70:312–6.
7. Bielory B, Bielory L. Atopic dermatitis and keratoconjunctivitis. Immunol Allergy Clin North Am 2010;30:323–36.
8. Power WJ, Tugal-Tutkun I, Foster CS. Long-term follow-up of patients with atopic keratoconjunctivitis. Ophthalmology 1998;105:637–42.
9. Jeng BH, Whitcher JP, Margolis TP. Pseudogerontoxon. Clin Experiment Ophthalmol 2004;32:433–4.
10. Nakata K, Inoue Y, Harada J, et al. A high incidence of Staphylococcus aureus colonization in the external eyes of patients with atopic dermatitis. Ophthalmology 2000;107:2167–71.
11. Easty D, Entwistle C, Funk A, et al. Herpes simplex keratitis and keratoconus in the atopic patient. A clinical and immunological study. Trans Ophthalmol Soc UK 1975;95:267–76.
12. Uchio E, Miyakawa K, Ikezawa Z, et al. Systemic and local immunological features of atopic dermatitis patients with ocular complications. Br J Ophthalmol 1998;82:82–7.
13. Jain V, Nair AG, Jain-Mhatre K, et al. Pellucid marginal corneal disease in a case of atopic keratoconjunctivitis. Ocul Immunol Inflamm 2010;18:187–9.
14. Yoneda K, Okamoto H, Wada Y, et al. Atopic retinal detachment. Report of four cases and a review of the literature. Br J Dermatol 1995;133:586–91.
15. Inada N, Shoji J, Kato H, et al. Clinical evaluation of total IgE in tears of patients with allergic conjunctivitis disease using a novel application of the immunochromatography method. Allergol Int 2009;58:585–9.
16. Tabbara KF, Nassar A, Ahmed SO, et al. Acquisition of vernal and atopic keratoconjunctivitis after bone marrow transplantation. Am J Ophthalmol 2008;146:462–5.
17. Matsuda A, Okayama Y, Terai N, et al. The role of interleukin-33 in chronic allergic conjunctivitis. Invest Ophthalmol Vis Sci 2009;50:4646–52.
18. O'Regan GM, Irvine AD. The role of filaggrin loss-of-function mutations in atopic dermatitis. Curr Opin Allergy Clin Immunol 2008;8:406–10.
19. Foster CS, Rice BA, Dutt JE. Immunopathology of atopic keratoconjunctivitis. Ophthalmology 1991;98:1190–6.
20. Calder VL, Jolly G, Hingorani M, et al. Cytokine production and mRNA expression by conjunctival T-cell lines in chronic allergic eye disease. Clin Exp Allergy 1999;29:1214–22.
21. Metz DP, Bacon AS, Holgate S, et al. Phenotypic characterization of T cells infiltrating the conjunctiva in chronic allergic eye disease. J Allergy Clin Immunol 1996;98:686–96.
22. Trocme SD, Leiferman KM, George T, et al. Neutrophil and eosinophil participation in atopic and vernal keratoconjunctivitis. Curr Eye Res 2003;26:319–25.
23. Matsuura N, Uchio E, Nakazawa M, et al. Predominance of infiltrating IL-4-producing T cells in conjunctiva of patients with allergic conjunctival disease. Curr Eye Res 2004;29:235–43.
24. Leonardi A, Curnow SJ, Zhan H, et al. Multiple cytokines in human tear specimens in seasonal and chronic allergic eye disease and in conjunctival fibroblast cultures. Clin Exp Allergy 2006;36:777–84.
25. Uchio E, Ono SY, Ikezawa Z, et al. Tear levels of interferon-gamma, interleukin (IL) -2, IL-4 and IL-5 in patients with vernal keratoconjunctivitis, atopic keratoconjunctivitis and allergic conjunctivitis. Clin Exp Allergy 1997;27:1328–1334.
26. Hingorani M, Calder V, Jolly G, et al. Eosinophil surface antigen expression and cytokine production vary in different ocular allergic diseases. J Allergy Clin Immunol 1998;102:821–30.
27. Cameron JA. Shield ulcers and plaques of the cornea in vernal keratoconjunctivitis. Ophthalmology 1995;102:985–93.
28. Trocme SD, Hallberg CK, Gill KS, et al. Effects of eosinophil granule proteins on human corneal epithelial cell viability and morphology. Invest Ophthalmol Vis Sci 1997;38:593–9.
29. Messmer EM, May CA, Stefani FH, et al. Toxic eosinophil granule protein deposition in corneal ulcerations and scars associated with atopic keratoconjunctivitis. Am J Ophthalmol 2002;134:816–21.
30. Baudouin C, Haouat N, Brignole F, et al. Immunopathological findings in conjunctival cells using immunofluorescence staining of impression cytology specimens. Br J Ophthalmol 1992;76:545–9.
31. Bonini S, Micera A, Iovieno A, et al. Expression of Toll-like receptors in healthy and allergic conjunctiva. Ophthalmology 2005;112:1528 [discussion 1548–29].
32. Leonardi A, Jose PJ, Zhan H, et al. Tear and mucus eotaxin-1 and eotaxin-2 in allergic keratoconjunctivitis. Ophthalmology 2003;110:487–92.
33. Ueta M, Uematsu S, Akira S, et al. Toll-like receptor 3 enhances late-phase reaction of experimental allergic conjunctivitis. J Allergy Clin Immunol 2009;123:1187–9.
34. Dogru M, Asano-Kato N, Tanaka M, et al. Ocular surface and MUC5AC alterations in atopic patients with corneal shield ulcers. Curr Eye Res 2005;30:897–908.
35. Dogru M, Okada N, Asano-Kato N, et al. Alterations of the ocular surface epithelial mucins 1, 2, 4 and the tear functions in patients with atopic keratoconjunctivitis. Clin Exp Allergy 2006;36:1556–65.
36. Hu Y, Matsumoto Y, Adan ES, et al. Corneal in vivo confocal scanning laser microscopy in patients with atopic keratoconjunctivitis. Ophthalmology 2008;115:2004–12.
37. Hingorani M, Calder VL, Buckley RJ, et al. The immunomodulatory effect of topical cyclosporine A in atopic keratoconjunctivitis. Invest Ophthalmol Vis Sci 1999;40:392–9.
38. Hingorani M, Moodaley L, Calder VL, et al. A randomized, placebo-controlled trial of topical cyclosporine A in steroid-dependent atopic keratoconjunctivitis. Ophthalmology 1998;105:1715–20.
39. Akpek EK, Dart JK, Watson S, et al. A randomized trial of topical cyclosporine 0.05% in topical steroid-resistant atopic keratoconjunctivitis. Ophthalmology 2004;111:476–82.
40. Joseph MA, Kaufman HE, Insler M. Topical tacrolimus ointment for treatment of refractory anterior segment inflammatory disorders. Cornea 2005;24:417–20.
41. Solomon A, Zamir E, Levartovsky S, et al. Surgical management of corneal plaques in vernal keratoconjunctivitis: a clinicopathologic study. Cornea 2004;23:608–12.
42. Ghoraishi M, Akova YA, Tugal-Tutkun I, et al. Penetrating keratoplasty in atopic keratoconjunctivitis. Cornea 1995;14:610–3.
43. Tanaka M, Dogru M, Takano Y, et al. Quantitative evaluation of the early changes in ocular surface inflammation following MMC-aided papillary resection in severe allergic patients with corneal complications. Cornea 2006;25:281–5.

16 *Giant Papillary Conjunctivitis*

JULIE H. TSAI

Introduction

Giant papillary conjunctivitis is an inflammatory condition seen in the upper tarsal conjunctiva, initially reported by Spring in 1974.[1] The author noted a papillary reaction, similar to that seen in patients with allergic conjunctivitis, though his findings were reported in soft contact lens wearers. Allansmith and colleagues further detailed the syndrome, suggesting that it may be immunologic in origin, with the proteinaceous deposits on the contact lenses serving as the antigen.[2] As the constellation of findings is predominantly associated with the use of contact lenses, the disease is also referred to as contact lens-induced papillary conjunctivitis (CLPC); however, the condition has also been reported in patients with ocular dermoids, ocular prostheses, exposed sutures following ocular procedures, extruded scleral buckles, filtering blebs, exposed corneal deposits, as well as tissue adhesives (Fig. 16.1).[3–10]

Epidemiology

Giant papillary conjunctivitis (GPC) is most often associated with wearing soft contact lenses, though it can occur with any type of contact lens. In a study of 221 patients, 85% were wearing soft contact lenses, with the remaining 15% of participants wearing rigid lenses.[11] One report noted an average interval of 10 months for the development of GPC for soft lens wearers, compared to 8.5 years for rigid lens wearers.[2] The type and material of the lens also contributes to the severity of the disease, with soft lens wearers suffering from more severe manifestations of disease than their counterparts in rigid gas-permeable lenses.[11] Silicone hydrogel lenses also appear to have similar effects with prolonged use, though the findings are seen more commonly in earlier designs.[12]

Researchers have also studied the association of other atopic conditions in patients with GPC, due to the similarities between GPC and other immunologically derived ocular disorders (e.g. vernal keratoconjunctivitis). Allergic rhinitis and hay fever are often estimated to range 10–20% in the general population, and in the subset of GPC patients, the incidence has been reported to be as low as 12% to over 26%.[11,13] One particular cohort reports that patients who suffer from allergies seem to have more severe signs and symptoms of GPC, compared to those who did not; however, the presence or absence of other allergic conditions did not have any effect on the ultimate treatment of those individuals or their long-term use of contact lenses.[11]

Pathophysiology

Neutrophils and lymphocytes are present in the epithelium and substantia propria of normal conjunctival tissue. Mast cells and plasma cells are also present, though they are sequestered to the substantia propria. In patients with GPC, these cells increase in number and are often found throughout the epithelium and the substantia propria, and are found in conjunction with other inflammatory cells, such as basophils and eosinophils.[14] These findings, along with elevation of cytokines and chemokines in the tear film of GPC patients, suggest a possible allergic mechanism for the development of disease. Interleukin-6 (IL-6) along with IL-6 soluble receptor (IL-6sr) have been noted to be elevated four- to eightfold compared to controls, and IL-6sr has been postulated to be an important mediator in the formation of the papillae.[15] Locally produced tear immunoglobulins (e.g. IgE, IgG, and even IgM in severe cases) are also found to be elevated in the tears of GPC patients, with the degree of elevation correlated to the severity of symptoms. It is interesting to note, that with discontinuation of lens wear and resolution of the signs and symptoms, these tear immunoglobulin levels return to normal.[12]

The proteinaceous deposits on the lens surface have classically been cited as the possible nidus for the development of inflammation and thus, the papillae associated with GPC. These various substances can cover 50% of the contact lens surface within 30 minutes of lens insertion, and 90% after 8 hours of wear time.[16,17] Even with the best cleaning regimens involving enzymatic treatment, a residual coating still exists, and as new coating material is constantly built on the surface of the lens, the overall lens coating increases.[18] The lens type and material also affect the rate and amount of accumulation of protein coating, as well as the total

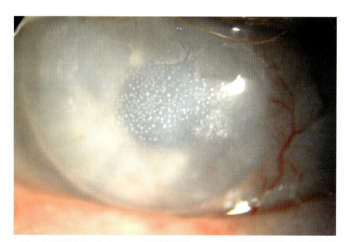

Figure 16.1 A slit lamp photography demonstrating contact lens deposits on a patient wearing a silicone hydrogel contact lens for therapeutic bandage lens use.

percentages of lipid, calcium and protein that deposit on the lens.[12] Differences in the polymer content, structure and charge determine the extent to which protein is deposited on the anterior lens surface.[19]

The nature of these deposits is similar in patients with and without GPC. In addition, there are no morphologic or biochemical findings that differentiate the coating on the contact lenses in these two groups; however, those affected with GPC generally have more coating on their contact lenses, and lenses of GPC patients can promote a clinical picture of injection, thickening and a papillary reaction on the upper tarsal conjunctiva in monkeys in a laboratory setting.[20] Cellular infiltrates seen in the biopsy samples from the monkeys are also similar to those seen in GPC; thus, the animal model strongly suggests that an antigen exists in the contact lens coating that may produce the same inflammatory reaction seen clinically as GPC.[20] These findings support the allergic hypothesis for GPC, as does the fact that immunoglobulins G, A and M (IgG, IgA, and IgM), were also found in the protein deposits on GPC-associated contact lenses; however, eosinophil major basic protein, a material elaborated from eosinophils found in allergic reactions, was not found to a significant degree on lenses of GPC patients.[21–24]

In contrast, the mechanical hypothesis is supported by the association between GPC and inert objects, such as cyanoacrylate adhesives, exposed sutures or scleral buckle elements, dermoids and orbital prostheses. Researchers have postulated that the irritation and friction from the lens damages conjunctival epithelial cells and causes release of chemotactic factors (e.g. neutrophil chemotactic factor).[24] Injection of these factors into the upper tarsal conjunctiva of rabbits produced a GPC-like reaction, suggesting that a combination of direct trauma and the resulting inflammatory cascade can stimulate a hypersensitivity reaction to lens-bound antigens.

Clinical Findings

A variety of symptoms have been reported by contact lens wearers with GPC, including but not limited to redness, burning, itching, foreign body sensation, excessive lens movement, decreased lens tolerance, and increased mucus production, particularly upon awakening in the morning. Often, in early disease, these symptoms may be out of proportion to the clinical findings; thus, a careful and selective history is necessary to elicit the reports of symptoms that many may consider normal discomfort associated with contact lens use.

The biomicroscopic findings of normal tarsal conjunctiva, include a vascular arcade of fine, radiating vessels running perpendicular to the lid margin and a smooth, moist and pink surface. This has been termed a 'satin' appearance.[2] Generally, the surface is devoid of papillae, or there may be a fine, fairly uniform papillary appearance detectable after the instillation of fluorescein dye and examination with a cobalt blue filter. These papillae, if present, are often smaller than 0.3 mm. Non-specific signs of inflammation, such as thickening of the tarsal conjunctiva with mild hyperemia, may be noted in early cases. In addition, bulbar conjunctival injection, superior corneal pannus, and corneal opacities may also be found on examination. As the

disease progresses, non-uniform papillary changes develop, and finally giant papillae are seen, defined as a papillary reaction greater than 0.3 mm (Fig. 16.2).

Further characterization of the size and location of the papillae is also helpful in correlating clinical findings with patient symptoms. Delineation of the upper tarsal plate into three zones, as well as two areas medially and laterally (Fig. 16.3), can be useful to the clinician in determining whether findings are within the normal variance or whether it represents disease. For example, large papillae in the junctional or transitional zone are not considered pathologic and

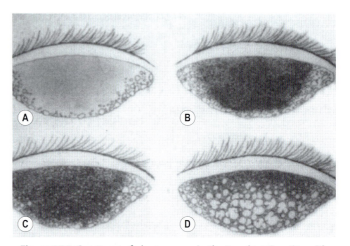

Figure 16.2 Spectrum of change seen in the tarsal conjunctiva with (**A**) a 'satin' or normal appearance of conjunctiva; (**B**) uniform papillae; (**C**) non-uniform papillae; and (**D**) giant papillae. (From Allansmith MR, Korb DR, Greiner JV, et al. Giant papillary conjunctivitis in contact lens wearers. Am J Ophthalmol 1977;82:697–708: with permission.)

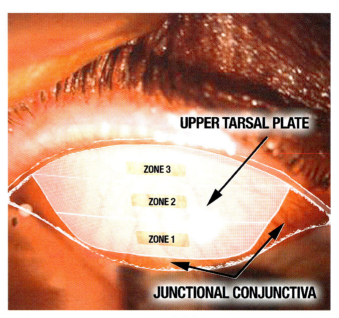

Figure 16.3 Zones of involvement in the upper tarsal conjunctiva: zone 1 lies along the tarsal border; zone 2 describes the central area of the tarsal plate; and zone 3 demarcates the area along the lid margin. The medial and lateral regions of the tarsal conjunctiva can be considered 'transition' zones, or junctional regions. (From Donshik PC, Elhers WG. Giant papillary conjunctivitis. Immunol Allergy Clin North Am 1997; 17:53–73: with permission.)

should be disregarded in the assessment of the upper tarsal conjunctiva.[12]

Diagnosis

Giant papillary conjunctivitis shares morphologic and histologic similarities with vernal conjunctivitis, but is best differentiated from this and other immunologically based conjunctival inflammation by the associated clinical history (e.g. contact lens wear, surgical intervention). Biomicroscopic findings may also be helpful, as the location and appearance of the papillae are associated with the type and material of the lens. Soft contact lens wearers often exhibit a generalized papillary response, whereas those wearing rigid gas-permeable lenses or silicone hydrogels manifest papillae in a more localized fashion. Korb and colleagues[25,26] have reported that papillae in soft and hard lens wearers differ in the location on the tarsal conjunctiva. Soft lens wearers usually form papillae nearest the upper margin of the tarsal plate (zones 1 and 2) and progress to diffuse involvement of all 3 zones, whereas rigid lens wearers and those using silicone hydrogel lenses develop papillae near the lid margin (zones 2 and 3) and persist in a more localized pattern.[12]

In addition, other associated signs and symptoms can aid in the diagnosis of GPC. These signs and symptoms are often classified into four stages:[2]

- *Stage 1, or preclinical disease*: minimal mucus discharge is usually noted upon awakening, and patients may report occasional itching after lens removal. Examination of the lenses reveals a mild protein coating. The tarsal conjunctiva may appear normal, or exhibit mild hyperemia with normal vascular structures.
- *Stage 2, or mild disease*: increased mucus production is noted, along with itching, increased lens awareness and marked coating of the contact lenses. Blurring of vision may occur. Mild to moderate injection of the tarsal conjunctiva is noted with some loss of the normal vascular pattern (i.e. superficial vessels are typically obscured, with deeper vessels still visible). The papillary reaction noted on examination may show variability in terms of the size of the papillae, which may be attributed to thickening of the underlying tissue. Some of the papillae measure 0.3 mm or greater at this stage, and can be best detected upon examination after instillation of fluorescein dye.
- *Stage 3, or moderate disease*: itching and mucus formation, along with lens coating, are more prominent at this point, and patients often report having difficulty with lens tolerability and keeping the lenses clean. Increased lens awareness and excessive lens movement with blinking often result in fluctuating quality of vision and reduction in lens wear time. The tarsal conjunctiva now shows marked thickening and injection, with obscuration of normal vascular pattern. The papillae have increased in both size and number, and the papillae appear more elevated secondary to changes in the underlying tissue (e.g. subconjunctival fibrosis and thickening).
- *Stage four, or severe disease*: patients are often unable to wear their lenses at all at this stage, with intense discomfort and cloudy vision upon initial insertion of the lenses. There is excessive lens movement, as well as poor centration of the contact lens. Increased mucus secretion is also reported, often to the point where patients note that their eyelids are stuck together in the mornings. The normal vascular pattern is completely obscured, and the papillae have enlarged to sizes of 1 mm or greater. Subconjunctival scarring and fluorescein staining of the apices of the papillae may be present (Fig. 16. 4).

It is important to note that, although these stages can aid in the characterization of the disease, patient presentation is often variable. Some patients may have minimal complaints but exhibit marked inflammatory changes on the tarsal conjunctiva; in contrast, patients with severe symptoms may present with only mild or early tarsal changes. Also, despite the fact that GPC is often noted bilaterally, the clinical findings may be grossly asymmetric. In some cases, the disparity between eyes is easily explained (e.g. poor lens fit), but in other cases, no specific etiology can be determined.[27]

Treatment

Giant papillary conjunctivitis treatment options are often directed at reducing or eliminating any mechanical stimulation and lens coating from the contact lenses or modulating the immune response to the antigenic proteins on the lens surface. Changing the lens cleaning regimen, decreasing the wear time, changing the material or design of the contact lens, or shortening the replacement interval, can all help to reduce the exposure to the antigenic proteins on the contact lens. Medications that may modulate the immune reaction include topical nonsteroidal anti-inflammatory agents, mast cell stabilizers, and topical corticosteroids. The ultimate goal in managing these patients is to allow them to continue wearing their contact lenses.

Depending on the severity of disease, several or all of the strategies for reducing lens coating or mechanical stimulation may need to be employed. One study noted that if only the cleaning regimen was changed, only 50% of affected patients were able to continue wearing the contact lenses.[11] A decrease in the wear time only resulted in 20% of patients who could continue to wear their lenses. Refitting the patients with new lenses resulted in a range of success rates: 68% of patients could tolerate wearing their lenses if they were refitted with the same type of lens; a change to a gas-permeable lens allowed for 82% of patients to return to contact lens wear; and frequent replacement of a daily wear lens resulted in a 91% success rate.[11]

The literature on immune response modulation for GPC has mainly focused on topical therapy, most commonly mast cell stabilizers and loteprednol etabonate (Lotemax®). Mast cell stabilizers have been shown to be effective, with one study finding a 70% success rate in patients with moderate to severe GPC that suffered a recurrence of symptoms despite changes in the contact lens polymer or design.[28,29] The use of a steroid, such as loteprednol, has been found to reduce the presence of papillae, itching, and lens intolerance.[30,31] However, chronic treatment with a steroid is generally not recommended in these cases.

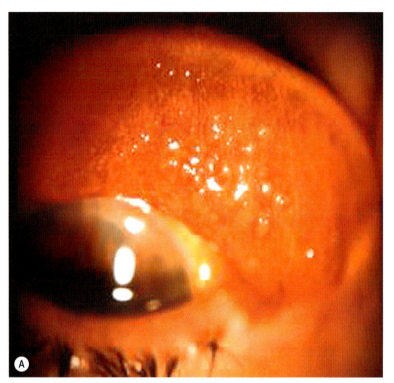 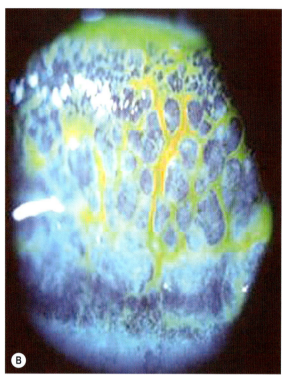

Figure 16.4 Stage 4 giant papillary conjunctivitis. (**A**) Clinical examination reveals marked injection and thickening of the conjunctiva, with large papillae. (**B**) Instillation of fluorescein highlights staining of the apices of the giant papillae when viewed using a cobalt blue filter. (From Donshik PC, Elhers WG. Giant papillary conjunctivitis. Immunol Allergy Clin North Am 1997;17:53–73: with permission.)

A combination of the two therapeutic options, therefore, seems most appropriate for initiating treatment for the patient suffering from GPC. For stage 1, or preclinical cases, more frequent observation (e.g. 4–6 month follow-up visits) may be all that is required, as these individuals are generally asymptomatic but will be predisposed to developing GPC. Treatment for stage 2 to stage 3 should begin with discontinuation of contact lenses anywhere from 2–4 weeks, with re-evaluation of the conjunctiva and refit with frequent replacement contact lenses. These can range from daily disposables to lenses that are replaced every 2 weeks. For those patients changing their lenses every 1–2 weeks, a lens cleaning regimen utilizing a hydrogen peroxide-based cleaner is preferred.[12] If there is a return of symptoms despite a change in the lens type and polymer, discontinue the lenses for another 2–4 weeks, refit with a daily disposable lens (or rigid gas-permeable lens) and add a mast cell stabilizer. These patients should generally be re-evaluated 3–4 times per year.

For severe, or stage 4 disease, discontinuation of contact lens wear may be required for at least 4 weeks, along with refitting the contact lens with either a daily disposable or rigid gas-permeable lens. The key for therapy at this stage is to determine if resolution of the associated findings of corneal and apical papillary staining has occurred; it is often noted that the appearance and size of the papillae may not change during the course of treatment for severe GPC. If the associated inflammatory signs have resolved, then attempts to refit the patient with a new lens may have a greater success rate. Specifically, if the patient is refitted with a daily wear contact lens and replaces the lens in an interval of 4 weeks or less, the rate of developing GPC drops to 4.5%. Individuals utilizing daily disposable lenses have not been reported to develop GPC.[32]

Summary

Giant papillary conjunctivitis continues to pose a challenge to both patients who have it and the physicians who treat this condition. With a clear understanding of the conjunctival anatomy, along with a suggestive clinical history (i.e. contact lens use) and thorough anterior segment examination, the physician should be able to confidently diagnose GPC and provide the appropriate level of care dependent upon disease severity. To date, the underlying etiology of GPC remains unclear, but further research may elucidate its cause, and ultimately lead to better treatment.

References

1. Spring TF. Reaction to hydrophilic lenses. Med J Aust 1974;1:449–50.
2. Allansmith MR, Korb DR, Greiner JV, et al. Giant papillary conjunctivitis in contact lens wearers. Am J Ophthalmol 1977;83:697–708.
3. Jolson AS, Jolson SC. Suture barb giant papillary conjunctivitis. Ophthalmic Surg 1984;15:139–40.
4. Vengayil S, Vanathi M, Dada T, et al. Filtering bleb-induced giant papillary conjunctivitis. Cont Lens Anterior Eye 2008;31:41–3.
5. Srinivasan BD, Jakobiec FA, Iwamoto T, et al. Giant papillary conjunctivitis with ocular prostheses. Arch Ophthalmol 1979;97:892–5.
6. Skrypuch OW, Willis NR. Giant papillary conjunctivitis from an exposed prolene suture. Can J Ophthalmol 1986;21:189–92.
7. Manners RM, Vardy SJ, Rose GE. Localised giant papillary conjunctivitis secondary to a dermolipoma. Eye (Lond) 1995;9(Pt 3):376–8.

8. Dunn JP, Jr., Weissman BA, Mondino BJ, et al. Giant papillary conjunctivitis associated with elevated corneal deposits. Cornea 1990;9: 357–8.

9. Carlson AN, Wilhelmus KR. Giant papillary conjunctivitis associated with cyanoacrylate glue. Am J Ophthalmol 1987;104: 437–8.

10. Robin JB, Regis-Pacheco LF, May WN, et al. Giant papillary conjunctivitis associated with an extruded scleral buckle. Case report. Arch Ophthalmol 1987;105:619.

11. Donshik PC. Giant papillary conjunctivitis. Trans Am Ophthalmol Soc 1994;92:687–744.

12. Donshik PC, Ehlers WH, Ballow M. Giant papillary conjunctivitis. Immunol Allergy Clin North Am 2008;28:83–103, vi.

13. Friedlaender MH. Some unusual nonallergic causes of giant papillary conjunctivitis. Trans Am Ophthalmol Soc 1990;88:343–9; discussion 349–51.

14. Allansmith MR, Korb DR, Greiner JV. Giant papillary conjunctivitis induced by hard or soft contact lens wear: quantitative histology. Ophthalmology 1978;85:766–78.

15. Shoji J, Inada N, Sawa M. Antibody array-generated cytokine profiles of tears of patients with vernal keratoconjunctivitis or giant papillary conjunctivitis. Jpn J Ophthalmol 2006;50:195–204.

16. Fowler SA, Allansmith MR. The surface of the continuously worn contact lens. Arch Ophthalmol 1980;98:1233–6.

17. Fowler SA, Allansmith MR. Evolution of soft contact lens coatings. Arch Ophthalmol 1980;98:95–9.

18. Fowler SA, Allansmith MR. The effect of cleaning soft contact lenses. A scanning electron microscopic study. Arch Ophthalmol 1981; 99:1382–6.

19. Minarik L, Rapp J. Protein deposits on individual hydrophilic contact lenses: effects of water and ionicity. Clao J 1989;15:185–8.

20. Ballow M, Donshik PC, Rapacz P, et al. Immune responses in monkeys to lenses from patients with contact lens induced giant papillary conjunctivitis. Clao J 1989;15:64–70.

21. Trocme SD, Kephart GM, Bourne WM, et al. Eosinophil granule major basic protein in contact lenses of patients with giant papillary conjunctivitis. Clao J 1990;16:219–22.

22. Richard NR, Anderson JA, Tasevska ZG, et al. Evaluation of tear protein deposits on contact lenses from patients with and without giant papillary conjunctivitis. Clao J 1992;18:143–7.

23. Jones B, Sack R. Immunoglobulin deposition on soft contact lenses: relationship to hydrogel structure and mode of use and giant papillary conjunctivitis. Clao J 1990;16:43–8.

24. Elgebaly SA, Donshik PC, Rahhal F, et al. Neutrophil chemotactic factors in the tears of giant papillary conjunctivitis patients. Invest Ophthalmol Vis Sci 1991;32:208–13.

25. Korb DR, Allansmith MR, Greiner JV, et al. Biomicroscopy of papillae associated with hard contact lens wearing. Ophthalmology 1981; 88:1132–66.

26. Korb DR, Greiner JV, Finnemore VM, et al. Biomicroscopy of papillae associated with wearing of soft contact lenses. Br J Ophthalmol 1983;67:733–6.

27. Palmisano PC, Ehlers WH, Donshik PC. Causative factors in unilateral giant papillary conjunctivitis. Clao J 1993;19:103–7.

28. Meisler DM, Berzins UJ, Krachmer JH, et al. Cromolyn treatment of giant papillary conjunctivitis. Arch Ophthalmol 1982;100: 1608–10.

29. Kruger CJ, Ehlers WH, Luistro AE, et al. Treatment of giant papillary conjunctivitis with cromolyn sodium. Clao J 1992;18:46–8.

30. Asbell P, Howes J. A double-masked, placebo-controlled evaluation of the efficacy and safety of loteprednol etabonate in the treatment of giant papillary conjunctivitis. Clao J 1997;23:31–6.

31. Bartlett JD, Howes JF, Ghormley NR, et al. Safety and efficacy of loteprednol etabonate for treatment of papillae in contact lens-associated giant papillary conjunctivitis. Curr Eye Res 1993;12:313–21.

32. Donshik PC, Porazinski AD. Giant papillary conjunctivitis in frequent-replacement contact lens wearers: a retrospective study. Trans Am Ophthalmol Soc 1999;97:205–16; discussion 216–20.

17 Treatment of Allergic Eye Disease

AMY T. KELMENSON, NAVEEN K. RAO, and MICHAEL B. RAIZMAN

Introduction

Ocular allergies are a common group of disorders that can be debilitating for patients and, at times, challenging for physicians to diagnose and treat. For the purpose of developing an appropriate treatment strategy, it can be useful to conceptually divide ocular allergies into six categories: seasonal allergic conjunctivitis (SAC), perennial allergic conjunctivitis (PAC), vernal keratoconjunctivitis (VKC), atopic keratoconjunctivitis (AKC), giant papillary conjunctivitis (GPC), and contact allergic conjunctivitis (CAC).

SAC is the most prevalent form of ocular allergy and is often accompanied by seasonal allergic rhinitis. Its seasonal incidence is closely tied to the cyclic release of environmental plant-derived airborne allergens. PAC is more likely to occur year-round, though most patients also experience seasonal exacerbations, and is thought to be caused by indoor allergens, such as animal dander and dust mites. Both SAC and PAC can cause significant morbidity, but rarely cause permanent visual impairment. VKC is a less common, self-limited variant of ocular allergy, that can present with unique corneal and conjunctival manifestations, described elsewhere in this text. AKC is a chronic condition associated with atopic dermatitis or eczema, often in individuals with a history of atopy. Both VKC and AKC are primary conjunctival disorders that can cause secondary corneal scarring and therefore, can be vision-threatening. Giant papillary conjunctivitis (GPC) is a reversible condition, most commonly associated with chronic mechanical irritation from contact lenses, exposed sutures, or prostheses. CAC occurs after sensitization to ocular medications and their preservatives.[1]

This chapter will focus on treatment of ocular allergic disease. The following sections address avoidance, medical therapy, and surgical therapy of ocular allergies. A brief review of new and experimental treatment modalities is included as well.

Avoidance

Avoiding known allergen triggers is critical to prevent or ameliorate the symptoms of ocular allergies. Many patients are aware of their allergen triggers, but in some cases allergy testing can be helpful. Possible strategies for avoiding allergens include, staying indoors during high pollen counts, using air conditioners and air filters in the home and car, keeping windows closed, and washing hair and clothes after being outdoors. Patients with perennial allergic conjunctivitis may benefit from covering bedding with plastic covers, removing carpets, and avoiding pets. At a minimum, pets should not be allowed in the bedroom. When eyes itch, the natural response is to rub. The temporary relief of itching achieved from rubbing is negated by a more exuberant inflammatory response.[2] Eye rubbing may bring large quantities of allergens in direct contact with the conjunctiva from the hands and may mechanically disrupt cell membranes, resulting in further release of inflammatory mediators.[2,3] The inflammation, in turn, may result in an itch – rub cycle that is difficult to break. In addition, chronic eye rubbing has been associated with the development of keratoconus. Encouraging patients to stop rubbing their eyes should be a fundamental goal. Cool artificial tears may provide some relief by diluting both inflammatory mediators and allergens on the ocular surface. Cool compresses and ice packs to the eyelids may reduce swelling and provide some additional relief. For many patients, non-medical treatments alone are not sufficient.[1]

Treatment of concurrent lid margin disease can be problematic, particularly in the case of AKC. Warm compresses, eyelids scrubs, and eyelid massage, mainstays of treatment for meibomian gland dysfunction and blepharitis, can exacerbate the chronic inflammation in AKC. Patients should be discouraged from using moisture on the lids, as this can worsen the eczematous changes of the lid skin, such as redness, thickening, and development of fissures. Instead, the use of dry warm compresses is preferred. Any subsequent lid massage should be limited to gentle pressure over the meibomian glands, rather than a vigorous back-and-forth motion. Adjunct use of oral tetracyclines, such as doxycycline or minocycline, and nutritional supplements, such as fish oil and flaxseed oil, can also be helpful.

Medical Therapy

When choosing a medical therapy for allergic conjunctivitis, it is important to remember that the efficacy of an individual medication will vary between patients. As discussed below, each medical therapy targets different mediators in the inflammatory cascade for allergic conjunctivitis (Figs 17.1, 17.2). Selection of an antiallergy medication should be based on the severity, symptoms and projected duration of a patient's allergic disease. For example, a patient with a severe allergic response may initially benefit from a topical corticosteroid, while a patient with moderate symptoms from complex allergies or who requires extended treatment, may do well with mast cell stabilizers or dual-action agents (mast cell stabilizer/antihistamine). Topical medications are listed in Table 17.1.

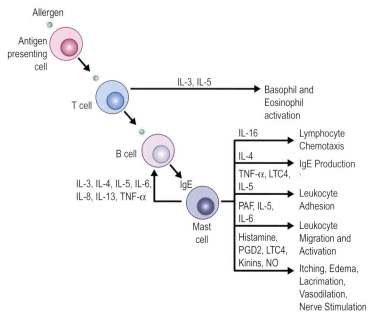

Figure 17.1 Mast cell activation pathways. (Adapted from: Mishra GP, Tamboli V, Jwala J, et al. Recent Patents and Emerging Therapeutics in the Treatment of Allergic Conjunctivitis. Recent Pat Inflamm Allergy Drug Discov 2011;5:26–36.)

VASOCONSTRICTORS

Over-the-counter topical decongestants containing vasoconstrictors with or without antihistamines are generally well tolerated and effective for patients with mild allergic symptoms.[4,5] Although the antihistamine component is weak, the vasoconstrictor component is very effective in reducing conjunctival hyperemia via alpha adrenoceptor stimulation. In the United States, either pheniramine or antazoline, the common antihistamines, is combined with naphazoline, a vasoconstrictor. Using these drops over time may result in tachyphylaxis, requiring patients to use the drops more frequently to obtain the same vasoconstrictor effect. Furthermore, discontinuation of vasoconstricting eyedrops may result in rebound hyperemia.[6] Depending on the underlying condition, artificial tears, corticosteroid drops, or long-term therapy with mast cell stabilizers and/or immunotherapy may help alleviate dependence on the vasoconstricting eyedrops.[6] Due to their mydriatic effect, topical decongestants are contraindicated in patients with narrow angles.

ANTIHISTAMINES

Antihistamines are medications that target the H_1 histamine receptor. First-generation antihistamines block peripheral H_1 receptors, but also cross the blood – brain barrier and block central nervous system H_1 and cholinergic receptors as well. This produces the unwanted side effect of sedation. Nonselective topical antihistamines include pheniramine, antazoline, chlorpheniramine, and cyclizine.

Second-generation antihistamines do not cross the blood – brain barrier. They selectively block peripheral H_1 receptors, reducing the occurrence of sedation while still effectively treating allergic symptoms. These more potent topical

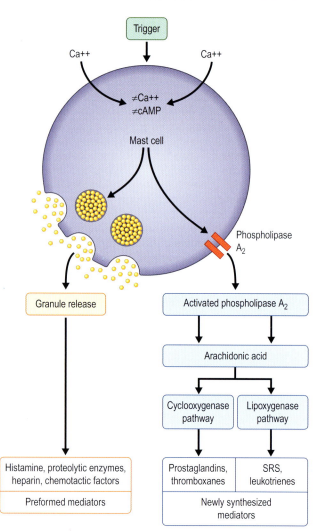

Figure 17.2 When activated, mast cells in the conjunctiva and eyelid release preformed mediators of inflammation from their granules and newly synthesized mediators from their cell membranes via the arachidonic acid cascade. (From Raizman MB. Update on Ocular Allergy. Focal Points Clinical Modules for Ophthalmologists 1994;12:1.)

antihistamines include levocabastine hydrochloride 0.05% and emedastine difumarate 0.05%. Most of the recent antihistamines have also been shown to have some mast cell stabilizing properties as well. Most topical antihistamines have a rapid onset of action, but have a short duration of action, requiring up to four times daily dosing. Selective antihistamines with mast cell stabilizing properties, such as olopatadine, azelastine, ketotifen, alcaftadine, epinastine, and bepotastine, have been shown to have a rapid onset but a longer duration of action when compared to the other topical antihistamines, lasting up to 16 hours.[7–10] Because of the improved efficacy of combined antihistamine/mast cell stabilizers, the pure antihistamine drops have largely been replaced by combination drops.

Systemic therapy with oral antihistamines (diphenhydramine, carbinoxamine, clemastine, chlorpheniramine, brompheniramine, oxatomide, cetirizine, levocetirizine, loratadine, desloratidine, ketotifen, and fexofenadine) may be beneficial for perennial, vernal, or atopic allergic keratoconjunctivitis, given the chronicity of the disease and the potential for patients to become sensitized to preservatives

Table 17.1 Topical Medications for the Treatment of Allergic Conjunctivitis

Route of administration indicates whether the medication is an ocular or dermal preparation. Note that systemic medications are not included in this table.

Class/Mechanism of Action	Medication	Route of Administration
Antihistamines		
Nonselective	pheniramine	ocular
	antazoline	ocular
	chlorpheniramine	ocular
	cyclizine	ocular
	epinastine	ocular
Selective	levocabastine	ocular
	azelastine	ocular
	emedastine	ocular
	alcaftadine	ocular
	bepotastine	ocular
	olopatadine	ocular
Mast cell stabilizers	cromoglycate	ocular
	lodoxamide	ocular
	pemirolast	ocular
	nedocromil	ocular
Dual-acting agents (H_1 receptor blockade and mast cell stabilization)	olopatadine	ocular
	azelastine	ocular
	ketotifen	ocular
	alcaftadine	ocular
	epinastine	ocular
	bepotastine	ocular
NSAIDs	ketorolac	ocular
	diclofenac	ocular
	flurbiprofen	ocular
Corticosteroids	prednisolone	ocular
	loteprednol	ocular
	fluoromethalone	ocular
	dexamethasone	ocular
	difluprednate	ocular
	rimexolone	ocular
	betamethasone	ocular/dermal
	hydrocortisone	dermal
	triamcinolone	dermal
	desonide	dermal
	clobetasone	dermal
Immunosuppressive agents	cyclosporine	ocular
	tacrolimus	ocular/dermal
	pimecrolimus	dermal

(From Mishra GP, Tamboli V, Jwala J, et al. Recent patents and emerging therapeutics in the treatment of allergic conjunctivitis. Recent Pat Inflamm Allergy Drug Discov 2011;5:26–36.)

in some commercial topical preparations. However, oral antihistamines are seldom used to treat isolated seasonal or perennial allergic conjunctivitis, but are frequently used to treat systemic allergy. They should be used with caution in patients with cardiac arrhythmias, or in combination with erythromycin, ketoconazole, itraconazole and troleandomycin. These medications may improve systemic symptoms, but ocular symptoms may worsen. Symptoms of dry eye may be induced or compounded by the propensity of antihistamines to reduce tear production. Topical antihistamines have muscarinic binding properties which, in theory, may also cause or worsen dry eye syndrome. The data on their effect on tear production are conflicting.[11] In general, there is little clinical evidence that topical antihistamines induce dryness. When oral antihistamines are needed to treat rhinitis, the addition of a topical antihistamine may help the ocular symptoms.

MAST CELL STABILIZERS

Traditional mast cell stabilizers are thought to limit the flux of calcium across the mast cell membrane, thus preventing degranulation and release of vasoactive substances. Medications in this group include sodium cromoglycate 4%, lodoxamide tromethamine 0.1%, and the newer mast cell stabilizers: pemirolast potassium 0.1%, and nedocromil sodium 2%.

Given that these medications inhibit the release of histamine rather than block histamine receptors, they are better at preventing than treating allergic signs and symptoms. Their effects may not be seen until 2 to 5 days after initiation of therapy, while their maximum benefit is achieved 15 days after initiating therapy. Therefore, if patients have allergic symptoms during a defined season, they should begin these medications about 2 weeks prior to their allergy season and continue throughout the entire season. Mast cell stabilizers represent the mainstay of therapy for vernal and atopic keratoconjunctivitis. Nedocromil, originally thought to be just a mast cell stabilizing agent, is recognized to have multiple actions resulting in rapid relief of symptoms. These actions include antihistaminic (H_1 antagonist) effects, reduction of ICAM-1 expression, and inhibitory effects on eosinophils and neutrophils.[12]

Numerous studies have demonstrated the safety and effectiveness of cromolyn sodium, nedocromil, lodoxamide, and pemirolast, in treating signs and symptoms of vernal and seasonal allergic conjunctivitis.[13–21] When comparing the older agents, lodoxamide is about 2500 times more potent than sodium cromoglycate in an animal model, although their efficacy in controlling the symptoms of allergic conjunctivitis is similar.[22] A long-term comparison of nedocromil versus cromolyn sodium found that nedocromil 2% produced a more rapid and marked improvement in symptoms over cromolyn 2% and decreased the need for steroid rescue.[23] Lodoxamide 0.1% may have additional benefits over cromolyn sodium because it has been found to also have potential antieosinophil action.[16,24]

Additional studies suggest that mast cell stabilizers may act through other mechanisms. Cromolyn sodium reportedly inhibits the chemotaxis, activation, degranulation, and cytotoxicity of neutrophils, eosinophils, and monocytes.[16,25] Lodoxamide and cromolyn sodium may also have effects on Th2 cells, which have been implicated in the pathogenesis of VKC.[26] In some patients, mast cell stabilizing drops may be more effective for chronic therapy than dual-acting agents (antihistamine/mast cell stabilizing agents).

DUAL-ACTING AGENTS

The dual-acting medications, including olopatadine hydrochloride 0.1% and 0.2%, azelastine hydrochloride 0.05%, ketotifen fumarate 0.025% (available over the counter), alcaftadine 0.25%, bepotastine 1.5%, and epinastine hydrochloride 0.05%, have antihistamine and mast cell stabilizing properties. Most of these drugs have additional modes of action, including eosinophil and basophil inhibition.[27,28] These medications are usually effective for the treatment and prevention of signs and symptoms of allergic conjunctivitis.[29–31] Olopatadine 0.2% and alcaftadine are the only antiallergy eyedrops approved for once-daily dosing. These dual-action medications are appropriate choices for patients with acute seasonal exacerbations, as well as those with chronic perennial symptoms; they are the mainstay of therapy for the majority of patients with allergic conjunctivitis.

NONSTEROIDAL ANTI-INFLAMMATORY DRUGS (NSAIDS)

Ketorolac tromethamine 0.5%, diclofenac, and flurbiprofen are nonsteroidal anti-inflammatory agents which decrease the activity of cyclooxygenase, an enzyme responsible for arachidonic acid metabolism. The inhibition of cyclooxygenase, in turn, reduces prostaglandin production, most notably the highly pruritic PGE_2 and PGI_2.[32] These drugs have been shown to reduce itching, ICAM-1 expression, and tryptase levels in tears associated with ocular allergy.[33–35] Topical ketorolac tromethamine, the only approved nonsteroidal anti-inflammatory drug for managing ocular allergies, has been shown to provide relief of the signs and symptoms of allergic conjunctivitis.[36,37] Some patients have transient stinging upon instillation. The newer agents discussed above have largely replaced the topical nonsteroidal anti-inflammatory agents.

Signs and symptoms of VKC have been reported to improve with the addition of oral aspirin (1.5 g–4.0 g per day), although routine administration at these high doses could produce serious side effects, especially given that many VKC patients are children.[38,39]

CORTICOSTEROIDS

Topical corticosterioids, including prednisolone, loteprednol, dexamethasone, fluorometholone, and rimexolone, are highly effective for the treatment of ocular allergy because they block most allergic inflammatory cascades (including the late-phase mediators). Corticosteroids diminish the signs and symptoms of ocular allergy by stabilizing capillary permeability, decreasing the influx of inflammatory cells, and inhibiting the activation and degranulation of inflammatory cells.[40] Intranasal corticosteroids, when used to treat allergic rhinitis, may also improve concurrent ocular symptoms.[41–43] Corticosteroids are particularly helpful in the treatment of VKC and AKC but are less often used for GPC or SAC. Given their propensity to induce cataracts, elevate intraocular pressure in susceptible individuals and potentiate ocular infections, their judicious use is indicated.[44]

It may be necessary to use corticosteroids in SAC for short periods, if the allergic response is severe and conservative therapy has failed. Loteprednol, an ester corticosteroid which is metabolized in the aqueous humor, is effective in treating seasonal allergic conjunctivitis. In a recent retrospective study, loteprednol 0.2% was well tolerated with no reports of adverse reactions in patients treated for SAC or PAC for at least 12 months.[45]

Moderate to severe cases of VKC or AKC that are unresponsive to mast cell stabilizers and antihistamines, may necessitate the short-term use of topical corticosteroids. Corneal involvement at any stage warrants the

consideration of corticosteroid therapy. Bonini and colleagues reported that 85% of patients in their long-term cohort of 195 VKC patients, required steroids at some point during the course of the disease.[46]

Allansmith found that 'pulse' therapy with topical dexamethasone (1%) given every 2 hours, eight times daily and gradually tapered over days to weeks, to be effective for breakthrough attacks of VKC inflammation.[47]

In the absence of corneal involvement, low-absorption corticosteroids, such as fluorometholone, loteprednol, and rimexolone, should be tried first. Dose and frequency are determined based on the level of inflammation, with a gradual taper occurring over 2 weeks. Only after first-line therapy fails should more potent agents, such as prednisolone, dexamethasone, or betamethasone be considered.[48] Supratarsal injection of short- or intermediate-acting corticosteroids has also been reported to confer relief in severe VKC.[49]

Active corneal signs may necessitate the initial use of more potent steroids, such as prednisolone or difluprednate. It is critical to recognize even the mildest forms of corneal disease, as delay in treatment could result in poor visual outcome. Although pathognomonic for VKC, shield ulcers often begin as a mild, non-specific subepithelial 'haze.'

Corticosteroid ointments may be helpful for treatment of atopic dermatitis in cases with significant eyelid skin involvement. Corticosteroid ointments used on the skin include betamethasone, hydrocortisone, triamcinolone, desonide, and clobetasone. Unfortunately, side effects, such as elevation of intraocular pressure, cataract formation, and skin atrophy, limit the use of corticosteroids on eyelid skin. It is critical to educate patients not to use corticosteroid ointments around the eyes for extended periods without close monitoring.

Long-term maintenance, topical steroid therapy should be avoided given the potential complications, including glaucoma, formation of cataracts, and increased susceptibility to infections. Corticosteroid therapy has been associated with 2% to 7% of VKC patients developing glaucoma and 14% developing cataracts.[46,50,51] If corticosteroids are necessary, patients should be given the lowest concentration for the shortest duration with appropriate follow-up.

ADDITIONAL TREATMENTS FOR VKC AND AKC
Immunosuppressive Agents

CYCLOSPORINE

Cyclosporine, an immunosuppressive drug commonly used to prevent organ-graft rejection, has demonstrated efficacy in controlling ocular inflammation. Cyclosporine works primarily by binding to the cytosolic protein cyclophilin and blocking Th2 lymphocyte proliferation and IL-2 production.[52] It also inhibits histamine release from mast cells and basophils and reduces IL-5 production, which may limit the infiltration of eosinophils into the conjunctiva.[53,54] Clinically, cyclosporine A administration results in a reduction in total T cells, a normalization of the CD4:CD8 ratio, a decrease in T-cell activation, and a reduction in T-cell cytokine expression, especially IL-2 and IFN. Cyclosporine A has been shown to have an immunomodulatory effect in atopic and vernal keratoconjunctivitis.[55-57] Leonardi and colleagues suggest that cyclosporine shows particular effectiveness in VKC by reducing conjunctival fibroblast proliferation and IL-1b production.[58]

Cyclosporine 1% to 2% ophthalmic emulsions in olive, maize, or castor oil have been shown to be effective in the treatment of VKC and AKC.[59-66] It has been demonstrated that cyclosporine 2%, used four times daily over 2 weeks, significantly decreases signs and symptoms in VKC patients and that it was effective in decreasing dependence of steroids in patients with AKC.[67,68] Several groups have examined the effectiveness of cyclosporine at concentrations as low as 0.05%, but results at these levels have been equivocal. Spadavecchia and colleagues suggest that 1% may be the lower bound for effective dosage as demonstrated in their cohort of school-age children.[69] Leonardi and colleagues found cyclosporine to have a significant steroid sparing effect, allowing VKC to be controlled with mast cell stabilizers alone.[70] Unlike corticosteroids, cyclosporine has not been associated with lens changes or increases in intraocular pressure.[71,72] However, many patients complain of burning and irritation associated with current formulations. Other adverse events, such as bacterial or viral infections, are rare.

At present, topical cyclosporine is commercially available in the United States, only as a 0.05% emulsion (Restasis). Higher concentrations must be formulated by hospital pharmacies. In Europe, phase III clinical trials have been completed for a new cyclosporine preparation, Vekacia, which is indicated for the treatment of VKC.

Tacrolimus and Pimecrolimus

Tacrolimus (FK506) is an immunosuppressant drug used for prevention of organ transplant rejection. It inhibits calcineurin and stops the synthesis and release of cytokines from T lymphocytes, preventing T-lymphocyte activation. Multiple recent studies have investigated topical tacrolimus 0.005–0.03% as a treatment for both vernal and atopic conjunctivitis with good results.[73-82] The studies have demonstrated efficacy comparable to that of corticosteroids for clinical signs and symptoms, as well as decrease in conjunctival inflammatory markers, such as eosinophils, neutrophils, and lymphocytes.[80] Tacrolimus therapy alone has been demonstrated to treat the symptoms and signs of VKC and AKC, such as burning, tearing, photophobia, injection, pain, and itching, as well as regression of GPC, resolution of shield ulcers, and healing of corneal epithelial disease.[75] It appears to be successful in the treatment AKC and VKC, even in patients who have been refractory to treatment with systemic and/or topical steroids, antihistamines, mast cell stabilizers, cyclosporine A, and even surgical resection/cryopexy of GPC.[74] There have not been any demonstrated adverse effects, except for burning upon instillation. Tacrolimus does not appear to elevate intraocular pressure; therefore it may be a good alternative to treatment with corticosteroids, especially for patients who are steroid responders.[76,81] Another calcineurin inhibitor, pimecrolimus, is more selective than tacrolimus and can also be used safely as an ointment for periocular atopic dermatitis. Tacrolimus and pimecrolimus ointment can be applied to

the lid skin safely for relief of periocular atopic dermatitis, without the side effects of corticosteroids, such as skin atrophy, elevation of intraocular pressure, and cataract formation.

Systemic tacrolimus has been investigated for treatment of VKC or AKC with success, but with greater potential for adverse effects due to systemic immunosupression.[82]

OTHER TREATMENTS

Agents that oppose leukotriene action are considered to be important in asthma and other atopic diseases, which may have steroid-independent components. These agents can be used alongside steroids and might allow the reduction of steroid use. Montelukast is a leukotriene receptor antagonist that has demonstrated high affinity, binding to the leukotriene receptor.[83] Clinical studies in patients with seasonal allergic rhinitis indicated that while symptoms of allergic rhinitis were improved with montelukast, there was no significant difference in ocular symptoms between montelukast and placebo.[84] However, montelukast has been demonstrated to be effective in atopic dermatitis, especially of the face, leading to alleviation of pruritus and atopic skin changes.[83]

Some patients experience relief when their eyes are closed, thus making occlusive therapies (patching, occlusive goggles or a tarsorrhaphy) helpful in some situations, probably by minimizing contact with airborne allergens.[85] While contact lens wear may also help limit exposure to airborne allergens, the presence of papillae on the tarsal conjunctiva can make contact lens wear uncomfortable. Additionally, the contact lenses themselves can worsen symptoms of ocular allergies, as discussed below, so this strategy is not routinely recommended.

SURGICAL TREATMENT

The treatment of VKC is frequently challenging and may require a multidisciplinary approach. Despite the development of new medications which are usually effective in treating acute phases of VKC, the disease can still be debilitating for some patients. Although VKC is self-limited with good prognosis, surgical treatment may become necessary for certain complications, including for large giant papillae, conjunctival scarring, and corneal shield ulcers.

For large symptomatic papillae, conjunctival transposition or autografts have been performed with some effect.[86] Cryotherapy of the tarsal conjunctiva often provides temporary relief, possibly by decreasing the number of inflammatory cells and reducing the inflammatory mediators released; however, the papillae and symptoms usually return. Bonini and colleagues have noted that cryogenic surgery performed to reduce papillary excrescences, may result in a pemphigoid-like appearance throughout the conjunctiva.[46] Belfair and colleagues have described the use of CO_2 laser in removing giant papillae in refractory VKC.[87,88] However, the long-term effectiveness of this modality is unclear. In general, conjunctival surgery is rarely required and should be avoided.

Corneal shield ulcers may respond to bandage soft contact lenses, patching, and tarsorrhaphy, in addition to the medical therapy described. Cases that do not respond to conservative measures or exhibit inflammatory deposits in the ulcer base may require surgical intervention.

Surgical debridement and superficial keratectomy can aid in the re-epithelialization of the cornea.[89] Daily debridement of the ulcer may promote more rapid healing. One study demonstrated rapid re-epithelialization of three central corneal lesions from VKC, that were treated with excimer laser phototherapeutic keratectomy. This was performed after active inflammation was controlled and the inflammatory plaque overlying the shield ulcer was removed.[90]

There have also been multiple reports of successful management of shield ulcers with use of amniotic membrane transplantation, either alone or in combination with cryotherapy of GPC, or prior debridement of the ulcer.[91–93]

Cameron has proposed a classification system for shield ulcers based on their clinical characteristics, response to treatment, and complications. Grade 1 ulcers had a clear base, responded favorably to medical treatment, and re-epithelialized with minimal scarring. Grade 2 ulcers had visible inflammatory debris in the base, responded poorly to medical therapy alone, and demonstrated delayed re-epithelialization with complications, such as bacterial keratitis. Grade 2 patients showed dramatic response to scraping the base of the ulcer, with re-epithelialization occurring by 1 week. Grade 3 ulcers had elevated plaque formation and responded best to surgical therapy.[88] Solomon and colleagues have also reported successful re-epithelialization of the cornea, after surgical scraping of vernal plaques in patients who had been nonresponsive to maximal medical therapy.[94] Sridhar and colleagues demonstrated additional benefits in combining amniotic membrane grafting, with surgical debridement in a small group of VKC patients.[93] Sangwan and colleagues suggest that limbal stem cell transplantation may also have promise in severe cases of VKC.[95]

Phototherapeutic keratectomy may also be useful in removing superficial corneal scars. Deep anterior lamellar keratoplasty might be necessary for deeper and visually compromising corneal scars. Restoring optical clarity of the cornea would be especially critical in a young child at risk for developing amblyopia. The chronic surrounding inflammation and the tendency toward trophic erosions can make corneal transplantation particularly challenging in this young population.

Additional Treatments for GPC

Contact lens wearers often do not want to discontinue wearing their lenses, despite having symptomatic GPC. After insertion, contact lenses become coated with a biofilm that can act as a base for antigen deposition and trigger GPC. Patients should maintain meticulous contact lens hygiene or switch to a daily disposable type of contact lens.[1] Mechanical removal of mucus and protein deposits from the lens surface by rubbing the contact lens can reduce the likelihood of irritation. Use of hydrogen peroxide-based contact lens cleaning solutions can be helpful as well. Similarly, regular cleaning of ocular prostheses can reduce mucus and protein build-up that can precipitate GPC.

Theoretically, when contact lenses are worn while eyedrops are used, the pharmacokinetics of the drug's active ingredient and preservative can be altered, allowing for prolonged ocular exposure to these chemicals.[96] Thus, putting in contacts at least 20 minutes after drop instillation is recommended. Allergic conjunctivitis can adversely affect tear film stability, which may be why patients with a history of ocular allergy often have contact-lens-related discomfort.[4,97]

New and Experimental Treatment Modalities

New therapies are being investigated which may be more effective and have safer side effect profiles than current treatment modalities.[4] Several patents filed in recent years aim to devise new strategies to treat ocular allergies. Whether these strategies prove to be clinically useful remains to be seen. Large-scale clinical studies have not yet been performed, and therefore, the use of the treatments listed below cannot be recommended at this time. The strategies below are listed for information only.

Yedger filed a patent describing use of lipid-conjugated peptides to treat conjunctivitis by inhibiting phospholipase A2.[98] Phospholipase A2 is an enzyme that catalyzes the breakdown of cell membrane phospholipids, leading to production of inflammatory mediators. By inhibiting phospholipase A2, the inventors report reduction in levels of ocular inflammatory mediators and reduction of corneal opacification. Kato and colleagues have reported on a novel selective glucocorticoid receptor agonist, ZK209614, which compared favorably with betamethasone in reducing conjunctival edema in rat and feline models of experimental allergic conjunctivitis.[98] While betamethasone caused steroid-induced elevation of intraocular pressure, ZK209614 did not cause a steroid response. Topical chlorogenic acid and glucosamine are being investigated for their inhibitory effects on transglutaminase. In a guinea pig model, chlorogenic acid was found to decrease conjunctival hyperemia and edema.[98] Cyclic AMP (cAMP) is a key cytokine regulating activity of neutrophils, eosinophils, and mast cells. Drugs which inhibit phosphodiesterase IV (PDE IV) dependent hydrolysis of cAMP are being investigated for their effects on suppressing activation of the inflammatory cascade. Toll-like receptors (TLR) have been identified on mast cells and circulating leukocytes, regulating the Th1:Th2 balance that can lead to allergic disease. Novel compounds which inhibit TLR and help to down-regulate this pathway are being investigated. Small interfering RNA aimed at blocking various targets in the intracellular mast cell signal transduction cascade are being studied.[98] Inhibitory molecules, targeting histamine H_4 receptors and Janus protein kinase-3 (JAK-3) are other areas of research. Monoclonal antibodies against the eotaxin receptor are being studied and may limit recruitment of eosinophils to the ocular surface. Sublingual immunotherapy (SLIT) is an effective hyposensitization treatment for allergic rhinitis, and its use for reducing subjective symptoms of allergic conjunctivitis, was the subject of a recent Cochrane Review meta-analysis of nearly 4000 participants with allergic rhinitis and allergic conjunctivitis. The study found that SLIT is moderately effective in reducing ocular allergy symptom scores.[99]

References

1. Rothman JS, Raizman MB, Friedlander MH. Seasonal and perennial allergic conjunctivitis. In: Krachmer JH, Mannis MJ, Holland EJ, editors. Cornea. 3rd ed. Philadelphia: Elsevier; 2011.
2. Greiner JV, Peace DG, Baird RS, et al. Effects of eye rubbing on the conjunctiva as a model of ocular inflammation. Am J Ophthalmol 1985;100:45–50.
3. Raizman MB, Rothman JS, Maroun F, et al. Effect of eye rubbing on signs and symptoms of allergic conjunctivitis in cat-sensitive individuals. Ophthalmology 2000;107:2158–61.
4. Greiner JV, Udell IJ. A comparison of the clinical efficacy of pheniramine solution and olopatadine hydrochloride ophthalmic solution in the conjunctival allergen challenge model. Clin Ther 2005;275:468–577.
5. Abelson MB, Allansmith MR, Friedlander MH. Effects of topically applied ocular decongestant and antihistamine. Am J Ophthalmol 1980;90:254–7.
6. Spector SL, Raizman MB. Conjunctivitis medicamentosa. J Allergy Clin Immunol 1994;94:134–6.
7. Albietz JM, Lenton LM. Management of the ocular surface and tear film before, during, and after laser in situ keratomileusis. J Refract Sur 2004;20:62–71.
8. Moss SE, Klein R, Klein BE. Prevalence of and risk factors for dry eye syndrome. Arch Ophthalmol 2000;118:1264–8.
9. Williams JI, Kennedy KS, Gow JA, et al. Prolonged effectiveness of bepotastine besilate ophthalmic solution for the treatment of ocular symptoms of allergic conjunctivitis. J Ocul Pharmacol Ther 2011;27:385–93.
10. Torkildsen G, Shedden A. The safety and efficacy of alcaftadine 0.25% ophthalmic solution for the prevention of itching associated with allergic conjunctivitis. Curr Med Res Opin 2011;27:623–31.
11. Lekhanont K, Park CY, Combs JC, et al. Effect of topical olopatadine and epinastine in the botulinum toxin B-induced mouse model of dry eye. J Ocul Pharmacol Ther 2007;23:83–8.
12. Corin RE. Nedocromil sodium: a review of the evidence for adual mechanism of action. Clin Exp Allergy 2000;30:461–8.
13. Foster CS. Evaluation of topical cromolyn sodium in the treatment of vernal keratoconjunctivitis. Ophthalmology 1988;95:194–201.
14. Abelson MB, Berdy GJ, Mundorf T, et al. Pemirolast potassium 0.1% ophthalmic solution is an effective treatment for allergic conjunctivitis: a pooled analysis of two prospective, randomized, double-masked, placebo-controlled, phase III studies. J Ocul Pharmacol Ther 2002;18:475–88.
15. Bonini S, Barney NP, Schiavone M, et al. Effectiveness of nedocromil sodium 2% eyedrops on clinical symptoms and tear fluid cytology of patients with vernal conjunctivitis. Eye 1992;6:648–52.
16. Bonini S, Schiavone M, Bonini S, et al. Efficacy of lodoxamide eye drops on mast cells and eosinophils after allergen challenge in allergic conjunctivitis. Ophthalmology 1997;104:849–53.
17. Foster CS. Evaluation of topical cromolyn sodium in the treatment of vernal keratoconjunctivitis. Ophthalmology 1988;95:194–201.
18. Blumenthal M, Casale T, Dockhorn R, et al. Efficacy and safety of nedocromil sodium ophthalmic solution in the treatment of seasonal allergic conjunctivitis. Am J Ophthalmol 1992;113:56–63.
19. El Hennawi M. A double blind placebo controlled group comparative study of ophthalmic sodium cromoglycate and nedocromil sodium in the treatment of vernal keratoconjunctivitis. Br J Ophthalmol 1994;78:365–9.
20. Kjellman NI, Stevens MT. Clinical experience with Tilavist: an overview of efficacy and safety. Allergy 1995;50:14–22.
21. Stockwell A, Easty DL. Group comparative trial of 2% nedocromil sodium with placebo in the treatment of seasonal allergic conjunctivitis. Eur J Ophthalmol 1994;4:12–23.
22. Johnson HG, White GJ. Development of new antiallergic drugs (cromolyn sodium, lodoxamide tromethamine). What is the role of cholinergic stimulation in the biphasic dose response? Monogr Allergy 1979;14:299–306.
23. Verin PH, Dicker ID, Mortemousque B. Nedocromil sodium eye drops are more effective than sodium cromoglycate eye drops for the long-term management of vernal keratoconjunctivitis. Clin Exp Allergy 1999;29:529–36.
24. Caldwell DR, Verin P, Hartwich-Young R, et al. Efficacy and safety of lodoxamide 0.1% vs. cromolyn sodium 4% in patients with vernal keratoconjunctivitis. Am J Ophthalmol 1992;113:632–7.
25. Kay AB, Walsh GM, Moqbel R, et al. Disodium cromoglycate inhibits activation of human inflammatory cells in vitro. J Allergy Clin Immunol 1987;80:1–8.
26. Avunduk AM, Avunduk MC, Kapicioglu Z, et al. Mechanisms and comparison of anti-allergic efficacy of topical lodoxamide and cromolyn sodium treatment in vernal keratoconjunctivitis. Ophthalmology 2000;107:1333–7.
27. Hasala H, Malm-Erjefält M, Erjefält J, et al. Ketotifen induces primary necrosis of human eosinophils. J Ocul Pharmacol Ther 2005;21:318–27.
28. Randley BW, Sedgwick J. The effect of azelastine on neutrophil and eosinophil generation of superoxide. J Allergy Clin Immunol 1989;83:400–5.
29. Whitcup SM, Bradford R, Lue J, et al. Efficacy and tolerability of ophthalmic epinastine: a randomized, double-masked, parallel-group, active and vehicle-controlled environmental trial in patients with seasonal allergic conjunctivitis. Clin Ther 2004;26:29–34.
30. Greiner JV, Michaelson C, McWhirter CL, et al. Single dose of ketotifen fumarate .025% vs 2 weeks of cromolyn sodium 4% for allergic conjunctivitis. Adv Ther 2002;19:185–93.
31. Spangler DL, Bensch G, Berdy GJ. Evaluation of the efficacy of olopatadine hydrochloride 0.1% ophthalmic solution and azelastine hydrochloride 0.05% ophthalmic solution in the conjunctival allergen challenge model. Clin Ther 2001;23:1272–80.
32. Woodward DF, Nieves AL, Hawley SB, et al. The pruritogenic and inflammatory effects of prostanoids in the conjunctiva. J Ocul Pharmacol Ther 1995;11:339–47.
33. Tinkelman DG, Rupp G, Kaufman H, et al. Double-masked, paired comparison clinical study of ketorolac tromethamine 0.5% ophthalmic solution compared with placebo eyedrops in the treatment of seasonal allergic conjunctivitis. Surv Ophthalmol 1993;38:133–40.
34. Ballas Z, Blumenthal M, Tinkelman DG, et al. Clinical evaluation of ketorolac tromethamine 0.5% ophthalmic solution for the treatment of seasonal allergic conjunctivitis. Surv Ophthalmol 1993;38:141–8.
35. Leonardi A, Busato F, Fregona IA, et al. Anti-inflammatory and antiallergic effects of ketorolac tromethamine in the conjunctival provocation model. Br J Ophthalmol 2000;84:1228–32.
36. Raizman MB. Results of a survey of patients with ocular allergy treated with topical ketorolac tromethamine. Clin Ther 1995;17:882–90.
37. Donshik PC, Pearlman D, Pinnas J, et al. Efficacy and safety of ketorolac tromethamine 0.5% and levocabastine 0.05%: a multicenter comparison in patients with seasonal allergic conjunctivitis. Adv Ther 2000;17:94–102.
38. Abelson MB, Butrus SI, Weston JH. Aspirin therapy in vernal conjunctivitis. Am J Ophthalmol 1983;95:502–5.
39. Chaudhary KP. Evaluation of combined systemic aspirin and cromolyn sodium in intractable vernal catarrh. Ann Ophthalmol 1990;22:314–8.
40. Abelson MB, Schaefer K. Conjunctivitis of allergic origin: immunologic mechanisms and current approaches to therapy. Surv Ophthalmol 1993;38:115–32.
41. Bernstein DI, Levy AL, Hampel FC, et al. Treatment with intranasal fluticasone propionate significantly improves ocular symptoms in patients with seasonal allergic rhinitis. Clin Exp Allergy 2004;34:952–7.
42. Hong J, Bielory B, Rosenberg JL. Efficacy of intranasal corticosteroids for the ocular symptoms of allergic rhinitis: A systematic review. Allergy Asthma Proc 2011;32:22–35.
43. Bielory L, Chun Y, Bielory BP, et al. Impact of mometasone furoate nasal spray on individual ocular symptoms of allergic rhinitis: a meta-analysis. Allergy 2011;66:686–93.
44. Friedlaender MH. Corticosteroid therapy of ocular inflammation. Int Ophthalmol Clin 1983;23:175–82.
45. Ilyas H, Slonim CB, Braswell GR, et al. Long-term safety of loteprednol etabonate 0.2% in the treatment of seasonal and perennial allergic conjunctivitis. Eye Contact Lens 2004;30:10–3.
46. Bonini S, Bonini S, Lambiase A, et al. Vernal keratoconjunctivitis revisited: a case series of 195 patients with long-term follow-up. Ophthalmology 2000;107:1157–63.
47. Allansmith MR. Vernal conjunctivitis. In: Duane's clinical ophthalmology, vol. 4. Philadelphia: JB Lippincott; 1992.

48. Leonardi A. Vernal keratoconjunctivitis: pathogenesis and treatment. Prog Retin Eye Res 2002;21:319–39.

49. Holsclaw DS, Whitcher JP, Wong IG, et al. Supratarsal injection of corticosteroid in the treatment of refractory vernal keratoconjunctivitis. Am J Ophthalmol 1996;121:243–9.

50. Leonardi A, Busca F, Motterle L, et al. Case series of 406 vernal keratoconjunctivitis patients: a demographic and epidemiological study. Acta Ophthalmol Scand 2006;84:406–10.

51. Tabbara KF. Ocular complications of vernal keratoconjunctivitis. Can J Ophthalmol 1999;34:88–92.

52. Lightman S. Therapeutic considerations: symptoms, cells and mediators. Allergy 1995;50(Suppl. 21):10–3; discussion: 34–38.

53. Tabbara KF. Ocular complications of vernal keratoconjunctivitis. Can J Ophthalmol 1999;34:88–92.

54. Sperr WR, Agis H, Czerwenka K, et al. Effects of cyclosporine A and FK-506 on stem cell factor-induced histamine secretion and growth of human mast cells. J Allergy Clin Immunol 1996;98:389–99.

55. Whitcup SM, Chan CC, Luyo DA, et al. Topical cyclosporine inhibits mast cell-mediated conjunctivitis. Invest Ophthalmol Vis Sci 1996;37:2686–93.

56. Hingorani M, Calder VL, Buckley RJ, et al. The immunomodulatory effect of topical cyclosporine A in atopic keratoconjunctivitis. Invest Ophthalmol Vis Sci 1999;40:392–9.

57. Leonardi A, Borghesan F, DePaoli M, et al. Procollagens and inflammatory cytokine concentrations in tarsal and limbal vernal keratoconjunctivitis. Exp Eye Res 1998;67:105–12.

58. Leonardi A, DeFranchis G, Fregona IA, et al. Effects of cyclosporine A on human conjunctival fibroblasts. Arch Ophthalmol 2001;119:1512–7.

59. BenEzra D, Pe'er J, Brodsky M, et al. Cyclosporine eyedrops for the treatment of severe vernal keratoconjunctivitis. Am J Ophthalmol 1986;101:278–82.

60. Bleik JH, Tabbara KF. Topical cyclosporine in vernal keratoconjunctivitis. Ophthalmology 1991;98:1679–84.

61. Holland EJ, Olsen TW, Ketcham JM, et al. Topical cyclosporine A in the treatment of anterior segment inflammatory disease. Cornea 1993;12:413–9.

62. Kaan G, Ozden O. Therapeutic use of topical cyclosporine. Ann Ophthalmol 1993;25:182–6.

63. Kiliç A, Gürler B. Topical 2% cyclosporine A in preservative-free artificial tears for the treatment of vernal keratoconjunctivitis. Can J Ophthalmol 2006;41:693–8.

64. Pucci N, Novembre E, Cianferoni A, et al. Efficacy and safety of cyclosporine eyedrops in vernal keratoconjunctivitis. Ann Allergy Asthma Immunol 2002;89:298–303.

65. Secchi AG, Tognon MS, Leonardi A. Topical use of cyclosporine in the treatment of vernal keratoconjunctivitis. Am J Ophthalmol 1990;110:641–5.

66. Pucci N, Caputo R, Mori F, et al. Long-term safety and efficacy of topical cyclosporine in 156 children with vernal keratoconjunctivitis. Int J Immunopathol Pharmacol 2010;23:865–71.

67. Hingorani M, Moodaley L, Calder VL, et al. A randomized, placebo-controlled trial of topical cyclosporine A in steroid-dependent atopic keratoconjunctivitis. Ophthalmology 1998;105:1715–20.

68. Lambiase A, Leonardi A, Sacchetti M, et al. Topical cyclosporine prevents seasonal recurrences of vernal keratoconjunctivitis in a randomized, double-masked, controlled 2-year study. J Allergy Clin Immunol 2011;128:896–7.

69. Spadavecchia L, Fanelli P, Tesse R, et al. Efficacy of 1.25% and 1% topical cyclosporine in the treatment of severe vernal keratoconjunctivitis in childhood. Pediatr Allergy Immunol 2006;17:527–32.

70. Leonardi A, Borghesan F, Faggian D, et al. Eosinophil cationic protein in tears of normal subjects and patients affected by vernal keratoconjunctivitis. Allergy 1995;50:610–3.

71. Pucci N, Novembre E, Cianferoni A, et al. Efficacy and safety of cyclosporine eyedrops in vernal keratoconjunctivitis. Ann Allergy Asthma Immunol 2002;89:298–303.

72. Perry HD, Donnenfeld ED, Kanellopoulos AJ, et al. Topical cyclosporine A in the management of postkeratoplasty glaucoma. Cornea 1997;16:284–8.

73. Kheirkhah A, Zavareh MK, Farzbod F, et al. Topical 0.005% tacrolimus eye drop for refractory vernal keratoconjunctivitis. Eye 2011;25:872–80.

74. Garcia DP, Alperte JI, Cristobal JA, et al. Topical tacrolimus ointment for the treatment of intractable atopic keratoconjunctivitis: a case report and review of the literature. Cornea 2011;30:462–5.

75. Tam PM, Young AL, Cheng LL, et al. Topical tacrolimus 0.03% monotherapy for vernal keratoconjunctivitis – case series. Br J Ophthalmol 2010;94:1405–6.

76. Remitz A, Virtanen HM, Reitamo S, et al. Tacrolimus ointment in atopic blepharoconjunctivitis does not seem to elevate intraocular pressure. Acta Ophthalmol 2011;89:295–6.

77. Attas-Fox L, Barkana Y, Iskhakov V, et al. Topical tacrolimus 0.03% ointment for intractable allergic conjunctivitis: an open-lable pilot study. Curr Eye Res 2008;33:545–9.

78. Kymionis GD, Goldman D, Ide T, et al. Tacrolimus ointment 0.03% in the eye for treatment of giant papillary conjunctivitis. Cornea 2008;27:228–9.

79. Miyazaki D, Tominaga T, Kakimaru-Hasegawa A, et al. Therapeutic effects of tacrolimus ointment for refractory ocular surface inflammatory diseases. Ophthalmology 2008;115:988–92.

80. Virtanen HM, Reitamo S, Kari M, et al. Effect of 0.03% tacrolimus ointment on conjunctival cytology in patients with severe atopic blepharoconjunctivitis: a retrospective study. Acta Ophthalmol Scand 2006;84:693–5.

81. Nivenius E, Van der Ploeg I, Jung K, et al. Tacrolimus ointment vs. steroid ointment for eyelid dermatitis in patients with atopic keratoconjunctivitis. Eye 2007;21:968–75.

82. Anzaar F, Gallagher MJ, Bhat P, et al. Use of systemic T-lymphocyte signal transduction inhibitors in the treatment of atopic keratoconjunctivitis. Cornea 2011;27:884–8.

83. Kägi MK. Leukotriene receptor antagonists – a novel therapeutic approach in atopic dermatitis? Dermatology 2001;203:280–3.

84. Ashrafzadeh A, Raizman MB. New modalities in the treatment of ocular allergy. Int Ophthalmol Clin 2003 Winter;43:105–10.

85. Jun J, Bielory L, Raizman MB. Vernal conjunctivitis. Immunol Allergy Clin North Am 2008;28:59–82.

86. Nishiwaki-Dantas MC, Dantas PE, Pezzutti S, et al. Surgical resection of giant papillae and autologous conjunctival graft in patients with severe vernal keratoconjunctivitis and giant papillae. Ophthal Plast Reconstr Surg 2000;16:438–42.

87. Belfair N, Monos T, Levy J, et al. Removal of giant vernal papillae by CO2 laser. Can J Ophthalmol 2005;40:472–6.

88. Cameron JA. Shield ulcers and plaques of the cornea in vernal keratoconjunctivitis. Ophthalmology 1995;102:985–93.

89. Ozbek Z, Burakgazi AZ, Rapuano CJ, et al. Rapid healing of vernal shield ulcer after surgical debridement: a case report. Cornea 2006;25:472–3.

90. Cameron JA, Antonios SR, Badr IA. Excimer laser phototherapeutic keratectomy for shield ulcers and corneal plaques in vernal keratoconjunctivitis. J Refract Surg 1995;11:31–5.

91. Rouher N, Pilon F, Dalens H, et al. Implantation of preserved human amniotic membrane for the treatment of shield ulcers and persistent corneal epithelial defects in chronic allergic conjunctivitis. J Fr Ophthalmol 2004;27:1091–7.

92. Chandra A, Maurya OP, Reddy B, et al. Amniotic membrane transplantation in ocular surface disorders. J Indian Med Assoc 2005;103:364–6.

93. Sridhar MS, Sangwan VS, Bansal AK, et al. Amniotic membrane transplantation in the management of shield ulcers of vernal keratoconjunctivitis. Ophthalmology 2001;108:1218–22.

94. Solomon A, Zamir E, Levartovsky S, et al. Surgical management of corneal plaques in vernal keratoconjunctivitis: a clinicopathologic study. Cornea 2004;23:608–12.

95. Sangwan VS, Murthy SI, Vemuganti GK, et al. Cultivated corneal epithelial transplantation for severe ocular surface disease in vernal keratoconjunctivitis. Cornea 2005;24:426–30.

96. Jain MR. Drug delivery through soft contact lenses. Br J Ophthalmol 1988;72:150–4.

97. Suzuki S, Goto E, Dogru M, et al. Tear film lipid layer alterations in allergic conjunctivitis. Cornea 2006;25:277–8.

98. Mishra GP, Tamboli V, Jwala J, et al. Recent patents and emerging therapeutics in the treatment of allergic conjunctivitis. Recent Pat Inflamm Allergy Drug Discov 2011;5:26–36.

99. Calderon MA, Penagos M, Sheikh A, et al. Sublingual immunotherapy for treating allergic conjunctivitis. Cochrane Database Syst Rev 2011;6:CD007685.

18 *Pterygium*

MINAS T. CORONEO and JEANIE J.Y. CHUI

Introduction

Pterygium (pleural: pterygia) is a prevalent ocular surface lesion, traditionally described as an encroachment of altered bulbar conjunctiva onto the cornea.[1] Its name originates from the diminutive of πτερυζ, (Greek, small wing) referring to its characteristic wing-like growth pattern.[2] Pterygium is an enigma and many theories have been proposed as to its pathogenesis. Historically, pterygia were considered to be degenerative lesions exemplified by degradation of Bowman's layer and elastosis. The current view is that pterygium is an aberrant wound healing process, characterized by centripetal growth of a leading edge of altered limbal epithelial cells, followed by a squamous metaplastic epithelium with goblet cell hyperplasia and an underlying stroma of activated, proliferating fibroblasts, neovascularization, inflammatory cells, and extracellular matrix remodeling.[3]

Pterygia and other sun-related eye diseases (the ophthalmohelioses) pose a significant health problem to many communities. In Australia, with a population of approximately 22 million, it has been estimated that approximately 60 000 general practice visits annually include care for pterygia.[4] The direct annual cost of pterygium in Australia is AU\$8.3 million and this is likely to be an underestimation. Pterygium is often prevalent in developing countries with scarce health resources and in this setting can be a blinding disease.[5,6] In biological terms, if conjunctival/limbal autografting is performed, 50% of the limbus and associated stem cells can be affected. Given the importance of stem cells in long-term corneal maintenance, pterygium is a condition of great significance.

Historically, the consequences of pterygium on the ocular surface have also been underestimated and the disease trivialized. Boxes 18.1 and 18.2 summarise associated vision loss and primary and secondary complications of pterygia. Systemic associations, such as polymorphous light eruption, porphyria cutanea tarda and skin malignancy[7] have not been well recognized, yet pterygium is almost certainly a significant biomarker for substantial ultraviolet ocular and body surface insolation. Progressive pterygia can lead to complications, such as astigmatism and increased higher-order aberrations. These aberrations are decreased significantly at 2 weeks after surgery and remain relatively stable, yet they remain at levels much higher than in normal eyes.[8] A possible cause may relate to the observation that invasion of the pterygium head deep to Bowman's membrane, predicts postoperative corneal opacity/scarring.[9] With ready availability of aberrometry and optical coherence tomography, a consideration is to operate before such changes are

---

Box 18.1 Pterygium Associated Visual Disturbances

Aberrations
  Astigmatism
    ▪ traction (± gaze evoked)
    ▪ tear pooling
  Higher order
Transcorneal extension
  ▪ direct
  ▪ corneal opacity → glare, reduced contrast sensitivity
Visual field loss
Tear film disturbances/dry eye
Restricted abduction – diplopia
Contact lens intolerance

Box 18.2 Ocular Assocations of Pterygium

Primary

- Dry eye syndrome
- Dellen formation
  - secondary to inflammation
  - cystic changes
- Foreign body sequestration
- Neoplasia
  - intraepithelial neoplasia
  - squamous cell carcinoma
  - melanoma
  - epithelioma
  - fibroblastic sarcoma
- Corneal neural changes
- Corneal endothelial changes

Secondary

- Recurrence ± granuloma
- Corneocleritis
  - bacterial
  - nectrotizing
- Symblepharon
- Corneoscleral perforation ± endophthalmitis
  - surgical
  - post beta irradiation, mitomycin C
  - in Sjögren's syndrome
- Amputation neuroma
- Ligneous conjunctivitis
- Subconjunctival fibrosis and free graft donor site
- Thiotepa
  - poliosis, dermal depigmentation, beware pregnancy
- Beta irradiation
  - iritis, episcleritis, conjunctivitis
  - cataract
  - conjunctival telangiectasia
  - delayed scleral necrosis
  - lacrimal drainage system damage
- Mitomycin C
  - delayed epithelialization, scleral thinning, ulceration, calcification, elevated intraocular pressure/glaucoma, iritis, cataract, corneal edema, punctual stenosis

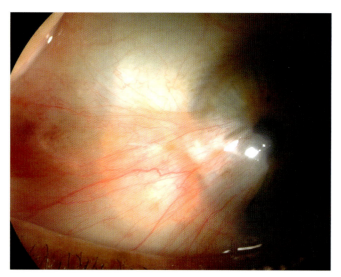

Figure 18.1 Primary pterygium.

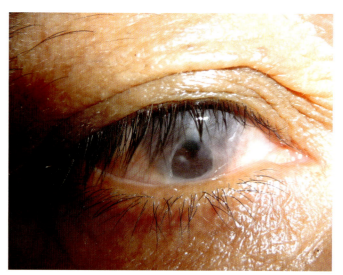

Figure 18.2 Double pterygium – concurrent temporal and nasal pterygium.

established. Given these findings, the era of refractive pterygium surgery may have arrived.

The association with dry eye is also well known. A twofold increased risk of dry eye symptoms exists in pterygium patients.[10] While a direct mechanical mechanism is obvious, advances in our understanding of the inflammatory basis of dry eye syndrome[11] suggest an indirect effect of inflammatory mediators in pterygium, resulting in a 'pseudo-dry-eye state.'

Clinical Features

APPEARANCE

The classic appearance of a pterygium is that of a wing-shaped fibrovascular lesion extending from the bulbar conjunctiva onto the cornea (Fig. 18.1). Pterygia may be primary or recurrent, unilateral or bilateral, and present nasally or temporally in either or both eyes. They occur invariably in the palpebral fissure, predominantly at the nasal limbus, while temporal pterygia are less common and rarely found in isolation (Fig. 18.2).[12] Anatomically, the pterygium may be divided into three parts. The 'head' consists of the apex enclosed by an avascular cap, the 'neck' refers to the region between the head and limbus overlying the cornea, and the 'body' is the portion overlying the sclera.[13] When observed by slit lamp, gray 'islets' may be present within the cap at the advancing edge of the pterygium (Fig. 18.3). First described by Fuchs, these 'flecks' or Fuchs' islets represent the most advanced parts of the pterygium, which coalesce over time with the migrating boundary, to form tongue-shaped extensions at the apex.[14] Iron deposition in the corneal epithelium, just apical to the head of the pterygium, is known as Stocker's line.[15]

SYMPTOMS

Dry eye symptoms such as redness, irritation and blurred vision are common in pterygium.[10] Reduced tear break-up time and abnormal tear-ferning have been reported with partial restoration of tear function once the pterygium is removed.[16] Pterygium-associated visual disturbances are summarized in Box 18.1.

Histopathology

Topographic studies of the pterygium show that it is an epithelium-covered protuberance of connective tissue projecting over the ocular surface with an apex that extends in the direction of growth.[17] The epithelium is characterized by centripetal growth of a leading edge of altered limbal epithelial cells,[18] followed by abnormal conjunctival epithelium, with features of goblet cell hyperplasia and squamous metaplasia (Fig. 18.4A).[19] The underlying connective tissue stroma consists of activated, proliferating fibroblasts and blood vessels.[20] Chronic mixed inflammatory infiltrates may be present, comprising lymphocytes, plasma cells, mast cells, Langerhans cells, monocytes and macrophages, with neutrophils present in acutely inflamed lesions (Fig. 18.4B). Immunoglobulin (IgG and IgE) deposition along the basement membrane,[21] aberrant expression of HLA-DR[22] and adhesion molecules (ICAM-1 and VCAM-1)[23] have also been reported. Extracellular matrix changes are prominent features of pterygium. These include dissolution of Bowman's layer at the migrating head and accumulation of elastotic material within the stroma (Fig. 18.4C).

Differential Diagnosis

The differential diagnosis of pterygium includes pinguecula, pseudopterygium, and various conjunctival tumors. Although there are some similarities, these entities may be distinguished by morphology and clinical behavior. Of note, it is critical to consider limbal/conjunctival malignancy given that both pterygium and pinguecula may harbor epithelial dysplasia.[24]

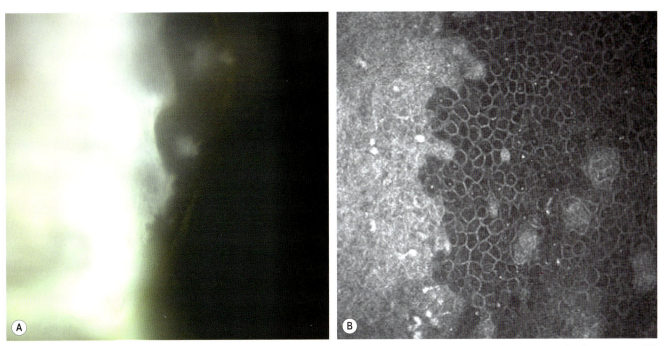

Figure 18.3 The apex of a pterygium showing the presence of Fuchs' flecks as observed by slit lamp (**A**) and by in vivo confocal microscopy (**B**). (Reprinted with permission from Chui J, Coroneo MT, Tat LT, et al. Ophthalmic pterygium a stem cell disorder with premalignant features. Am J Pathol 2011;178:817–27.)

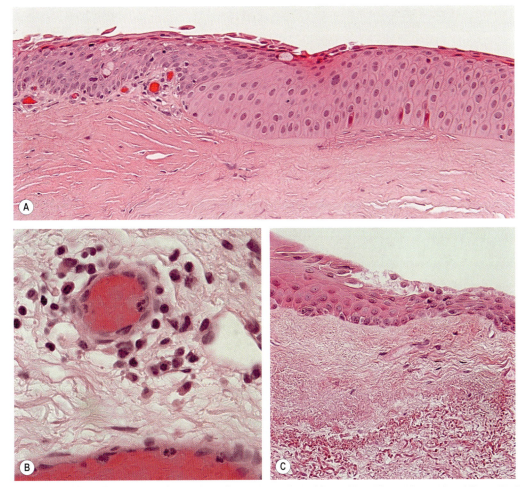

Figure 18.4 Hematoxylin and eosin-stained paraffin sections of the head of a pterygium, showing an abrupt transition from corneal to conjunctival-like epithelium with underlying fragmentation of Bowman's membrane (**A**). Mixed perivascular inflammatory infiltrate within the pterygium stroma (**B**). Pterygium stroma demonstrating prominent elastotic changes (**C**). Original magnification: ×200 (**A**), ×1000 oil emersion (**B**) and ×400 (**C**). (Figures A and C have been reprinted with permission from Chui J, Coroneo MT, Tat LT, et al. Ophthalmic pterygium a stem cell disorder with premalignant features. Am J Pathol 2011;178:817–27.)

PINGUECULA

Pinguecula (pleural: pingueculae) appears as an elevated yellow white plaque in the conjunctiva adjacent to the nasal or temporal limbus. They are distinguished from pterygia by their lack of corneal invasion, possibly due to an intact limbal barrier. Although most pinguecula are slow growing with a benign course, it is recognized that some may evolve into pterygia.[14] The histological changes of pinguecula are similar to those in pterygium and comprise predominantly subepithelial elastosis, hyaline degeneration, eosinophilic and basophilic concretions,[25] squamous and metaplastic changes of the epithelium.[26]

PSEUDOPTERYGIUM AND OTHER INFLAMMATORY CONDITIONS

Pseudopterygium originates from conjunctival adhesions to corneal defects as a result of trauma, previous surgery or inflammation. A key feature that differentiates pseudopterygia from true pterygia, is that the former may occur anywhere on the corneal circumference, whereas the latter are typically limited to the 3- and 9-o'clock position. The pseudopterygium has a broad, flat leading edge at its point of attachment, with the bulk of the lesion not adherent to the underlying cornea.[27] Conditions that may be associated with pseudopterygium include Fuchs' superficial marginal keratitis and Terrien's marginal degeneration.[28] Other inflammatory conditions to be considered include phlyctenular keratoconjunctivitis, nodular episcleritis and actinic granulomas.

CONJUNCTIVAL TUMORS

Benign and malignant tumors of the conjunctiva may be confused with pterygia. These include limbal dermoid, papilloma, amyloidosis, lymphoma of the conjunctiva, non-pigmented nevi, melanoma, conjunctival intraepithelial neoplasia and squamous cell carcinoma.[29] Of special consideration are pre-neoplastic lesions, such as ocular surface squamous neoplasia[30] and primary acquired melanosis,[31] which may coexist with pterygia.[32] A high index of suspicion should be maintained when managing pterygia with an atypical appearance. Given these lesions may not be clinically obvious, histological examination of all excised pterygia is recommended.

Epidemiology

Pterygium is present worldwide with prevalence rates depending on the age group and geographical location. In Cameron's survey of the world's distribution of pterygia,[33] higher rates were observed in those living in peri-equatorial countries, including hot, dry and dusty climates. This is supported by an Australian study that showed a prevalence up to 15.2% in Aborigines living in the northern territories, compared to 4.5% in those living in the southern states. A positive correlation was seen with lifetime sun exposure.[34] However, the high incidence of pterygium in Tibetans (14.5%)[35] and Mongolians (17.8%)[36] living in high altitudes but away from the equator, contradicts these pterygia

epidemiology studies. The high incidence in Eskimos in Greenland (8.6%)[37] and watermen in Chesapeake Bay (16.7%)[38] results from reflected sunlight off snow or water. From these studies, it is clear that cumulative ultraviolet (UV) light exposure is a major risk factor for pterygia. Other risk factors include family history, increasing age, male gender, and rural residency, while wearing glasses or a hat have a protective effect.[39,40] Certain groups, such as welders[41], laborers and outdoor workers have increased incidence of pterygium, as a result of their occupational exposure.[42] Pterygia are also more common in sawmill workers exposed to dusty environments, where chronic irritation and microtrauma is hypothesized to play a role in these cases.[43] More recently, exposure to arsenic[44] and petrochemicals[45] have also been linked to pterygia.

Pathogenesis

The pathogenesis of pterygium is poorly understood. The popular view of pterygium as a degenerative condition was based on histological evidence of the extracellular matrix degradation. However, this is contradicted by its invasive growth habit and propensity to recur when excised. In reality, both degenerative and hyperplastic processes are present in pterygium,[1] with multiple mechanisms contributing to its formation (Fig. 18.5). These mechanisms may be divided into inherited factors, environmental triggers (UV light, viral infections) and factors that perpetuate its growth (cytokines, growth factors and matrix metalloproteinases). Cumulative DNA damage and activation of anti-apoptotic factors may also contribute to the proliferative

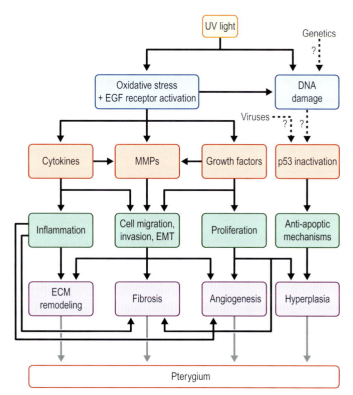

Figure 18.5 Multiple mechanisms in the pathogenesis of pterygium.

phenotype of pterygium, while the contribution of stem cells and neurogenic inflammation will also be discussed.

ULTRAVIOLET LIGHT

The role of chronic UV exposure in the pathogenesis of pterygium is well supported by epidemiological studies and its clinical associations with other UV-related conditions, such as photo-aged skin, cataracts, climatic droplet keratopathy, squamous cell and basal cell carcinomas.[32] The curious growth habit of the pterygium and it predilection for the medial limbus is explained by our model of peripheral light focusing effect of the anterior chamber, which concentrates incidental light by 20× onto the medial limbus (Fig. 18.6).[46] Chronic focal UV damage to this region is hypothesized to activate limbal stem cells, leading to formation of a pterygium.[47] Also intriguing is autofluorescence of pterygia under UV light (300–400 nm) (Fig. 18.7),[48] which may precede visible signs of an ocular surface lesion (Fig. 18.8).[49] The cause for autofluorescence is unknown but we speculate that it may represent altered collagen or cellular activity as a result of solar damage.[48] Additionally, pterygia share certain histological features with photo-aged

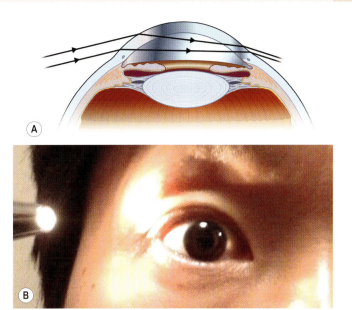

Figure 18.6 Peripheral light focusing effect of the anterior chamber. A model (**A**) predicting the pathway taken by incident light through the anterior chamber to form a limbal focus demonstrated in vivo (**B**).

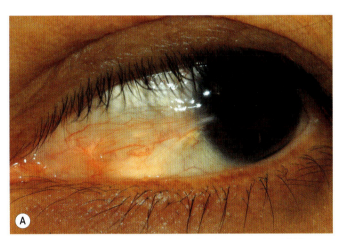
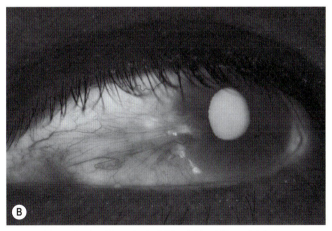

Figure 18.7 Autofluorescence in a primary pterygium. The lesion observed under visible light (**A**) and under UV light (**B**).

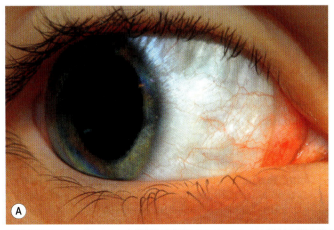
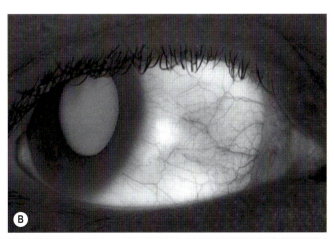

Figure 18.8 Photograph in visible light documenting a clinically normal medial limbal area in an 11-year-old patient (**A**). UV fluorescence photography of the same patient showing an area of fluorescence at the nasal limbus (**B**).

skin including epidermal proliferation, inflammatory infiltrates, activated fibroblasts and extracellular matrix remodeling.[3] To follow, we will discuss UV activated molecular mechanisms that are involved in the pathogenesis of pterygium.

OXIDATIVE STRESS AND GROWTH FACTOR RECEPTOR SIGNALING

UV-induced oxidative stress has been implicated in the pathogenesis of pterygium. Supportive evidence include the presence of 8-hydroxydeoxyguanosine (a DNA photo-oxidation product)[50] and malondialdehyde (a product of lipid peroxidation),[51] inducible nitric oxide synthase and nitric oxide (NO)[52] in pterygium tissue. Reactive oxygen species (ROS), such as NO may act as a pro-angiogenic factor by mediating vascularization,[53] endothelial proliferation and migration,[54] MMP-2 activation,[55] and potentially, MMP expression patterns in pterygia. Other ROS, such as hydrogen peroxide are known to activate epidermal growth factor receptors (EGFRs) and subsequent downstream signaling via the mitogen-activated protein kinase (MAPK) pathways, such as extracellular signal-regulated kinase (ERK), c-jun amino-terminal kinase (JNK) and p38.[56] In pterygium cell cultures, UV activated JNK and p38 induces expression of pro-inflammatory cytokines,[57] while activation of ERK is responsible for induction of MMP-1.[58,59]

PRO-INFLAMMATORY CYTOKINES AND IMMUNOLOGICAL MECHANISMS

Epidemiological studies have hinted that chronic inflammation from desiccation, chemical exposure and microtrauma may play a role in the pathogenesis of pterygia. Wong suggested a mechanism where inflammation at the junction of the conjunctival blood vessels and Bowman's membrane degraded proteins which then act as angiogenic factors.[60] The presence of mixed chronic inflammatory infiltrates including T lymphocytes, plasma cells, mast cells, Langerhans cells, monocytes, and macrophage supports the conclusion that immunological mechanisms[21] might be involved. Although immune infiltrates may contribute to inflammation in pterygia, their presence are likely a consequence of cytokines and other pro-inflammatory mediators present in pterygium (Box 18.3).[3] Interleukins (IL-1, IL-6, IL-8) and tumor necrosis factor-alpha (TNF-α) are known

to be induced by UV light[61] and NF-κB, signaling that is activated in pterygia.[62,63] Their presence mediates influx of immune cells and induction of MMP expression in pterygia, while IL-4 may mediate fibrosis in recurrent lesions.[64] Another UV-inducible enzyme that is overexpressed in pterygia is cycloxygenase-2 (COX-2), which converts arachidonic acid into prostaglandin.[65] Its expression is associated with the anti-apoptotic factor survivin.[66] COX-2 induces MMP-1 and MMP-9 in organ-cultured corneas,[67] and may also contribute to elevated MMP expression in pterygia. S100 proteins are calcium-binding proteins that have roles in wound healing, inflammation and cancer,[68] and have recently been described to be elevated in pterygium tissue[69] and in the tears of patients with pterygia.[70] The functional significance of S100 proteins in pterygia requires further study. However, their up-regulation may reflect induction by UV, cytokines or other environmental stressors.[71,72] Stem cell factor (SCF) is also elevated in the plasma and ocular tissues of patients with pterygia.[73,74] SCF attracts and induces maturation of mast cells,[73] and their presence may promote fibrosis and neovascularization in pterygia.[75] Langerhans cells have also been observed in pterygium tissue by immunohistochemical[76] and in vivo confocal microscopy.[77] It is speculated that a higher level of antigenic and mitogenic exposure,[76] or the presence of cytokines in pterygia, might have aided in their recruitment and maturation.[77] The role of Langerhans cells in pterygium pathogenesis requires further study but it was hypothesized that Langerhans cells may be involved in T-cell recruitment.[78]

It is interesting to note that while clinical evidence supports the notion that persistent inflammation may lead to postoperative recurrence,[79] the quantity of infiltrating T cells in pterygia specimens did not correlate with clinical parameters, such as severity of inflammation or preoperative use of topical steroids or non-steroidal anti-inflammatory drugs.[80] Additionally, recurrence was not predicted by histological appearance.[81] This implies that inflammation does not act alone and that other factors may also contribute to recurrence of a pterygium.

FIBROANGIOGENIC GROWTH FACTORS

Growth factors and their receptors have been reported in pterygia (Table 18.1). They serve to induce proliferation and/or migration of epithelial cells, fibroblasts or vascular cells, which contribute to hyperplasia, fibrosis and angiogenesis in pterygium.[3,81]

Pro-fibrotic cytokines and growth factors expressed in pterygia include IL-1, TNF-α, CTGF, EGF family, FGF-2, PDGF, and TGF-β.[82] Of these, TGF-β is particularly important since it induces myofibroblast differentiation, epithelial mesenchymal transition and alters synthesis of extracellular matrix components.[83] Aberrant TGF-β signaling[84,85] is thought to contribute to fibrosis in pterygia, and its suppression by amniotic membrane[86] may explain the efficacy of this treatment.

Elevated pro-angiogenic factors (IL-8, TNF-α, FGF-2, HB-EGF and VEGF) combined with lack of angiogenic inhibitors (PEDF and thrombospondin-1) encourage prominent neovascularization in pterygia.[82] VEGF, a major pro-angiogenic factor, is elevated in the tears, plasma and ocular tissues of patients with pterygia.[74,87] VEGF expression in

---

Box 18.3 Cytokines and Inflammatory Mediators in Pterygium

- Interleukin-1
- Interleukin-4
- Interleukin-6
- Interleukin-8
- Tumor necrosis factor-α
- Stem cell factor
- Cycoloxygenase-2
- Defensins α1 and α2
- Erythropoietin Receptor
- S100A6, A8 and A9

Table 18.1 Growth Factors and Their Receptors in Pterygium

Growth Factor and Related Proteins	Receptors
Epidermal growth factor	EGFR
Heparin binding growth factor	ErbB2
	ErbB3
Fibroblast growth factor-2	FGFR-1
Nerve growth factor	TRKA
Ciliary neurotrophic factor	NGFR
Neurotrophin 4	
Platelet derived growth factor	PDGFR-β
Transforming growth factor-β	TGF-βRI
	TGF-βRII
	TGF-βRIII
Vascular endothelial growth factor	VEGFR1
	VEGFR2
Insulin-like growth factor binding proteins (IGFBP)	
IGFBP2	
IGFBP3	
IGFBP8 (connective tissue growth factor)	

Box 18.4 Gene Association Studies on Patients with Pterygia

Associated with Pterygia

- hOGG1 (Exon 7, 1245C>G)
- GSTM1 (Null genotype)
- XRCC6 (Promoter, −991C>T)
- XRCC1 (Arg399 Glu)

Not Associated with Pterygia

- TP53 (Exon 4, 119C>G)
- CDKN1A (Exon 2, 98C>A)
- TNF (Promoter, −308G>A)
- IL1B (Promoter, −511C>T, Exon 5, +3954C>T)
- IL1RN (Intron 2, variable number tandem repeat of 86bp, Alleles 1, 2, 3, 4 and 5)
- TGFB1 (Promoter, −509C>T)
- XRCC6 (Promoter, −57G>C)
- hOGG1 (Ser326Cys)
- APE1 (Asp148Glu)

Relationship Unclear

- VEGFA (Promoter, −460T>C)

pterygia may be driven by multiple stimuli (UV, hypoxia, cytokines and growth factors) and probably represents a common pro-angiogenic pathway.[3,82]

More recently, neurotrophins and their receptors have been investigated in pterygia, where nerve growth factor (NGF), ciliary neurotrophic factor and neurotrophin-4/5 were reported to be elevated. In addition, the high- and low-affinity NGF receptors (TRKA and NGFR, respectively) have also been described in epithelial cells and blood vessels of pterygia.[88–90] A pro-angiogenic role for neurotrophins is suggested by the correlation of NGF – TRKA staining with microvessel density in pterygia.[89]

MATRIX METALLOPROTEINASES AND EXTRACELLULAR MATRIX REMODELING

Matrix metalloproteinases (MMPs) are zinc-dependent endopeptidases that degrade components of the extracellular matrix and cell surface molecules. These enzymes are counterbalanced by endogenous inhibitors, called tissue inhibitors of metalloproteinases (TIMPs). MMPs participate in ocular physiology, pathophysiology, and are key mediators of photo-aging, where they regulate proliferation, cell migration, inflammation and angiogenesis.[91] Overexpression of MMPs relative to TIMPs is thought to contribute to the invasive phenotype of pterygia, where MMP expression may be induced by UV light, cytokines (IL-1 and TNF-α) and growth factors (EGF and TGF-α).[3,82] Of interest is the association of MMP-2 and -9 with disease progression,[92] suggesting that MMPs may be an attractive target for management of this disease.

Additional to extracellular matrix breakdown, altered synthesis of matrix components have been reported in pterygia, including tropoelastin,[93] glycosaminoglycans,[94] hyaluronic acid,[95] periostin,[64] fibulin-2 and fibulin-3.[96] Altered matrix components may increase the bioavailability of heparin-binding growth factors and cytokines (e.g. IL-8, FGF-2, HB-EGF, VEGF, PDGF and TGF-β) which are normally sequestered by the extracellular matrix and released upon its degradation.[97]

INHERITED FACTORS

Although environmental exposure plays a major role in the pathogenesis of pterygia, inherited factors may influence its development. Supporting this concept are families with pterygia where ocular disease often presents at a younger age and with an autosomal dominant inheritance pattern.[98,99] Individuals with xeroderma pigmentosum,[100] single nucleotide polymorphisms in 8-oxoguanine glycosylase 1 (hOGG1),[101] X-ray repair cross-complementing-1 (XRCC1)[102] or X-ray repair cross-complementing-6 (XRCC6),[103] have been associated with pterygium development, suggesting defective DNA repair may contribute to the pathogenesis of this condition. Genetic variants in glutathione S-transferase M1 (GSTM1)[104] and cytochrome P4501A1 (CYP1A1),[105] enzymes that metabolize polycyclic aromatic hydrocarbons, are reported to be associated with pterygia. (See Box 18.4 for details on gene association studies in pterygia.) The CYP1A1 MspI polymorphism, in particular, is associated with accumulation of Benzo[a] pyrene 7,8 diol-9,10-epoxide (BPDE)-like DNA adducts in pterygium tissue,[105] implying interactions between genetic and environmental factors in this condition.

VIRAL INFECTIONS

Based on Knudson's hypothesis of cancer as a result of cumulative DNA mutations, Detorakis et al. proposed a role for oncogenic viruses in the pathogenesis of pterygia in their two-hit model.[106] The 'first hit' is attributed to a genetic predisposition for pterygia or acquired DNA damage from UV exposure. The 'second hit' may be additional UV exposure or caused by infections, such as human papillomavirus (HPV) or herpes simplex virus (HSV).[106] Evidence supporting HPV in the pathogenesis of pterygia include the detection of HPV subtypes 1, 2, 6, 11, 16, 18, 37, 52, 54 and HPV90 in pterygium tissue. However, the prevalence rate (0–100%) varies widely between studies.[107] These findings might be explained by variable HPV infection rates between populations[108] or methodological differences. A possible contributing mechanism might be the inactivation of p53 by viral oncoprotein (HPV 16/18 E6).[109] Studies on HSV have been restricted to two centers with prevalence of 22% in Greece[110] and 5% in Taiwan,[111] and co-infection with HPV was associated with postoperative recurrence in one study.[110] Given the limited and inconsistent data, viral infection is likely not an absolute requirement for pterygium formation.

GENETIC AND EPIGENETIC CHANGES

Some authors favor the idea that cumulative DNA damage[106,112] might be involved in the pathogenesis of pterygia. Additional to the presence of 8-hydroxydeoxyguanosine (8-OHdG)[50] and BPDE-like DNA adducts[105] in pterygia of susceptible individuals, a number of genetic changes have been described including loss of heterozygosity, microsatellite instability,[113] and mutations in Kirsten-ras[114] and p53 genes.[109,115,116] Of these, only p53 mutations have been studied extensively.

The tumor suppressor protein p53, is often referred to as the 'guardian of the genome'. P53 is normally found in low levels due to its short half-life. In the presence of DNA damage, it stabilizes, translocates to the nucleus, inducing cell cycle arrest, DNA repair or apoptosis.[117] Normal p53 function prevents accumulation of genetic aberrations and this gene is frequently mutated in cancers.[118] Dushku and Reid proposed that inactivating mutations of p53 impairs programmed cell death and allows genetic mutations to accumulate, leading to the formation of pterygia.[112] Using immunohistochemical methods, they observed elevated p53 in pterygia without concurrent apoptosis.[112] Subsequently, others also reported elevated p53 staining in pterygia, relative to normal conjunctival tissues, but not all pterygia stained for p53,[119] nor was p53 expression related to recurrence.[120] DNA sequencing studies revealed four cases of monoallelic deletion[116] and eight cases of point mutations.[115] When DNA sequencing was paired with protein detection, it was observed that accumulation of p53 protein is not necessarily accompanied by p53 mutations,[121] while deletion mutations may result in loss of p53 expression.[115] Furthermore, viral oncoprotein inactivation of p53 has been suggested.[109] Therefore, further studies are required to establish the true prevalence of p53 mutations and their role in the pathogenesis of pterygia.

Although little is known regarding the mechanisms involved, there is emerging evidence that epigenetic changes are present in pterygia. These include hypermethylation of the promoter of p16 (CDKN2A),[122] E-cadherin (CDH1),[123] transglutaminase 2 (TGM-2),[124] and hypomethylation for MMP2 and CD24.[124] The activity of DNA methyltransferases might be responsible. Chen et al. reported that 29% of pterygia expressed DNA methyltransferase 3b, a factor associated with hypermethylation of the p16 promoter and down-regulation of p16 protein.[122] The role of aberrant methylation in pterygia requires further exploration.

ABNORMAL PROLIFERATION AND ANTI-APOPTOTIC MECHANISMS

Abnormal proliferation and anti-apoptotic factors have been documented in pterygia, which might explain their propensity for recurrence and the presence of a high proportion of dysplasia in some case series.[24] Supporting evidence include elevated expression of anti-apoptotic proteins (BCL-2[125] and survivin[66]) and cell cycle related molecules associated with proliferation (cyclin D1, Ki67 and proliferating cell nuclear antigen)[126,127] and suppression of p27 (KIP1)[128] in pterygium epithelial cells. Elevated DNA content is also reported in the fibrovascular layer,[129] with pterygium fibroblasts exhibiting a transformed phenotype of reduced serum dependence and anchorage independent growth in culture,[130] altered lipid metabolism[131] and expression of insulin-like growth factor binding proteins, which are also known to be altered in cancers.[132,133]

STEM CELLS

Epithelial Stem Cells

Chronic focal UV exposure was originally hypothesized to alter limbal stem cells, therefore, leading to an infiltrative phenotype that gave rise to a pterygium.[18,47] Studies have now shown pterygium and limbal epithelium shared biomarkers, including cytokeratins,[18] vimentin,[18] telomerase,[134] tumor protein p63,[135] ATP-binding cassette, subfamily G, member 2[90] and nerve growth factor receptor.[90] Our recent identification of stem-like cells corresponding to the clinical observation of Fuchs' flecks at the advancing head of the pterygium (Fig. 18.9) lends further support to this theory.[32] It is interesting to note that despite the presence of stem-like cells, pterygia also display features of focal limbal stem cell deficiency, including absent limbal palisades, conjunctival ingrowth and vascularization of the cornea. These changes respond to treatment by limbal autografts once the pterygium is excised.[136,137] Therefore, one might speculate that pterygia primarily represent a dysfunction of limbal stem cells and the stem cell niche.

Epithelial Mesenchymal Transition

Epithelial mesenchymal transition (EMT), a process where epithelial cells take on characteristics of mesenchymal cells, has been described in pterygia. Specifically, two studies have shown pterygium epithelial cells concurrently expressed epithelial (cytokeratin 14) and mesenchymal markers (alpha-smooth muscle actin and vimentin), and signaling molecules associated with EMT (beta-catenin, snail and slug).[138,139] This leads us to speculate that pterygium fibroblasts may have originated from limbal epithelium via EMT under the influences of TGF-β and FGF-2 or UV exposure.[82] Alternatively, pterygium fibroblasts are hypothesized to be recruited from myofibroblasts in the periorbital fibroadipose tissue posterior to Tenon's capsule.[140]

Bone Marrow-Derived Progenitor Cells

Bone marrow-derived progenitor cells expressing hematopoietic (CD34, AC133 or c-kit) or mesenchymal (STRO-1) markers have been reported in pterygium and are hypothesized to contribute to the fibrovascular stroma.[141] Supporting this concept is the presence of bone marrow-derived

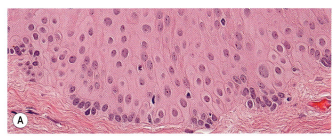

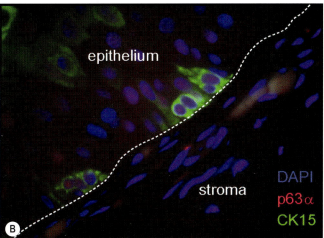

Figure 18.9 Clusters of stem-like cells at the head of a pterygium. H&E (**A**) and immunofluorescent labelled stem-like cells expressing p63α and CK15 (**B**). (Figures reprinted with permission from Chui J, Coroneo MT, Tat LT, et al. Ophthalmic pterygium a stem cell disorder with premalignant features. Am J Pathol 2011;178:817–27.)

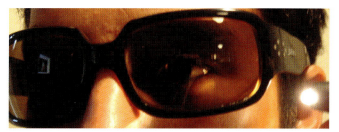

Figure 18.10 Demonstartion of peripheral light focusing while the pateint is wearing wraparound sunglasses with a broad side arm.

cells in the normal corneal stoma,[142] together with animal models showing recruitment of bone marrow-derived cells to areas of active fibrosis,[143] and neovascularization.[144] Ocular tissue hypoxia-induced cytokines are thought to act as chemoattractants to the eye.[144] Lee et al. showed that patients with pterygia had elevated circulating CD34 and c-kit positive progenitor cells and plasma VEGF, stem cell factor and Substance P.[74]

NEUROGENIC INFLAMMATION

The above theories do not explain some aspects of pterygia, such as its centripetal growth pattern, that gives rise to its characteristic wing-like appearance. To address this issue, a neurogenic model was proposed, whereby corneal nerves may influence the centripetal migration of corneal epithelium and pterygium cells.[82,145] This model is based on several observations: (1) normal corneal epithelial turnover as summarized in the XYZ hypothesis;[146] (2) the radial arrangement of corneal nerves and their close relationship with corneal epithelium and keratocytes;[147] (3) involvement of sensory neurons in wound healing and inflammation;[148] (4) the presence of myelinated and unmyelinated nerve fibers within the connective tissue mass of pterygia.[149]

The limbus is the focal point of chronic UV exposure, where limbal epithelium, stromal cells, blood vessels and the perilimbal nerve plexus may be damaged by UV light. The neuronal response to UV injury may also be an important trigger for the development of pterygia. UV exposure

may induce release of sensory neuropeptides, such as substance P (SP) and calcitonin gene-related peptide (CGRP), which participate in neurogenic inflammation through their roles as vasodilators, immune cell chemoattractants, and by inducing cytokine production from resident corneal cells to amplify the inflammatory response.[148] In pterygia, SP and its receptor (NK1R) are expressed by epithelial cells, fibroblasts and infiltrating immune cells, and have been shown to induce migration of pterygium fibroblasts and vascular endothelium, suggesting a fibroangiogenic role.[145] The above evidence, together with the distribution of corneal nerves,[147] suggests that corneal nerves might play a role in the development of pterygia.

Management

The ultimate aim of treating a pterygium is to restore the ocular surface anatomy, function, cosmesis, and alleviate all associated symptoms. This is not always achievable but having this goal may provide a therapeutic framework on which to base interventions. The aim should be for perfection, especially if surgery is contemplated. The eye has been termed the aesthetic center of the face and, in communicating, a great deal of attention is paid to ocular appearance and movement.[150]

PREVENTION

While prevention of ocular UV damage has remained an elusive goal, prevention of recurrence both short and long term remains a concern, particularly for high-risk groups, such as surfers. Advice about appropriate eye protection requires some consideration. It is unlikely that, in a brief consultation, advice about adequate wrap-around sunglasses and a brimmed hat is likely to change habits of a lifetime. We have found that demonstrating the peripheral light focusing effect (Fig. 18.10), especially while patients are wearing sunglasses, helps them understand the reasons for these recommendations. Specific advice about suppliers of appropriate sunglasses, particularly for patients with refractive error, is important since peripheral light can be difficult to block even with what might be considered an appropriate degree of side protection. Providing brief but pointed reading material is also helpful. In younger patients with early disease, demonstrating the lesions with anterior segment photography and fluorescence photography[49] (see Fig. 18.8) has also been helpful. Serial photographs taken over many years can either reassure the patient that the condition is stable or help in making a decision to operate when growth is demonstrated.

MEDICAL

There is little doubt that inflammation, acute and chronic, remains a crucial component for development of pterygia. The standard treatments of lubricants and topical anti-inflammatory drugs, such as nonsteroidal agents (NSAIDs) or steroids can be useful[151] but often limited, particularly in advanced disease. While effective in the short term, NSAIDs in particular but also the newer low-dose formulation of dexamethasone (0.01%) can be effective,[152] particularly in patients with recurrent disease in whom surgery is not desired. However, a more recent strategy is the use of topical cyclosporine 0.05%, which provides relatively safe medium- to long-term anti-inflammatory treatment and management of moderate to severe dry eye.[153] Its use in the management of pterygium was proposed in 2006[154] and it has since been used to prevent recurrences in the postoperative period.[155,156] Given the setting of dry eye that appears common in patients with pterygia, it is safe and efficacious, although more formal studies are in process. Cyclosporine, apart from its anti-inflammatory effects, has multiple modes of action that may benefit treatment of pterygia. It is reassuring for some patients to undergo medical treatment before surgery is contemplated, particularly in patients with recurrent disease.

SURGICAL

A recent review of surgical treatment of pterygia,[157] demonstrates that a wide variety of approaches exist, owing to the difficulty in curing this condition. This is hardly surprising given the relatively recent understanding of the pathophysiology (see Fig. 18.5) that involves stem cells and healing responses via complex pathways. Two key concepts in our approach are the use of reconstructive procedures and the control of the postoperative and any ongoing inflammatory response. Furthermore, there is a significant surgeon factor in outcomes that raises the issue of training, since the best chance of cure is at the first procedure and the risk of recurrence appears to increase with subsequent surgery. In our opinion, this should not be a procedure for the occasional surgeon.

The gold-standard technique is excision with autoconjunctival, reconstructive grafting, which provides low recurrence and complication rates, as well as excellent cosmesis[158,160] but takes time and skill to perform. The procedure, first described in 1947[161] and subsequently popularized,[161] while seemingly straightforward, can be carried out with variations that could explain differences in reported recurrence rates. This procedure provides an excellent example of how reconstructive techniques are invariably superior to destructive surgical modalities.

Certain aspects of pterygium surgery deserve attention and are discussed below:

1. Transplantation of bulbar conjunctiva as opposed to limbal – conjunctival transplantation remains controversial. The general view is that it makes little difference if limbus is included and since there is the risk of limbal compromise at the donor site, many surgeons prefer to use conjunctival grafts. However, one study demonstrating that limbal transplantation was more effective than free conjunctival transplantation for treatment of recurrent pterygia.[163] The long-standing concept that corneal epithelial stem cells reside mainly in the limbus has been challenged;[164] it has been shown that basal cells of bulbar conjunctival epithelium share a similar expression pattern of stem cell-associated markers to the limbal epithelium.[165] This may help explain why a limbal area appears to reform when conjunctival grafts are used.

2. Management of Tenon's capsule also remains controversial. There is a long-held belief that Tenon's capsule gives rise to recurrences and should therefore, be widely excised.[159,160,166] Hirst described a technique known as, pterygium extended removal followed by extended conjunctival transplantation, which involves an extensive tenonectomy, followed by a large autoconjunctival graft. In his prospective series[159,160] the recurrence rate for primary pterygium was 0.4% and there were no recurrences in the recurrent pterygium group. This was a single-surgeon series and intensive postoperative inflammatory treatment was used. Another approach for recurrent pterygia is to 'seal the gap.' After extensive excision of the pterygium and associated cicatrix, the medial fornix is reconstructed and the exposed areas are covered by conjunctival amniotic membrane grafts.[167] A 6% recurrence rate was reported and one patient suffered from diplopia. An important part of these techniques is the adequate covering of underlying tissue by epithelial or membranous structures. This raises the possibility that the wound healing response is being modulated, in part by epithelial – stromal interactions[168] and perhaps, with adequate graft cover, such extensive excisions are not necessary, particularly if the inflammatory response is controlled.

3. Inflammation is central to pterygium pathogenesis and surgical response, as well as the extent of signs, symptoms, growth and recurrence. In one study,[169] inadequate use of postoperative topical steroids was associated with nearly triple the recurrence rate. Interestingly, in Hirst's studies[159,160] with low recurrence rates used topical steroids were used every 2 hours for the first 3 weeks with treatment extended to 9 weeks. More recently, topical cyclosporine has been used postoperatively following the high-recurrence rate bare sclera technique. This prospective, randomized study showed that topical cyclosporine 0.05% halved the recurrence rate from 44% in the control to 22% in the treatment group.[156] It remains to be seen whether cyclosporine is as effective in the more sophisticated surgical techniques but it has a safer side effect profile.

4. Adjunctive antifibrotic treatment, such as mitomycin and beta irradiation, aims to modify the wound healing response by suppression of proliferation of tissues in the postoperative phase. By their nature, these are mostly destructive techniques, and all have had complications associated with their use. Unfortunately, serious complications, such as scleral necrosis can take more than a decade to manifest, yet it can take a generation for surgeons to change techniques. Accordingly, these techniques were the primary therapy to reduce pterygium

recurrence for more than 50 years in Australia, yet it is only recently that practice patterns have changed after long-term studies reported a high rate of scleral necrosis and a moderately high recurrence rate.[170,171] Since mitomycin is a 'radiomimetic' agent, there are concerns about its long-term safety, given the reports of serious complications with beta radiation use. While the short-term complications may be dose-dependent and doses have been adjusted downward following reports of blinding complications[170] the long-term safety issue remains. Also, the potential role of damage to stem cells by adjunctive treatment is of interest, since these cells are critical to the long-term maintenance of ocular surface integrity.

Another aspect of the use of adjunctive treatments is the potential compromise of ocular tissue if future surgery is needed. Damaged scleral/episcleral vasculature can create problems, particularly for future conjunctival autografting techniques. Cameron noted that the aim of using irradiation was to destroy episcleral vessels, that could potentially provide nutrition for a recurrent pterygium.[33] We have reported cases in which graft failure occurred following previous beta radiation or mitomycin used as adjunctive therapy in the initial surgical management for pterygia.[172] This is of concern as adjunctive techniques can be associated with moderate recurrence rates. These observations resulted in our developing the use of adjuvant hyperbaric oxygen therapy to support autografts in the management of recurrent pterygium.[173] This technique was associated with a very low recurrence rate and rapid healing of the graft (Fig. 18.11). It should be noted that hyperbaric oxygen is also useful in the management of scleral melts associated with pterygium procedures.[174]

A number of randomized clinical trials have examined recurrence rates after using amniotic membrane grafts to cover the excision defect, as compared to conjunctival autografting.[175] These studies have all demonstrated a significantly lower pterygium recurrence rate in the conjunctival autograft group. Furthermore, amniotic membrane is not readily available in parts of the world where pterygia are common. The expense of amniotic membrane may be a problem in some parts of the world.

More recently, pterygium neovascularization, a process driven by elevated expression of multiple proangiogenic growth factors and cytokines, as well as a decrease in angiogenic inhibitors,[82] has been proposed as a target in both primary and in particular, recurrent pterygia. An attractive therapeutic target is VEGF, a potent proangiogenic growth factor that induces corneal neovascularization in the absence of inflammation. VEGF antagonists, such as humanized monoclonal antibodies targeting VEGF (Bevacizumab and Ranibizumab), have become readily available. VEGF has been known to be present in pterygia for over a decade,[52] being initially described in the epithelium of the head of the pterygium. A number of subsequent studies have confirmed this finding and have described VEGF in both basal and superficial epithelium, as well as in vascular endothelium and macrophages.[3,57,176] VEGF levels were found to be significantly higher in recurrent, compared with primary pterygium.[177] Since increased vascularity

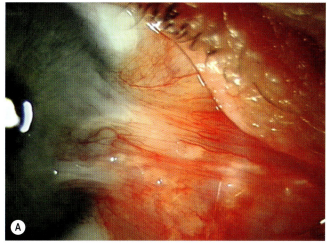

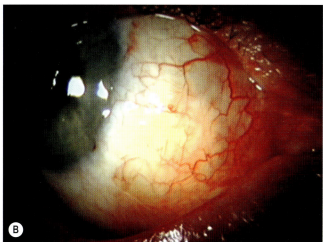

Figure 18.11 A large recurrent pterygium after multiple previous excisions and applications of beta radiation (**A**). The patient suffered form horizontal diplopia because of scarring that involved the medial rectus. Postoperative image of the same patient (**B**). The recurrent pterygium was widely excised, the medial rectus freed and a large autoconjunctival – limbal graft applied. The patient underwent hyperbaric oxygen treatment in the postoperative period. The remarkable aspect of this treatment is the rapid healing and reduction of graft inflammation, as well as the minimal (if any) graft shrinkage. This case illustrates the large extent of grafting that is possible.

contributes to poor cosmesis and requests for early intervention, a logical tactic is to develop antiangiogenic/anti-VEGF therapy to induce regression of blood vessels and possibly retard pterygium progression.

Several small clinical studies have been conducted[178,179] to treat primary and recurrent pterygia. Treatments have been delivered intra- or postoperatively with either topical therapy or intralesional injections. Results have been mixed, with some reports of an early but unsustained response.[178] There is little effect on recurrence rate, according to published reports.[179] Given the complexity of angiogenesis, it may be necessary to use combination angiostatic therapies to target multiple pathways.[180] An indication that this might be necessary is the recent finding that COX-2 and VEGF are highly expressed in macrophages infiltrating human pterygia. This finding suggests a bridge between the immune process and the tumor-like characteristics of a pterygium because both COX-2 and VEGF are important in skin carcinogenesis, induced by UV light damage.[176] Topical NSAIDs, inhibitors of COX, have been found to be useful in the management of pterygia[151,181] and thus, could be used in combination with VEGF inhibitors.

Corticosteroids are another inhibitor of neovascularization. Preliminary data on anecortave acetate suggest an inhibitory effect on recurrent pterygium[182] but it was not compared with other anti-inflammatory treatments.

Another approach has been to target another component of the pterygium pathogenesis cascade, matrix metalloproteinases, with an inhibitor such as doxycycline. This drug has been shown to inhibit, the growth of cultured pterygium epithelia cells[183] but clinical data are not yet available.

5. A useful approach to the surgical time factor has been the advent of the 'cut and paste technique,' utilizing tissue glue to rapidly attach graft tissue during the procedure.[184] A concern with these techniques is their safety with large grafts which in our view they provide excellent functional and cosmetic results. Of particular concern is the integrity of the limbal sutures, since if these break or dislodge, the graft can retract and compromise outcomes. A hybrid technique involving two limbal sutures and tissue gluing of the rest of the graft has been described (Ezra Maguen, personal communication) and may prove to be an excellent compromise for large grafts.

Recently, a promising technique that uses a simple method of 'tissue welding' wherein the graft is opposed to host conjunctiva with a tying forceps and a weld achieved by touching the forceps with a hand-held cautery has been described.[185] Again, the strength of these welds, particularly in large grafts, must be assessed in larger multicenter studies.

6. Another aspect of pterygium surgery is the pain associated with surgery.[186,187] The procedure can be one of the most painful ophthalmic procedures currently performed, hardly surprising given the extent of the ocular surface involved, particularly when an autograft is harvested. While the procedure is frequently carried out under topical anesthesia, we prefer peribulbar blocks, particularly for recurrent cases. Alternatively, long-acting topical anesthetics or gel preparations may be used.[188]

Another useful strategy is the use of a contact lens placed at the end of surgery and left in place during the acute healing phase.[189] We routinely use a Balafilcon A extended-wear contact lens for a week after surgery and have found that this lens is less conducive to ocular surface cell adherence.[190]

7. Unsuspected neoplasia is present in ≈10–30% of specimens[32] and it has been suggested that all pterygia specimens should be submitted for histopathologic examination.[30,32] For cases in which neoplasia is detected, more frequent postoperative surveillance is recommended; however, such cases can be treated with topical interferon with or without retinoic acid, a very effective medical treatment for this condition.[191,192]

8. In very advanced cases, especially if there is bilateral disease (Fig. 18.12), there may be a relative shortage of conjunctival tissue that can be used in reconstruction.

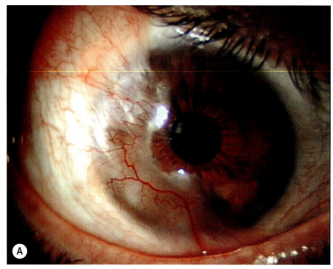

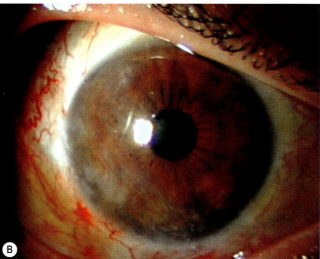

Figure 18.12 Preoperative image of a patient with extensive disease after surgery for multiple recurrences (**A**). The second eye was similarly affected. Postoperative image of the same pateint (**B**). The pateint underwent excison of the recurrent pteygium and grafting using a conjunctival equivalent derived from autologous cultivated conjunctival epithelial cells grown on human amniotic membrane.

While other types of mucus or amniotic membrane can be used, reconstruction using a serum-free derived autologous cultivated conjunctival equivalent derived from ex vivo expansion of conjunctival epithelial cells on human amniotic membranes has been successfully utilized.[193] While this technique can only be carried out in specialized units, improvements in stem cell transplantation holds promise for greater use of this technique. Potentially, it could obviate the need for creating autoconjunctival grafts.

Author's Technique

Following adequate anesthesia (typically a peribulbar block with long-acting anesthetic) a few drops of brimonidine are applied as a vasoconstrictor. Brimonidine does not dilate the pupil like adrenaline. Half-strength povidone is applied and careful lash-excluding draping is carried out. The head of the pterygium is excised using a 23-gauge needle-tip technique[194] (Fig. 18.13A). This technique

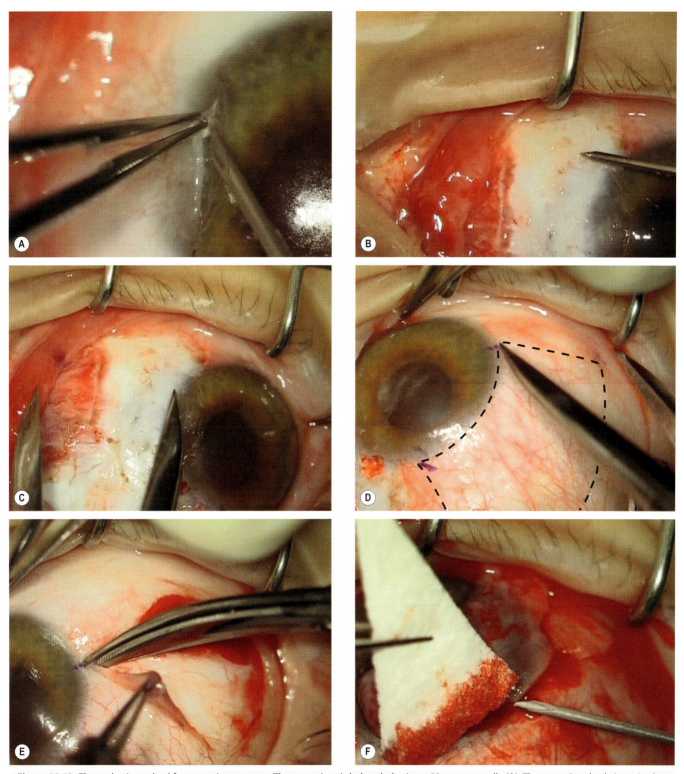

Figure 18.13 The author's method for pterygium surgery. The pterygium is beheaded using a 23-gauge needle (**A**). The pterygium body is excised to the caruncle and bleeding controlled with a diathermy (**B**). The size of the defect created by pterygium excision is measured with calipers and, in particular, the horizontal extent is measured with the eye in forced abduction (**C**). Graft size is marked at the superior limbus and bulbar conjunctiva. The graft has a trapezoidal shape, being wider in the forniceal than limbal aspect (**D**). A thin conjunctival graft is dissected with spring scissors (**E**), then folded down over the cornea and kept on tension with the short end of a Stroll wedge. The limbus is dissected to approximately 50% of the vertical extent of the palisades of Vogt using a 23-gauge needle tip (**F**).

Continued on following page

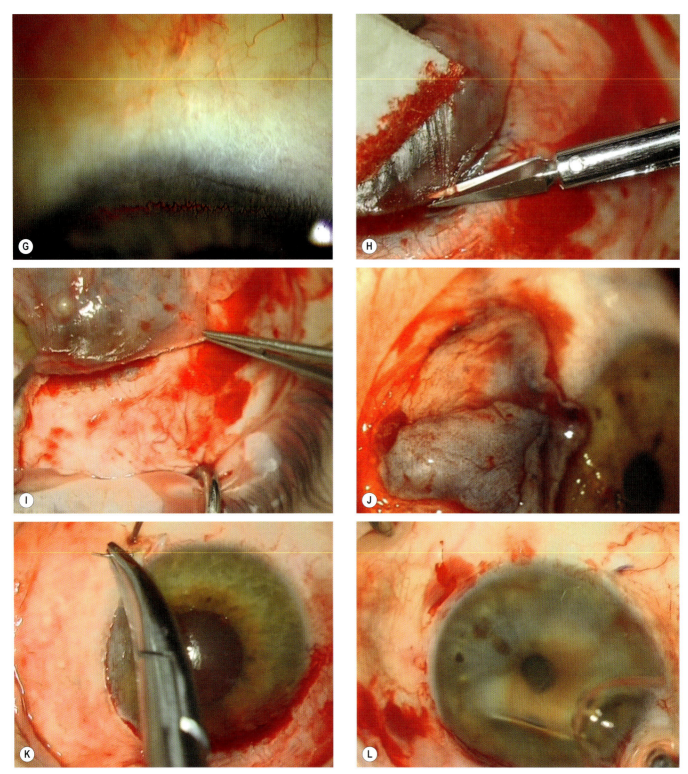

Figure 18.13 (Continued) The superior limbus, some months after surgery, showing the horizontal line through the palisades of Vogt that delineates the inferior aspect of the graft donor site (**G**). In this way the limbus is 'split,' allowing some limbal cells to be taken in the graft and the remainder to stay in their normal location. This method avoids limbal failure at the donor site. Amputation of the limbal – conjunctival graft at the limbal edge using Vannas' scissors. The graft is held under tension with the edge of a Stroll wedge (**H**). The limbal edges of the graft are picked up at the limbal edges with non-toothed tying forceps. At this stage the epithelial surface is in contact with the corneal surface and the graft has to be slid across to the site of pterygium excision and inverted so that the epithelial aspect is superficial. The limbal edge of the graft is aligned with the limbal aspect of the defect (**I**). Graft orientation can be checked with trypan blue, as this dye stains Tenon's capsule preferentially to the epithelial surface (**J**). The graft is sutured in place, commencing with limbal sutures using an absorbable 10-0 Polyglycolic Acid (PolySyn GA-966, Sharpoint) suture. Small bites of episclera/sclera are taken at the limbus and all knots are buried (**K**). At the end of the procedure, an extended wear Balafilcon A contact lens (PureVision, Bausch and Lomb) is placed on the ocular surface and left in place for 1 week (**L**).

minimizes the amount of corneal tissue excised and even though a relatively rough stromal surface is left behind, epithelial smoothing results in an even ocular surface. This also allows complete removal of abnormal tissue from the cornea, since residual tissue left on the cornea is a cause of concern for many patients. For a right-handed surgeon operating on a left eye, the microscope can be moved so pterygium head dissection is carried out from the side.

The body of the pterygium is then excised, taking care to:

1. Excise tissue for about 1 mm above and below these sites where the pterygium crosses the limbus. This is because abnormal pterygium epithelial cells have been described in these locations[18] and also because some recurrences appear to arise from these sites.
2. Excise inflamed tissue, sometimes as far as the caruncle (Fig. 18.13B). This is essential in obtaining good cosmesis. Care is taken to remain superficial and to avoid the check ligaments and capsule in a primary pterygium. Any excess Tenon's capsule underlying this excised area is also trimmed but 'fishing for Tenon's' by pulling on exposed connective tissue is avoided.

Bleeding is minimized with a minimalist use of an intra-ocular diathermy (Fig. 18.13B). Care is taken to check for bleeding in the cut edges of the conjunctiva, particularly in the region of the caruncle. The size of the defect is measured (Fig. 18.13C) and the graft size is marked (Fig. 18.13D). Not infrequently, the area to be dissected extends to the superior fornix. Using a squint hook to pull upwards on the superior blade of the speculum can enhance exposure in this area. Westcott-style spring scissors are used to create a thin flap (Fig. 18.13E). Such scissors can vary in size, tip configuration and blade sharpness, we favor those made by Martin (35-822-11), which are wrapped and sterilized separately from other instruments. The scissors are replaced if judged to be blunt. An assistant's help in holding up the proximal aspect of the graft is useful, particularly for large grafts. The dissected graft is then folded down over the cornea (Fig. 18.13F). Excessive Tenon's can be trimmed from this exposed under-surface of the graft, using a toothed forceps to engage the Tenon's excess. Also, any buttonholes can be repaired, as the knot will be located on the under-surface of the graft. The short end of a Stroll wedge is used to pull the graft inferiorly and the limbus is dissected (Fig. 18.13F). There is often bleeding because of perforating vessels in this area and this is controlled with a second wedge. This maneuver allows a splitting of the limbus (Fig. 18.13G and H). The graft is then detached from the remaining limbus (Fig. 18.13I). The cut edges have a crenellated appearance, believed to be due to the morphology of the palisades of Vogt. The graft (Fig. 18.13J) is slid across a balanced salt-lubricated cornea, flipped over and placed in the defect created by the pterygium excision. Trypan blue can be used to check graft orientation, as this dye stains Tenon's capsule preferentially to the epithelial surface (Fig. 18.13K). The graft is sutured in place commencing with limbal sutures (Fig. 18.13L). An extended-wear contact lens is placed at the end of the procedure. Care is taken to make sure that the contact lens covers the limbal aspect of the graft. The post-operative eye drop regimen consists of chloramphenicol, prednefrin forte and preservative-free diclofenac used four times daily and usually tapered after 1 week. Topical treatment is typically 4–6 weeks. If excessive inflammation occurs, topical treatment is prolonged and topical cyclosporine may be introduced.

For recurrent pterygia, a forced duction is used to help determine the extent of fibrosis of tissues between the recurrence site and medial rectus muscle. In severe cases the medial rectus muscle is isolated and appropriate dissection with excision of Tenon's capsule carried out, forced duction tests being repeated to make sure that all fibrotic bands are cut. Such cases require extensive grafts. In cases of unilateral pterygium with inadequate superior bulbar conjunctiva, donor tissue can be taken from the other eye. This is discussed with the patient preoperatively. All such cases receive hyperbaric oxygen for a week after surgery.[173] This technique has evolved and has a recurrence rate of ≈1%.

Training of Surgeons

A critical issue in the management of this prevalent disease is surgeon training. It is recognized that the widespread use of phacoemulsification has deprived generations of ophthalmologists of the ability to suture. Even with glue techniques, conjunctival graft suturing remains important, since the cost of glues makes this technique prohibitive in some settings and there are concerns about glue efficacy in very large grafts. For these reasons, we have developed a porcine eye model, for both teaching the creation and suturing of conjunctival grafts and for developing improved graft techniques.[195]

The Future

Advances in our understanding of the basic pathophysiology of a pterygium are likely to result in more sophisticated pharmacological interventions.[82] It appears that the use of topical cyclosporine, with its multiple actions, is an early manifestation of this approach. There is a great need to develop animal models for this disease not only to improve our understanding of pathophysiology but also to better test surgical techniques. The current model,[183] based on transplantation of cultured human pterygium epithelial cells into athymic nude mice, may not adequately represent human disease, and size may limit its use as a surgical model.[196] Stem cell culture and/or graft techniques have the potential to replace the need for conjunctival graft dissection. Use of sophisticated laser techniques might allow faster, more accurate graft creation and better attachment techniques will also help to shorten surgical time.

Development and use of a grading scale for pterygium, perhaps using more advanced imaging techniques, such as optical coherence tomography,[9,197] might aid in the evaluation of various techniques. Standardization and optimization of postoperative treatment regimes, will also allow better comparison of different techniques.

More sophisticated public health campaigns based on detection of early UV damage[49] and perhaps self-monitoring using readily available cameras, may raise awareness of this disease and the need for adequate sun protection. The use of ultraviolet-blocking contact lenses, for the first time, has meant that the limbus can be protected from ultraviolet light.[7] The inadequacy of current sunglass designs has been acknowledged in the new sunglass standards and provides a challenge for manufacturers to design better protection devices.[7] The role of diet, known to confer protection against ultraviolet skin damage, as well as dry eye, requires investigation.[198] There is also a need to overcome the trivialization of this disease, which in parts of the world, is a blinding condition and which even when managed adequately, has long-term consequences for the cornea.

References

1. Duke-Elder S. Diseases of the outer eye. Part 1. In: Duke-Elder S, editor. System of Ophthalmology: volume 8 Diseases of the outer eye. London: Kimpton UK; 1965. p. 569–85.
2. Murube J. Pterygium: descriptive nomenclature of the past. Ocul Surf 2008;6(3):104–7. Epub 2008/09/11.
3. Di Girolamo N, Chui J, Coroneo MT, et al. Pathogenesis of pterygia: role of cytokines, growth factors, and matrix metalloproteinases. Prog Retin Eye Res 2004;23(2):195–228. Epub 2004/04/20.
4. Wlodarczyk J, Whyte P, Cockrum P, et al. Pterygium in Australia: a cost of illness study. Clin Exp Ophthalmol 2001;29(6):370–5. Epub 2002/01/10.
5. Sopoaga F, Buckingham K, Paul C. Causes of excess hospitalizations among Pacific peoples in New Zealand: implications for primary care. J Prim Health Care 2010;2(2):105–10. Epub 2010/08/10.
6. Ramke J, Brian G, du Toit R. Eye disease and care at hospital clinics in Cook Islands, Fiji, Samoa and Tonga. Clin Exp Ophthalmol 2007;35(7):627–34. Epub 2007/09/27.
7. Coroneo M. Ultraviolet radiation and the anterior eye. Eye Contact Lens 2011;37(4):214–24. Epub 2011/06/15.
8. Shibata N, Kitagawa K, Sakamoto Y, et al. Changes in corneal higher order aberration after pterygium excision. ARVO Meeting Abstracts 2010;51(5):2399.
9. Ashizawa J, Hori Y, Saishin Y, et al. Use of Fourier-domain optical coherence tomography to assess pterygium surgery. ARVO Meeting Abstracts 2010;51(5):2408.
10. Lee AJ, Lee J, Saw SM, et al. Prevalence and risk factors associated with dry eye symptoms: a population based study in Indonesia. Br J Ophthalmol 2002;86(12):1347–13451. Epub 2002/11/26.
11. Stern ME, Pflugfelder SC. Inflammation in dry eye. Ocul Surf 2004;2(2):124–30. Epub 2007/01/12.
12. Dolezalova V. Is the occurrence of a temporal pterygium really so rare? Ophthalmologica 1977;174(2):88–91. Epub 1977/01/01.
13. Tan DTH. Pterygium. In: Holland EJ, Mannis MJ, editors. Ocular surface disease: medical and surgical management. 1st ed. Springer-Verlag; 2002. p. 65–89.
14. Fuchs E. Ueber das Pterygium. Graefes Arch for Ophthalmol 1892;38(2):1–89.
15. Hansen A, Norn M. Astigmatism and surface phenomena in pterygium. Acta Ophthalmol (Copenh) 1980;58(2):174–81. Epub 1980/04/01.
16. Li M, Zhang M, Lin Y, et al. Tear function and goblet cell density after pterygium excision. Eye 2007;21(2):224–8. Epub 2005/12/13.
17. Seifert P, Eckert J, Spitznas M. Topological-histological investigation of the pterygium. Graefes Arch Clin Exp Ophthalmol 2001;239(4):288–93. Epub 2001/07/14.
18. Dushku N, Reid TW. Immunohistochemical evidence that human pterygia originate from an invasion of vimentin-expressing altered limbal epithelial basal cells. Curr Eye Res 1994;13(7):473–81. Epub 1994/07/01.
19. Chan CM, Liu YP, Tan DT. Ocular surface changes in pterygium. Cornea 2002;21(1):38–42. Epub 2002/01/24.
20. Seifert P, Sekundo W. Capillaries in the epithelium of pterygium. Br J Ophthalmol 1998;82(1):77–81.
21. Pinkerton OD, Hokama Y, Shigemura LA. Immunologic basis for the pathogenesis of pterygium. Am J Ophthalmol 1984;98(2):225–8.
22. Ioachim-Velogianni E, Tsironi E, Agnantis N, et al. HLA-DR antigen expression in pterygium epithelial cells and lymphocyte subpopulations: an immunohistochemistry study. Ger J Ophthalmol 1995;4(2):123–9. Epub 1995/03/01.
23. Tekelioglu Y, Turk A, Avunduk AM, et al. Flow cytometrical analysis of adhesion molecules, T-lymphocyte subpopulations and inflammatory markers in pterygium. Ophthalmologica 2006;220(6):372–8. Epub 2006/11/11.
24. Clear AS, Chirambo MC, Hutt MS. Solar keratosis, pterygium, and squamous cell carcinoma of the conjunctiva in Malawi. Br J Ophthalmol 1979;63(2):102–9. Epub 1979/02/01.
25. Hogan MJ, Alvarado J. Pterygium and pinguecula: electron microscopic study. Arch Ophthalmol 1967;78(2):174–86. Epub 1967/08/01.
26. Dong N, Li W, Lin H, et al. Abnormal epithelial differentiation and tear film alteration in pinguecula. Invest Ophthalmol Vis Sci 2009;50(6):2710–5. Epub 2009/02/03.
27. Soliman W, Mohamed TA. Spectral domain anterior segment optical coherence tomography assessment of pterygium and pinguecula. Acta Ophthalmol 2012;90(5):461–5. Epub 2010/11/03.
28. Keenan JD, Mandel MR, Margolis TP. Peripheral ulcerative keratitis associated with vasculitis manifesting asymmetrically as fuchs superficial marginal keratitis and terrien marginal degeneration. Cornea 2011;30(7):825–7. Epub 2010/12/15.
29. Seitz B, Fischer M, Holbach LM, et al. [Differential diagnosis and prognosis of 112 excised epibulbar epithelial tumors]. Klin Monbl Augenheilkd 1995;207(4):239–46. Epub 1995/10/01. Differential diagnose und Prognose bei 112 exzidierten epibulbaren epithelialen Tumoren.
30. Hirst LW, Axelsen RA, Schwab I. Pterygium and associated ocular surface squamous neoplasia. Arch Ophthalmol 2009;127(1):31–2. Epub 2009/01/14.
31. Perra MT, Colombari R, Maxia C, et al. Finding of conjunctival melanocytic pigmented lesions within pterygium. Histopathology 2006;48(4):387–93. Epub 2006/02/21.
32. Chui J, Coroneo MT, Tat LT, et al. Ophthalmic pterygium a stem cell disorder with premalignant features. Am J Pathol 2011;178(2):817–27. Epub 2011/02/02.
33. Cameron ME. Pterygium throughout the world. Springfield, Ill.: Thomas; 1965.
34. Moran DJ, Hollows FC. Pterygium and ultraviolet radiation: a positive correlation. Br J Ophthalmol 1984;68(5):343–6. Epub 1984/05/01.
35. Lu P, Chen X, Kang Y, et al. Pterygium in Tibetans: a population-based study in China. Clin Exp Ophthalmol 2007;35(9):828–33. Epub 2008/01/05.
36. Lu J, Wang Z, Lu P, et al. Pterygium in an aged Mongolian population: a population-based study in China. Eye 2009;23(2):421–7. Epub 2007/10/20.
37. Norn MS. Spheroid degeneration of cornea and conjunctiva. Prevalence among Eskimos in Greenland and caucasians in Copenhagen. Acta Ophthalmol (Copenh) 1978;56(4):551–62. Epub 1978/01/01.
38. Taylor HR, West SK, Rosenthal FS, et al. Corneal changes associated with chronic UV irradiation. Arch Ophthalmol 1989;107(10):1481–4. Epub 1989/10/01.
39. Threlfall TJ, English DR. Sun exposure and pterygium of the eye: a dose-response curve. Am J Ophthalmol 1999;128(3):280–7. Epub 1999/10/08.
40. McCarty CA, Fu CL, Taylor HR. Epidemiology of pterygium in Victoria, Australia. Br J Ophthalmol 2000;84(3):289–92. Epub 2000/02/24.
41. Karai I, Horiguchi S. Pterygium in welders. Br J Ophthalmol 1984;68:347-9. Epub 1984/05/01.
42. Wong TY, Foster PJ, Johnson GJ, et al. The prevalence and risk factors for pterygium in an adult Chinese population in Singapore: the Tanjong Pagar survey. Am J Ophthalmol 2001;131(2):176–83. Epub 2001/03/03.
43. Okoye OI, Umeh RE. Eye health of industrial workers in Southeastern Nigeria. West Afr J Med 2002;21(2):132–7. Epub 2002/10/31.
44. Lin W, Wang SL, Wu HJ, et al. Associations between arsenic in drinking water and pterygium in southwestern Taiwan. Environ Health Perspect 2008;116(7):952–5. Epub 2008/07/17.
45. Omoti AE, Waziri-Erameh JM, Enock ME. Ocular disorders in a petroleum industry in Nigeria. Eye 2008;22(7):925–9. Epub 2007/04/03.

46. Coroneo MT, Müller-Stolzenburg NW, Ho A. Peripheral light focusing by the anterior eye and the ophthalmohelioses. Ophthalmic Surg 1991;22:705-11.

47. Coroneo MT. Pterygium as an early indicator of ultraviolet insolation: a hypothesis. Br J Ophthalmol 1993;77(11):734–9. Epub 1993/11/01.

48. Ooi JL, Sharma NS, Sharma S, et al. Ultraviolet fluorescence photography: patterns in established pterygia. Am J Ophthalmol 2007;143(1):97–101. Epub 2006/11/23.

49. Ooi JL, Sharma NS, Papalkar D, et al. Ultraviolet fluorescence photography to detect early sun damage in the eyes of school-aged children. Am J Ophthalmol 2006;141(2):294–8. Epub 2006/02/07.

50. Tsai YY, Cheng YW, Lee H, et al. Oxidative DNA damage in pterygium. Mol Vis 2005;11:71–5.

51. Lu L, Wang R, Song X. [Pterygium and lipid peroxidation]. Zhonghua Yan Ke Za Zhi 1996;32(3):227–9.

52. Lee DH, Cho HJ, Kim JT, et al. Expression of vascular endothelial growth factor and inducible nitric oxide synthase in pterygia. Cornea 2001;20(7):738–42. Epub 2001/10/06.

53. Kon K, Fujii S, Kosaka H, et al. Nitric oxide synthase inhibition by N(G)-nitro-L-arginine methyl ester retards vascular sprouting in angiogenesis. Microvasc Res 2003;65(1):2–8.

54. Ziche M, Morbidelli L, Masini E, et al. Nitric oxide mediates angiogenesis in vivo and endothelial cell growth and migration in vitro promoted by substance P. J Clin Invest 1994;94(5):2036–44.

55. Brown DJ, Lin B, Chwa M, et al. Elements of the nitric oxide pathway can degrade TIMP-1 and increase gelatinase activity. Mol Vis 2004;10:281–8.

56. Peus D, Vasa RA, Meves A, et al. H_2O_2 is an important mediator of UVB-induced EGF-receptor phosphorylation in cultured keratinocytes. J Invest Dermatol 1998;110(6):966–71.

57. Di Girolamo N, Wakefield D, Coroneo MT. UVB-mediated induction of cytokines and growth factors in pterygium epithelial cells involves cell surface receptors and intracellular signaling. Invest Ophthalmol Vis Sci 2006;47(6):2430–7. Epub 2006/05/26.

58. Di Girolamo N, Coroneo MT, Wakefield D. UVB-elicited induction of MMP-1 expression in human ocular surface epithelial cells is mediated through the ERK1/2 MAPK-dependent pathway. Invest Ophthalmol Vis Sci 2003;44(11):4705–14. Epub 2003/10/28.

59. Di Girolamo N, Coroneo M, Wakefield D. Epidermal growth factor receptor signaling is partially responsible for the increased matrix metalloproteinase-1 expression in ocular epithelial cells after UVB radiation. Am J Pathol 2005;167(2):489–503. Epub 2005/07/29.

60. Wong WW. A hypothesis on the pathogenesis of pterygiums. Ann Ophthalmol 1978;10(3):303–8. Epub 1978/03/01.

61. Kennedy M, Kim KH, Harten B, et al. Ultraviolet irradiation induces the production of multiple cytokines by human corneal cells. Invest Ophthalmol Vis Sci 1997;38(12):2483–91. Epub 1997/12/31.

62. Siak JJ, Ng SL, Seet LF, et al. The nuclear-factor kappaB pathway is activated in pterygium. Invest Ophthalmol Vis Sci 2011;52(1):230–6. Epub 2010/09/03.

63. Torres J, Enriquez-de-Salamanca A, Fernandez I, et al. Activation of MAPK signaling pathway and NF-kappaB activation in pterygium and ipsilateral pterygium-free conjunctival specimens. Invest Ophthalmol Vis Sci 2011;52(8):5842–52. Epub 2011/06/21.

64. Kuo CH, Miyazaki D, Yakura K, et al. Role of periostin and interleukin-4 in recurrence of pterygia. Invest Ophthalmol Vis Sci 2010;51(1):139–43. Epub 2009/08/08.

65. Chiang CC, Cheng YW, Lin CL, et al. Cyclooxygenase 2 expression in pterygium. Mol Vis 2007;13:635–8. Epub 2007/05/23.

66. Maxia C, Perra MT, Demurtas P, et al. Relationship between the expression of cyclooxygenase-2 and survivin in primary pterygium. Mol Vis 2009;15:458–63. Epub 2009/02/28.

67. Ottino P, Bazan HE. Corneal stimulation of MMP-1, -9 and uPA by platelet-activating factor is mediated by cyclooxygenase-2 metabolites. Curr Eye Res 2001;23(2):77–85.

68. Eckert RL, Broome AM, Ruse M, et al. S100 proteins in the epidermis. J Invest Dermatol 2004;123(1):23–33. Epub 2004/06/12.

69. Riau AK, Wong TT, Beuerman RW, et al. Calcium-binding S100 protein expression in pterygium. Mol Vis 2009;15:335–42. Epub 2009/02/19.

70. Zhou L, Beuerman RW, Ang LP, et al. Elevation of human alpha-defensins and S100 calcium-binding proteins A8 and A9 in tear fluid of patients with pterygium. Invest Ophthalmol Vis Sci 2009;50(5):2077–86. Epub 2009/01/27.

71. Lee YM, Kim YK, Eun HC, et al. Changes in S100A8 expression in UV-irradiated and aged human skin in vivo. Arch Dermatol Res 2009;301(7):523–9. Epub 2009/05/26.

72. Lim SY, Raftery MJ, Goyette J, et al. Oxidative modifications of S100 proteins: functional regulation by redox. J Leukoc Biol 2009;86(3):577–87. Epub 2009/02/25.

73. Nakagami T, Watanabe I, Murakami A, et al. Expression of stem cell factor in pterygium. Jpn J Ophthalmol 2000;44(3):193–7. Epub 2000/07/29.

74. Lee JK, Song YS, Ha HS, et al. Endothelial progenitor cells in pterygium pathogenesis. Eye 2007;21(9):1186–93. Epub 2006/05/30.

75. Ribatti D, Nico B, Maxia C, et al. Neovascularization and mast cells with tryptase activity increase simultaneously in human pterygium. J Cell Mol Med 2007;11(3):585–9. Epub 2007/07/20.

76. Chen YT, Tseng SH, Tsai YY, et al. Distribution of vimentin-expressing cells in pterygium: an immunocytochemical study of impression cytology specimens. Cornea 2009;28(5):547–52. Epub 2009/05/08.

77. Zhivov A, Beck R, Guthoff RF. Corneal and conjunctival findings after mitomycin C application in pterygium surgery: an in-vivo confocal microscopy study. Acta Ophthalmol 2009;87(2):166–72. Epub 2008/06/10.

78. John-Aryankalayil M, Dushku N, Jaworski CJ, et al. Microarray and protein analysis of human pterygium. Mol Vis 2006;12:55–64. Epub 2006/02/01.

79. Kheirkhah A, Casas V, Sheha H, et al. Role of conjunctival inflammation in surgical outcome after amniotic membrane transplantation with or without fibrin glue for pterygium. Cornea 2008;27(1):56–63. Epub 2008/02/05.

80. Awdeh RM, DeStafeno JJ, Blackmon DM, et al. The presence of T-lymphocyte subpopulations (CD4 and CD8) in pterygia: evaluation of the inflammatory response. Adv Ther 2008;25(5):479–87. Epub 2008/05/17.

81. Rohrbach IM, Starc S, Knorr M. [Predicting recurrent pterygium based on morphologic and immunohistologic parameters]. Ophthalmologe 1995;92(4):463–8. Epub 1995/08/01. Vorhersage von Pterygiumrezidiven aufgrund morphologischer und immunhistologischer Parameter.

82. Chui J, Di Girolamo N, Wakefield D, et al. The pathogenesis of pterygium: current concepts and their therapeutic implications. Ocul Surf 2008;6(1):24–43. Epub 2008/02/12.

83. Saika S, Yamanaka O, Sumioka T, et al. Fibrotic disorders in the eye: targets of gene therapy. Prog Retin Eye Res 2008;27(2):177–96. Epub 2008/02/05.

84. Kria L, Ohira A, Amemiya T. Immunohistochemical localization of basic fibroblast growth factor, platelet derived growth factor, transforming growth factor-beta and tumor necrosis factor-alpha in the pterygium. Acta Histochem 1996;98(2):195–201. Epub 1996/04/01.

85. Kria L, Ohira A, Amemiya T. Growth factors in cultured pterygium fibroblasts: immunohistochemical and ELISA analysis. Graefes Arch Clin Exp Ophthalmol 1998;236(9):702–8. Epub 1998/10/23.

86. Lee SB, Li DQ, Tan DT, et al. Suppression of TGF-beta signaling in both normal conjunctival fibroblasts and pterygial body fibroblasts by amniotic membrane. Curr Eye Res 2000;20(4):325–34. Epub 2000/05/12.

87. Aspiotis M, Tsanou E, Gorezis S, et al. Angiogenesis in pterygium: study of microvessel density, vascular endothelial growth factor, and thrombospondin-1. Eye 2007;21(8):1095–101. Epub 2006/07/11.

88. Hong S, Choi JY, Lee HK, et al. Expression of neurotrophic factors in human primary pterygeal tissue and selective TNF-alpha-induced stimulation of ciliary neurotrophic factor in pterygeal fibroblasts. Exp Toxicol Pathol 2008;60(6):513–20. Epub 2008/07/01.

89. Ribatti D, Nico B, Perra MT, et al. Correlation between NGF/TrkA and microvascular density in human pterygium. Int J Exp Pathol 2009;90(6):615–20. Epub 2009/09/18.

90. Di Girolamo N, Sarris M, Chui J, et al. Localization of the low-affinity nerve growth factor receptor p75 in human limbal epithelial cells. J Cell Mol Med 2008;12(6B):2799–811. Epub 2009/02/13.

91. Wong TT, Sethi C, Daniels JT, et al. Matrix metalloproteinases in disease and repair processes in the anterior segment. Surv Ophthalmol 2002;47(3):239–56. Epub 2002/06/08.

92. Yang SF, Lin CY, Yang PY, et al. Increased expression of gelatinase (MMP-2 and MMP-9) in pterygia and pterygium fibroblasts with disease progression and activation of protein kinase C. Invest Ophthalmol Vis Sci 2009;50(10):4588–96. Epub 2009/05/08.

93. Wang IJ, Hu FR, Chen PJ, et al. Mechanism of abnormal elastin gene expression in the pinguecular part of pterygia. Am J Pathol 2000;157(4):1269–76. Epub 2000/10/06.

94. Kaneko M, Takaku I, Katsura N. Glycosaminoglycans in pterygium tissues and normal conjunctiva. Jpn J Ophthalmol 1986;30(2):165–73. Epub 1986/01/01.

95. Fitzsimmons TD, Molander N, Stenevi U, et al. Endogenous hyaluronan in corneal disease. Invest Ophthalmol Vis Sci 1994;35(6):2774–82. Epub 1994/05/01.

96. Perez-Rico C, Pascual G, Sotomayor S, et al. Tropoelastin and fibulin overexpression in the subepithelial connective tissue of human pterygium. Am J Ophthalmol 2011;151(1):44–52. Epub 2010/11/26.

97. Tumova S, Woods A, Couchman JR. Heparan sulfate proteoglycans on the cell surface: versatile coordinators of cellular functions. Int J Biochem Cell Biol 2000;32(3):269–88. Epub 2000/03/15.

98. Zhang JD. An investigation of aetiology and heredity of pterygium. Report of 11 cases in a family. Acta Ophthalmol (Copenh) 1987;65(4):413–6.

99. Hecht F, Shoptaugh MG. Winglets of the eye: dominant transmission of early adult pterygium of the conjunctiva. J Med Genet 1990;27(6):392–4. Epub 1990/06/01.

100. Goyal JL, Rao VA, Srinivasan R, et al. Oculocutaneous manifestations in xeroderma pigmentosa. Br J Ophthalmol 1994;78(4):295–7. Epub 1994/04/01.

101. Kau HC, Tsai CC, Hsu WM, et al. Genetic polymorphism of hOGG1 and risk of pterygium in Chinese. Eye 2004;18(6):635–9. Epub 2004/01/13.

102. Chen PL, Yeh KT, Tsai YY, et al. XRCC1, but not APE1 and hOGG1 gene polymorphisms is a risk factor for pterygium. Mol Vis 2010;16:991–6. Epub 2010/06/26.

103. Tsai YY, Bau DT, Chiang CC, et al. Pterygium and genetic polymorphism of DNA double strand break repair gene Ku70. Mol Vis 2007;13:1436–40. Epub 2007/09/05.

104. Tsai YY, Lee H, Tseng SH, et al. Null type of glutathione S-transferase M1 polymorphism is associated with early onset pterygium. Mol Vis 2004;10:458–61.Epub 2004/07/27.

105. Tung JN, Wu HH, Chiang CC, et al. An association between BPDE-like DNA adduct levels and CYP1A1 and GSTM1 polymorphisma in pterygium. Mol Vis 2010;16:623–9. Epub 2010/08/12.

106. Detorakis ET, Drakonaki EE, Spandidos DA. Molecular genetic alterations and viral presence in ophthalmic pterygium. Int J Mol Med 2000;6(1):35–41. Epub 2000/06/14.

107. Di Girolamo N. Association of human papilloma virus with pterygia and ocular-surface squamous neoplasia. Eye (Lond) 2012;26(2):202–11. Epub 2011/12/03.

108. Piras F, Moore PS, Ugalde J, et al. Detection of human papillomavirus DNA in pterygia from different geographical regions. Br J Ophthalmol 2003;87(7):864–6. Epub 2003/06/19.

109. Tsai YY, Chang CC, Chiang CC, et al. HPV infection and p53 inactivation in pterygium. Mol Vis 2009;15:1092–7. Epub 2009/06/09.

110. Detorakis ET, Sourvinos G, Spandidos DA. Detection of herpes simplex virus and human papilloma virus in ophthalmic pterygium. Cornea 2001;20(2):164–7. Epub 2001/03/15.

111. Chen YF, Hsiao CH, Ngan KW, et al. Herpes simplex virus and pterygium in Taiwan. Cornea 2008;27(3):311–3. Epub 2008/03/26.

112. Dushku N, Reid TW. P53 expression in altered limbal basal cells of pingueculae, pterygia, and limbal tumors. Curr Eye Res 1997;16(12):1179–92. Epub 1998/01/14.

113. Spandidos DA, Sourvinos G, Kiaris H, et al. Microsatellite instability and loss of heterozygosity in human pterygia. Br J Ophthalmol 1997;81(6):493–6.

114. Detorakis ET, Zafiropoulos A, Arvanitis DA, et al. Detection of point mutations at codon 12 of KI-ras in ophthalmic pterygia. Eye 2005;19(2):210–4. Epub 2004/07/03.

115. Tsai YY, Cheng YW, Lee H, et al. P53 gene mutation spectrum and the relationship between gene mutation and protein levels in pterygium. Mol Vis 2005;11:50–5.

116. Reisman D, McFadden JW, Lu G. Loss of heterozygosity and p53 expression in Pterygium. Cancer Lett 2004;206(1):77–83.

117. Lakin ND, Jackson SP. Regulation of p53 in response to DNA damage. Oncogene 1999;18(53):7644–55.

118. Drouin R, Therrien JP. UVB-induced cyclobutane pyrimidine dimer frequency correlates with skin cancer mutational hotspots in p53. Photochem Photobiol 1997;66(5):719–26.

119. Onur C, Orhan D, Orhan M, et al. Expression of p53 protein in pterygium. Eur J Ophthalmol 1998;8(3):157–61.

120. Chowers I, Pe'er J, Zamir E, et al. Proliferative activity and p53 expression in primary and recurrent pterygia. Ophthalmology 2001;108(5):985–8.

121. Schneider BG, John-Aryankalayil M, Rowsey JJ, et al. Accumulation of p53 protein in pterygia is not accompanied by TP53 gene mutation. Exp Eye Res 2006;82(1):91–8. Epub 2005/07/12.

122. Chen PL, Cheng YW, Chiang CC, et al. Hypermethylation of the p16 gene promoter in pterygia and its association with the expression of DNA methyltransferase 3b. Mol Vis 2006;12:1411–6. Epub 2006/12/07.

123. Young CH, Chiu YT, Shih TS, et al. E-cadherin promoter hypermethylation may contribute to protein inactivation in pterygia. Mol Vis 2010;16:1047–53. Epub 2010/07/03.

124. Riau AK, Wong TT, Lan W, et al. Aberrant DNA methylation of matrix remodeling and cell adhesion related genes in pterygium. PLoS One 2011;6(2):e14687. Epub 2011/03/02.

125. Tan DT, Tang WY, Liu YP, et al. Apoptosis and apoptosis related gene expression in normal conjunctiva and pterygium. Br J Ophthalmol 2000;84(2):212–6. Epub 2000/02/03.

126. Tsironi S, Ioachim E, Machera M, et al. Presence and possible significance of immunohistochemically demonstrable metallothionein expression in pterygium versus pinguecula and normal conjunctiva. Eye 2001;15(Pt 1):89–96. Epub 2001/04/25.

127. Ueda Y, Kanazawa S, Kitaoka T, et al. Immunohistochemical study of p53, p21 and PCNA in pterygium. Acta Histochem 2001;103(2):159–65. Epub 2001/05/23.

128. Kase S, Takahashi S, Sato I, et al. Expression of p27(KIP1) and cyclin D1, and cell proliferation in human pterygium. Br J Ophthalmol 2007;91(7):958–61. Epub 2006/12/21.

129. Tan DT, Liu YP, Sun L. Flow cytometry measurements of DNA content in primary and recurrent pterygia. Invest Ophthalmol Vis Sci 2000;41(7):1684–6. Epub 2000/06/14.

130. Chen JK, Tsai RJ, Lin SS. Fibroblasts isolated from human pterygia exhibit transformed cell characteristics. In Vitro Cell Dev Biol Anim 1994;30A(4):243–8. Epub 1994/04/01.

131. Peiretti E, Dessi S, Mulas MF, et al. Fibroblasts isolated from human pterygia exhibit altered lipid metabolism characteristics. Exp Eye Res 2006;83(3):536–42. Epub 2006/05/16.

132. Wong YW, Chew J, Yang H, et al. Expression of insulin-like growth factor binding protein-3 in pterygium tissue. Br J Ophthalmol 2006;90(6):769–72. Epub 2006/02/21.

133. Solomon A, Grueterich M, Li DQ, et al. Overexpression of insulin-like growth factor-binding protein-2 in pterygium body fibroblasts. Invest Ophthalmol Vis Sci 2003;44(2):573–80. Epub 2003/01/31.

134. Shimmura S, Ishioka M, Hanada K, et al. Telomerase activity and p53 expression in pterygia. Invest Ophthalmol Vis Sci 2000;41(6):1364–9. Epub 2000/05/08.

135. Sakoonwatanyoo P, Tan DT, Smith DR. Expression of p63 in pterygium and normal conjunctiva. Cornea 2004;23(1):67–70. Epub 2004/01/01.

136. Dekaris I, Gabric N, Karaman Z, et al. Pterygium treatment with limbal-conjunctival autograft transplantation. Coll Antropol 2001;25(Suppl):7–12. Epub 2002/01/31.

137. Tan D. Conjunctival grafting for ocular surface disease. Curr Opin Ophthalmol 1999;10(4):277–81. Epub 2000/01/06.

138. Kato N, Shimmura S, Kawakita T, et al. Beta-catenin activation and epithelial-mesenchymal transition in the pathogenesis of pterygium. Invest Ophthalmol Vis Sci 2007;48(4):1511–7. Epub 2007/03/29.

139. Kase S, Osaki M, Sato I, et al. Immunolocalisation of E-cadherin and beta-catenin in human pterygium. Br J Ophthalmol 2007;91(9):1209–12. Epub 2007/03/16.

140. Touhami A, Di Pascuale MA, Kawatika T, et al. Characterisation of myofibroblasts in fibrovascular tissues of primary and recurrent pterygia. Br J Ophthalmol 2005;89(3):269–74.

141. Ye J, Song YS, Kang SH, et al. Involvement of bone marrow-derived stem and progenitor cells in the pathogenesis of pterygium. Eye 2004;18(8):839–43. Epub 2004/03/06.

142. Yamagami S, Ebihara N, Usui T, et al. Bone marrow-derived cells in normal human corneal stroma. Arch Ophthalmol 2006;124(1):62–9.

143. Ishii G, Sangai T, Sugiyama K, et al. In vivo characterization of bone marrow-derived fibroblasts recruited into fibrotic lesions. Stem Cells 2005;23(5):699–706.

144. Takahashi T, Kalka C, Masuda H, et al. Ischemia- and cytokine-induced mobilization of bone marrow-derived endothelial progenitor cells for neovascularization. Nat Med 1999;5(4):434–8.

145. Chui J, Di Girolamo N, Coroneo MT, et al. The role of substance P in the pathogenesis of pterygia. Invest Ophthalmol Vis Sci 2007;48(10):4482–9. Epub 2007/09/28.

146. Thoft RA, Friend J. The X, Y, Z hypothesis of corneal epithelial maintenance. Invest Ophthalmol Vis Sci 1983;24(10):1442–3.

147. Muller LJ, Marfurt CF, Kruse F, et al. Corneal nerves: structure, contents and function. Exp Eye Res 2003;76(5):521–42.

148. Benrath J, Eschenfelder C, Zimmerman M, et al. Calcitonin gene-related peptide, substance P and nitric oxide are involved in cutaneous inflammation following ultraviolet irradiation. Eur J Pharmacol 1995;293(1):87–96.

149. van der Zypen F, van der Zypen E, Daicker B. [Ultrastructural studies on the pterygium. II. Connective tissue, vessels and nerves of the conjunctival part (author's transl)]. Albrecht Von Graefes Arch Klin Exp Ophthalmol 1975;193(3):177–87. Epub 1975/01/01. Zur Ultrastruktur des Pterygium. II. Bindegewebe, Gefass- und Nervensystem des konjunktivalen Anteils.

150. Coroneo MT, Rosenberg ML, Cheung LM. Ocular effects of cosmetic products and procedures. Ocul Surf 2006;4(2):94–102. Epub 2006/05/10.

151. Frucht-Pery J, Siganos CS, Solomon A, et al. Topical indomethacin solution versus dexamethasone solution for treatment of inflamed pterygium and pinguecula: a prospective randomized clinical study. Am J Ophthalmol 1999;127(2):148–52. Epub 1999/02/25.

152. Jonisch J, Steiner A, Udell IJ. Preservative-free low-dose dexamethasone for the treatment of chronic ocular surface disease refractory to standard therapy. Cornea 2010;29(7):723–6. Epub 2010/05/22.

153. Utine CA, Stern M, Akpek EK. Clinical review: topical ophthalmic use of cyclosporin A. Ocul Immunol Inflamm 2010;18(5):352–61. Epub 2010/08/26.

154. Schechter BA. Efficacy of topical cyclosporine 0.05% in the prevention of ocular surface inflammation secondary to pterygia. Am Acad Ophthalmol Annual Meeting 2006;Poster #81.

155. Ozulken K, Koc M, Ayar O, et al. Topical cyclosporine A administration after pterygium surgery. Eur J Ophthalmol 2011. Epub 2011/07/05.

156. Turan-Vural E, Torun-Acar B, Kivanc SA, et al. The effect of topical 0.05% cyclosporine on recurrence following pterygium surgery. Clin Ophthalmol 2011;5:881–5. Epub 2011/07/16.

157. Hirst LW. The treatment of pterygium. Surv Ophthalmol 2003;48(2):145–80. Epub 2003/04/11.

158. , Starc S, Knorr M, Steuhl KP, et al. Autologous conjunctiva-limbus transplantation in treatment of primary and recurrent pterygium. Ophthalmologe 1996;93:219–23.

159. Hirst LW. Prospective study of primary pterygium surgery using pterygium extended removal followed by extended conjunctival transplantation. Ophthalmology 2008;115(10):1663–72. Epub 2008/06/17.

160. Hirst LW. Recurrent pterygium surgery using pterygium extended removal followed by extended conjunctival transplant: recurrence rate and cosmesis. Ophthalmology 2009;116(7):1278–86. Epub 2009/07/07.

161. Tagle RB. A new operative technic of conjunctival grafting in the pterygium. Arch Ophthalmol 1947;38(3):409.

162. Kenyon KR, Wagoner MD, Hettinger ME. Conjunctival autograft transplantation for advanced and recurrent pterygium. Ophthalmology 1985;92(11):1461–70. Epub 1985/11/01.

163. Al Fayez MF. Limbal versus conjunctival autograft transplantation for advanced and recurrent pterygium. Ophthalmology 2002;109(9):1752–5. Epub 2002/09/05.

164. Sun TT, Tseng SC, Lavker RM. Location of corneal epithelial stem cells. Nature 2010;463(7284):E10–11; discussion E1. Epub 2010/02/26.

165. Qi H, Zheng X, Yuan X, et al. Potential localization of putative stem/progenitor cells in human bulbar conjunctival epithelium. J Cell Physiol 2010;225(1):180–5. Epub 2010/05/12.

166. Barraquer JI. Etiology, pathogenesis, and treatment of the pterygium. In: Transactions of the New Orleans Academy of Ophthalmology: Symposium on Medical and Surgical Diseases of the Cornea. St. Louis: Mosby; 1980:167–78.

167. Liu J, Fu Y, Xu Y, et al. New grading system to improve the surgical outcome of multirecurrent pterygia. Arch Ophthalmol 2012;130(1):39–49. Epub 2012/01/11.

168. Notara M, Shortt AJ, Galatowicz G, et al. IL6 and the human limbal stem cell niche: a mediator of epithelial–stromal interaction. Stem Cell Res 2010;5(3):188–200. Epub 2010/09/04.

169. Yaisawang S, Piyapattanakorn P. Role of post-operative topical corticosteroids in recurrence rate after pterygium excision with conjunctival autograft. J Med Assoc Thai 2003;86(Suppl 2):S215–23. Epub 2003/08/22.

170. Hirst LW. Mitomycin C in the treatment of pterygium. Clin Exp Ophthalmol 2006;34(3):197–8. Epub 2006/05/05.

171. Troutbeck R, Hirst L. Review of treatment of pterygium in Queensland: 10 years after a primary survey. Clin Exp Ophthalmol 2001;29(5):286–90. Epub 2001/11/27.

172. Assaad NN, Coroneo MT. Conjunctival autograft failure in eyes previously exposed to beta-radiation or mitomycin. Arch Ophthalmol 2008;126(10):1460–1. Epub 2008/10/15.

173. Assaad NN, Chong R, Tat LT, et al. Use of adjuvant hyperbaric oxygen therapy to support limbal conjunctival graft in the management of recurrent pterygium. Cornea 2011;30(1):7–10. Epub 2010/09/18.

174. Green MO, Brannen AL. Hyperbaric oxygen therapy for beta-radiation-induced scleral necrosis. Ophthalmology 1995;102(7):1038–41. Epub 1995/07/01.

175. Ozer A, Yildirim N, Erol N, et al. Long-term results of bare sclera, limbal-conjunctival autograft and amniotic membrane graft techniques in primary pterygium excisions. Ophthalmologica 2009;223(4):269–73. Epub 2009/04/03.

176. Park CY, Choi JS, Lee SJ, et al. Cyclooxygenase-2-expressing macrophages in human pterygium co-express vascular endothelial growth factor. Mol Vis 2011;17:3468–80. Epub 2012/01/06.

177. Detorakis ET, Zaravinos A, Spandidos DA. Growth factor expression in ophthalmic pterygia and normal conjunctiva. Int J Mol Med 2010;25(4):513–6. Epub 2010/03/04.

178. Bahar I, Kaiserman I, McAllum P, et al. Subconjunctival bevacizumab injection for corneal neovascularization in recurrent pterygium. Curr Eye Res 2008;33(1):23–8. Epub 2008/01/25.

179. Shenasi A, Mousavi F, Shoa-Ahari S, et al. Subconjunctival bevacizumab immediately after excision of primary pterygium: the first clinical trial. Cornea 2011;30(11):1219–22. Epub 2011/10/01.

180. Friedlander M. Combination angiostatic therapies: targeting multiple angiogenic pathways. Retina 2009;29(6 Suppl):S27–9. Epub 2009/07/09.

181. Frucht-Pery J, Solomon A, Siganos CS, et al. Treatment of inflamed pterygium and pinguecula with topical indomethacin 0.1% solution. Cornea 1997;16:42–7.

182. Santos CI, Zeiter JH, Speaker MG. Efficacy and safety of topical 1.0% anecortave acetate (AL-3789) as anti-neovascular therapy for recurrent pterygium. Invest Ophthalmol Vis Sci 1999;40(4):S1778.

183. Cox CA, Amaral J, Salloum R, et al. Doxycycline's effect on ocular angiogenesis: an in vivo analysis. Ophthalmology 2010;117(9):1782–91. Epub 2010/07/08.

184. Koranyi G, Seregard S, Kopp ED. The cut-and-paste method for primary pterygium surgery: long-term follow-up. Acta Ophthalmol Scand 2005;83(3):298–301. Epub 2005/06/14.

185. Xu F, Li M, Yan Y, et al. A novel technique of sutureless and glue-less conjunctival autografting in pterygium surgery by electrocautery pen. Cornea 2012;Epub ahead of print 2012/05/15.

186. Wishaw K, Billington D, O'Brien D, et al. The use of orbital morphine for postoperative analgesia in pterygium surgery. Anaesth Intensive Care 2000;28(1):43–5. Epub 2000/03/04.

187. Caccavale A, Romanazzi F, Imparato M, et al. Ropivacaine for topical anesthesia in pterygium surgery with fibrin glue for conjunctival autograft. Cornea 2010;29(4):375–6. Epub 2010/02/19.

188. Young AL, Leung GY, Cheng LL, et al. Randomised controlled trial on the effectiveness of lidocaine gel vs tetracaine drops as the sole topical anaesthetic agent for primary pterygium surgery. Eye (Lond) 2009;23(7):1518–23. Epub 2008/11/08.

189. Arenas E, Garcia S. A scleral soft contact lens designed for the postoperative management of pterygium surgery. Eye Contact Lens 2007;33(1):9–12. Epub 2007/01/17.

190. Di Girolamo N, Chui J, Wakefield D, et al. Cultured human ocular surface epithelium on therapeutic contact lenses. Br J Ophthalmol 2007;91(4):459–64. Epub 2006/09/22.

191. Skippen B, Tsang HH, Assaad NN, et al. Rapid response of refractory ocular surface dysplasia to combination treatment with topical all-trans retinoic acid and interferon alfa-2b. Arch Ophthalmol 2010;128(10):1368–9. Epub 2010/10/13.

192. Krilis M, Tsang H, Coroneo M. Treatment of conjunctival and corneal epithelial neoplasia with retinoic acid and topical interferon

alfa-2b: Long term follow up. Ophthalmology 2012. Epub ahead of print 2012/06/19.

193. Ang LP, Tan DT, Cajucom-Uy H, et al. Autologous cultivated conjunctival transplantation for pterygium surgery. Am J Ophthalmol 2005;139(4):611–9. Epub 2005/04/06.

194. Coroneo MT. Beheading the pterygium. Ophthalmic Surg 1992;23(10):691–2. Epub 1992/10/01.

195. Kuo M. Novel techniques for conjunctival autograft creation. [BSc (Med) Honours Thesis]: University of New South Wales; 2012.

196. Di Girolamo N, Wakefield D, Coroneo MT. Doxycycline's and ocular angiogenesis. Ophthalmology 2011;118(4):789–90; author reply 90-1. Epub 2011/04/05.

197. Kieval JZ, Karp CL, Shousha MA, et al. Ultra-high resolution optical coherence tomography for differentiation of ocular surface squamous neoplasia and pterygia. Ophthalmology 2011. Epub 2011/12/14.

198. Coroneo MT, Coroneo H. Feast your eyes: the eye health cookbook. West Lakes, South Australia: Seaview Press; 2010.

19 *Ocular Surface Neoplasias*

FASIKA A. WORETA and CAROL L. KARP

Introduction

The three most common ocular surface tumors arising from the conjunctiva and cornea can be classified as ocular surface squamous neoplasia, melanocytic tumors, and lymphoid tumors. These lesions have malignant potential and therefore, warrant a high index of suspicion for diagnosis and appropriate management. The clinical features, diagnostic work-up, and management of these lesions will be reviewed in this chapter.

Ocular Surface Squamous Neoplasia

Ocular surface squamous neoplasia (OSSN) is an umbrella term used to describe cancerous epithelial lesions of the cornea and conjunctiva, ranging from dysplasia to carcinoma-in-situ to invasive squamous cell carcinoma.[1] The term conjunctival and corneal epithelial neoplasia (CIN) describes varying degrees of dysplasia confined to the surface epithelium, and when it is full thickness is called carcinoma-in-situ. When invading the basement membrane, the term squamous cell carcinoma applies.

Epidemiology

Ocular surface squamous neoplasia (OSSN) has an estimated incidence in the United States of 0.03 per 100000 persons.[2] Higher incidences have been reported in other parts of the world with more sun exposure, with an estimated incidence of 1.9 per 100000 persons in Australia[3] and 3.5 per 100000 persons in Uganda.[4] It is the most common, non-pigmented ocular surface tumor.[5] OSSN occurs more commonly in middle-aged or elderly individuals. Lee and Hirst reported an average age of occurrence of 56 years, with a range of 4 to 96 years.[3] Patients with xeroderma pigmentosum and human immunodeficiency virus develop OSSN at younger ages.[6,7] It is also more common in fair-skinned individuals and males, with a fivefold higher incidence in Caucasian males.[2]

Etiology

The pathophysiology of OSSN is likely multifactorial and the most important risk factors identified in the literature are discussed later.

SOLAR ULTRAVIOLET RADIATION

Numerous epidemiologic studies have identified ultraviolet B (UV-B) light as a major etiologic factor in the pathogenesis of OSSN.[1,2,8,9] Newton et al. demonstrated a 49% decline in the rate of OSSN for each 10-degree increase in latitude, due to the decrease in solar ultraviolet radiation with increasing latitude.[9]

In a case control study, Lee at al. identified fair skin, pale irises, a propensity to sunburn, and prolonged sun exposure in early life as risk factors for OSSN.[8]

UV-B light is known to cause DNA damage through formation of pyrimidine dimers.[10] Patients with xeroderma pigmentosum, who are more susceptible to the effects of sunlight, due to a defect in DNA repair mechanisms, have increased incidences of OSSN.[6] It has been proposed the effect of UV-B radiation may be due to the overexpression of the p53 tumor suppressor gene.[11]

HUMAN IMMUNODEFICIENCY VIRUS (HIV) INFECTION

The increased frequency of OSSN since the advent of the acquired immunodeficiency syndrome (AIDS) epidemic, strongly suggests the role of the human immunodeficiency virus (HIV) in increasing the risk of developing OSSN.[7,12] In a study in Malawi, 79% of patients diagnosed with OSSN were found to be HIV positive. In HIV patients, OSSN occurs at a younger age and tends to be more aggressive.[12] This emphasizes the importance of testing for HIV in younger patients diagnosed with OSSN, as it may be the first presenting sign of the disease.[7,12]

HUMAN PAPILLOMAVIRUS (HPV) INFECTION

Whereas, the role of HPV in the pathogenesis of cervical cancer has been well established, the role of HPV as an etiologic factor in OSSN remains unclear. Various studies have demonstrated an association between HPV subtypes and OSSN,[13,14] while other studies have failed to show any association.[15,16] Further evidence confusing the etiologic role of HPV includes the presence of unilateral OSSN in patients with bilateral conjunctival HPV DNA, the presence of HPV in normal conjunctival tissue, and the persistence of HPV infection many years after eradication of OSSN.[13,17,18] It is possible HPV may not act alone but may require a cofactor, such as HIV or UV-B light, in order to cause disease.[17,19]

OTHER ETIOLOGIC FACTORS

Other risk factors reported in the literature include heavy smoking and exposure to petroleum derivatives.[20,21] It has also been reported in association with pterygium.[22] Finally, there have been case reports of OSSN in immunosuppressed patients with neoplasia (lymphoma, leukemia) and following organ transplantation.[23]

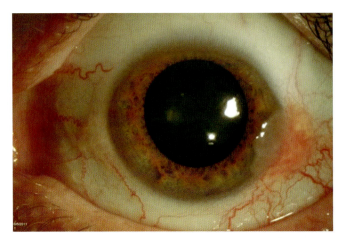

Figure 19.1 Conjunctival epithelail neoplasia (CIN). Classic clinical appearance of CIN, located at the limbus in the interpalpebral zone. Note the gelatinous/papillary appearance.

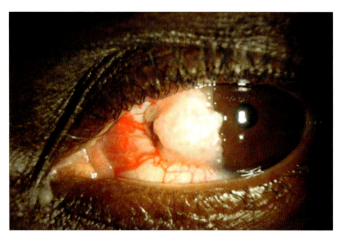

Figure 19.2 Squamous cell carcinoma of the conjunctiva. Note large feeder vessels.

Clinical Features

Ocular surface squamous neoplasia, most commonly presents with foreign body sensation, irritation, redness, or a growth on the ocular surface.[1] Lesions are typically unilateral and slow growing. More than 95% of these lesions occur in the mitotically active limbal region, within the sun-exposed interpalpebral zone.[24,25] More rarely, it can involve the cornea or bulbar conjunctiva alone. It also can occasionally involve the forniceal or palpebral conjunctiva or involve the bulbar conjunctiva or cornea alone. The lesion may be fleshy and markedly elevated, sessile, or minimally elevated.

The classic macroscopic appearance of OSSN is a gelatinous limbal mass with feeder vessels. It can be also have a papilliform appearance with a strawberry-like papillary growth at the limbus or demonstrate leukoplakic changes. (Fig. 19.1).[1,26] Nodular and diffuse are two other appearances that have been described. The nodular form is well circumscribed and rapidly growing, while the diffuse form may mimic a chronic conjunctivitis and has a tendency for metastasis to regional lymph nodes.[1]

Corneal lesions appear as opalescent, gray lesions that have characteristic fimbriated margins and are often associated with small isolated clusters of gray or white tissue. Lesions isolated to the cornea are rare, thought to arise from the limbus and conjunctiva.

It may be difficult to distinguish CIN from squamous cell carcinoma (SCC) based on clinical examination. SCC may be larger and more elevated with a feeder vessel, and adherent to the underlying tissues (Fig. 19.2).[27,28] CIN lesions tend to be freely mobile over the sclera.

Differential Diagnosis

Ocular surface squamous neoplasia is most commonly misdiagnosed as pinguecula, pterygium, actinic keratosis and squamous papilloma, or episcleritis.[29] Hirst et al. found in a histopathologic review of 533 pterygium specimens, 9.8% were found to have evidence of dysplasia.[30] This supports the notion that all excised pterygium specimens should be submitted for pathology at the time of removal. The differential diagnosis includes other benign entities, such as pyogenic granuloma, inflammatory pannus, phlyctenulosis, and pseudoepitheliomatous hyperplasia. Amelanotic melanoma, sebaceous cell carcinoma, and keratoacanthoma can also rarely simulate OSSN.[29,31] Keratoacanthoma can be distinguished by its rapid growth over several months.

Diagnostic Evaluation

DIAGNOSTIC CYTOLOGY

Exfoliative Cytology

Papanicolaou smear cytology is widely accepted as a valuable diagnostic tool in the detection of cervical cancer and has also been described to be useful in the diagnosis of external ocular tumors.[32] A cytobrush or spatula is used to scrape the surface of the suspicious lesion and the cells are sent on a slide to pathology, fixed with 95% alcohol, and stained using a Papanicolaou technique. A major disadvantage is that the superficial nature of the sample may lead to missing the tumor cells. In addition, with this technique, it is not possible to determine the degree of tissue invasion or localize the tumor.[26]

Impression Cytology

Impression cytology is another technique that can be used to obtain cells from the surface of the conjunctival lesion, with its use first described in limbal tumors in 1954.[33] In this technique, a filter paper composed of cellulose acetate, millipore filter paper, or a biopore membrane device, is placed on the ocular surface using gentle pressure and subsequently fixed and stained with the Papanicolaou stain. Nolan and Hirst reported a sensitivity for the diagnosis of OSSN with impression cytology of only 78%.[34] Unlike exfoliative cytology, this method allows for localization of the lesion with preservation of cell-to-cell relationships. Similar to exfoliative cytology, only superficial cells are obtained and thus, the presence of invasion cannot be determined.

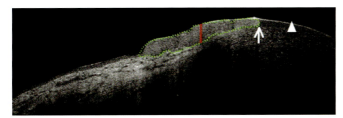

Figure 19.3 UHR-OCT of ocular surface squamous neoplasia. Note hyperreflective thickening of the epithelium (*green dotted lines and red line*) with sudden transition (*arrow*) to normal epithelium (*arrowhead*), characteristic of OSSN.

The advantage of both impression and exfoliative cytology is that they there are relatively simple, painless, and minimally invasive methods, which can be performed in the office after the application of topical anesthesia. They may also be a simple method for the detection of recurrences.[32]

CONFOCAL MICROSCOPY

There have been several reports of in vivo confocal microscopy as a useful tool in the diagnosis of OSSN.[35,36] Confocal microscopy allows for real-time, noninvasive imaging at the cellular level by optical microscopic sectioning of the ocular surface. Malandrini and colleagues described a case of CIN, with a clear distinction between the healthy and pathological epithelium on confocal microscopy. The epithelial cells near the lesion were larger in size, more irregularly shaped, and demonstrated brighter nuclei.[35]

ULTRA-HIGH RESOLUTION OPTICAL COHERENCE TOMOGRAPHY

More recently, ultra-high resolution optical coherence tomography (UHR- OCT) has been described as a noninvasive diagnostic tool to evaluate ocular surface lesions. This technology allows for morphologic visualization of the corneal architecture, with an axial resolution of 2–3 μm. Kieval et al. found that UHR-OCT of pterygia and OSSN lesions demonstrated a high degree of correlation to histopathological specimens.[37] The UHR-OCT of OSSN showed thickened epithelium with an abrupt transition from normal to neoplastic tissue (Fig. 19.3). UHR-OCT of pterygia demonstrated a normal thin epithelium, with thickening of the underlying subepithelial mucosal layers. The sensitivity and specificity for differentiating between OSSN and pterygia using UHR-OCT with an epithelial thickness cutoff of 142 μm was 94% and 100%, respectively.[37]

BIOPSY

Histopathologic diagnosis, either by incisional or excisional biopsy, is the only definitive method for the diagnosis of OSSN.

Pathology

Pre-invasive OSSN lesions are classified as mild, moderate, or severe, based on the extent of replacement of the

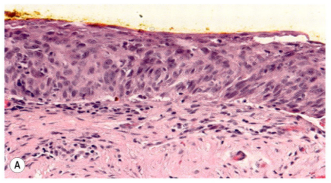

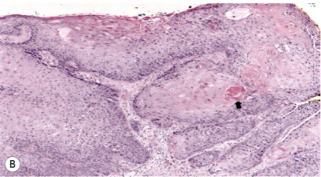

Figure 19.4 (**A**) Conjunctival intraepithelial neoplasia. Hematoxylin and eosin stain, 400× magnification. The conjunctival epithelium displays disordered maturation with loss of polarity. The abnormal cells demonstrate cellular atypia, and mitotic figures. Note hyperkeratosis (thickening of keratin layer) and parakeratosis (retention of nuclei). (**B**) Squamous cell carcinoma of the conjunctiva. Hematoxylin and eosin stain, 100× magnification. The conjunctival epithelium displays full-thickness disordered maturation, with invasion of cells into the underlying substantia propria. Foci of dyskeratosis and keratin pearl formation are present (*arrow*). (Courtesy of S. Dubovy, M.D., Bascom Palmer Eye Institute.)

epithelium by dysplastic cells that lack normal maturation (Fig. 19.4A). The cells are usually long and elongated. Mild dysplasia (CIN grade I) is when the dysplasia is confined to the lower one-third of the epithelium. In moderate dysplasia (CIN grade II), the abnormal cells extend to the middle third of the epithelium. Severe dysplasia (CIN grade III) involves the full-thickness epithelium with total loss of the normal cellular polarity and is also known as CIS. The epithelial basement membrane is intact.

In invasive SCCA, the dysplastic cells invade the basement membrane of the epithelium into the substantia propria of the conjunctiva. When the cornea is involved, the lesions do not invade Bowman's layer unless it has been previously disrupted by ocular surgery.

Most conjunctival SCCA's are well differentiated, demonstrating individually keratinzed cells (dyskeratosis) and concentric collections of keratinized cells (horn cells). Well-differentiated tumors demonstrate varying degrees of cellular pleomorphism with hyperchromatic nuclei, prominent nucleoli and the presence of mitotic figures. Hyperparakeratosis and parakeratoses are also present (Fig. 19.4B).[26,27]

Histopathologic variants with more aggressive behavior are spindle cell carcinoma, mucoepidermoid carcinoma, and adenoid squamous cell carcinoma.[26]

Treatment

SURGICAL EXCISION WITH CRYOTHERAPY

Surgical excision, alone or in combination with medical therapy, is the most established treatment for OSSN. With surgical excision alone, the rate of recurrence is high, ranging from 5% to 33% with negative margins and up to 56% with positive surgical margins.[26] A 'no touch' technique, in which touching the tumor with any instruments is avoided, reduces the risk of tumor seeding.[38] Wide margins of 4–6 mm should be obtained. If the lesion extends into the sclera or cornea, a superficial keratectomy or partial-thickness sclerectomy may be needed.

Absolute alcohol epitheliectomy of the involved cornea is also recommended.

To delineate the margins of the lesion, rose bengal staining or UHR-OCT can be used. However, there is evidence that the microscopic signs of OSSN may extend beyond the macroscopic border the tumor,[17] and many surgeons prefer adjuvant cryotherapy to the limbus and conjunctival margins at the time of excision.

Cryotherapy is thought to work initially by its thermal effect and also by obliteration of the microcirculation, resulting in ischemic infarction and a double freeze–slow thaw technique is recommended.[1] The rates of recurrence with excision and cryotherapy have been reported to be lower than with excision alone, at about 12%.[19,39] Excess cryotherapy should be avoided, since side effects include iritis, abnormal intraocular pressure, sector iris atrophy, hyphema, ablation of the peripheral retina, corneal neovascularization, and limbal stem cell deficiency.[1,19]

Since wide excisions are recommended, surgical excision often results in large defects, necessitating the use of a conjunctival autograft, an oral mucosal graft, or an amniotic membrane transplant. A number of studies have described successful reconstruction of the ocular surface with preserved amniotic membrane after excision of CIN, SCC, primary acquired melanosis, and melanoma.[40,41] Amniotic membrane is a helpful technique, since defects of any size can be closed, and the membrane has additional properties of promoting epithelialization, and reducing neovascularization, scarring and fibrosis.[40] In addition, the use of fibrin glue, instead of sutures to secure the membrane reduces inflammation.[42] The use of a conjunctival autograft of adequate size from either the same or opposite eye is an option. Care needs to be taken to avoid large areas of stem cell removal, which may lead to scarring, symblepharon, and limbal stem cell deficiency. Thick buccal or labial grafts are generally reserved for cases with extensive symblephara and might potentially interfere with the ability to observe for recurrence of the underlying tumor.[40]

In summary, the preferred technique for OSSN removal involves excision of the tumor with wide margins, absolute alcohol epitheliectomy of the involved cornea, cryotherapy using a double freeze–slow thaw cycle to the limbus and conjunctival margins, and amniotic membrane transplantation (Fig. 19.5).

TOPICAL CHEMOTHERAPY

Due to high recurrence rates of OSSN, medical therapies have been increasingly used. Mitomycin-C (MMC),

5-fluorouracil (5-FU) and interferon α-2b (IFN-α-2b) are useful in the treatment of the OSSN.

A potential advantage of medical therapy is the ability to treat the entire ocular surface, theoretically treating microscopic and subclinical disease. It is useful as primary treatment in patients who are not surgical candidates and for patients with recurrent, annular, or diffuse disease. In addition to its role in the primary treatment of OSSN, it can also be used as an adjunct to surgery, providing chemo-reduction prior to excision. Postoperatively, it is indicated when there are positive margins after excision and when there is tumor recurrence.

ANTIMETABOLITES

MMC is an alkylating agent that inhibits DNA synthesis by the production of free radicals. It is used as a topical drop at concentration of 0.02% or 0.04% four times daily for 7 to 14 days in cycles. One week is allowed between cycles to minimize ocular toxicity. Excellent responses raging from 87.5% to 100% have been reported.[43,44] Side effects include conjunctival hyperemia, blepharospasm, corneal punctate erosions, punctal stenosis, and limbal stem cell deficiency.[44] Punctal plugs should be used to prevent punctal stenosis. Refrigeration is required and at our institution (Bascom Palmer Eye Institute) the cost is about US$225 per bottle.

5-FU is a pyrimidine analogue that inhibits the incorporation of thymidine into DNA, during the S-phase of the cell cycle. It is prescribed as a 1% topical solution applied four times daily for 4 to 7 days, with 30–35 days off for a total of two to five cycles.[45] It has also been used for 4 weeks continuously.[46] 5-FU may lead to ocular surface irritation and thus, 4 to 7 days a month dosing is preferred by the authors. Unlike MMC, it does not require refrigeration and is less costly (about US$75 per bottle).

INTERFERON α-2B

Interferon α is a family of proteins, secreted by leukocytes, with antiviral and antineoplastic properties. It has been used in the treatment of many cancers, including cervical intraepithelial neoplasia,[47] cutaneous squamous cell carcinoma,[48] and renal cell carcinoma.[49] It has also been used to treat viral lesions, including hepatitis B and C, and condyloma acuminata.[50] INF α-2b is a recombinant protein that has been used in the treatment of OSSN with success rates of above 80%.[51,52] It can be given as topical eye drops or a subconjunctival injection, and a combination of both may be used.

Topical INF α-2b is much better tolerated than MMC and 5-FU. Interferon drops are very gentle and well tolerated. Reported side effects include mild conjunctival hyperemia and follicular conjunctivitis.[53] Topical INF α-2b (1 million IU/mL) is dosed four times daily and given continuously until the tumor resolves. It is not cycled like MMC and 5-FU and the cost is about US$225 per month for the eye drops. On average, the time on the medication is 3 months. Figure 19.6 demonstrates the case of a 54-year-old male with OSSN, which resolved after 12 weeks of treatment with topical INF α-2b.

Interferon can also be given as subconjunctival injections. These may be given once to thrice weekly. Side

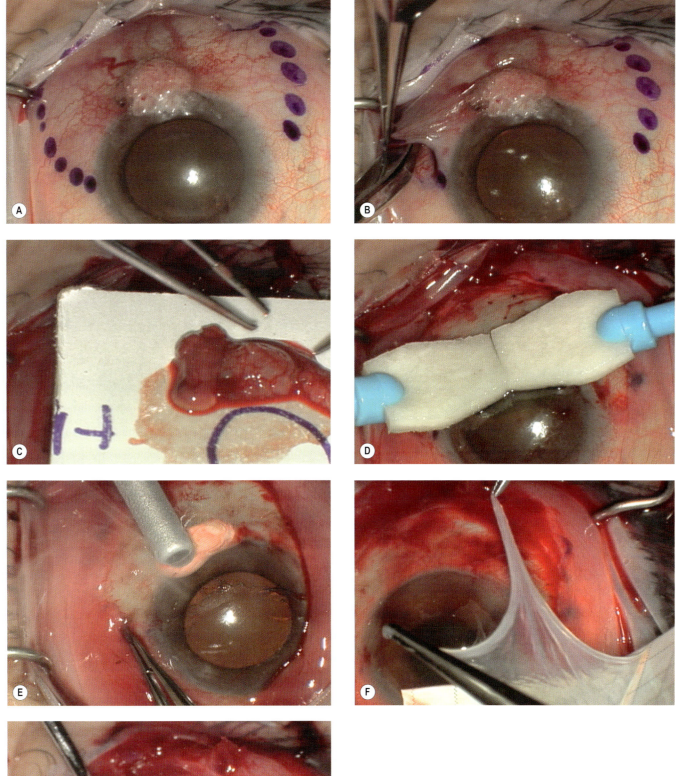

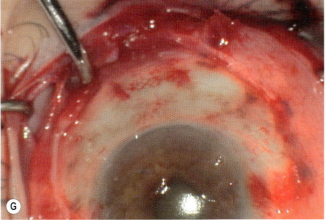

Figure 19.5 Surgical technique for excision of ocular surface squamous neoplasia, cryotherapy, and amniotic membrane transplant. (**A**) Tumor outlined in marking pen with 4–6 mm margins. (**B**) Conjunctival tumor being excised using Westcott scissors using a 'no touch' technique. (**C**) Tumor placed in proper orientation on marked cardboard. (**D**) Absolute dehydrated alcohol applied to corneal surface for 60 seconds. (**E**) Application of cryotherapy to limbus and conjunctival margins. (**F**) Amniotic membrane placed and glued over defect with stromal side down. (**G**) Final appearance after amniotic membrane glued in place.

effects of subconjunctival delivery include fever, chills, headache, myalgias, and arthralgias, which may last a few hours after the injection. Acetaminophen at a dose of 1000 milligrams every 6 hours is helpful. The time to tumor resolution is generally faster with subconjunctival injections (average 1.4 months), as compared to resolution topical INF α-2b drops (average 2.8 months).[51,52] The sub-conjunctival dose is 0.5 mL (3 million IU/0.5 mL solution) repeated one to three times a week until clinical resolution occurs.

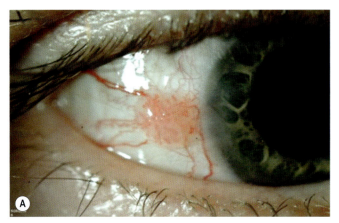

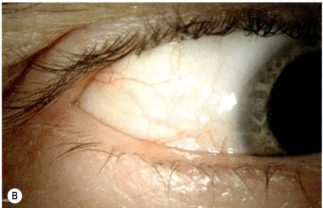

Figure 19.6 (**A**) Clinical appearance of ocular surface neoplasia before treatment. (**B**) After treatment with topical interferon α-2b drops four times daily for 12 weeks, complete resolution was achieved.

A comparison of MMC, 5-FU, and INF-α-2b are summarized in Table 19.1.

Prognosis

Ocular surface squamous neoplasia is considered a low-grade malignancy with a good prognosis, as the tumor is generally slow growing. Local recurrences are common, with most occurring within the first 2 years.[1] Intraocular invasion and metastasis are extremely rare. Intraocular invasion is thought to occur by tumor cells entering the eye at the limbus and invading the trabecular meshwork, anterior chamber, ciliary body, iris and choroid.[54] Sites of metastasis include the parotid gland, submandibular and submaxillary glands, preauricular, cervical lymph nodes, lungs, and bone and are related to a delay in management.[55]

Melanoctyic Tumors

Conjunctival melanoma is a tumor that arises from the melanocytes in the basal layer of the conjunctival epithelium. Other melanocytic lesions of the ocular surface include conjunctival nevi, racial melanosis, ocular melanocytosis, and primary acquired melanosis. Clinical features of each are summarized in Table 19.2.

CONJUNCTIVAL NEVUS

A conjunctival nevus is a pigmented or nonpigmented mass, which is mobile, circumscribed, and elevated. It is the most common conjunctival tumor, accounting for 28% of all conjunctival tumors and 52% of those classified as melanocytic tumors.[5] Nevi usually present in childhood or early adolescence, most commonly located in the bulbar conjunctiva, caruncle, or plica semiluminaris. Intralesional cysts are commonly visible at the slit lamp (Fig. 19.7). Growth may occur with hormonal changes, such as during puberty or pregnancy, but otherwise the lesion size remains stable. In a study of 410 patients with conjunctival nevi, 1% showed evolution into melanoma over an interval of 7 years.[56]

Table 19.1   Comparison of Mitomycin C (MMC), 5-Fluoruracil (5-FU), and Interferon α-2b (INF α-2b) for Use in Treatment of Ocular Surface Squamous Neoplasia

	MMC	5-FU	INF α-2b	INF α-2b
Formulation	Topical drops	Topical drops	Topical drops	Intralesional injection
Compounding required	Yes	Yes	Yes	No
Dose	0.02% or 0.04%	1%	1 million IU/mL	3 million IU/0.5 mL
Cost	≈US$225/cycle	≈US $75/cycle	≈US $225/month	Covered by insurance (~US $89)
Refrigeration	Yes	No	Yes	Yes
Expiration time	14 days	10 days	30 days	N/A
Side effects	Significant hyperemia Pain Punctal stenosis Corneal toxicity Possible limbal stem cell deficiency	Moderate hyperemia Pain Punctal stenosis	Mild hyperemia Mild follicular conjunctivitis	Transient fevers, chills, headache, myalgias

Table 19.2   A comparison of Ocular Surface Melanocytic Lesions

Melanocytic Lesion	Time of Onset	Clinical Features	Natural History	Malignant Potential
Nevus	Youth	Well-circumscribed, mobile, focal lesion, appearance of cysts within lesion	May enlarge with puberty or pregnancy, otherwise stable	1% risk of conjunctival melanoma
Racial melanosis	Middle age	Flat, diffuse, non-circumscribed lesion Bilateral Occurs in darkly pigmented individuals	May gradually increase in size and pigment over time	None
Ocular melanocytosis	Congenital	Flat, gray-brown pigmentation of episclera	Stable in appearance	1:400 lifetime risk of uveal melanoma
Primary acquired melanosis	Middle age	Flat, diffuse, patchy lesion with nonhomogeneous pigmentation Unilateral Occurs in patients with fair complexion	May wax and wane in pigmentation and growth pattern	0% if no or mild atypia 13–46% risk of conjunctival melanoma with severe atypia
Melanoma	Middle to old age	Elevated brown or non-pigmented lesion, immobile, feeder vessels may be present	Demonstrates growth	Overall mortality 25%

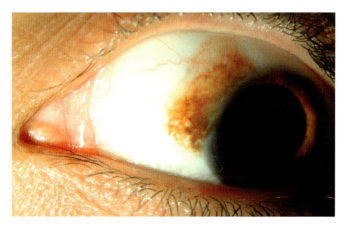

Figure 19.7 Conjunctival nevus. Note slight elevation with subtle cysts present within the lesion.

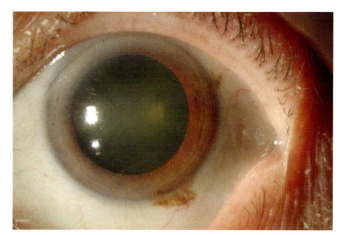

Figure 19.8 Primary acquired melanosis (PAM) in a Caucasian patient. Note two areas of PAM at the limbus.

PRIMARY ACQUIRED MELANOSIS

Conjunctival primary acquired melanosis (PAM) accounts for 11% of all conjunctival tumors and 21% of melanocytic lesions.[5] It presents as a unilateral, patchy area of conjunctival pigmentation in middle-aged or elderly adults with fair skin (Fig. 19.8). The pigmentation can wax or wane over time.[28] PAM with atypia can only be distinguished from PAM without atypia by histologic examination. In a study of 311 eyes with PAM, lesions without atypia or mild atypia showed 0% progression to melanoma and lesions with severe atypia showed progression to melanoma in 13%.[57] In addition, those with a greater extent of PAM in clock hours had a greater risk for transformation into melanoma. In the Armed Formed Institute of Pathology series of 41 patients with PAM, progression to melanoma occurred in 0% with PAM without atypia and in 46% if the PAM showed microscopic evidence of atypia.[58]

MELANOMA

Epidemiology

Conjunctival melanoma is a rare tumor, accounting for 2–5% of ocular melanomas.[59] It accounts for 13% of all conjunctival tumors and 25% of all melanocytic tumors.[5]

The estimated incidence in the United States is 0.5 per million.[60] There is evidence that the incidence of conjunctival melanoma has been increasing in the United States, Sweden, and Finland.[61–63] Based on data from the Surveillance, Epidemiology, and End Results (SEER) study by the National Cancer Institute, the incidence of conjunctival melanoma has increased from 0.22 cases per million, per year in 1973–1979, to 0.46 in 1990–1999.[62] This increase was most notable in white men.

Conjunctival melanoma is more common in middle-aged and elderly people, with the majority of patients between 40 and 70 years of age.[59] It has been reported rarely in children, with age 10 being the youngest age of diagnosis.[59,64] It is also uncommon in non-white populations. In a series of 382 patients with conjunctival melanoma, 94% patients were white, 3% were black, and 3% were Hispanic or Asian.[64]

Etiology

Unlike cutaneous melanoma, there is no clear evidence regarding the association of UV exposure and conjunctival melanoma. A study in Sweden demonstrated an increase in the incidence of conjunctival melanoma in sun-exposed

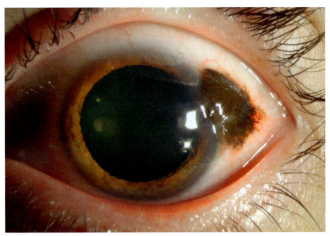

Figure 19.9 Conjunctival melanoma arising from primary acquired melanosis.

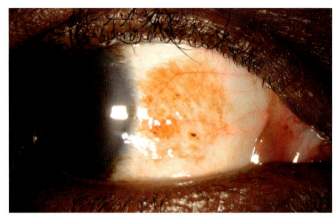

Figure 19.10 Racial melanosis. Note darkly pigmented skin of the patient, characteristic conjunctival folds as the limbus and pigmentation on the nasal conjunctiva of the right eye. Symmetric pigmentation was present in the left eye.

areas (bulbar, limbal and caruncular conjunctiva) over time, while the incidence in non-sun-exposed areas (tarsal and forniceal conjunctiva) remained constant.[61] Conjunctival melanoma can arise from a conjunctival nevus (7%), primary acquired melanosis (74%), or de novo (19%).[64]

Clinical Features

The clinical appearance of conjunctival melanoma is variable. It generally occurs as a brown to tan elevated lesion that is relatively immobile (Fig. 19.9). Prominent feeder vessels might be present. As the lesion frequently arises from PAM, surrounding flat PAM might be present. The most frequently involved locations are the bulbar conjunctiva and limbus. Less commonly, the fornix, palpebral conjunctiva, and caruncle may be involved.[64] The majority of melanomas are pigmented (59%), but up to 20% are non-pigmented (amelanotic) and 21% are mixed.[64] The cornea may be involved by growth of the tumor cells from the limbus, but the tumor cells generally do not penetrate Bowman's layer.

Differential Diagnosis

The differential diagnosis of conjunctival melanoma includes other pigmented lesions, such as nevi, racial melanosis, ocular melanocytosis, and PAM. Nevi rarely present in the palpebral conjunctiva or fornix and thus, any lesions presenting in these area should be removed. Unlike PAM, racial melanosis occurs in darkly pigmented individuals and is bilateral. The pigmentation is usually around the limbus, often for 360 degrees (Fig. 19.10). Ocular melanocytosis is a congenital pigmentation of the sclera and periocular skin that can be mistaken for primary acquired melanosis. However, the gray-brown pigment is located beneath the conjunctival tissue. Patients with this condition have a 1:400 risk of developing uveal melanoma in their lifetime.[65]

Epithelial lesions, such as squamous papilloma and OSSN, can acquire pigment in darkly pigmented individuals

and resemble melanoma.[66] Rarely, there can be extraocular extension from a ciliary body melanoma or melanocytoma to the epibulbar surface.[67] Metastatic cutaneous melanoma to the conjunctiva has also been reported.[68] Other lesions in the differential include staphylomas, hematic cysts, foreign bodies, blue nevus, subconjunctival hematomas, ochronosis deposits in patients with alkaptonuria and adrenochrome pigment in the inferior fornix in patients previously on epinephrine eyedrops.[69,70]

Diagnostic Work-Up

Any pigmented lesion presenting in adulthood demonstrating growth or change in pattern of pigmentation or vascularity should undergo excisional biopsy.[59] Slit lamp clinical photos are helpful in monitoring for any changes.

Definitive diagnosis of conjunctival melanoma can only be made with surgical excision histopathology. Incisional biopsy should not be performed on a suspected conjunctival melanoma, as it has been associated with increased risk of tumor recurrence, likely due to seeding of cells.[71] Ultrasound biomicroscopy can be useful in detecting the presence of intraocular invasion and in measuring tumor dimensions.[72] Anterior segment OCT can detect intralesional cysts in conjunctival nevi.[73]

All patients with melanoma should be referred to an oncologist for a complete systemic work-up. Magnetic resonance imaging of the brain and orbits is important in cases of suspected orbital extension and to rule out brain metastasis.[74] Sentinel lymph node biopsy to detect micrometastatic disease, is currently being investigated, but long-term survival benefit of this has not yet been established. Some advocate the use of sentinel lymph node biopsy when the risk of metastasis is high, such as with non-limbal tumors and with a tumor thickness greater than 2 mm.[75]

Pathology

Conjunctival melanoma is composed of malignant melanocytic cells with nuclear atypia, prominent nucleoli, and abundant cytoplasm. Jakobiec and colleagues described four types of atypical melanocytes found in conjunctival melanomas: small polyhedral cells; large, round epithelioid cells with eosinophilic cytoplasm; spindle cells; and balloon cells.[27,76] The abnormal cells initially begin in the basal area of the epithelium, but then invade the stroma where they gain access to conjunctival lymphatic vessels.[27] There may be microscopic evidence of a pre-existing nevus or PAM.

PAM without atypia is defined as increased pigmentation of the conjunctival epithelium, with or without an increase in the melanocytes. The melanocytes are confined to the basal layer of the epithelium and do not show any cytologic atypia. In PAM with mild atypia, the melanocytes show cellular atypia but are still confined to the basal layer of the epithelium. PAM with severe atypia is defined by the presence of epithelioid cells and/or extension of the atypical melanocytes into the more superficial layers of the epithelium (pagetoid spread) (Fig. 19.11).[77]

Histopathologic features predictive of worse prognosis include pagetoid spread, the presence of epithelioid cells, histologic evidence of lymphatic invasion, and high numbers of mitotic figures.[58,59,70] As demonstrated with cutaneous melanomas, depth of invasion is a major prognostic factor. Immunohistochemical markers, such as S100, Melan A, or HMB-45, can be used to aid in the diagnosis.[78]

Treatment

The primary treatment for conjunctival melanoma is surgical excision, with wide margins (4–6 m), using a 'no touch'

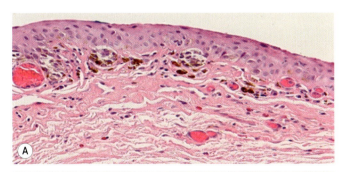

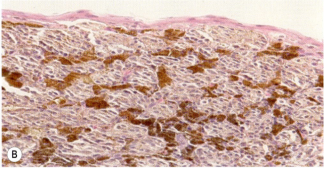

Figure 19.11 (**A**) Primary acquired melanosis with atypia. Hematoxylin and eosin stain, 400× magnification. Note the basilar layer of the conjunctival epithelium is pigmented. There are atypical melanocytes present within the epithelium, but there is no invasion of the basement membrane. (**B**) Conjunctival melanoma. Note invasion of atypical melanocytes into the substantia propria (hematoxylin and eosin, 400×). (Courtesy of S. Dubovy, M.D., Bascom Palmer Eye Institute.)

technique, a partial sclerectomy if the tumor is adherent to the sclera, absolute alcohol epitheliectomy of the involved cornea, and cryotherapy using a double freeze–slow thaw cycle to the limbus and conjunctival margins. Excision with cryotherapy versus excision alone has been shown to reduce local recurrence rate from 68% to 18%.[79] To avoid seeding of tumor cells, it is critical to use fresh instruments after tumor removal. The resulting defect can be closed with amniotic membrane transplantation. Lesions that extend into the globe require enucleation and lesions that extend in the orbit may require exenteration.

Small areas of PAM limited to 1–2 clock hours with bulbar or limbal location can be observed. Biopsy-proven PAM without atypia also can be observed with serial slit lamp examination with clinical photos. Map biopsies are preferred for extensive areas of PAM occupying more than 4–6 clock hours. If atypia is found on histology, medium-sized PAM lesions should be removed surgically using the 'no touch' technique with cryotherapy. For more extensive PAM lesions involving large areas of the limbus or diffusely, involving the palpebral conjunctiva, cryotherapy using a double freeze–slow thaw technique should be used to treat the inexciseable pigment.

Diffuse, multifocal, or recurrent conjunctival melanomas may be more difficult to treat with surgical excision. In these cases, topical chemotherapy using MMC or IFN-α-2b can be used. The majority of the data available is with MMC.[80] There are few studies on the use of IFN,[81,82] and further studies are needed. For PAM with atypia, topical MMC has similar recurrence rates as reported following local excision and cryotherapy.[83]

Metastatic disease to the regional lymph nodes may be treated with lymph node dissection and adjuvant therapy in the form of radiation or chemotherapy. Disseminated conjunctival melanoma is treated with systemic chemotherapy combined with interferon.[59] Figure 19.12 summarizes the algorithm for the management of pigmented lesions of the conjunctiva.

Prognosis

Local recurrence is common after surgery, with recurrence rates estimated to be as high as 43% to 50% at 10 years.[71,84] Any recurrence of tumor, whether pigmented or not, should be surgically excised and treated with cryotherapy. Shields and colleagues found that regional or distant tumor metastasis was present in 16% of patients at 5 years, 26% at 10 years, and 32% at 15 years.[71] The most common regional lymph nodes to be involved are the preauricular, submandibular, and deeper cervical lymph nodes. The most common sites of distant metastasis are the brain, liver, and lungs. The 10-year mortality rate has been reported to range from 13% to 30%.[71,85] Unfavorable prognosis is associated with non-limbal tumors, the presence of positive tumor margins on pathology, and de novo melanoma.[64] Shields and colleagues found that the 10-year mortality rate of tumors with de novo origin (35%) was four times greater than the mortality rate of those with melanoma arising from nevus or PAM (9%).[64]

Due to the high rate of metastases, patients should be monitored regularly for metastatic disease. Physical

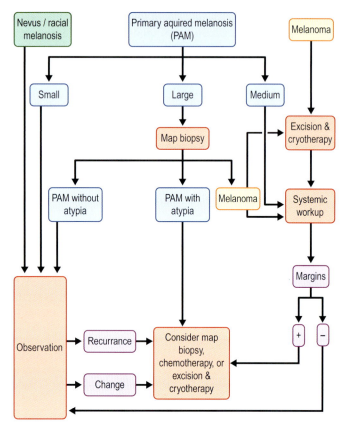

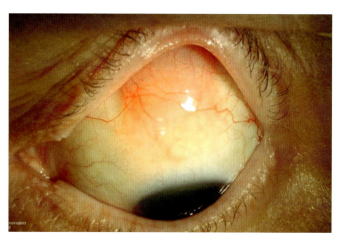

Figure 19.13 Conjunctival lymphoma. Note the salmon-colored, elevated lesion in the superior bulbar conjunctiva, hidden underneath the lid.

Figure 19.12 Algorithm for the management of pigmented lesions of the conjunctiva. (Source: Oellers P, Karp C. Diagnosis and management of pigmented lesions of the conjunctiva. Techniques in Ophthalmology 2011;9:57–62.)

examination should include palpation of the lymph nodes of the head and neck. An annual chest X-ray and brain MRI are advised.[74]

CONJUNCTIVAL LYMPHOMA

Epidemiology

Conjunctival lymphomas are the third most common conjunctival malignancy after melanoma, accounting for 1.5% of all conjunctival tumors.[86] Ocular adnexal lymphoma is most common in the orbit (64%), followed by the conjunctiva (28%), and the eyelids (8%).[87] It accounts for 2% of all cases of non-Hodgkin's lymphoma (NHL) and 8% of all cases of NHL at extranodal sites.[88] The average age of presentation for conjunctival lymphoma is in the sixth decade of life.[89] Bilateral presentation occurs 20% to 38% of the time and systemic involvement is present in 20% to 31% of cases.[90] The majority of ocular adnexal lymphomas are mucosa-associated lymphoid tissue (MALT) lymphomas, a subtype of extranodal marginal zone lymphomas.

Etiology

The normal conjunctiva has a submucosal reservoir of lymphoid tissue. MALT lymphoma is thought to arise as a result of chronic antigen stimulation of this tissue, due to persistent infection or inflammation. The potential infectious association with conjunctival lymphoma is intriguing. Several organisms have been implicated, including *Helicobacter pylori* (*H. pylori*), *Chlamydia psittaci* (*C. psittaci*), hepatitis C, and human T-cell lymphotrophic virus.

The association between gastric MALT lymphoma and *H. pylori* infection has been well established. Recently, *H. pylori* has been detected in conjunctival MALT lymphomas as well.[91] Although this relationship is not yet well established, further investigation is warranted.

An association between the intracellular bacterium *C. psittaci* and ocular adnexal lymphoma has also been reported.[92,93] This has led to a strong interest in the use of doxycycline in treating ocular adnexal lymphomas, which has been demonstrated with some success.[93] Other studies have demonstrated no association with *C. psittaci*[94] or a variable association in different geographic areas.[92]

Clinical Features

Conjunctival lymphoma can present in one of two ways. Most commonly, it presents as a diffuse, slightly elevated, pink, fleshy mass with the classic description of 'salmon patch' (Fig. 19.13). It is most commonly located in the forniceal or midbulbar conjunctiva, hidden under the eyelid in the superior and inferior quadrants.[90] It is usually painless with an insidious onset. Less commonly, conjunctival lymphoma presents as a chronic follicular conjunctivitis.

Differential Diagnosis

Benign lymphoid hyperplasia cannot be differentiated from lymphoma on clinical appearance alone and therefore, biopsy should be performed. The differential diagnosis includes nodular scleritis, chronic conjunctivitis, ectopic lacrimal gland, lipoma, herniated orbital fat, amyloid deposition, benign ocular tumors, such as squamous papilloma and lymphangiectasis, and malignant ocular tumors, such as OSSN and amelantoic melanoma.

Diagnostic Work-Up

The diagnosis of suspected conjunctival lymphoma should be confirmed by biopsy. Two biopsies should be taken for evaluation. One sample is placed in formalin and evaluated using light microscopy with the standard hematoxylin and eosin stain. The other sample must be fresh tissue to perform immunohistochemistry, flow cytometry, and molecular genetic analysis.

All patients with a positive biopsy should be referred to an oncologist for a systemic work-up, including a complete blood cell count with differential, imaging of the chest and abdomen, and possibly bone marrow biopsy.

Pathology

Lymphoid tumors are composed of solid sheets of lymphocytes and may be classified as benign reactive hyperplasia, atypical lymphoid hyperplasia, or malignant lymphoma.[27,90] The vast majority of conjunctival lymphomas are non-Hodgkin's B-cell tumors. Two-thirds of tumors are the MALT/EBZL subtype.[95] Other histologic subtypes include follicular cell, lymphoplasmacytic, mantle cell, and diffuse large B-cell lymphoma. MALT, follicular cell, and lymphoplasmacytic lymphomas are low-grade tumors with an indolent course, while mantle cell and diffuse large B-cell lymphomas are considered high-grade tumors with an aggressive course.[96]

Under light microscopy, MALT lymphoma demonstrates a diffuse cellular infiltrate composed of small round lymphocytes, atypical lymphocytes with cleaved nuclei, monocytoid cells, and plasma cells (Fig. 19.14). Neoplastic cells expand the margin zone and may proliferate within germinal centers, creating numerous poorly formed secondary

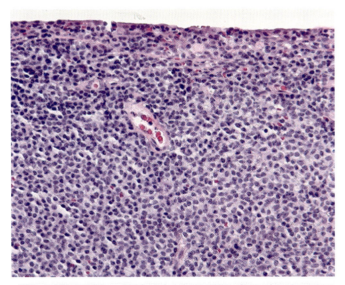

Figure 19.14 Conjunctival lymphoma. Hematoxylin and eosin stain, 400× magnification. Pathology demonstrates sheets of monotonous-appearing, small, round lymphocytes. Note bland nuclei and no mitotic figures (low-grade characteristics). Immunohistochemistry and flow cytometry confirmed the diagnosis of mucosa-associated lymphoid tissue (MALT) lymphoma. (Courtesy of S. Dubovy, M.D., Bascom Palmer Eye Institute.)

follicles.[97] Follicular cell lymphoma demonstrates well-formed follicles with a germinal center arrangement.

Immunophenotypic analysis and flow cytometry can provide information regarding cell population type by identifying markers, such as the CD20 antigen on B cells. Molecular genetic analysis can be useful in identifying overexpression of heavy rearrangements, as well as translocations specific to tumor types.[96] The genetic analysis is critical for differentiating a monoclonal versus benign polyclonal population.

Treatment

When localized to the conjunctiva, the standard of treatment is external beam radiation. Radiotherapy has been proven to be effective for all different subtypes of conjunctival lymphoma, with local control rates ranging from 91% to 100%.[89] Recommended radiation doses are approximately 30–40 Gy, with the dosage based on tumor grade or type.[98] The major adverse effects of radiation include dry eye, conjunctivitis, cataract, and radiation retinopathy.

Surgical excision with cryotherapy for localized disease can be considered when lesions are small and circumscribed.[90] Intralesional injections of interferon α-2b have been reported with success.[99] In a recent interventional pilot study of three patients with relapsed conjunctival lymphoma, Ferreri and colleagues demonstrated disease remission after intralesional rituximab injections for localized disease.[100]

When systemic involvement is present, first-line treatment is typically rituximab alone or in combination with chemotherapy. Rituximab is a recombinant mouse/human chimeric anti-CD20 antibody, that is being investigated as a first-line treatment of CD20-positive lymphomas with systemic involvement. By binding the CD20 antigen on B cells, rituximab triggers apoptosis and antibody-mediated cytotoxicity. Salepci et al. reported a case of bilateral conjunctival MALT lymphoma, which relapsed after radiation treatment. Remission was achieved with six weekly cycles on intravenous rituximab.[101] Ferreri and colleagues demonstrated lymphoma regression in five patients with newly diagnosed ocular adnexal MALT lymphoma treated with intravenous rituximab as a single agent. However, four of five patients demonstrated relapse at a median time of 5 months, suggesting a lower efficacy than reported for gastric MALT lymphoma.[102]

Rituximab in combination with chemotherapy may achieve greater success. In a study of nine patients with newly diagnosed ocular adnexal lymphomas, first-line therapy with rituximab and chlorambucil achieved complete remission in 89% of patients, with a median follow-up of 2 years.[103] The International Extranodal Lymphoma Study Group is currently conducting a multicenter trial to determine whether the addition of rituximab to chlorambucil will improve the outcome of MALT lymphoma in comparison to treatment with chlorambucil or rituximab alone.[104]

Another agent being investigated in the treatment of systemic lymphomas is ibritumomab tiuxetan (trade name Zevalin™). Zevalin is a combination of a mouse Ig1 monoclonal antibody with the chelator tiuxetan, to which the radioactive isotope yttrium-90 is added. It binds to the C20 antigen of B cells and the radiation from the isotope kills cells. Zevalin was FDA approved in 2002, to treat patients with relapsed or refractory, low-grade or follicular non-Hodgkin's lymphoma. In a pilot study of 12 patients with ocular adnexal lymphoma, treated with rituximab followed by Zevalin, 83% of patients achieved a complete response, with no evidence of recurrence at median follow-up time of 20 months.[105] Adverse effects included pancytopenia, fatigue, nausea, and headache. The most serious adverse effect is the increased incidence of secondary myelodysplastic syndrome and acute myelogenous leukemia, as a recent study showed a 5-year cumulative incidence of 8.29% of these cancers after treatment with Zevalin.[106]

Due to the association between *C. psittaci* and ocular adnexal lymphomas, doxycycline has emerged as a promising management option. In a multicenter prospective trial of 27 patients with untreated or relapsed ocular adnexal MALT, Ferreri and colleagues investigated the effect of 100 mg of doxycycline twice daily for 3 weeks on lymphoma remission. Doxycycline treatment produced an overall response rate of 48% among the entire patient population, and a 64% response rate in those with ocular adnexal lymphomas positive for Cp DNA. At 2 years, 67% of those with Cp DNA-positive lymphomas had no evidence of recurrence. In addition, doxycycline eliminated *C. psittaci* infection in all patients with positive Cp DNA. The International Extranodal Lymphoma Study Group has initiated a large international prospective trial to investigate the effect of the doxycycline.[107] The major advantage of doxycycline treatment is that it is relatively safe and inexpensive.

Prognosis

Conjunctival lymphoma has the best prognosis of the ocular adnexal lymphomas, with systemic lymphoma developing in only 20% to 31% of patients. In lymphomas of the orbit and eyelid, systemic involvement is present in 35% and 70%, respectively.[90] Since systemic involvement can occur up to several years after ocular diagnosis, patients should be monitored for systemic involvement every 6 months for 5 years and yearly thereafter.

The prognosis is best for MALT lymphomas compared with follicular, diffuse large B-cell, mantle cell and lymphoplasmacytic lymphomas. Spontaneous regression of MALT lymphomas 1 to 5 years following biopsy has been reported.[108]

MISCALLENOUS TUMORS

Kaposi's Sarcoma

Prior to the advent of highly active antiretroviral therapy (HAART), Kaposi's sarcoma (KS) was one of the most common acquired immunodeficiency syndrome (AIDS)-related illnesses.[109] It is a vascular tumor that most commonly affects the skin, but can also involve the mucous membranes and internal organs. Conjunctival and adnexal KS were among the first ocular lesions described in individuals with AIDS and can be an AIDS-defining illness.[110]

In 1995, Chang and colleagues identified a new herpes virus in KS lesions from patients with AIDS, now known as the human herpesvirus 8 (HHV-8).[111] HHV-8 is found in 95% of patients with Kaposi's sarcoma and is thought to be important in the pathogenesis of KS.[112]

Although most commonly presenting as an eyelid tumor, KS can also develop in the conjunctiva. Conjunctival KS is most commonly seen in the lower fornix, followed by the bulbar conjunctiva and the upper fornix.[113] Clinically, it appears as a painless, reddish vascular mass that may resemble a hemorrhagic conjunctivitis.

Pathology demonstrates malignant spindle-shaped cells with elongated oval nuclei surrounding a complex arrangement of capillary channels and vascular spaces without endothelium.[113]

Conjunctival KS typically has an indolent course, with the goal of treatment being palliation of symptoms and preservation of vision.[114] If small, circumscribed, and localized to the bulbar conjunctiva, surgical excision may be performed.

KS tumors are radiosensitive and local radiation can produce palliation of symptoms.[115] Intralesional α-2b has also been reported to be effective in case reports.[116] Systemic treatment includes chemotherapy and immune reconstitution with highly active antiretroviral therapy.[113]

Conjunctival Metastatic Tumors

Metastatic tumors to the conjunctiva are rare. In a report of 1643 tumors of the conjunctiva, 13 cases of conjunctival metastasis were described.[5] The most commonly reported primary cancers associated with metastasis are breast, lung, and cutaneous melanoma. Laryngeal cancer has also been reported.[68] Rarely, bilateral conjunctival infiltrates may be the first sign of relapsed acute leukemia.[117]

Most patients presenting with conjunctival metastasis have a previously diagnosed primary malignancy, as conjunctival metastasis occurs at advanced stages of disease. Occasionally, it may be the first presenting sign of an underlying systemic cancer that has not yet been diagnosed.[118] The mean survival time after diagnosis of conjunctival metastasis is on the order of months.[68]

Sebaceous Cell Carcinoma

Sebaceous cell carcinoma is a malignant neoplasm arising from meibomian glands, Zeiss glands, or the sebaceous glands of caruncle. It accounts for 1–5.5% of all eyelid malignancies, occurring typically between the ages of 60 to 70.[119]

Sebaceous cell carcinoma is known for masquerading as a number of benign and malignant conditions, such as chronic blepharoconjunctivitis, chalazion, basal cell carcinoma, or squamous cell carcinoma, often leading to a delay in diagnosis.

The conjunctival epithelium can be secondarily involved in 40% to 80% of cases by pagetoid (intraepithelial) spread. When there is diffuse intraepithelial involvement of the bulbar, forniceal, or tarsal conjunctiva, sebaceous cell carcinoma can mimic a chronic unilateral blepharoconjunctivitis. In rare cases, it may arise within the conjunctival epithelium, without any underlying glandular carcinoma.[31]

Due to the increased morbidity and mortality associated with delayed diagnosis, the clinician should have a low threshold for performing biopsy in cases of unilateral chronic blepharoconjunctivitis unresponsive to conventional treatment.

Pathology of sebaceous cell carcinoma demonstrates atypical sebaceous cells with large nuclei, prominent nucleoli and foamy cytoplasm. The presence of lipid can be demonstrated with oil-red O or Sudan black staining of frozen sections.

The mainstay of treatment is complete surgical excision with wide margins, using frozen sections at the time of surgery. Map biopsies from the bulbar and tarsal conjunctiva should be performed to determine the presence and extent of intraepithelial spread prior to surgical management. Cryotherapy should be applied to the involved conjunctiva. In cases of extensive conjunctival involvement, exenteration may be warranted.

The most common site of metastasis is the regional lymph nodes, reported in 8% to 14% of cases.[120] Increased awareness, leading to earlier detection and treatment has improved mortality rates from 24% in the past to less than 10%.[120]

Secondary Conjunctival Involvement from Adjacent Tumors

The conjunctiva may be involved by extraocular extension of intraocular tumors and by extension of eyelid and orbital tumors. Extrascleral extension of a ciliary body melanoma into subconjunctival tissue can simulate a conjunctival melanoma.[28] Rhabdomyosarcoma of the orbit, the most common orbital malignancy of childhood, can also demonstrate extension into subconjunctival tissue from the anterior orbit and thus, can present as a conjunctival mass.[121] It can also rarely present localized to the conjunctiva without orbital involvement.[122]

References

1. Lee GA, Hirst LW. Ocular surface squamous neoplasia. Surv Ophthalmol 1995;39:429–50.
2. Sun EC, Fears TR, Goedert JJ. Epidemiology of squamous cell conjunctival cancer. Cancer Epidemiol. Biomarkers Prev 1997;6:73–7.
3. Lee GA, Hirst LW. Incidence of ocular surface epithelial dysplasia in metropolitan Brisbane. A 10-year survey. Arch Ophthalmol 1992;110:525–7.
4. Ateenyi-Agaba C. Conjunctival squamous-cell carcinoma associated with HIV infection in Kampala, Uganda. Lancet 1995;345:695–6.
5. Shields CL, Demirci H, Karatza E, et al. Clinical survey of 1643 melanocytic and nonmelanocytic conjunctival tumors. Ophthalmology 2004;111:1747–54.
6. Gaasterland DE, Rodrigues MM, Moshell AN. Ocular involvement in xeroderma pigmentosum. Ophthalmology 1982;89:980–6.
7. Karp CL, Scott IU, Chang TS, et al. Conjunctival intraepithelial neoplasia. A possible marker for human immunodeficiency virus infection? Arch Ophthalmol 1996;114:257–61.
8. Lee GA, Williams G, Hirst LW, et al. Risk factors in the development of ocular surface epithelial dysplasia. Ophthalmology 1994;101:360–4.
9. Newton R, Ferlay J, Reeves G, et al. Effect of ambient solar ultraviolet radiation on incidence of squamous-cell carcinoma of the eye. Lancet 1996;347:1450–1.
10. Trosko JE, Krause D, Isoun M. Sunlight-induced pyrimidine dimers in human cells in vitro. Nature 1970;228:358–9.
11. Dushku N, Hatcher SL, Albert DM, et al. p53 expression and relation to human papillomavirus infection in pingueculae, pterygia, and limbal tumors. Arch Ophthalmol 1999;117:1593–9.
12. Spitzer MS, Batumba NH, Chirambo T, et al. Ocular surface squamous neoplasia as the first apparent manifestation of HIV infection in Malawi. Clin Exp Ophthalmol 2008;36:422–5.
13. McDonnell JM, McDonnell PJ, Sun YY. Human papillomavirus DNA in tissues and ocular surface swabs of patients with conjunctival epithelial neoplasia. Invest Ophthalmol Vis Sci 1992;33:184–9.
14. Scott IU, Karp CL, Nuovo GJ. Human papillomavirus 16 and 18 expression in conjunctival intraepithelial neoplasia. Ophthalmology 2002;109:542–7.
15. Eng HL, Lin TM, Chen SY, et al. Failure to detect human papillomavirus DNA in malignant epithelial neoplasms of conjunctiva by polymerase chain reaction. Am J Clin Pathol 2002;117:429–36.
16. Guthoff R, Marx A, Stroebel P. No evidence for a pathogenic role of human papillomavirus infection in ocular surface squamous neoplasia in Germany. Curr Eye Res 2009;34:666–71.
17. Basti S, Macsai MS. Ocular surface squamous neoplasia: a review. Cornea 2003;22:687–704.
18. McDonnell JM, Wagner D, Ng ST, et al. Human papillomavirus type 16 DNA in ocular and cervical swabs of women with genital tract condylomata. Am J Ophthalmol 1991;112:61–6.
19. Kiire CA, Srinivasan S, Karp CL. Ocular surface squamous neoplasia. Int Ophthalmol Clin 2010;50:35–46.
20. Napora C, Cohen EJ, Genvert GI, et al. Factors associated with conjunctival intraepithelial neoplasia: a case control study. Ophthalm Surg 1990;21:27–30.
21. Pe'er J. Ocular surface squamous neoplasia. Ophthalmol Clin N Am 2005;18:1–13, vii.
22. Degrassi M, Piantanida A, Nucci P. Unexpected histological findings in pterygium. Optometry and Vision Science 1993;70:1058–60.
23. Shields CL, Ramasubramanian A, Mellen PL, et al. Conjunctival squamous cell carcinoma arising in immunosuppressed patients (organ transplant, human immunodeficiency virus infection). Ophthalmology 2011;118:2133–7 e1.
24. Farah S, Baum TD, Conlon R, et al. Tumors of the cornea and conjunctiva. In: Albert DM, Jakobiec FA, editors. Principles and practice of ophthalmology. 2nd ed. Philadelphia: W.B. Saunders Co.: 2000. p. 1002–19.
25. Warner MA, Mehta MN, Jakobiec FA. Squamous neoplasms of the conjunctiva. In: Krachmer JH, Mannis MJ, Holland EJ, editors. Cornea. 3rd ed. Philadelphia: Elsevier/Mosby; 2005. p. 461–75.
26. Pe'er J, Frucht-Pery J. Ocular surface squamous neoplasia In: Singh AD, editor. Clinical ophthalmic oncology. Philadelphia: Saunders Elsevier; 2007. p. 136–40.
27. Shields JA, Shields CL. Eyelid, conjunctival, and orbital tumors : an atlas and textbook. 2nd ed. Philadelphia: Lippincott Williams & Wilkins; 2008. p. xiii, 805.
28. Shields CL, Shields JA. Tumors of the conjunctiva and cornea. Surv Ophthalmol 2004;49:3–24.
29. Rudkin AK, Dodd T, Muecke JS. The differential diagnosis of localised amelanotic limbal lesions: a review of 162 consecutive excisions. Br J Ophthalmol 2011;95:350–4.
30. Hirst LW, Axelsen RA, Schwab I. Pterygium and associated ocular surface squamous neoplasia. Arch Ophthalmol 2009;127:31–2.
31. Margo CE, Grossniklaus HE. Intraepithelial sebaceous neoplasia without underlying invasive carcinoma. Surv Ophthalmol 1995;39:293–301.
32. Gelender H, Forster RK. Papanicolaou cytology in the diagnosis and management of external ocular tumors. Arch Ophthalmol 1980;98:909–12.
33. Larmande A, Timsit E. Importance of cytodiagnosis in ophthalmology: preliminary report of 8 cases of tumors of the sclero-corneal limbus. Bulletin des sociétés d'ophtalmologie de France 1954;5:415–9.
34. Nolan GR, Hirst LW. Impression cytology in the diagnosis of ocular surface squamous neoplasia. Br J Ophthalmol 2001;85:888.

35. Malandrini A, Martone G, Traversi C, et al. In vivo confocal microscopy in a patient with recurrent conjunctival intraepithelial neoplasia. Acta Ophthalmol 2008;86:690–1.

36. Duchateau N, Hugol D, D'Hermies F, et al. Contribution of in vivo confocal microscopy to limbal tumor evaluation. Journal français d'ophtalmologie 2005;28:810–6.

37. Kieval JZ, Karp CL, Shousha MA, et al. Ultra-high resolution optical coherence tomography for differentiation of ocular surface squamous neoplasia and pterygia. Ophthalmology 2011;119:481–6.

38. Shields JA, Shields CL, De Potter P. Surgical management of conjunctival tumors. The 1994 Lynn B. McMahan Lecture. Arch Ophthalmol 1997;115:808–15.

39. Peksayar G, Soyturk MK, Demiryont M. Long-term results of cryotherapy on malignant epithelial tumors of the conjunctiva. Am J Ophthalmol 1989;107:337–40.

40. Gündüz K, Uçakhan OO, Kanpolat A, et al. Nonpreserved human amniotic membrane transplantation for conjunctival reconstruction after excision of extensive ocular surface neoplasia. Eye 2006; 20:351–7.

41. Espana EM, Prabhasawat P, Grueterich M, et al. Amniotic membrane transplantation for reconstruction after excision of large ocular surface neoplasias. Br J Ophthalmol 2002;86:640–5.

42. Hick S, Demers PE, Brunette I, et al. Amniotic membrane transplantation and fibrin glue in the management of corneal ulcers and perforations: a review of 33 cases. Cornea 2005;24:369–77.

43. Prabhasawat P, Tarinvorakup P, Tesavibul N, et al. Topical 0.002% mitomycin C for the treatment of conjunctival-corneal intraepithelial neoplasia and squamous cell carcinoma. Cornea 2005;24: 443–38.

44. Sepulveda R, Pe'er J, Midena E, et al. Topical chemotherapy for ocular surface squamous neoplasia: current status. Br J Ophthalmol 2010; 94:532–5.

45. Yeatts RP, Engelbrecht NE, Curry CD, et al. 5-Fluorouracil for the treatment of intracpithelial neoplasia of the conjunctiva and cornea. Ophthalmology 2000;107:2190–5.

46. Midena E, Angeli CD, Valenti M, et al. Treatment of conjunctival squamous cell carcinoma with topical 5-fluorouracil. Br J Ophthalmol 2000;84:268–72.

47. Chakalova G, Ganchev G. Local administration of interferon-alpha in cases of cervical intraepithelial neoplasia associated with human papillomavirus infection. Journal of B.U.ON. 2004;9:399–402.

48. Edwards L, Berman B, Rapini RP, et al. Treatment of cutaneous squamous cell carcinomas by intralesional interferon alfa-2b therapy. Arch Dermatol 1992;128:1486–9.

49. Decatris M, Santhanam S, O'Byrne K. Potential of interferon-alpha in solid tumours: part 1. BioDrugs 2002;16:261–81.

50. Bergman SJ, Ferguson MC, Santanello C. Interferons as therapeutic agents for infectious diseases. Infect Dis Clin N Am 2011;25: 819–34.

51. Galor A, Karp CL, Chhabra S, et al. Topical interferon alpha 2b eyedrops for treatment of ocular surface squamous neoplasia: a dose comparison study. Br J Ophthalmol 2010;94:551–4.

52. Karp CL, Galor A, Chhabra S, et al. Subconjunctival/perilesional recombinant interferon alpha-2b for ocular surface squamous neoplasia: a 10-year review. Ophthalmology 2010;117:2241–6.

53. Karp CL, Moore JK, Rosa Jr RH. Treatment of conjunctival and corneal intraepithelial neoplasia with topical interferon alpha-2b. Ophthalmology 2001;108:1093–8.

54. Stokes JJ. Intraocular extension of epibulbar squamous cell carcinoma of the limbus. Transactions – American Academy of Ophthalmology and Otolaryngology. Am Acad Ophthalmol Otolaryngol 1955;59:143–6.

55. Tabbara KF, Kersten R, Daouk N, et al. Metastatic squamous cell carcinoma of the conjunctiva. Ophthalmology 1988;95: 318–21.

56. Shields CL, Fasiuddin AF, Mashayekhi A, et al. Conjunctival nevi: clinical features and natural course in 410 consecutive patients. Arch Ophthalmol 2004;122:167–75.

57. Shields JA, Shields CL, Mashayekhi A, et al. Primary acquired melanosis of the conjunctiva: risks for progression to melanoma in 311 eyes. The 2006 Lorenz E. Zimmerman lecture. Ophthalmology 2008;115:511–9 e2.

58. Folberg R, McLean IW, Zimmerman LE. Primary acquired melanosis of the conjunctiva. Hum Pathol 1985;16:129–35.

59. Seregard S. Conjunctival melanoma. Surv Ophthalmol 1998;42: 321–50.

60. Hu DN, Yu G, McCormick SA, et al. Population-based incidence of conjunctival melanoma in various races and ethnic groups and comparison with other melanomas. Am J Ophthalmol 2008;145: 418–23.

61. Triay E, Bergman L, Nilsson B, et al. Time trends in the incidence of conjunctival melanoma in Sweden. Br J Ophthalmol 2009;93: 1524–8.

62. Yu GP, Hu DN, McCormick S, et al. Conjunctival melanoma: is it increasing in the United States? Am J Ophthalmol 2003;135: 800–6.

63. Tuomaala S, Eskelin S, Tarkkanen A, et al. Population-based assessment of clinical characteristics predicting outcome of conjunctival melanoma in whites. Invest Ophthalmol Vis Sci 2002;43: 3399–408.

64. Shields CL, Markowitz JS, Belinsky I, et al. Conjunctival melanoma: outcomes based on tumor origin in 382 consecutive cases. Ophthalmology 2011;118:389–95 e1–e2.

65. Singh AD, De Potter P, Fijal BA, et al. Lifetime prevalence of uveal melanoma in white patients with oculo(dermal) melanocytosis. Ophthalmology 1998;105:195–8.

66. Folberg R, Jakobiec FA, Bernardino VB, et al. Benign conjunctival melanocytic lesions. Clinicopathologic features. Ophthalmology 1989;96:436–61.

67. Char DH. Surgical management of melanocytoma of the ciliary body with extrascleral extension. Am J Ophthalmol 1994;118: 404–5.

68. Kiratli H, Shields CL, Shields JA, et al. Metastatic tumours to the conjunctiva: report of 10 cases. Br J Ophthalmol 1996;80:5–8.

69. Brownstein S. Malignant melanoma of the conjunctiva. Cancer Control 2004;11:310–6.

70. Pe'er J, Folberg R. Conjunctival melanoma. In: Singh AD, Damato BE, Pe'er J, et al, editors. Clinical ophthalmic oncology. Philadelphia: Saunders Elsevier; 2007.

71. Shields CL, Shields JA, Gunduz K, et al. Conjunctival melanoma: risk factors for recurrence, exenteration, metastasis, and death in 150 consecutive patients. Arch Ophthalmol 2000;118:1497–507.

72. Ho VH, Prager TC, Diwan H, et al. Ultrasound biomicroscopy for estimation of tumor thickness for conjunctival melanoma. J Clin Ultrasound 2007;35:533–7.

73. Shields CL, Belinsky I, Romanelli-Gobbi M, et al. Anterior segment optical coherence tomography of conjunctival nevus. Ophthalmology 2011;118:915–9.

74. Shields CL, Shields JA. Ocular melanoma: relatively rare but requiring respect. Clin Dermatol 2009;27:122–33.

75. Tuomaala S, Kivela T. Metastatic pattern and survival in disseminated conjunctival melanoma: implications for sentinel lymph node biopsy. Ophthalmology 2004;111:816–21.

76. Jakobiec FA, Folberg R, Iwamoto T. Clinicopathologic characteristics of premalignant and malignant melanocytic lesions of the conjunctiva. Ophthalmology 1989;96:147–66.

77. Folberg R, McLean IW. Primary acquired melanosis and melanoma of the conjunctiva: terminology, classification, and biologic behavior. Hum Pathol 1986;17:652–4.

78. Iwamoto S, Burrows RC, Grossniklaus HE, et al. Immunophenotype of conjunctival melanomas: comparisons with uveal and cutaneous melanomas. Arch Ophthalmol 2002;120:1625–9.

79. De Potter P, Shields CL, Shields JA, et al. Clinical predictive factors for development of recurrence and metastasis in conjunctival melanoma: a review of 68 cases. Br J Ophthalmol 1993;77:624–30.

80. Kurli M, Finger PT. Topical mitomycin chemotherapy for conjunctival malignant melanoma and primary acquired melanosis with atypia: 12 years' experience. Graefe's Arch Clin Exp Ophthalmol 2005;243:1108–14.

81. Finger PT, Sedeek RW, Chin KJ. Topical interferon alfa in the treatment of conjunctival melanoma and primary acquired melanosis complex. Am J Ophthalmol 2008;145:124–9.

82. Herold TR, Hintschich C. Interferon alpha for the treatment of melanocytic conjunctival lesions. Graefe's Arch Clin Exp Ophthalmol 2010;248:111–5.

83. Pe'er J, Frucht-Pery J. The treatment of primary acquired melanosis (PAM) with atypia by topical Mitomycin C. Am J Ophthalmol 2005;139:229–34.

84. Norregaard JC, Gerner N, Jensen OA, et al. Malignant melanoma of the conjunctiva: occurrence and survival following surgery and radiotherapy in a Danish population. Graefe's Arch Clin Exp Ophthalmol 1996;234:569–72.

85. Seregard S, Kock E. Conjunctival malignant melanoma in Sweden 1969–91. Acta Ophthalmologica 1992;70:289–96.
86. Grossniklaus HE, Green WR, Luckenbach M, et al. Conjunctival lesions in adults. A clinical and histopathologic review. Cornea 1987;6:78–116.
87. Knowles DM, Jakobiec FA, McNally L, et al. Lymphoid hyperplasia and malignant lymphoma occurring in the ocular adnexa (orbit, conjunctiva, and eyelids): a prospective multiparametric analysis of 108 cases during 1977 to 1987. Hum Pathol 1990;21:959–73.
88. Bairey O, Kremer I, Rakowsky E, et al. Orbital and adnexal involvement in systemic non-Hodgkin's lymphoma. Cancer 1994;73: 2395–9.
89. Tsai PS, Colby KA. Treatment of conjunctival lymphomas. Semin Ophthalmol 2005;20:239–46.
90. Shields CL, Shields JA, Carvalho C, et al. Conjunctival lymphoid tumors: clinical analysis of 117 cases and relationship to systemic lymphoma. Ophthalmology 2001;108:979–84.
91. Lee SB, Yang JW, Kim CS. The association between conjunctival MALT lymphoma and *Helicobacter pylori*. Br J Ophthalmol 2008; 92:534–6.
92. Chanudet E, Zhou Y, Bacon CM, et al. *Chlamydia psittaci* is variably associated with ocular adnexal MALT lymphoma in different geographical regions. J Pathol 2006;209:344–51.
93. Ferreri AJ, Ponzoni M, Guidoboni M, et al. Bacteria-eradicating therapy with doxycycline in ocular adnexal MALT lymphoma: a multicenter prospective trial. J Natl Cancer Inst 2006;98: 1375–82.
94. Rosado MF, Byrne GE, Jr., Ding F, et al. Ocular adnexal lymphoma: a clinicopathologic study of a large cohort of patients with no evidence for an association with *Chlamydia psittaci*. Blood 2006; 107:467–72.
95. Auw-Haedrich C, Coupland SE, Kapp A, et al. Long term outcome of ocular adnexal lymphoma subtyped according to the REAL classification. Revised European and American Lymphoma. Br J Ophthalmol 2001;85:63–9.
96. Bardenstein DS. Orbital and adnexal lymphoma. In: Singh AD, Damato BE, Pe'er J, et al, editors. Clinical ophthalmic oncology. Philadelphia: Saunders Elsevier; 2007.
97. Cahill M, Barnes C, Moriarty P, et al. Ocular adnexal lymphoma-comparison of MALT lymphoma with other histological types. Br J Ophthalmol 1999;83:742–7.
98. Martinet S, Ozsahin M, Belkacemi Y, et al. Outcome and prognostic factors in orbital lymphoma: a Rare Cancer Network study on 90 consecutive patients treated with radiotherapy. Int J Rad Oncol Biol Phys 2003;55:892–8.
99. Blasi MA, Tiberti AC, Valente P, et al. Intralesional interferon-alpha for conjunctival mucosa-associated lymphoid tissue lymphoma long-term results. Ophthalmology 2012;119:494–500.
100. Ferreri AJ, Govi S, Colucci A, et al. Intralesional rituximab: a new therapeutic approach for patients with conjunctival lymphomas. Ophthalmology 2011;118:24–8.
101. Salepci T, Seker M, Kurnaz E, et al. Conjunctival malt lymphoma successfully treated with single agent rituximab therapy. Leukemia Res 2009;33:e10–13.
102. Ferreri AJ, Ponzoni M, Martinelli G, et al. Rituximab in patients with mucosal-associated lymphoid tissue-type lymphoma of the ocular adnexa. Haematologica 2005;90:1578–9.
103. Rigacci L, Nassi L, Puccioni M, et al. Rituximab and chlorambucil as first-line treatment for low-grade ocular adnexal lymphomas. Ann Hematol 2007;86:565–8.
104. International Exranodal Lymphoma Study Group. Multicenter randomized trial of chlorambucil versus chlorambucil plus rituximab versus rituximab in extranodal marginal zone b-cell lymphoma of mucosa associated lymphoid tissue (MALT Lymphoma). Available from http://clinicaltrials.gov/ct2/show/NCT00210353.
105. Esmaeli B, McLaughlin P, Pro B, et al. Prospective trial of targeted radioimmunotherapy with Y-90 ibritumomab tiuxetan (Zevalin) for front-line treatment of early-stage extranodal indolent ocular adnexal lymphoma. Annals of Oncology 2009;20:709–14.
106. Guidetti A, Carlo-Stella C, Ruella M, et al. Myeloablative doses of yttrium-90-ibritumomab tiuxetan and the risk of secondary myelodysplasia/acute myelogenous leukemia. Cancer 2011: 117:5074–84.
107. International Extranodal Lymphoma Study Group. A clinico-pathological study to investigate the possible infective causes of non-Hodgkin lymphoma of the ocular adnexae. Available from http://clinicaltrials.gov/ct2/show/NCT01010295.
108. Matsuo T, Yoshino T. Long-term follow-up results of observation or radiation for conjunctival malignant lymphoma. Ophthalmology 2004;111:1233–7.
109. Dal Maso L, Serraino D, Franceschi S. Epidemiology of AIDS-related tumours in developed and developing countries. Eur J Cancer 2001;37:1188–201.
110. Holland GN, Gottlieb MS, Yee RD, et al. Ocular disorders associated with a new severe acquired cellular immunodeficiency syndrome. Am J Ophthalmol 1982;93:393–402.
111. Chang Y, Cesarman E, Pessin MS, et al. Identification of herpesvirus-like DNA sequences in AIDS-associated Kaposi's sarcoma. Science 1994;266:1865–9.
112. Moore PS, Chang Y. Detection of herpesvirus-like DNA sequences in Kaposi's sarcoma in patients with and without HIV infection. N Engl J Med 1995;332:1181–5.
113. Jeng BH, Holland GN, Lowder CY, et al. Anterior segment and external ocular disorders associated with human immunodeficiency virus disease. Surv Ophthalmol 2007;52:329–68.
114. Kohanim S, Daniels AB, Huynh N, et al. Local treatment of Kaposi sarcoma of the conjunctiva. Int Ophthalmol Clin 2011;51: 183–92.
115. Ghabrial R, Quivey JM, Dunn JP, Jr., et al. Radiation therapy of acquired immunodeficiency syndrome-related Kaposi's sarcoma of the eyelids and conjunctiva. Arch Ophthalmol 1992;110:1423–6.
116. Qureshi YA, Karp CL, Dubovy SR. Intralesional interferon alpha-2b therapy for adnexal Kaposi sarcoma. Cornea 2009;28:941–3.
117. Font RL, Mackay B, Tang R. Acute monocytic leukemia recurring as bilateral perilimbal infiltrates. Immunohistochemical and ultrastructural confirmation. Ophthalmology 1985;92:1681–5.
118. Shields JA, Gunduz K, Shields CL, et al. Conjunctival metastasis as the initial manifestation of lung cancer. Am J Ophthalmol 1997; 124:399–400.
119. Kass LG, Hornblass A. Sebaceous carcinoma of the ocular adnexa. Surv Ophthalmol 1989;33:477–90.
120. Shields JA, Demirci H, Marr BP, et al. Sebaceous carcinoma of the eyelids: personal experience with 60 cases. Ophthalmology 2004; 111:2151–7.
121. Shields JA, Shields CL. Rhabdomyosarcoma: review for the ophthalmologist. Surv Ophthalmol 2003;48:39–57.
122. Joffe L, Shields JA, Pearah JD. Epibulbar rhabdomyosarcoma without proptosis. J Pediatr Ophthalmol 1977;14:364–7.

20 Conjunctivochalasis

KRISTIANA D. NEFF

Introduction

Conjunctivochalasis (CCh) is a characteristically bilateral condition where redundant, nonedematous conjunctiva causes a spectrum of clinical findings ranging from exacerbation of an unstable tear film to mechanical disruption of tear flow. The origination of the term conjunctivochalasis came from W. L. Hughes in 1942; however, descriptions of this same entity were noted as early as 1908 by Elschnig and by Braunschweig and Wollenberg in 1921 and 1922, respectively.[1] They described the more severe spectrum of findings in CCh of subconjunctival hemorrhage, pain, and exposure keratopathy. Later work described the more mild symptomatology of CCh, including dry eye to the more moderate symptoms of excess lacrimation by impeding tear clearance.[2]

Because CCh can be asymptomatic, it is often overlooked as a normal variant of aging. However, it is an important clinical diagnosis that must be considered in the evaluation of patients with ocular irritation and tearing. CCh typically presents as loose inferior conjunctiva, that disrupts the inferior tear meniscus; however, it is thought to also involve the superior conjunctiva in some cases.[3,4] Aside from the most common symptoms of irritation and lacrimation, other associated complaints include blurred vision, discharge, dryness, ocular fatigue, subconjunctival hemorrhage, and eye stiffness on awakening.[5] The severity of CCh symptoms tends to worsen with both downgaze and digital pressure.

Slit lamp biomicroscopy can show prolapse of the conjunctiva over the lower lid margin in the temporal, medial or nasal regions, or any combination of these regions (Fig. 20.1). This conjunctival prolapse can impede tear outflow through the inferior punctum, resulting in epiphora. Mechanical trauma can also cause recurrent subconjunctival hemorrhage in this sector (Fig. 20.2).

The diagnostic dilemma in managing CCh lies in the fact that other more common etiologies of tearing and ocular irritation must be ruled out as causative or contributory agents to the tear flow disruption or tear instability. The same symptom constellation can be seen in isolated dry eye syndrome, isolated CCh or a mixed presentation of these diseases. Lid pathology, as well as systemic entities, such as ocular allergy and thyroid eye disease can also present with similar symptoms. One must be able to determine how much the presence of redundant conjunctiva contributes to the patient's irritation. This can be particularly challenging in cases of mild CCh.

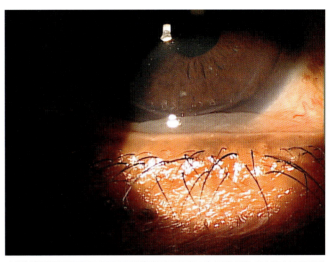

Figure 20.1 Inferior conjunctivochalasis in a patient with symptoms of tearing, ocular irritation and intermittent pain. The extent of conjunctival prolapse over the inferior lid margin at the limbus is most extensive in the middle region of the lid margin in this case.

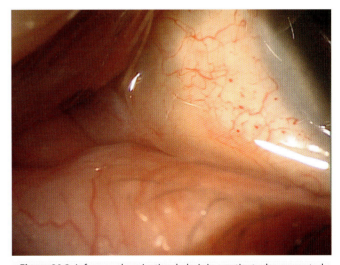

Figure 20.2 Inferonasal conjuctivochalasis in a patient who presented with recurrent subconjuctival hemorrhage in the nasal conjunctiva. The patient also had symptoms of epiphora and foreign body sensation. The extent of conjunctivochalasis is most exensive inferonasally where the redundant conjunctiva is blocking the inferior puncta and undergoing mechanical trauma with each blink.

Epidemiology

Conjunctivochalasis has been identified to be an age-dependent phenomenon by several studies.[4,6–8] It has been seen in patients as early as the first decade of life and tends to increase in prevalence and severity with age. The Zhang study estimated the prevalence to be 44.08% in a senile Chinese population, while Mimura noted an even higher prevalence in a hospital-based Japanese population. There was no increase in grade of severity of CCh based on gender in Mimura's study. The location of CCh is most frequently found in the nasal and temporal regions of inferior conjunctiva, versus middle zone of inferior conjunctiva or superior conjunctiva.[4,7,8] Conjunctivochalasis has also been noted to be more frequent in patients with thyroid disease and with contact lens wear.[6,9]

Pathophysiology

Information regarding the pathogenesis of conjunctivochalasis is minimal and often conflicting. The earliest publications suggested senile changes involving the subcutaneous, elastic or supporting tissue, in the conjunctiva. Eye rubbing, mechanical irritation or trauma to conjunctiva, and abnormal eyelid position, were all implicated in development of CCh; however, no true etiology has been determined. More recent studies have offered a more mechanistic approach to evaluating the pathogenesis of CCh.

Francis et al., in a prospective clinical and histopathological study of 29 CCh patients, showed that 22 of 29 specimens displayed normal conjunctival histology, while only four specimens showed inflammatory changes and three specimens showed elastosis (Fig. 20.3).[10] They hypothesized, based on these results, that the pathogenesis of CCh is therefore, multifactorial, including local trauma, ultraviolet radiation and delayed tear clearance as inciting factors. Watanabe et al. demonstrated microscopic lymphangiectasia of the subconjunctiva in 39 of 44 specimens taken from patients with severe CCh, with no evidence of inflammation.[11] They also noted loss of typical fiber patterns with fragmented elastic fibers and sparse assemblages of collagen fibers in all 44 specimens. Their conclusion was that mechanical forces between the lower eyelid and conjunctiva gradually impaired lymphatic flow, resulting in lymphatic dilation and clinical CCh. Immunostaining by Yokoi et al. supported the negligible role of inflammation in CCh, by comparing conjunctival samples in CCh patients to those of known normal and known inflammatory ocular surface disease.[5]

Although there is little histopathologic support of inflammation playing a role in CCh, mechanistic evidence suggests a shift in the normal balance of conjunctival matrix

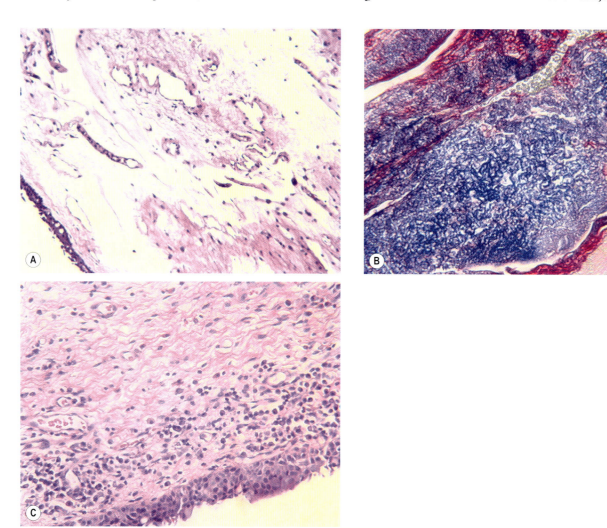

Figure 20.3 Histologic findings in sections of patients undergoing conjunctivochalasis resection. (**A**) Normal conjunctiva (10×, haematoxylin and eosin). (**B**) Marked elastotic degeneration of conjunctiva (20×, Van Gieson). (**C**) Subepithelial conjunctival infiltrate consisting mainly of plasma cells and lymphocytes (20×, haematoxylin and eosin). (Reprinted with permission from: Francis IC, Chan DG, Kim P, et al. Case-controlled clinical and histopathological study of conjunctivochalasis. Br J Ophthalmol. 2005;89(3):302–5.)

metalloproteinases (MMPs) and tissue inhibitors (TIMPs). These enzymes serve to degrade extracellular matrix, possibly contributing to the pathogenesis of CCh.[12] Specifically, Li, et al. showed overexpression of MMP-1 and MMP-3 mRNA in tissue cultured conjunctivochalasis fibroblasts, versus normal human conjunctival fibroblasts. No difference was noted in MMP-2, TIMP-1, TIMP-2, and urokinase plasminogen activator in the same study. Further studies then showed that inflammatory mediators tumor necrosis factor-α (TNF-α) and interleukin-1β (IL-1β) may increase expression of MMP-1 and MMP-3 in conjunctivochalasis fibroblasts.[13] Other proinflammatory cytokines, tear IL-6 and IL-8, were shown to be increased in the tear film of CCh patients.[14] It has been suggested that this interaction of MMPs and their inhibitors, which normally participate in connective tissue degradation and remodeling, may offer some insight into the clinical manifestation of loose, redundant conjunctiva.

Symptoms

Conjunctivochalasis is one of the most common under-diagnosed and misdiagnosed ocular surface diseases. The difficulty in diagnosing CCh is that the symptoms are non-specific and the onset is insidious. Initial symptoms include foreign body sensation, burning, 'dryness' and discomfort. These non-specific symptoms together with the intermittent clinical findings of conjunctival edema often lead to misdiagnosis. The majority of patients with CCh have been diagnosed with the more common ocular surface disease conditions, such as dry eye, anterior blepharitis, meibomian gland disease or allergic eye disease, prior to the correct diagnosis. Another problem in the diagnosis of CCh, is that many clinicians do not recognize the significance of the conjunctival findings or are unaware of CCh as a significant clinical entity.

As the clinical findings progress and the conjunctival redundancy increases, the puncta can be blocked, thus leading to the later symptoms of epiphora. It is at this later stage that many patients are first diagnosed.

Grading Systems

Several grading systems have been developed to describe conjunctivochalasis. The first group to categorize CCh was Höh et al., who looked at the number of lid-parallel conjunctival folds (LIPCOF).[15] They noted the number of LIPCOF had a high predictive value for diagnosis of kerato-conjunctivitis sicca (Table 20.1). At present, the most widely used grading system was proposed by Meller and Tseng in 1998 (Table 20.2) who adapted the scale by Höh and associates and included the extent of CCh, changes with downgaze and digital pressure, and presence of punctual occlusion.[2] This system has been utilized in the majority of studies to define extent of CCh. The newest grading

Table 20.1 Classification of Conjunctivochalasis Using the Lid-Parallel Folds (LIPCOF) Method Grading of Conjunctivochalasis*

Grade	Number of Folds and Relationship to the Tear Meniscus Height
0	No persistent fold
1	Single, small fold
2	More than two folds and not higher than the tear meniscus
3	Multiple folds and higher than the tear meniscus

*Modified from Höh et al.[15] with permission of the authors and Ophthalmologe.
(Reprinted with permission from: Meller D, Tseng SCG. Conjunctivochalasis: literature review and possible pathophysiology. Surv Ophthalmol 1998;43:225–32. Copyright Elsevier, 1998.)

Table 20.2 Proposed New Grading System for Conjunctivochalasis*

Location	Folds Versus Tear Meniscus Height	Punctal Occlusion	Change in Downgaze	Changes by Digital Pressure
0	A	O+	G↑	P↑
1	B	O−	G←→	P←→
2	C		G↓	P↓
3				
0: none	A: < tear meniscus	O+ = nasal location with punctal occlusion	G↑ = height/extent of chalasis increases in downgaze	P↑ = height/extent of chalasis increases on digital pressure
1: one location	B: = tear meniscus	O− = nasal location without punctal occlusion	G←→ = no difference	P←→ = no difference
2: two locations	C: > tear meniscus		G↓ = height/extent of chalasis decreases in downgaze	P↓ = height/extent of chalasis decreases on digital pressure
3: whole lid				

*The new grading system defines the extension of redundant conjunctiva as grade 1 = 1 location, 2 = 2 locations, 3 = whole lid. For 1 and 2, it is further specified as T, M, N if conjunctivochalasis is found in the temporal, the middle (or inferior to the limbus), and the nasal aspect of the lower lid, respectively. For each location (T, M, and N), further notation is given to indicate if the height of folds is less that (A), equal to (B), or greater than (C) the tear meniscus height. If it is found in the nasal (N) location, the extent of chalasis is further determine as to whether it occludes the inferior puncta. For each location, it is further graded as G⇑ if its height is greater than, as G⇔ if equal to, and as G⇓ if less than the tear meniscus height. Likewise it is further graded as P⇑, P⇔, and P⇓ if it is worse, no difference, or better with digital pressure (P), respectively.
(Reprinted with permission from: Meller D, Tseng SCG. Conjunctivochalasis: literature review and possible pathophysiology. Surv Ophthalmol. 1998;43:225–32. Copyright Elsevier, 1998.)

Table 20.3 Modified Meller and Tseng's Grading System for Conjunctivochalasis Used in the Present Study*

	Basic Grading Criteria		Supplement Grading Criteria		
	Folds Versus Tear Meniscus	Symptoms (S)	Punctal Occlusion and Tear Meniscus Height	Height/Extent of Chalasis Changes in Downgaze	BUT (B)
0	No persistent fold	No	Without occlusion	No difference	≥10 s
1	Single small fold	No	Without occlusion and tear meniscus height ≤0.3 mm	No difference	≥10 s
2	Two or more folds and not higher than the tear meniscus	Mild	Nasal location with partial occlusion and discontinuous tear meniscus	Mildly increases in downgaze	6–9 s
3	Multiple folds and higher than the tear meniscus	Medium	Nasal location with complete occlusion and discontinuous tear meniscus	Significant increase in downgaze	4–5 s
4	Multiple folds, higher than the tear meniscus, and causing exposure problems	Severe	Nasal location with complete occlusion and no tear meniscus	Severe increase in downgaze	≤3 s

*Symptoms indicate dryness, foreign body sensation, and epiphora, evaluated by the patients themselves; BUT: break-up time (seconds).
This grading system for conjunctivochalasis obeys the following rule: if the clinical appearance of a certain patients corresponds to F2 + S2, or F2+ any two of O2, G2, and B2, the patient will be diagnosed as Grade II conjunctivochalasis, and so forth with Grade 0, Grade I, Grade III, or Grade IV. Grade II, Grade III, and Grade IV are also defined as 'clinically significant conjunctivochalasis'.
(Reprinted with permission from: Zhang X, Li Q, Zou H, et al. BMC Public Heath. 2011;11:198.)

system proposed by Zhang et al. in 2011 (Table 20.3) further modified Meller and Tseng's approach by including three symptoms (epiphora, feeling of dryness, and foreign body sensation) and unstable tear film-break up time (BUT).[8] The authors felt these modifications were necessary to flesh out those 'asymptomatic, normal older people' they felt added to the very high prevalence rates of CCh noted in some epidemiologic studies. The validity of this scale needs to be proven in future studies.

Therapeutic Options

No intervention for asymptomatic conjunctivochalasis is required. Once a patient becomes symptomatic, medical therapy is initiated with trials of lubrication or topical corticosteroids. Any other components of ocular surface disease, such as allergic conjunctivitis, meibomian gland disease, dry eye syndrome, and allergic eye disease, should concurrently be addressed. As the clinical findings may fluctuate, several clinical exams may be required to confirm the diagnosis. When other ocular surface disease has been ruled out and conservative medical management fails to control the patient's symptoms, surgical intervention is then indicated.

Surgical options include a variety of methods to reduce the amount of redundant conjunctival folding. The most commonly employed procedure involves simple conjunctival excision of the redundant tissue. Conjunctival resection was initially described using a crescentic excision of conjunctiva 5 mm posterior to the limbus and closed with absorbable suture.[1]

The author's preferred conjunctival resection technique involves customizing the resection to each individual's specific degree of conjunctival laxity. The areas of redundant conjunctiva are identified, and a limbal peritomy is created, 1 mm posterior to the limbus in the involved sectors. The freed conjunctiva is then advanced centrally with the help of radial relaxing incisions, allowing the surgeon to visualize the extent of excess tissue folding. The visualized tissue redundancy extending past the limbal peridomy is then

excised. Fibrin glue can then be utilized to appose the wound margins. This sutureless technique can be adapted to all cases of conjunctivochalasis, from mild to severe. It is important to eliminate only excess tissue, so as to avoid contracture of the inferior fornix. For the majority of cases, the redundant conjunctival is most visible inferiorly and this is the area that is resected. However, in many cases the redundant tissue involves all the bulbar conjunctiva and the resection is carried out for 360 degrees.

Several other techniques have shown to decrease or resolve symptoms of CCh; however, there have not been prospective comparative analysis to determine the relative efficacy of these different surgical procedures. These other procedures include conjunctival fixation to sclera with three 6-0 Vicryl sutures[16] and elliptical excision of redundant conjunctiva.[3] Serrano and Mora modified the excision technique by creating a peritomy, just posterior to the limbus with two radial, relaxing incisions to avoid scarring or retraction of the inferior fornix.[17] Amniotic membrane transplantation for CCh has been described as a treatment with either suture fixation of the amniograft[18–20] or fixation through the use of fibrin glue.[21] However, CCh is a condition of redundant conjunctiva, so most clinicians feel that the addition of other tissue, such as amniotic membrane is not warranted. Fibrin glue has also been used as an adjunctive step to conjunctival resection and has been shown to be effective (Fig. 20.4).[22]

The more minimally invasive superficial thermocautery of the inferior conjunctiva, has also shown to improve symptoms of CCh and improve conjunctival laxity.[23,24] Nakasato and colleagues described a novel technique where ligation testing was used to predict appropriate candidates to undergo thermocautery of the inferior bulbar conjunctiva. This allowed them to treat symptomatic patients with CCh in an outpatient setting and to stratify patients into groups that were more likely to respond to therapy. The ligation test technique describes an 8-0 silk suture formed into a loop, with forceps used to grasp redundant conjunctiva through the loop 3–4 mm inferior to the limbus until the CCh disappears. The loop is then tightened to ligate the excess tissue. Once anesthesia has worn off, patients were

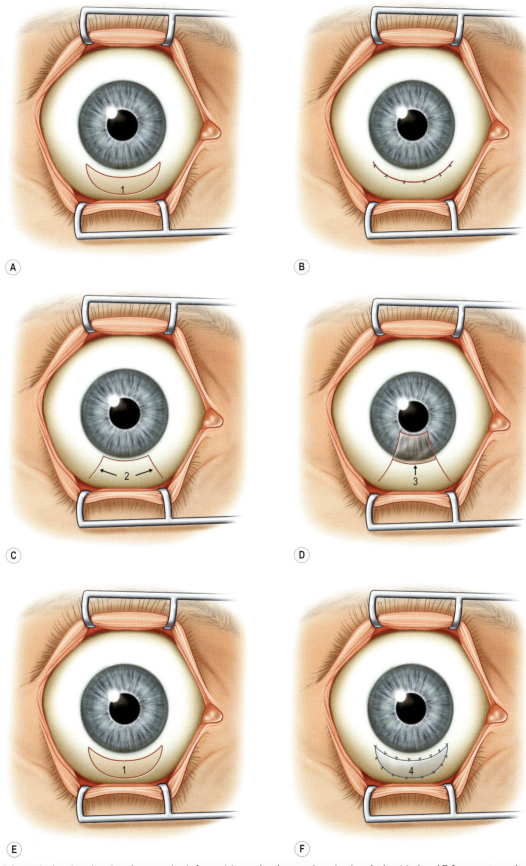

Figure 20.4 Schematic drawing showing three methods for excising redundant conjunctiva (*marked as 1 in A and E*) for symptomatic conjunctivochalasis. (**A**) Crescentic resection with (**B**) use of absorbable suture for closure. (**C**) Sectoral limbal peritomy with radial relaxing incisions. (**D**) The redundant conjunctiva (*marked as 3 in D*) is pulled toward the limbus, excised, and the remaining conjunctiva sutured in position. (**E**) Crescentic resection with (**F**) use of amniotic membrane for resurfacing the inferior bulbar conjunctival defect (*marked as 4 in F*). This can be accomplished with suture fixation or with the use of fibrin tissue glue. (Reprinted with permission from: Meller D, Tseng SCG. Conjunctivochalasis: literature review and possible pathophysiology. Surv Ophthalmol. 1998;43(3):225–32. Copyright Elsevier, 1998.)

evaluated for improvement or resolution of CCh symptoms, and if some improvement is noted, they were selected for thermocautery treatment. Following thermocautery, disappearance of symptoms was noted in 92.3% of treated eyes, and symptoms improved in the remaining 7.7% of eyes.[23] Because the severity of CCh increases with digital pressure and downward gaze, lid tightening procedures tend to worsen the symptoms of CCh-related dry eye.[7] Extensive conjunctival resections should also be avoided in order to minimize complications, such as contraction of the fornices, cicitricial entropion, and restriction of extraocular movement. When sutures are employed in the technique, increased foreign body sensation, suture-induced granulomas, and prolonged inflammatory reactions can be seen. Other early complications include chemosis, hyperemia, subconjunctival hemorrhage, and infection. Late complications, such as scar formation and residual or recurrent CCh are possible.

Conclusion

Conjunctivochalasis is a prevalent disease process in the older population. It should not be overlooked as an etiology of ocular irritation and tearing. In some cases, CCh can cause significant symptoms that may require surgical treatment. Treatment should proceed in a stepwise fashion, starting with non-invasive, medical therapies, followed by surgical intervention if medical management fails to control the patient's symptoms.

References

1. Hughes WL. Conjunctivochalasis. Am J Ophthalmol 1942;25: 48–51.
2. Meller D, Tseng SCG. Conjunctivochalasis: literature review and possible pathophysiology. Surv Ophthalmol 1998;43:225–32.
3. Liu D. Conjunctivochalasis. A cause of tearing and its management. Ophthal Plast Reconstr Surg 1986;2:25–8.
4. Di Pascuale MA, Espana EM, Kawakita T, et al. Clinical characteristics of conjunctivochalasis with or without aqueous tear deficiency. Br J Ophthalmol 2004;88:388–92.
5. Yokoi N, Komuro A, Nishii M, et al. Clinical impact of conjunctivochalasis on the ocular surface. Cornea [Clinical Trial] 2005; 24(Suppl. 8):S24–31.
6. Mimura T, Usui T, Yamamoto H, et al. Conjunctivochalasis and contact lenses. Am J Ophthalmol 2009;148:20–5 e1.
7. Mimura T, Yamagami S, Usui T, et al. Changes of conjunctivochalasis with age in a hospital-based study. Am J Ophthalmol 2009;147:171–7 e1.
8. Zhang X, Li Q, Zou H, et al. Assessing the severity of conjunctivochalasis in a senile population: a community-based epidemiology study in Shanghai, China. BMC Pub Health 2011;11:198.
9. de Almeida SF, de Sousa LB, Vieira LA, et al. Clinic-cytologic study of conjunctivochalasis and its relation to thyroid autoimmune diseases: prospective cohort study. Cornea 2006;25:789–93.
10. Francis IC, Chan DG, Kim P, et al. Case-controlled clinical and histopathological study of conjunctivochalasis. Br J Ophthalmol 2005; 89:302–5.
11. Watanabe A, Yokoi N, Kinoshita S, et al. Clinicopathologic study of conjunctivochalasis Cornea 2004;23:294–8.
12. Li DQ, Meller D, Liu Y, et al. Overexpression of MMP-1 and MMP-3 by cultured conjunctivochalasis fibroblasts. Invest Ophthalmol Vis Sci 2000;41:404–10.
13. Meller D, Li DQ, Tseng SCG. Regulation of collagenase, stromelysin, and gelatinase B in human conjunctival and conjunctivochalasis fibroblasts by interleukin-1beta and tumor necrosis factor-alpha. Invest Ophthalmol Vis Sci 2000;41:2922–9.
14. Erdogan-Poyraz C, Mocan MC, Bozkurt B, et al. Elevated tear interleukin-6 and interleukin-8 levels in patients with conjunctivochalasis. Cornea 2009;28:189–93.
15. Höh H, Schirra F, Kienecker C, et al. Lid-parallel conjunctival folds are a sure diagnostic sign of dry eye. Ophthalmologe 1995;92:802–8.
16. Otaka I, Kyu N. A new surgical technique for management of conjunctivochalasis. Am J Ophthalmol 2000;129:385–7.
17. Serrano F, Mora LM. Conjunctivochalasis: a surgical technique. Ophthalmic Surg 1989;20:883–4.
18. Meller D, Maskin SL, Pires RT, et al. Amniotic membrane transplantation for symptomatic conjunctivochalasis refractory to medical treatments. Cornea 2000;19:796–803.
19. Georgiadis NS, Terzidou CD. Epiphora caused by conjunctivochalasis: treatment with transplantation of preserved human amniotic membrane. Cornea 2001;20:619–21.
20. Maskin SL. Effect of ocular surface reconstruction by using amniotic membrane transplant for symptomatic conjunctivochalasis on fluorescein clearance test results. Cornea 2008;27:644–9.
21. Kheirkhah A, Casas V, Blanco G, et al. Amniotic membrane transplantation with fibrin glue for conjunctivochalasis. Am J Ophthalmol 2007;144:311–3.
22. Brodbaker E, Bahar I, Slomovic AR. Novel use of fibrin glue in the treatment of conjunctivochalasis. Cornea 2008;27:950–2.
23. Nakasato S, Uemoto R, Mizuki N. Thermocautery for Inferior conjunctivochalasis. Cornea 2012;31:514–9.
24. Kashima T, Akiyama H, Miura F, et al. Improved subjective symptoms of conjunctivochalasis using bipolar diathermy method for conjunctival shrinkage. Clin Ophthalmol 2011;5:1391–6.

21 *Superior Limbic Keratoconjunctivitis*

SHAWN C. RICHARDS and RICHARD S. DAVIDSON

Introduction

Superior limbic keratoconjunctivitis (SLK) is a rare disorder of the superior cornea and conjunctiva, that was first fully described by Frederick Theodore in 1963.[1] He suggested the term SLK to describe a series of patients with the following presenting signs: (1) inflammation of the superior tarsal conjunctiva, (2) inflammation of the superior bulbar conjunctiva, (3) fine punctate staining of the superior cornea, limbus, and the adjacent conjunctiva, and (4) filaments on the superior limbus or upper fourth of the cornea.

Presentation

Patients with SLK can present with a variety of non-specific complaints. The most common symptoms are irritation, burning, foreign body sensation, redness, photophobia, mucoid discharge from the eyes, and even an inflammatory ptosis. These symptoms are usually much more severe if the patient has corneal filaments. Often, the irritation is mild in the morning but worsens throughout the day.[2] The symptoms can be vague and intermittent and often are mistaken for other ocular surface disease, such as dry eye and blepharitis. Due to the fact that the clinical findings are often missed because the superior conjunctival is frequently not examined, SLK patients can be misdiagnosed or not diagnosed for many years.

In untreated patients, the natural course of the disease is one of episodic relapses and gradual improvement over several years, with eventual resolution of symptoms. Most patients are affected bilaterally (Fig. 21.1), but asymmetric and unilateral disease occurs. The female to male ratio is variable but is roughly 2:1.[3] Presentation typically occurs in the fourth or fifth decades of life.[4] A familial association has rarely been reported but is not the norm.

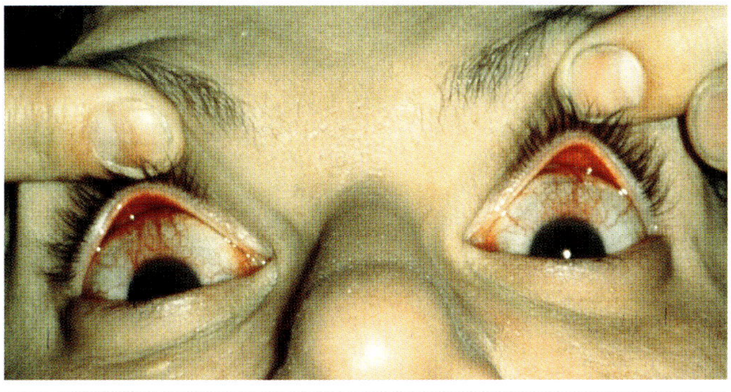

Clinical Examination

The classic physical finding associated with SLK is superior bulbar conjunctival injection. Vital stains, such as rose bengal or lissamine green are the most effective way to highlight abnormal conjunctiva (Fig. 21.2). These stains are especially beneficial in cases where the conjunctival injection may be subtle. Caution should be taken though, as vital staining of the superior bulbar conjunctiva does not guarantee a diagnosis of SLK. Bainbridge et al. looked at 93 consecutive patients who presented to an eye clinic for any reason, that were subsequently stained with rose bengal. While none of them carried a diagnosis of SLK, 25% of them exhibited staining of the superior bulbar conjunctiva.[2] This study reinforces the fact that a diagnosis of SLK should only be made after a thorough patient history is obtained and physical examination is performed. Other clinical findings of SLK include injection and redundancy of the superior bulbar conjunctiva, filaments of the superior cornea and conjunctiva, and a papillary reaction on the superior tarsal conjunctiva. The inferior tarsal conjunctiva is typically normal. Corneal hypoesthesia is also sometimes present.[1] The presence of filaments on the superior cornea should alert the clinician to the diagnosis of SLK, as this is

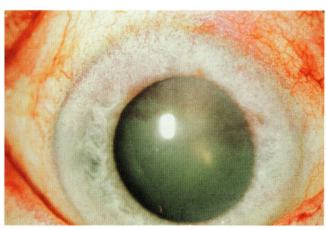

Figure 21.1 Bilateral presentation of a patient with SLK.

Figure 21.2 Rose bengal staining of superior bulbar conjunctiva and cornea, which is suggestive of a diagnosis of SLK.

the most common cause of this finding. When evaluating a patient for SLK, the upper lid should be everted to look for the common papillary reaction that is often seen in this condition. Key to the diagnosis of SLK is the willingness of the clinician to examine the superior bulbar conjunctiva. Many clinicians do not elevate the upper lid to examine the superior part of the eye. If the upper lid is not elevated, the diagnosis of SLK is missed. It is prudent to include lid elevation as part of the examination steps in any patient with ocular surface symptoms. Another factor in missing the diagnosis of SLK, is the fact that the superior bulbar conjunctival injection may be subtle. If the clinician looks at the superior conjunctiva with the biomicroscope on high magnification only, subtle findings may be unrecognized. It is useful in the SLK patient to simultaneously elevate both upper lids and look at the superior conjunctiva with the unaided eye. This simple technique may often be the most useful way to see the conjunctival injection.

Etiology

While there have been many theories about the etiology of SLK, some uncertainty remains. Some have suggested a viral cause, but cultures have been universally negative. In other studies, bacterial cultures have been shown to be positive but mostly for normal ocular flora. An autoimmune etiology has also been proposed, but this is also less likely, due to the lack of immunoglobulin deposition noted on direct immunofluorescence, a lack of increase in eosinophils, and the variable response to topical steroids. The most popular theory is that of mechanical trauma.

Abnormalities in the interaction of the superior tarsal and bulbar conjunctiva lead to constant abnormal movement of the superior bulbar conjunctiva during blinking. This abnormality could be due to tight apposition of the tarsal conjunctiva against the globe in the setting of thyroid eye disease, exophthalmos, scarring of the superior tarsal conjunctiva,[5] inflammation, or dryness. This theory is supported by the strong association of SLK with both thyroid dysfunction, which is found in 33% of patients suffering from SLK, and dry eye disease, which is found in 25% of patients diagnosed with SLK.[3] Further credence is given to the mechanical theory by the discovery that transforming growth factor-beta2 and tenascin are up-regulated in the conjunctiva of patients with SLK, as compared to controls. Expression of both of these is known to be affected by mechanical stress and injury.[6]

Other biochemical abnormalities have been identified in patients with SLK. For example, expression of certain cytokeratins (CKs) has been found to be altered when compared to controls. Decreased expression of a marker for nonkeratinized stratified squamous epithelium, CK13, has been noted, along with increased expression of CK14. Also, increased expression of CK10, a marker for keratinization, has been positively correlated with disease severity.[7] These results suggest that an abnormality of differentiation in the conjunctival epithelium plays a role in the disease. In other studies, an overexpression of matrix metalloproteinases 1 and 3 (MMP-1 and MMP-3) has been noted, but it is unclear exactly what role this plays in the pathogenesis of the disease.[8]

Diagnosis

Diagnosis of SLK is based primarily on the clinical findings described earlier. The redundancy of the superior bulbar conjunctiva can be demonstrated by using a cotton-tipped applicator to pull the conjunctiva down over the superior cornea. This should be done after application of topical anesthesia and is not possible with normal conjunctiva. Impression cytology may give additional certainty to the diagnosis but is rarely necessary. With impression cytology, impressions of the superior bulbar conjunctiva demonstrate severe squamous metaplasia, with an absence of goblet cells. Impressions of the superior tarsal conjunctiva show mild squamous metaplasia with many inflammatory cells, while impressions of the inferior tarsal conjunctiva are essentially normal.[9]

Confocal microscopy has recently been investigated as an adjunctive diagnostic tool when SLK is suspected clinically. Two variables that were studied were mean individual epithelial cell area (MIECA) and nucleocytoplasmic (N/C) ratio. As compared to normal controls, SLK patients were found to have a significantly increased MIECA and a decreased N/C ratio. Additionally, the inflammatory cell density in SLK patients was increased, compared to controls. This increase significantly correlated with superior bulbar conjunctival rose bengal scores, as measured by impression cytology, giving additional credence to confocal microscopy as a reliable diagnostic tool.[10]

Treatment

Over the past several decades, a variety of treatments for SLK have been explored with varying reports of success. Initially, topical medical treatments should be attempted. Aggressive lubrication of the ocular surface should be used, either alone or in conjunction with punctal occlusion. Autologous serum tears may be more beneficial than commercial artificial tears, providing objective and subjective improvement in 82% of cases.[11] Topical steroids are often used, and have resulted in symptomatic improvement in some cases, but the overall results have been variable. Topical cyclosporine A, used four times daily has had very good success, with symptom resolution in 100% of patients in one report.[12] Topical ketotifen fumarate has also met with promising success in symptom resolution, though objective signs have not always improved.[13] In addition, topical administration of vitamin A and mast cell stabilizers has led to symptom resolution in a high percentage of patients.[14,15]

If topical treatments are unsuccessful, injection of medication may be indicated. In one study, a supratarsal triamcinolone injection was found to decrease symptoms, as well as corneal and conjunctival staining in all patients who received the treatment.[16]

Chun and Kim used large-diameter contact lenses to decrease trauma to the superior bulbar conjunctiva, which resulted in improvement of symptoms in 38% of patients. Those SLK patients who did not improve were given an injection of botulinum toxin A to the pretarsal orbicularis muscle. This resulted in resolution of symptoms in 100% of patients.[4]

Surgical Treatment

As the hallmark of SLK is redundancy of the superior bulbar conjunctiva, the surgical treatments target that structural abnormality. Many different methods have been employed to attempt to tighten the redundant superior bulbar conjunctiva. Initial attempts using silver nitrate were effective, but caution needs to be taken as severe ocular burns can result, especially when using a solid applicator.[17] In fact, a solid silver nitrate application should never be utilized in the management of SLK. Some clinicians have advocated the use of thermocautery to tighten the superior bulbar conjunctiva. Udell et al. found that this led to symptom resolution in 73% of patients, in addition to an increase in the density of goblet cells after resolution.[18] Liquid nitrogen cryotherapy, using the double freeze–thaw technique, was found to resolve symptoms in 57% of eyes after one treatment and 100% of eyes after one repeat treatment.[19] Conjunctival fixation sutures placed in the superior fornix, have been reported to result in complete symptom resolution as well.[20]

Resection of the superior bulbar conjunctiva has been used in cases where medical treatment and/or conjunctival tightening have proven unsuccessful. This technique has been the most successful and predictable. For most clinicians this is the preferred and initial surgical treatment. Conjunctival resection has not only been shown to alleviate symptoms but also results in resolution of the squamous metaplasia of the affected conjunctiva. The surgical technique can be performed with topical anesthesia for most cases. The abnormal conjunctiva is outlined with a marking pen. Subconjunctival balanced salt solution is injected to assist in the separation of the conjunctiva and Tenon's fascia from the sclera. Resection of the conjunctiva and Tenon's is completed with a scissor. The conjunctival defect is then closed partially, by advancing the resected conjunctival border anteriorly. The conjunctiva can be sutured or fixated with tissue glue. The clinician must be careful not to resect too much conjunctiva. In rare cases, the redundant conjunctiva can recur, necessitating further conjunctival resection.

Conclusion

While SLK is an uncommon disorder, it should be suspected in all patients who present with eye irritation, burning, or foreign body sensation, especially in those who have failed conventional dry eye/blepharitis treatments. Careful examination of the superior conjunctiva, aided by vital staining, is imperative as part of the clinical examination. Several different medical and surgical treatments have proven successful in decreasing symptoms. Conjunctival resection is a very successful treatment for those patients requiring surgical intervention.

References

1. Theodore FH. Superior limbic keratoconjunctivitis. Eye Ear Nose Throat Mon 1963;42:25–8.
2. Bainbridge JW, Mackie IA, Mackie I. Diagnosis of Theodore's superior limbic keratoconjunctivitis. Eye (Lond) 1998;12(Pt 4):748–9.
3. Nelson JD. Superior limbic keratoconjunctivitis (SLK). Eye (Lond) 1989;3(Pt 2):180–9.
4. Chun YS, Kim JC. Treatment of superior limbic keratoconjunctivitis with a large-diameter contact lens and botulium toxin A. Cornea 2009;28:752–8.
5. Raber IM. Superior limbic keratoconjunctivitis in association with scarring of the superior tarsal conjunctiva. Cornea 1996;15:312–6.
6. Matsuda A, Tagawa Y, Matsuda H. TGF-beta2, tenascin, and integrin beta1 expression in superior limbic keratoconjunctivitis. Jpn J Ophthalmol 1999;43:251–6.
7. Matsuda A, Tagawa Y, Matsuda H. Cytokeratin and proliferative cell nuclear antigen expression in superior limbic keratoconjunctivitis. Curr Eye Res 1996;15:1033–8.
8. Sun YC, Hsiao CH, Chen WL, et al. Overexpression of matrix metalloproteinase-1 (MMP-1) and MMP-3 in superior limbic keratoconjunctivitis. Invest Ophthalmol Vis Sci 2011;52:3701–5.
9. Gris O. Conjunctival resection with and without amniotic membrane graft for the treatment of superior limbic keratoconjunctivitis. Cornea 2010;29:1025–30.
10. Kojima T, Matsumoto Y, Ibrahim OM, et al. In vivo evaluation of superior limbic keratoconjunctivitis using laser scanning confocal microscopy and conjunctival impression cytology. Invest Ophthalmol Vis Sci 2010;51:3986–92.
11. Goto E, Shimmura S, Shimazaki J, et al. Treatment of superior limbic keratoconjunctivitis by application of autologous serum. Cornea 2001;20:807–10.
12. Sahin A, Bozkurt B, Irkec M. Topical cyclosporine a in the treatment of superior limbic keratoconjunctivitis: a long-term follow-up. Cornea 2008;27:193–5.
13. Udell IJ, Guidera AC, Madani-Becker J. Ketotifen fumarate treatment of superior limbic keratoconjunctivitis. Cornea 2002;21:778–80.
14. Confino J, Brown SI. Treatment of superior limbic keratoconjunctivitis with topical cromolyn sodium. Ann Ophthalmol 1987;19:129–31.
15. Ohashi Y, Watanabe H, Kinoshita S, et al. Vitamin A eyedrops for superior limbic keratoconjunctivitis. Am J Ophthalmol 1988;105:523–7.
16. Shen YC, Wang CY, Tsai HY, et al. Supratarsal triamcinolone injection in the treatment of superior limbic keratoconjunctivitis. Cornea 2007;26:423–6.
17. Laughrea PA, Arentsen JJ, Laibson PR. Iatrogenic ocular silver nitrate burn. Cornea 1985–1986;4:47–50.
18. Udell IJ, Kenyon KR, Sawa M, et al. Treatment of superior limbic keratoconjunctivitis by thermocauterization of the superior bulbar conjunctiva. Ophthalmology 1986;93:162–6.
19. Fraunfelder FW. Liquid nitrogen cryotherapy of superior limbic keratoconjunctivitis. Am J Ophthalmol 2009;147:234–8.
20. Yamada M, Hatou S, Mochizuki H. Conjunctival fixation sutures for refractory superior limbic keratoconjunctivitis. Br J Ophthalmol 2009;93:1570–1.

22 *Oculodermal Surface Disease*

ANA CAROLINA VIEIRA and MARK J. MANNIS

A variety of disorders affect both the skin and the ocular surface. This chapter will focus on the oculodermal disorders that primarily affect the ocular surface, their clinical findings and principles of management. Stevens–Johnson syndrome and ocular cicatricial pemphigoid will be covered in greater detail in Chapters 30 and 31, respectively.

Rosacea

Acne rosacea is a chronic inflammatory condition that affects the central facial skin and may involve the eyes in up to 58% of patients.[1,2] Albeit common, rosacea is often overlooked, even though ocular rosacea is classified as one of the defined clinical subtypes of the disease. Early diagnosis and treatment are crucial in order to avoid disfiguring facial involvement, ocular morbidity and the emotional distress that untreated disease may cause.[3]

EPIDEMIOLOGY

Rosacea affects 16 million Americans and is commonly recognized to be more prevalent in fair-skinned patients of Celtic or Scandinavian origin.[4] Women are more commonly affected than men, and the onset is typically between the ages of 30 and 50 years.[4]

ETIOLOGY

The precise etiology of rosacea is uncertain. Among the various theories of causation are inflammatory, infectious, dietary, and psychological theories. Several studies support an inflammatory mechanism. An elevated concentration of interleukin-1 and greater activity of gelatinase B (MMP-9) were found in the tear fluids of patients with ocular rosacea.[5] Vascular dilation and incompetence may also contribute to the signs and symptoms of the disease.[6] Microbial organisms such as *Helicobacter pylori* and *Demodex folliculorum* have been identified as possible causative factors of the disease.[6] Molecular studies suggest that an altered innate immune response may be involved in the pathogenesis of this disorder, inducing high levels of cathelicidin, an antimicrobial peptide with vasoactive and pro-inflammatory actions.[7]

DIAGNOSIS

There is no objective diagnostic test specific to rosacea. The diagnosis is clinical, and the disease is often underdiagnosed since patients may be unaware of their symptoms, and physicians may not recognize the early findings, especially early ocular disease.[3]

A standard classification proposed by the National Rosacea Society Expert Committee was published in 2002.

This classification system describes primary and secondary features of rosacea and defines four subtypes of the disease (erythematotelangiectatic, papulopustular, phymatous, and ocular). Evolution from one subtype to another may or may not occur. The features of rosacea are listed in Table 22.1.[4]

CLINICAL FINDINGS

Rosacea develops gradually and begins with transient flushing that may be triggered by certain factors that are specific to each individual. The most common triggers are listed in Table 22.2. As disease progresses, transitory erythema and telangiectasia of the skin become apparent. Chronic,

Table 22.1 Primary and Secondary Features of Rosacea

Primary Features	Description
Flushing (transient erythema)	Frequent blushing or flushing
Non-transient erythema	Persistent redness of the facial skin
Papules and pustules	Red papules with or without pustules. Nodules.
Telangiectasia	Telangiectases are common but not necessary for a rosacea diagnosis

Secondary Features	Description
Burning or stinging sensations	
Elevated plaques	
Dry appearance	Dry appearance of central facial skin
Edema	Facial edema
Ocular manifestations	
Peripheral location	
Phymatous changes	

The presence of one or more of the primary signs with an axial facial distribution is indicative of rosacea. One or more of the secondary features may or may not be present.[4]
(Adapted from the Standard Classification of Rosacea, proposed by the National Rosacea Society Expert Committee (Wilkin J, Dahl M, Detmar M et al. Standard classification of rosacea: Report of the National Rosacea Society Expert Committee on the classification and staging of rosacea. J Am Acad Dermatol 2002;46:584–7)

Table 22.2 Most Common Trigger Factors of Rosacea

Foods and Drinks	Environmental	Emotional
Spicy food	Sun exposure	Anger
Chocolate	Heat	Stress
Soy sauce	Excessive cold	Embarrassment
Dairy products	Wind	**Others**
Alcohol	Humidity	Exercise
Hot drinks		Menopause

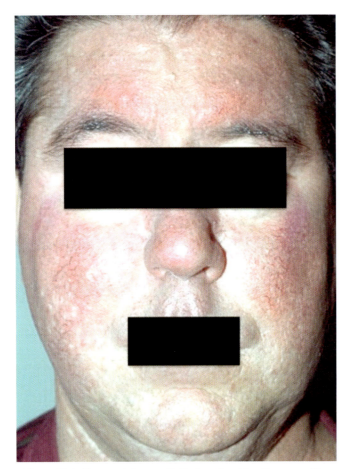

Figure 22.1 Characteristic roseatic findings involving the convexities of the central face (cheeks, chin, nose and forehead).

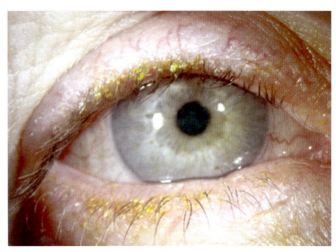

Figure 22.2 Blepharitis in a patient with ocular rosacea. Note the lid telangiectasia.

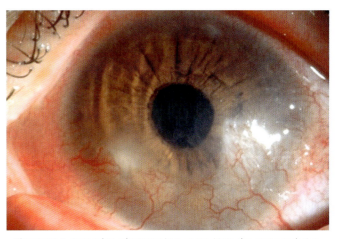

Figure 22.3 Corneal involvement in rosacea. Note the neovascularization with triangular infiltrates.

untreated disease may present with persistent erythema, telangiectasia, papules, pustules and sebaceous gland hypertrophy localized primarily on the convexities of the central face (cheeks, chin, nose and forehead) (Fig. 22.1).[4]

OCULAR ROSACEA

Ocular involvement has been reported in up to 58% of patients with rosacea and corneal involvement in 33%.[3] As many as 90% of patients with ocular rosacea may have only very subtle skin changes, and in 20% of the cases, the ocular signs may precede skin involvement, making the diagnosis particularly challenging.[1]

The ocular rosacea patient may complain of foreign body sensation, 'bloodshot' appearance, dryness, photophobia and tearing. Decreased visual acuity may be present in cases with corneal involvement.

The findings in ocular rosacea are often non-specific, the most common being meibomian gland dysfunction and blepharitis (Fig. 22.2). A history of recurrent hordeolum and chalazia is common. Chronic conjunctivitis characterized by interpalpebral conjunctival hyperemia may be present. When corneal involvement is present, it typically begins with peripheral neovascularization, which may coalesce into characteristic triangular subepithelial marginal infiltrates (Fig. 22.3). These 'spade-shaped' inflammatory infiltrates can progress to the central cornea and lead to ulceration and perforation.[2] Other reported ocular findings include dendritic keratopathy, iritis, episcleritis, scleritis and even scleral perforation (Fig. 22.4).[3,8]

TREATMENT

The initial management of rosacea is the identification and avoidance of trigger factors. With manifest early skin disease, the dermatologic manifestations of rosacea may be controlled with topical medications, such as metronidazole cream (0.75% and 1% formulations), azelaic acid gel 15% and sulfacetamide/sulfur.[9,10] Other topical treatments include clindamycin, erythromycin, pimecrolimus, tacrolimus and tretinoin.[10] When topical treatment alone is insufficient, systemic therapy should be initiated. Oral tetracyclines (500 mg twice daily) and doxycycline (40–100 mg daily from 8 to 16 weeks) have safely improved both skin and ocular rosacea. In 2006, the FDA approved a daily formulation of 40 mg doxycycline monohydrate (Oracea®, Galderma) for the treatment of rosacea. In unresponsive cases and those when tetracyclines are

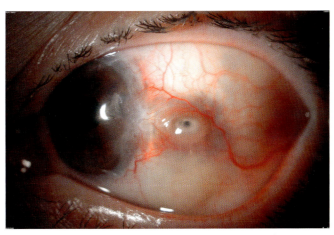

Figure 22.4 A rare case of spontaneous scleral perforation in a patient with ocular rosacea.

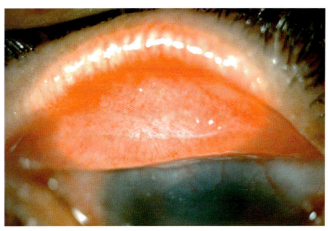

Figure 22.5 Subepithelial fibrosis at the tarsal conjunctiva in a patient with OCP.

contraindicated, oral azythromycin (500 mg/day for 2 weeks) is considered an option. Oral isotretinoin (0.3 to 1.0 mg/kg/day) is recommended in more severe intractable cases. Vascular laser therapy and intense pulsed light can be used for treatment of resistant skin telangiectasias and persistent erythema.[9,10]

The management of mild ocular rosacea includes warm compresses and lid hygiene. Antibiotic ointments prescribed daily, at bedtime, may decrease eyelid flora and help soften collarettes. Moderate ocular rosacea should be treated with oral tetracycline or doxycycline in addition to local ocular therapy. As in the management of skin rosacea, tetracyclines may be initially administered 500 mg twice daily, or 250 mg four times daily for 3–4 weeks, and then tapered according to monitored clinical response. Doxycycline may be prescribed in a regimen of 40–100 mg once or twice daily for 6–12 weeks.[10] Many patients present with flare-ups once the medication is discontinued and may, therefore, require long-term maintenance therapy at a titrated maintenance dose. Topical azithromycin can be useful as an off-label treatment for posterior blepharitis in ocular rosacea, particularly in patients intolerant to oral antibiotics mentioned earlier.

In cases of severe ocular surface inflammation, episcleritis, iritis and keratitis, topical steroids may prove beneficial but must be monitored for steroid-induced side effects.[10] If corneal thinning or perforation occurs, surgical intervention may be necessary. Placement of cyanoacrylate glue, lamellar patch grafts, and penetrating keratoplasty are management options.

Ocular Cicatricial pemphigoid

Mucous membrane pemphigoid (cicatricial pemphigoid) consists of a group of chronic and progressive autoimmune subepithelial blistering diseases that may affect the oral, ocular, pharyngeal, laryngeal, genital and anal mucosa.[11] Characteristically, cicatricial pemphigoid demonstrates linear deposits of IgG, IgA, or C3 in the epithelial basement membrane on immunofluorescence microscopy or immunoperoxidase analysis.[11]

Mucous membrane pemphigoid (MMP) that involves primarily the ocular surface, as chronic and progressive cicatrizing conjunctivitis is referred to as ocular cicatricial pemphigoid (OCP). However, ocular manifestations are present in 60% to 77% of all MMP patients.[11,12]

EPIDEMIOLOGY

Ocular cicatricial pemphigoid is considered a relatively rare disease, and its incidence is estimated to be between 1 in 15000 and 1 in 60000 ophthalmic patients.[11] The average age at diagnosis is between 60 and 70 years. Women are more commonly affected than men (2:1 ratio). No geographical or racial predilection has been reported.[11,12]

CLINICAL FINDINGS

The findings in OCP are usually bilateral but may be asymmetric. Patients initially complain of non-specific symptoms: irritation, tearing, burning, foreign body sensation and excessive mucus production. Early signs include recurrent papillary conjunctivitis and fine subepithelial scarring at the tarsal conjunctiva (Fig. 22.5).[11] Episodes of aggravation of the conjunctival inflammation followed by quiescent phases are observed throughout the course of the disease. With progression, worsening of the cicatrizing conjunctivitis, foreshortening of the conjunctival fornices and symblepharon formation (Fig. 22.6) occur. In more advanced cases, ankyloblepharon, cicatricial entropion, keratinization of the eyelid margins and trichiasis may develop.[11]

Corneal function is compromised in advanced disease as a result of chronic exposure, abnormal lid/globe contact and trauma from aberrant eyelashes. Dry eye also contributes to disruption of the corneal surface and is secondary to a combination of diminished aqueous tear production, mucin deficiency due to loss of conjunctival goblet cells and an accompanying predisposition to blepharitis. Corneal findings range from localized or diffuse punctate epitheliopathy to ulceration, opacification, neovascularization (Fig. 22.7) keratinization, and perforation that may lead to

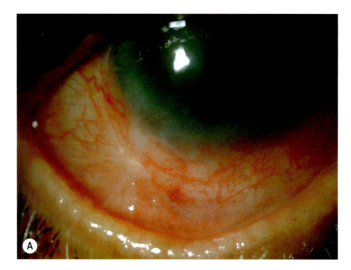

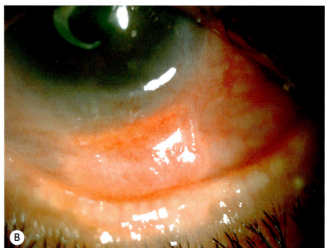

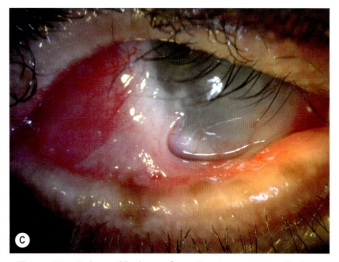

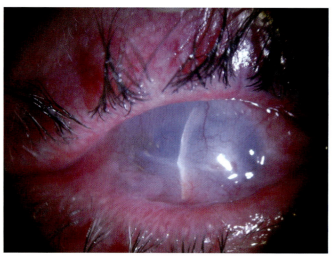

Figure 22.7 Severe corneal involvement in OCP.

Figure 22.6 Early symblepharon formation in a patient with OCP. (**A**) Right eye. (**B**) Left eye. (**C**) A more advanced case of OCP with trichiasis and symblepharon.

blindness. The compromised ocular surface is also at increased risk of bacterial and fungal keratitis.[11]

STAGING SYSTEMS

There are two widely accepted staging systems: one described by Mondino et al. and another by Foster et al.[13,14] Table 22.3 describes both systems. Since the disease is asymmetric, each eye should be evaluated separately.

TREATMENT

Dapsone is commonly used as the initial therapeutic agent in mild to moderate OCP.[15,16] For severe or more rapidly progressive disease, more aggressive therapy with systemic corticosteroids and cytotoxic agents such as cyclophosphamide is recommended.[11,15] Systemic treatments with methotrexate, cyclosporine A, azathioprine, mycophenolate mofetil and intravenous immunoglobulin therapy have also been used effectively.[11] Recommended doses are listed in Table 22.4. However, despite immunosuppression, some patients progress to end-stage ocular surface disease and eventual blindness.

Local adjunct management includes preservative-free lubricant drops, and punctal occlusion may also improve dry eye. Topical tacrolimus and subconjunctival mitomycin C have also been employed to decrease conjunctival inflammation and reverse the formation of symblepharon respectively. Topical corticosteroids do not effectively control the progression of disease and should, therefore, be avoided as the sole treatment of acute flare-ups or as a sole prolonged therapeutic approach.[11] Aberrant eyelashes may be treated with epilation or cryotherapy. Scleral contact lenses may be useful in protecting the ocular surface from trichiatic lashes and maintaining a wet corneal surface, permitting epithelial defects to heal.[17]

The ocular complications of advanced OCP may require surgical intervention including tarsorrhaphy, keratoplasty, limbal grafting and/or amniotic membrane transplantation, and keratoprosthesis. However, since surgical intervention may lead to exacerbation of conjunctival inflammation, surgical procedures should be performed as

Table 22.3 Description of Staging Systems for OCP[13,14]

	Stage I	Stage II	Stage III	Stage IV
Mondino et al.[13]	<25% shortening of conjunctival fornices	25–50% shortening of conjunctival fornices	50–75% shortening of conjunctival fornices	End-stage cicatricial pemphigoid
Foster et al.[14]	Chronic conjunctivitis with subepithelial fibrosis	Shortening of the inferior fornix	Symblepharon formation	End-stage OCP, surface keratinization, ankyloblepharon

Table 22.4 List of Main Systemic Immunosuppressive Agents Used for the Control of Ocular Cicatricial Pemphigoid

Immunossuppressive Agent	Dose
Dapsone*	50–200 mg/day
Prednisone	1 mg/kg/day
Cyclophosphamide	1–2 mg/kg/day
Azathioprine	1–2 mg/kg/day
Methotrexate+	5–10 mg/week
Mycophenolate mofetil	2–3 g/day

*Contraindicated in patients with glucose-6-phosphate dehydrogenase (G6PDH) deficiency due to risk of severe hemolytic anemia.
+Should be used with alternate-day folic acid (5 mg) to reduce the risk of adverse effects.

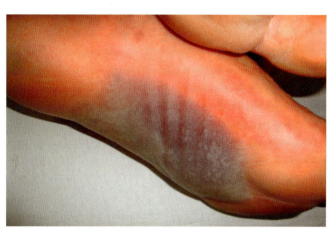

Figure 22.8 Epidermal detachment at plantar area in a patient with SJS.

necessary in the acute phase of the disease and only when the inflammatory component of the disease has been controlled by medication and remission has been achieved in the chronic stage. The prognosis for corneal grafting and keratoprosthesis surgery is extremely guarded in these patients.

Stevens–Johnson Syndrome and Toxic Epidermal Necrolysis

Stevens–Johnson Syndrome (SJS) and toxic epidermal necrolysis (TEN) constitute a group of acute, immune-mediated inflammatory diseases involving mucosal membranes and the skin. SJS is considered the less severe of the two conditions. Both are characterized by epidermal necrosis and mucosal involvement that can be induced by certain drugs or infections. A genetic predisposition has also been implicated.[18] Both diseases are rare, with an estimated incidence of approximately 1.2–6 and 0.4–1.2 cases per million persons, respectively.[19] Gender distribution is almost equal. Even with appropriate therapy, high mortality rates are observed in severe SJS and in TEN, and survivors suffer from long-term ocular surface complications that can lead to functional blindness.[20]

ETIOLOGY

The drugs most commonly associated with SJS and TEN are nevirapine, abacavir, lamotrigine, allopurinol, phenytoin, phenobarbital, carbamazepine, sulfonamide and beta-lactam antibiotics, tetracyclines, quinolones and NSAIDs. Infections associated with SJS and TEN include *Mycoplasma pneumoniae*, *Mycobacterium tuberculosis*, group A streptococci, hepatitis B virus, herpes simplex virus, Epstein–Barr virus, enterovirus and HIV.[18]

CLINICAL FINDINGS

In 1993, a consensus definition was established, and the clinical criteria for SJS were defined as widespread macules or flat atypical target lesions and epidermal detachment on less than 10% of the body surface area (Fig. 22.8).[18] Involvement of more than 30% of the body surface area was classified as TEN. Epidermal detachment between 10% and 30% was classified as SJS/TEN overlap.[18] Initial manifestations are usually fever and malaise. Cutaneous erythema, vesicular eruption and hemorrhagic erosions of mucous membranes follow these initial findings.

The ocular mucosa is involved in 69–82% of cases of SJS and in 50–88% of cases of TEN during the acute phase.[19] Chronic ocular complications are present in up to 35% of patients.[21] Other mucous membranes may be affected, with the oral mucosa most commonly involved (Fig. 22.9). Internal organ involvement is uncommon.

OCULAR MANIFESTATIONS

The acute stage of ocular surface disease is is usually in the first 2 weeks after onset of symptoms. The initial ocular findings are lid edema, conjunctival inflammation and necrosis. Fifteen to seventy-five percent of the patients develop bilateral membranous conjunctivitis (Fig. 22.10) that is often difficult to control.[21] Corneal involvement including epithelial defects and corneal infiltrates develop in approximately 25% of hospitalized patients.[21]

Despite intensive treatment during the acute stage, persistent inflammation of the ocular surface might continue even after hospital discharge. This prolonged inflammation might lead to destruction of limbal stem cells and

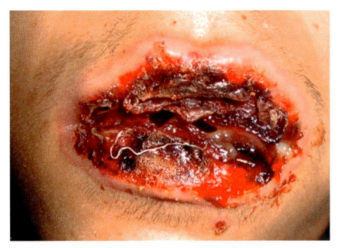

Figure 22.9 Hemorrhagic erosions of oral mucosa in SJS.

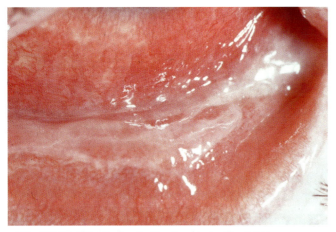

Figure 22.10 SJS with pseudomembranous conjunctivitis.

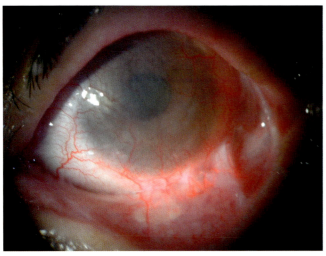

Figure 22.11 Symblepharon formation and complete corneal opacification and neovascularization in SJS.

secondary conjunctivalization and vascularization of the cornea, leading to profound visual loss.

Chronic inflammation may also lead to extensive scarring and symblepharon formation (Fig. 22.11), ankyloblepharon and alterations of the lid margins including trichiasis, entropion, and punctal occlusion. Sight-threatening corneal sequelae result from blink-related microtrauma caused by these cicatricial complications.[18] The destruction of goblet cells causing severe mucin deficiency dry eye and keratinization of the ocular surface are other common long-term complications.

TREATMENT

Identification and withdrawal of the inducing drug is crucial. If an infection is the cause, adequate antimicrobial treatment must be initiated promptly. A multidisciplinary approach is required in the management of the affected patient. In the acute stage, immunosuppressive therapy with corticosteroids, cyclosporine and intravenous immunoglobulins are controversial but are commonly employed.[18,19] Immunosuppressive intervention may reduce inflammation, but may increase the risk of infection. Additional treatment is based on supportive care, including repletion of fluid loss, prevention of infection is necessary, and in the severest of cases, patients are managed similar to burn patients.

Ocular mucosal lesions require close monitoring. Topical prophylactic antibiotics and corticosteroids may be used for acute management. Ocular maintenance includes the frequent use of preservative-free lubricant drops and ointment. Corneal epithelial defects may be treated using bandage contact lenses. Intravenous steroid pulse therapy has shown promising results in preventing ocular complications.[20]

Transplantation of cryopreserved amniotic membrane within 2 weeks of the onset of symptoms has shown promising results in promoting healing and reducing ocular surface inflammation and scarring.[21]

Prevention of symblepharon formation may reduce long-term complications. Removal of pseudomembranes, lysis of symblepharon using a glass rod and debridement of loose epithelium may improve the prognosis for the chronic stage.[21]

Scleral contact lenses may also be beneficial, providing mechanical protection from the lid margins and eyelashes and maintaining a moist cornea by preserving a pre-corneal tear reservoir.

Treatment of long-term complications may require transplantation of limbal stem cells prior to keratoplasty. Because limbal stem cell deficiency is usually bilateral in SJS/TEN, transplantation of allogeneic limbal stem cells is frequently necessary, requiring systemic immunosuppression, and is associated with a guarded prognosis.[22]

Keratoprosthesis is another option for visual rehabilitation in more severe cases; however, the results in SJS are worse than in non-autoimmune disorders.[22]

Ectodermal Dysplasias

The ectodermal dysplasias constitute a group of rare inherited disorders affecting the development of structures of ectodermal origin: hair, teeth, nails and sweat glands. This defect can lead to a range of conditions with variable inheritance patterns. More than 120 different ectodermal dysplasias have been described.

ECTRODACTYLY–ECTODERMAL DYSPLASIA-CLEFT LIP (EEC) SYNDROME

The EEC syndrome is characterized by ectrodactyly (lobster claw deformity of hands and feet), ectodermal dysplasia and cleft lip and palate (Fig. 22.12). It is an autosomal dominant condition, with incomplete penetrance and variable expressivity, caused by mutations in the *p63* gene.[23,24]

Ocular Involvement and Therapy

The most common ocular manifestations are partial or complete absence of the meibomian glands and abnormalities of the lacrimal drainage system with resulting keratopathy.[23] Anomalies of the lacrimal drainage system are present in up to 87% of patients and include absence or atresia of the puncta, incomplete development of the canaliculi, lacrimal sac or nasolacrimal ducts. Corneal involvement includes punctate keratopathy, stromal infiltration, opacification, thinning, pannus formation, neovascularization, and limbal stem cell deficiency.[24] Recurrent erosions and corneal perforations have also been reported.[25] Other ocular manifestations have been observed in EEC syndrome including telecanthus, micro/anophthalmia, trichiasis, entropion, madarosis (paucity of lashes and eyebrows) and blepharoconjunctivitis.[25] Linear deposition of antibasement membrane autoantibodies, similar to that seen in mucous membrane pemphigoid, was observed in four of six EEC syndrome patients with cicatrizing conjunctivitis.[26]

The treatment of ocular disease is aimed at symptomatic relief and preservation of vision. Tear substitutes provide protection of the ocular surface. Prophylactic antibiotics and topical corticosteroids reduce infection and inflammation, respectively. Epithelial defects may be managed with bandage contact lenses. Corneal perforations may require gluing or a corneal patch grafting. Visual rehabilitation may also employ limbal stem cell transplantation and keratoplasty. Drainage system anomalies may require surgical treatment, which may range from probing to dacryocystorhinostomy.

ANKYLOBLEPHARON–ECTODERMAL DEFECTS-CLEFT LIP/PALATE (AEC) SYNDROME

The AEC syndrome, or Hay–Wells syndrome, is a rare autosomal dominant syndrome associated with mutations in the *p63* gene.[27] It is characterized by ankyloblepharon, cleft lip/palate and ectodermal defects such as sparse hair, nail and dental changes, impairment in sweating and skin erosions. Such cutaneous erosions, especially in the scalp, are characteristic features of neonates with this disorder and are often complicated by infections.[27]

Ocular Involvement

Ankyloblepharon is present in 100% of cases. Other common ocular findings are blepharitis, conjunctivitis, disorders of the lacrimal system and madarosis of eyelashes and eyebrows.[27]

KERATITIS–ICTHYOSIS–DEAFNESS (KID) SYNDROME

The KID syndrome is a rare congenital disorder characterized by keratitis, deafness, and skin manifestations that are better classified as erythrokeratoderma than as ichthyosis.[28] Autosomal recessive and dominant cases have been reported.[28] Mutations in the GJB2 gene coding for connexin 26, a component of gap junctions in epithelial cells, have been observed.[29]

Early in life, neonates develop a transient generalized erythema. The skin findings gradually progress into hyperkeratotic plaques located on the forehead, cheeks, perioral area, and scalp, and the patient develops a leonine facies.[28,30] Hyperkeratosis may also be found on the trunk, elbows, knees and palmoplantar areas. During early infancy, the patient may develop keratitis and moderate to severe neurosensorial hearing impairment. There is also a predisposal to squamous cell carcinoma and increased risk of infections.[28,30]

Ocular Involvement and Therapy

Bilateral asymmetric corneal involvement with superficial and deep vascularization is present in more than 80% of patients (Fig. 22.13). Recurrent corneal erosions, corneal

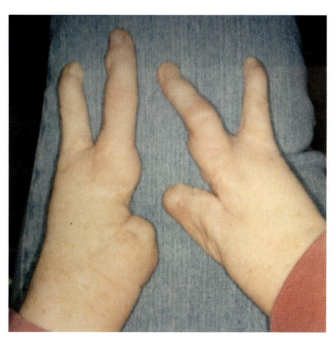

Figure 22.12 Lobster claw deformity of the hands in EEC syndrome.

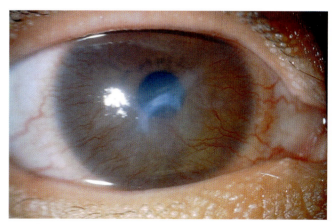

Figure 22.13 Corneal findings in KID syndrome.

scarring, decreased tear production and limbal stem cell deficiency are other common signs.[31] Lid margin alterations include meibomian gland dysfunction, trichiasis and keratinization. Sparse eyebrows and eyelashes are also frequently present.[31]

Preservation of useful vision may be a challenge. Therapy includes lubricant drops and ointment, topical corticosteroids and cyclosporine, and oral doxycycline. Bandage contact lenses may be used for treatment of recurrent epithelial erosions.[32] Recommended surgical procedures include amniotic membrane transplantation, superficial keratectomy and limbal allograft transplantation. Lamellar and penetrating keratoplasty as well as keratoprosthesis may be attempted for visual rehabilitation.[32]

References

1. Ghanem VC, Mehra N, Wong S, et al. The prevalence of ocular signs in acne rosacea: comparing patients from ophthalmology and dermatology clinics. Cornea 2003;22:230–3.
2. Alvarenga LS, Mannis MJ. Ocular rosacea. Ocul Surf 2005;3:41–58.
3. Cohen AF, Tiemstra JD. Diagnosis and treatment of rosacea. J Am Board Fam Pract 2002;15:214–7.
4. Wilkin J, Dahl M, Detmar M, et al. Standard classification of rosacea: Report of the National Rosacea Society Expert Committee on the classification and staging of rosacea. J Am Acad Dermatol 2002;46:584–7.
5. Afonso AA, Sobrin L, Monroy DC, et al. Tear fluid gelatinase B activity correlates with IL-1alfa concentration and fluorescein clearance in ocular rosacea. Invest Ophthalmol Vis Sci 1999;40:2506–12.
6. Crawford GH, Pelle MT, James WD. Rosacea: I. Etiology, pathogenesis, and subtype classification. J Am Acad Dermatol 2004;51:327–41.
7. Meyer-Hoffert U, Schröder JM. Epidermal proteases in the pathogenesis of rosacea. J Investig Dermatol Symp Proc 2011;15:16–23.
8. Vieira AC, Mannis MJ. Spontaneous scleral perforation in ocular rosacea. Vision Pan-America 2009;8(1):149–51.
9. Odom R, Dahl M, Dover J, et al. Standard management options for rosacea, Part 1: Overview and broad spectrum of care. Cutis 2009;84:43–7.
10. Odom R, Dahl M, Dover J, et al. Standard management options for rosacea, Part 2: options according to subtype. National Rosacea Society Expert Committee on the Classification and Staging of Rosacea. Cutis 2009;84:97–104.
11. Kirzhner M, Jakobiec FA. Ocular cicatricial pemphigoid: a review of clinical features, immunopathology, differential diagnosis, and current management. Semin Ophthalmol 2011;26:270–7.
12. Chang JH, McCluskey PJ. Ocular cicatricial pemphigoid: manifestations and management. Curr Allergy Asthma Rep 2005;5:333–8.
13. Mondino BJ, Brown SI. Ocular cicatricial pemphigoid. Ophthalmol 1981;88:95–100.
14. Foster CS. Cicatricial pemphigoid. Trans Am Opthalmol Soc 1986;84:527–663.
15. Chan LS, Ahmed AR, Anhalt GJ, et al. The first international consensus on mucous membrane pemphigoid: definition, diagnostic criteria, pathogenic factors, medical treatment, and prognostic indicators. Arch Dermatol 2002;138:370–9.
16. Bruch-Gerharz D, Hertl M, Ruzicka T. Mucous membrane pemphigoid: clinical aspects, immunopathological features and therapy. Eur J Dermatol 2007;17:191–200.
17. Schornack MM, Baratz KH. Ocular cicatricial pemphigoid: the role of scleral lenses in disease management. Cornea 2009;28:1170–2.
18. Mockenhaupt M. The current understanding of Stevens–Johnson syndrome and toxic epidermal necrolysis. Expert Rev Clin Immunol 2011;7:803–15.
19. Fu Y, Gregory DG, Sippel KC, et al. The ophthalmologist's role in the management of acute Stevens–Johnson syndrome and toxic epidermal necrolysis. Ocul Surf 2010;8:193–203.
20. Araki Y, Sotozono C, Inatomi T. Successful treatment of Stevens–Johnson syndrome with steroid pulse therapy at disease onset. Am J Ophthalmol 2009;147:1004–11.
21. Gregory DG. The ophthalmologic management of acute Stevens–Johnson syndrome. Ocul Surf 2008;6:87–95.
22. Sayegh RR, Ang LP, Foster CS, et al. The Boston keratoprosthesis in Stevens–Johnson syndrome. Am J Ophthalmol 2008;145:43–444.
23. Kaercher T. Ocular symptoms and signs in patients with ectodermal dysplasia syndromes. Graefes Arch Clin Exp Ophthalmol 2004;242:495–500.
24. Di Iorio E, Kaye SB, Ponzin D, et al. Limbal stem cell deficiency and ocular phenotype in ectrodactyly-ectodermal dysplasia-clefting syndrome caused by p63 mutations. Ophthalmoogy 2012;119:74–83.
25. McNab A, Potts M, Welham R. The EEC syndrome and its ocular manifestations. Br J Ophthalmol 1989;73:261–4.
26. Saw V, Dart J, Sitaru C, et al. Cicatrising conjunctivitis with anti-basement membrane autoantibodies in ectodermal dysplasia. Br J Ophthalmol 2008;92:1403–10.
27. Fete M, vanBokhoven H, Clements S, et al. Conference report: international research symposium on ankyloblepharon-ectodermal defects-cleft lip and/or palate (AEC) syndrome. Am J Med Genet A 2009;149A:1885–93.
28. Abdollahi A, Hallaji Z, Esmaili N, et al. KID syndrome. Dermatol Online J 2007;13:11.
29. Schütz M, Auth T, Gehrt A. The connexin26 S17F mouse mutant represents a model for the human hereditary keratitis–ichthyosis–deafness syndrome. Hum Mol Genet 2011;20:28–39.
30. Gonzales ME, Tlougan BE, Price HN, et al. Keratitis, icthyosis and deafness (KID) syndrome. Dermatol Online J 2009;15:11.
31. Meesmer EM, Kenyon KR, Rittinger O, et al. Ocular manifestations of keratitis–icthyosis–deafness syndrome. Ophthalmol 2005;112:e1–e6.
32. Djalilian AR, Kim JY, Saeed HN, et al. Histopathology and treatment of corneal disease in keratitis, ichthyosis, and deafness (KID) syndrome. Eye (Lond) 2010;24:738–40.

23 Ocular Graft-versus-Host Disease

PATRICIA A. PLE-PLAKON and SHAHZAD I. MIAN

Introduction

Hematopoietic stem cell transplantation (HSCT) is an increasingly common treatment for hematologic, immunologic, metabolic and neoplastic diseases. Graft-versus-host disease (GVHD) is a complication of allogeneic HSCT where an immunologic response by donor cells against host tissues occurs due to incompatibility between the recipient and donor cells. The prevalence of GVHD varies between 10% and 90% depending on age, donor cell compatibility, host environment, and prophylaxis protocols.[1,2] Human leukocyte antigen (HLA) markers are the most important factors, triggering the immune response and leading to the onset of GVHD. Tissues most commonly targeted by donor cells include, the gastrointestinal system, liver, lungs, skin and eyes.

GVHD has traditionally been characterized as acute and chronic, based on the time of onset. Acute GVHD occurs within the first 100 days after HSCT, while chronic GVHD occurs after that time. Ocular complications are most commonly associated with chronic GVHD.

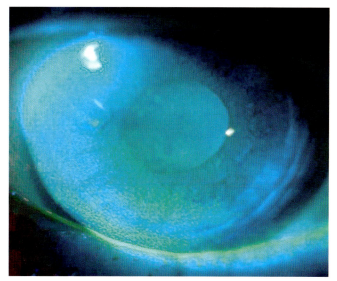

Figure 23.1 Patient with ocular GVHD with diffuse corneal and lid margin fluorescein staining.

Clinical Manifestations

Ocular GVHD affects 60–90% of patients with chronic systemic GVHD and may be the initial presentation of systemic GVHD.[3,4] Ocular manifestations vary widely from mild findings, to severe ocular sequelae and can affect the eyelid, lacrimal gland, conjunctiva, tear film, cornea, lens, vitreous, retina and optic nerve.[3,5–7] The most common presentation includes diseases of the ocular surface and lacrimal gland, with symptoms of dryness, irritation, blurred vision, photophobia, redness, and mucous discharge. Dry eye syndrome (DES) or keratoconjunctivitis sicca (KCS) occurs in 70% of GVHD patients. Patients, especially those with severe disease, frequently demonstrate conjunctival edema, chemosis, and pseudomembrane formation. Disease progression may lead to punctate keratopathy, corneal epithelial erosions, and corneal infections and ulcerations (Fig. 23.1). In addition to keratoconjunctivitis sicca, frequent manifestations of ocular GVHD include, conjunctival inflammation and fibrosis, cicatricial lagophthalmos, sterile conjunctivitis and uveitis.[6,8] It may also manifest with lacrimal gland dysfunction, spontaneous lacrimal punctual occlusion (SLPO), cicatricial ectropion or entropion, trichiasis, meibomian gland dysfunction, calcareous corneal degeneration, corneal perforation, synechiae, cataract, retinal vasculitis, retinal hemorrhage and optic neuropathy.[5–7,9–12] Ocular GVHD can have clinical manifestations similar to those of autoimmune and collagen vascular diseases affecting the eye, but ocular GVHD does not typically affect the posterior chamber.

Appropriate and timely treatment of ocular GVHD is critical, as a delay can lead to more serious manifestations, including chronic filamentary keratitis, corneal scarring, ulceration, and corneal perforation. This can result in significant morbidity and potentially permanent vision loss.

Pathophysiology

The immune response in GVHD is based on the role of donor T-lymphocytic cells in mounting an attack against host tissues. The primary cells responsible for this attack are the donor T-helper type 1 cells in acute GVHD and the donor T-helper type 2 cells in chronic GVHD. While the mechanism behind chronic GVHD has not been fully elucidated, there is a decreased tolerance to self-antigens and inflammatory reactions in multiple organ systems.

Conjunctivitis is commonly observed as a localized ocular reaction in GVHD. Although the mechanism is not fully understood, flow cytometry has demonstrated the proliferation of T cells in subconjunctival immunogenic inflammation.[13] Histopathology has revealed lymphocyte exocytosis and satellitosis, dyskeratotic cells, epithelial cell necrosis, subepithelial microvesicle formation and eventually, total separation of the epithelium in the conjunctiva of patients with GVHD.[6,14] Epithelial attenuation and goblet cell depletion have also been observed.[9]

In GVHD, donor lymphocytes infiltrate the lacrimal gland, leading to widespread fibrosis and aqueous tear deficiency.[15] Histopathology of the lacrimal gland in patients with chronic GVHD and DES reveals PAS-positive material accumulation in the acini and ductules, predominant T-cell infiltration in periductal areas, increased number and activation of stromal fibroblasts and excessive extracellular matrix fibrosis.[16] There is also prominent fibrosis of the glandular interstitium, similar to the chronic skin GVHD changes with generalized sclerodermal lichenoid.[9] Postmortem autopsy studies of the lacrimal gland in patients with GVHD have shown stasis of lacrimal gland secretions, epithelial cell debris within the lumina of lacrimal glands and periductal inflammation and fibrosis.[15] Additionally, immunohistochemical studies show primarily CD4 and CD8 T-cell infiltration in periductal areas of lacrimal glands of patients with chronic GVHD.[15]

Meibomian gland dysfunction (MGD) can also lead to dry eye symptoms in patients with GVHD. The meibomian glands secrete the lipid component of the tear film in order to retard tear evaporation. A recent study reported that 63% of chronic GVHD patients had MGD, with significant correlation in severity of DES symptoms.[6]

Diagnosis

A thorough patient history and ocular examination are necessary for the clinical diagnosis of ocular GVHD. Essential components of the history include extent of systemic GVHD, as well as systemic medications. The diagnostic criteria for ocular GVHD were established by the National Institutes of Health Consensus Development Project on Criteria for Clinical Trials in Chronic Graft-versus-Host Disease in 2005. The Diagnosis and Staging Working Group has stated that a mean Schirmer value of 5 mm at 5 minutes or new onset of keratoconjunctivitis sicca by slit lamp examination, with a mean Schirmer value of 6–10 mm, is sufficient for the diagnosis of chronic GVHD, if accompanied by involvement of at least one other organ system.[17]

Conjunctival biopsy may also aid in the diagnosis of ocular GVHD. Histopathology may reveal lymphocyte exocytosis and satellitosis, dyskeratotic cells, epithelial cell necrosis, subepithelial microvesicle formation and eventual total separation of the epithelium in the conjunctiva of patients with GVHD.[6,14]

Classification

Multiple classification systems have been used to categorize ocular GVHD. In 1989, Jabs et al. proposed a clinical staging system for conjunctival involvement in ocular GVHD (Table 23.1).[14] In 1998, Kiang et al. characterized the course of ocular GVHD into four stages (Table 23.2).[18]

An alternative classification system was proposed by Robinson et al. in 2004.[19] In this system, clinically relevant grading criteria for conjunctival GVHD are based on conjunctival pathology, observed in chronic GVHD patients (Table 23.3).

Table 23.1 Clinical Staging System for Conjunctivitis in Ocular GVHD

Stage I	Hyperemia
Stage II	Hyperemia with chemosis and/or serosanguineous exudates
Stage III	Pseudomembranous/membranous conjunctivitis

(Adapted from Jabs DA, Wingard J, Green WR, et al. The eye in bone marrow transplantation. III. Conjunctival graft-vs-host disease. Arch Ophthalmol 1989;107:1343–8.)

Table 23.2 Stages of Ocular GVHD

Stage 1	Subclinical stage	Tearing, mild nonspecific discomfort and photophobia. Mild chemosis, possible rose bengal staining. Lasting from a few days up to 1 month before other systemic symptoms of GVHD occur or the patient progresses to a more severe form of ocular GVHD.
Stage 2	Active stage	Mucopurulent conjunctivitis, pseudomembranous conjunctivitis, punctate keratitis or corneal abrasion. Patients usually have systemic manifestations of GVHD.
Stage 3	Convalescent stage	Secondary sicca. Irregular eyelid margins with obstructed meibomian gland orifices, tarsal and forniceal scarring and punctate corneal epitheliopathy
Stage 4	Necrotizing stage	Corneal melting and possible corneal perforation.

(Adapted from Kiang E, Tesavibul N, Yee R, et al. The Use of Topical Cyclosporine A in Ocular Graft-Versus-Host Disease. Bone Marrow Transplantation 1998;22:147–51.)

Table 23.3 Clinical Grading Criteria For Conjunctival GVHD

Grade 1	Conjunctival hyperemia occurring on the bulbar or palpebral conjunctiva in at least one eyelid
Grade 2	Palpebral conjunctival fibrovascular changes occurring along the superior border of the upper eyelid, or the lower border of the tarsal plate of the lower eyelid, with or without conjunctival epithelial sloughing, involving <25% of the total surface area in at least one eyelid
Grade 3	Palpebral conjunctival fibrovascular changes occurring along the superior border of the upper eyelid, or the lower border of the tarsal plate of the lower eyelid, involving 25–75% of the total surface area in at least one eyelid
Grade 4	Palpebral conjunctival fibrovascular changes involving >75% of the total surface area with or without a cicatricial entropion in at least one eyelid

(Adapted from Robinson MR, Lee SS, Rubin BI, et al. Topical Corticosteroid Therapy for Cicatricial Conjunctivitis Associated with Chronic Graft-Versus-Host Disease. Bone Marrow Transplantation 2004;33:1031–5.)

Management

The management of ocular GVHD includes primary prevention, as well as secondary treatment. Therapeutic approaches include medical, both local and systemic, and surgical therapies.

PREVENTION

Prevention of disease plays an important role in decreasing the morbidity associated with ocular GVHD. Environmental modifications and decreased exposure to low-humidity settings may reduce DES symptoms. Cool mist humidifiers can be particularly helpful for environmental modifications at home, including bedside use while sleeping. Minimizing ultraviolet light exposure and regular surveillance with ophthalmologic evaluation, can monitor for the development of infection, cataract, and intraocular pressure elevation. Therefore, a thorough ocular examination is recommended prior to HSCT. Prophylactic use of topical cyclosporine 0.05% might also reduce severity of disease.[20]

IMMUNOSUPPRESSION

Systemic immunosuppressive medications can be effective in preventing manifestations of GVHD, but this benefit must also be weighed against the associated risks of infection, hepatotoxicity, nephrotoxicity, hypertension, and even death. Agents include tacrolimus, mycophenolate mofetil, cyclosporine, methotrexate, sirolimus, antithymocyte globulin, thalidomide, UV light therapy and corticosteroids. These systemic therapies are often reserved for severe or refractory cases, due to long-term adverse events with chronic use. First-line treatments are instead targeted towards specific organ systems with ocular immunosuppressive agents. Local therapy has been effective while minimizing systemic adverse events.

LOCAL MEDICAL TREATMENT

Successful treatment modalities include lubrication, reduction of tear evaporation, minimizing ocular surface inflammation, and immunosuppression.

Lubrication and Reduction of Tear Evaporation

Preservative-free artificial tears and ophthalmic lubricating ointments are effective approaches in providing lubrication and diluting inflammatory mediators in the tear film.[2,21] Punctal occlusion can effectively decrease tear drainage from the ocular surface, with either silicone plugs or permanent thermal cauterization. Moisture chamber goggles may also prove beneficial in reducing tear evaporation and increasing patient comfort.

Treatment of Meibomian Gland Dysfunction

Dry eyes may be exacerbated by dysfunction of meibomian and Zeis glands, both of which normally serve to produce the outer lipid layer of the tear film. The lipid layer is crucial in minimizing evaporation of tears from the corneal surface. Treatment involves warm compresses, lid hygiene, and oral tetracyclines.

Topical Corticosteroids

Topical corticosteroids can reduce ocular surface inflammation in patients with GVHD. The mechanism of action is through lymphocyte apoptosis and blockage of cell-mediated inflammation. Topical corticosteroids are often combined with prophylactic topical antibiotics and tapered to avoid potential adverse side effects. Close follow-up is essential to monitor for corticosteroid-induced side effects. They are contraindicated in patients with corneal infiltrates, epithelial defects or stromal thinning.

Topical Cyclosporine A

Topical cyclosporine A is an anti-inflammatory agent, which produces local inhibition of T lymphocytes and cytokine production in the conjunctiva. As a result, cyclosporine can minimize destruction of lacrimal gland tissue and reduce keratitis sicca. Numerous studies have reported improvement in dry eye symptoms, corneal sensitivity, tear evaporation rate, tear break-up time, vital staining scores, goblet cell density, conjunctival squamous metaplasia grade and inflammatory cell numbers after treatment with topical cyclosporine 0.05%.[20,22–24] This has been used primarily in patients of chronic GVHD and KCS with minimal improvement, despite lubrication and topical steroids.

Autologous Serum Eye Drops

Autologous serum tears 20–50% have been used safely and effectively in the treatment of DES in patients with ocular GVHD. Unlike artificial tears, they contain albumin, epidermal growth factor, fibronectin, vitamin A, neurotrophic growth factor, and hepatocyte growth factor, all of which can assist in maintaining a healthy and stable tear film. Preliminary studies suggest that autologous serum acts to suppress apoptosis in both corneal and conjunctival epithelium.[25] A potential concern with this treatment modality is the risk of contamination, leading to infection.

Contact Lenses

Scleral contact lenses have also been used with success in patients with severe or refractory dry eye disease. These larger contact lenses function to create a tear-filled vault on the corneal surface without corneal contact. These include Jupiter lenses, as well as the custom-designed PROSE (Prosthetic Replacement of the Ocular Surface Ecosystem) lenses from the Boston Foundation for Sight (Fig. 23.2). Studies

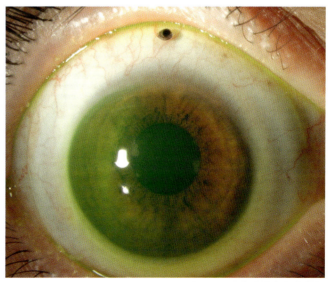

Figure 23.2 PROSE (Prosthetic Replacement of the Ocular Surface Ecosystem) lens from the Boston Foundation for Sight on ocular surface in a patient with severe dry eye syndrome.

have demonstrated improvement in both subjective symptoms and quality of life measures.[26]

Emerging Treatment Modalities

Other treatments have recently been reported to have therapeutic efficacy in ocular GVHD. These emerging agents include the topical immunomodulator tranilast (rizaben), topical tacrolimus, and retinoic acid, although large-scale studies are needed to further assess outcomes.

SURGICAL TREATMENT

In the most severe cases of ocular GVHD, maximal medical therapy may fail in reducing symptoms and protecting the ocular surface. Tarsorrhaphy or amniotic membrane grafting may be pursued to protect the corneal surface. The tarsorrhaphy may be performed with suture, glue adhesive, or botulinum toxin (Botox®, Allergan, Irvine, California) although suture tends to be the best technique as most patients with severe GVHD require a permanent tarsorrhaphy. Amniotic membrane may be placed with suture or fibrin glue in one or multiple layers, or in conjunction with a carrier, such as with ProKera® (Biotissue, Miami, Florida) or AmbioDisc® (AmbioDry™, Marietta, Georgia). Severe vision-threatening complications, such as descemetocele formation and corneal perforation, may ultimately develop despite maximal medical therapy. These complications require surgical treatment. In small descemetoceles or corneal perforations, cyanoacrylate glue patching may be beneficial. A large descemetocele will require anterior lamellar keratoplasty (DALK) or penetrating keratoplasty (PK). In cases with large corneal perforations, penetrating keratoplasty must be performed on an emergent basis with strong consideration of placement of a concurrent tarsorrhaphy and/or amniotic membrane graft.

Conclusion

Appropriate diagnosis and management of ocular GVHD is important in order to maintain visual acuity and quality of life in patients who have undergone HSCT. Ophthalmologists play a paramount role in the prevention and treatment of ocular complications. A multidisciplinary approach that incorporates collaboration with other medical services is essential for GVHD patients. This includes collaboration with the hematology and oncology service and stem cell transplantation team to optimize patient care.

References

1. Ferrara JL, Levine JE, Reddy P, et al. Graft-versus-host disease. Lancet 2009;373:1550–61.
2. Ferrara J, Antin J. The pathophysiology of graft-versus-host disease. In: Forman SJ, editor. Hematopoietic cell transplantation. Oxford: Blackwell; 1999. p. 305–15.
3. Kim SK. Update on ocular graft versus host disease. Curr Opin Ophthalmol 2006;17:344–8.
4. Couriel D, Carpenter PA, Cutler C, et al. Ancillary therapy and supportive care of chronic graft-versus-host disease: national institutes of health consensus development project on criteria for clinical trials in chronic graft-versus-host disease: V. Ancillary Therapy and Supportive Care Working Group Report. Biol Blood Marrow Transplant 2006;12:375–96.
5. Mencucci R, Rossi Ferrini C, Bosi A, et al. Ophthalmological aspects in allogenic bone marrow transplantation: Sjögren-like syndrome in graft-versus-host disease. Eur J Ophthalmol 1997;7:13–8.
6. Ogawa Y, Okamoto S, Wakui M, et al. Dry eye after haematopoietic stem cell transplantation. Br J Ophthalmol 1999;83:1125–30.
7. Franklin RM, Kenyon KR, Tutschka PJ, et al. Ocular manifestations of graft-vs-host disease. Ophthalmology 1983;90:4–13.
8. Ratanatharathorn V, Ayash L, Lazarus HM, et al. Chronic graft-versus-host disease: clinical manifestation and therapy. Bone Marrow Transplant 2001;28:121–9.
9. Krachmer JH. Cornea. 3rd ed. Philadelphia: Elsevier Mosby; 2011.
10. Deeg HJ. Graft-versus-host disease and the development of late complications. Transfus Sci 1994;15:243–54.
11. Lavid FJ, Herreras JM, Calonge M, et al. Calcareous corneal degeneration: report of two cases. Cornea 1995;14:97–102.
12. Kamoi M, Ogawa Y, Dogru M, et al. Spontaneous lacrimal punctal occlusion associated with ocular chronic graft-versus-host disease. Curr Eye Res 2007;32:837–42.
13. Cousins SW, Streilein JW. Flow cytometry detection of lymphocyte proliferation in eyes with immunogenic inflammation. Invest Ophthalmol Vis Sci 1990;31:2111–22.
14. Jabs DA, Wingard J, Green WR, et al. The eye in bone marrow transplantation. III. Conjunctival graft-vs-host disease. Arch Ophthalmol. 1989;107:1343–8.
15. Ogawa Y, Kuwana M. Dry eye as a major complication associated with chronic graft-versus-host disease after hematopoietic stem cell transplantation. Cornea 2003;22:S19–27.
16. Balaram M, Rashid S, Dana R. Chronic ocular surface disease after allogeneic bone marrow transplantation. Ocul Surf 2005;3:203–11.
17. Filipovich AH, Weisdorf D, Pavletic S, et al. Diagnosis and scoring of chronic graft-versus-host disease. NIH consensus development conference on criteria for clinical trials in chronic graft-versus-host disease: Diagnosis and Staging Working Group report. Biol Blood Marrow Transplant 2005;11:945–56.
18. Kiang E, Tesavibul N, Yee R, et al. The use of topical cyclosporine A in ocular graft-versus-host disease. Bone Marrow Transplant 1998;22:147–51.
19. Robinson MR, Lee SS, Rubin BI, et al. Topical corticosteroid therapy for cicatricial conjunctivitis associated with chronic graft-versus-host disease. Bone Marrow Transplant 2004;33:1031–5.
20. Malta JB, Soong HK, Shtein RM, et al. Treatment of ocular graft-versus-host disease with topical cyclosporine 0.05%. Cornea 2010;29:1392–6.
21. Kim SK, Couriel D, Ghosh S, et al. Ocular graft vs. host disease experience from MD Anderson Cancer Center: Newly described clinical spectrum and new approach to the management of stage III and IV ocular GVHD. Biol Blood Marrow Transplant 2006;12(2S1):49.
22. Rao SN, Rao RD. Efficacy of topical cyclosporine 0.05% in the treatment of dry eye associated with graft-versus-host disease. Cornea 2006;25:674–8.
23. Lelli GJ, Jr, Musch DC, Gupta A, et al. Ophthalmic cyclosporine use in ocular GVHD. Cornea 2006;25:635–8.
24. Wang Y, Ogawa Y, Dogru M, et al. Ocular surface and tear function after topical cyclosporine treatment in dry eye patients with chronic graft-versus-host disease. Bone Marrow Transplant 2008;41:293–302.
25. Kojima T, Higuchi A, Goto E, et al. Autologous serum eye drops for the treatment of dry eye diseases. Cornea 2008;27:S25–30.
26. Jacobs DS, Rosenthal P. Boston scleral lens prosthetic device for treatment of severe dry eye in chronic graft-versus-host disease. Cornea 2007;26:1195–9.

24 *Ligneous Conjunctivitis*

ANDREA Y. ANG, KRISTIANA D. NEFF, GARY S. SCHWARTZ, and EDWARD J. HOLLAND

Introduction

Ligneous conjunctivitis is a rare form of chronic conjunctivitis, characterized by the recurrent development of fibrin-rich, wood-like membranes, mainly on the tarsal conjunctiva. It is the main clinical manifestation of systemic plasminogen deficiency and typically presents in childhood. Less frequently, similar membranes may occur in other mucous membranes, including the ear, oral and respiratory tracts, gastrointestinal tracts, female genital tracts, and renal collecting system. Rarely, it can cause congenital occlusive hydrocephalus or juvenile colloid milium. Histopathological findings indicate that impaired wound healing, mainly of injured mucosal tissue, is due to markedly decreased plasmin-mediated extracellular fibrinolysis.

The first description of ligneous conjunctivitis appeared in 1847, with Bouisson[1] describing a 46-year-old man with bilateral pseudomembranous conjunctivitis. In 1933, the term 'ligneous,' meaning 'woody,' was introduced by Borel[2] to describe the characteristic wood-like consistency of the pseudomembranes. However, the link between ligneous conjunctivitis and plasminogen deficiency was not established until 1997 by Mingers et al.[3] As many patients develop similar pseudomembranes in other mucous membranes of the body, Mingers et al.[3] suggested the term 'pseudomembranous disease' to describe the systemic nature of this disease. Although the lesions have been referred to as pseudomembranous in the literature, the lesions are actually true membranes, as they bleed upon removal. It is characterized by multiple recurrences after local excision, and management involves the adjunctive use of topical and systemic replacement of plasminogen.

Epidemiology

Ligneous conjunctivitis is rare, and the prevalence of this disorder has not been firmly established. Ligneous conjunctivitis, associated with plasminogen deficiency is typically an autosomal recessive disorder that results from a homozygous or compound heterozygous defect. A study of 9611 blood donors in Scotland revealed a prevalence of 2.9 per 1000 heterozygous type I plasminogen deficiency subjects.[4] The theoretical prevalence of homozygotes or compound heterozygotes has been calculated in the range of 1.6 per 1 million people.[5] Females appear to be affected more than males, with a ratio of 1.27:1 to 1.39:1.[5,6]

The largest study of patients with severe type I plasminogen deficiency included 50 patients.[6] The median age of clinical presentation was 9.75 months (range, 3 days to 61 years), demonstrating that ligneous conjunctivitis can occur in older individuals, despite it being classically associated with infants and children. The most common manifestation in this group was ligneous conjunctivitis (80%), followed by ligneous gingivitis (34%), with 14% of patients suffering from both. Less common extraocular manifestations included involvement of the ears, upper and lower respiratory tract (sinus, larynx, bronchi, lungs; 30%), the female genital tract (8%), the gastrointestinal tract (duodenal ulcer; 2%), congenital occlusive hydrocephalus (8%), and juvenile colloid milium of the skin (2%). Two of the patients with congenital occlusive hydrocephalus had Dandy–Walker malformation. Several studies have shown extraocular manifestations of severe plasminogen deficiency without ocular involvement.[5,6]

Etiology

There has been definitive evidence to support that ligneous conjunctivitis is the result of plasminogen deficiency.[7–10] The case of ligneous conjunctivitis reported by Mingers et al. was also the first report of plasminogen deficiency in humans.[3] There are two types of plasminogen deficiency: type I (hypoplasminogenemia) is a quantitative deficiency and type II (dysplasminogenemia) is a qualitative deficiency. Type I deficiency is the type most associated with ligneous conjunctivitis. Development of ligneous lesions is most commonly caused by sporadic mutations in the plasminogen gene; however, compound-heterozygous or homozygous mutations have been reported.[3,5,6,9,10] Tefs et al. found the K19E mutation to be the most common genetic cause of type I plasminogen deficiency (34%) in a series of 50 patients.[6] Knowledge of the genetics of the disease allows for prenatal diagnosis in known carrier families, which can be crucial in cases of obstructive congenital hydrocephalus.[11]

Plasmin is a serine protease and is the predominant fibrinolytic enzyme in the human circulation, it is also found in the extracellular matrix.[12] Plasminogen is converted to plasmin by plasminogen activators in the blood.

Plasmin plays an important role in hemostasis as well as being an integral component of wound healing in its role in degrading fibrin. The gene for plasminogen is located on chromosome 6, and is produced predominantly by the liver. With plasminogen deficiency, wound-healing capability is diminished and is most pronounced in mucous membranes, such as the conjunctiva.[12] The impaired wound-healing capacity causes an arrest at the stage of granulation tissue formation and excessive fibrin deposition. Thus, fibrin-rich membranes or mucus strands accumulate, stimulating inflammatory cells and fibroblasts, while desiccation of the fibrin leads to the ligneous consistency of the conjunctival lesions. Similar pathophysiologic mechanisms occur in extraocular manifestations of plasminogen deficiency.

While in extravascular spaces, fibrinolysis with low to nonexistent levels of plasminogen activity is impaired. However, intravascularly this is not the case, as can be inferred from the fact that thrombotic phenomena are absent in patients with ligneous conjunctivitis and plasminogen deficiency. It has been suggested that nonplasmin-induced fibrinolysis is intensified in patients with plasminogen deficiency and ligneous conjunctivitis, through elevated polymorphonuclear elastase levels, among other factors.[10]

Due to the appearance, histopathology, clinical course, and response to treatment, the authors also believe that ligneous conjunctivitis results from an exaggerated inflammatory response to tissue injury. This injury may arise from infection or physical trauma, including surgery. These factors may incite a genetic predisposition, such as plasminogen deficiency to develop this response. Schuster and Seregard also postulated that conjunctivitis is the most common manifestation of plasminogen deficiency, due to frequent exposure to ocular irritants.[5] These irritants may start or perpetuate local inflammation and create ligneous membranes. Many cases of antecedent viral or bacterial infections have been described in the literature, including staphylococcal, streptococcal, and *Haemophilus* conjunctivitis.[13–15] In these cases, it appears that ligneous conjunctivitis in genetically susceptible individuals develops as an abnormal response to the conjunctival trauma elicited by the infecting organisms.

Trauma, especially from surgery, is also thought to be a cause of ligneous conjunctivitis. The authors have reported a case of a 24-year-old woman with ligneous conjunctivitis of the left upper eyelid, who underwent a conjunctival autograft from her left lower to left upper eyelid. Ligneous conjunctivitis subsequently developed at the previously unaffected donor site and became resistant to treatment in the original site of disease in the palpebral conjunctiva of the upper lid.[16] Later studies reported the same negative experience in previously unaffected fellow eyes.[17] In these cases, ligneous conjunctivitis appears to develop as an abnormal response of the immune system to the conjunctival trauma.

Pathophysiology/Histopathology

Histologic examination of ligneous membranes shows superficial or subepithelial deposits of eosinophilic amorphous hyaline, amyloid-like material with a variable proportion of granulation tissue with accompanying inflammatory cells (lymphocytes, plasma cells, and granulocytes) (Fig. 24.1).[5] This amorphous hyaline-like material has been shown to contain mainly fibrin and other plasma proteins, such as albumin and immunoglobulins (mainly IgG).[5] Ligneous lesions may also contain variable amounts of mucopolysaccharides in adjacent granulation tissue.[5] Abnormal vascular permeability has also been suggested as the source of the various components of the ligneous lesion. Melikian postulated that a serofibrinous transudate from the conjunctival neovascularization undergoes subsequent coagulation, with the resulting formation of granulation tissue and accumulation of the hyaline material, which becomes hardened in forming the ligneous membranes.[18]

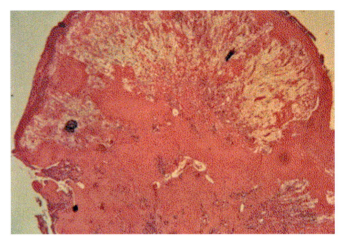

Figure 24.1 Histopathological appearance of a ligneous lesion. Large eosinophilic deposits are present in the stroma. (Reproduced from Schuster V, Seregard S. Ligneous conjunctivitis. Survey of Ophthalmology 2003;48:369–88. Figure 4.)

Immunohistochemical evaluation of ligneous conjunctivitis lesions was first performed in 1988.[19] In this study, a cellular infiltrate was seen that was composed mainly of T lymphocytes, which was seen again in later studies.[17] The ratio of T-helper/inducer:T-suppressor/cytotoxic cells was approximately 3:1. Immunofluorescent techniques demonstrated that the major components of the hyaline material in the substantia propria were immunoglobulins. IgG was the most prominent, with staining for both light and heavy chains, but primarily for κ-light chains.

Topical cyclosporine A has been reported to be more effective than other topical agents (short of plasminogen preparations) in the treatment of this disorder in several studies.[15,16,19] Cyclosporine A interferes with IL-2 production, therefore, preventing the activation and recruitment of the T-cell response. Immunohistochemical analysis of a lesion resected after 6 months of topical cyclosporine A therapy, supports the immune role of this entity.[19] A significant decrease in the total number of T lymphocytes was found, with the greatest decrease occurring in the T-suppressor/cytotoxic cell subpopulation. Also of interest was the absence of IL-2 receptors on the T cells. Finally, a decrease in the number of B lymphocytes and plasma cells occurred. These results indicate the local effect of cyclosporine A on the immune response. The marked reduction of T-suppressor/cytotoxic cells was a secondary effect, as these cells are recruited by activated T cells. The clinical response and histopathologic confirmation of the effect of cyclosporine A further support the inflammatory nature of this disease.

Diagnosis

The diagnosis of ligneous conjunctivitis is based on the clinical picture (ocular and/or extraocular membranous lesions), the typical histological findings, and a possible positive family history. In most patients with ligneous conjunctivitis, hypoplasminogenemia may be found.[5] In the report of Tefs et al. of 50 patients with plasminogen deficiency, plasminogen activity ranged from 4% to 51%.[6] If the responsible mutation has been identified in an affected family, then prenatal diagnosis of children at risk is possible.[5]

Clinical Findings

OCULAR FEATURES

Patients typically present with a chronic conjunctivitis. Discharge or membranes are not seen in the early stages. The earliest true ligneous lesion appears as a highly vascularized, raised, friable lesion. This lesion can be removed easily with forceps, although it tends to bleed on removal. With continued inflammation, a white, thickened, avascular mass appears above the neovascular membrane (Fig. 24.2). Attempts at removal of this lesion without appropriate anti-inflammatory therapy, often results in recurrence of the lesion to its original size within days. These lesions are most often seen on the palpebral conjunctiva of the upper and lower lids but may also be found on the bulbar conjunctiva, including the limbus. Bulbar conjunctival involvement may occur either from extension of a palpebral lesion or de novo. Limbal lesions may extend over the surface of the cornea and, in the most severe cases, lead to corneal neovascularization and scarring. Corneal involvement occurs in 26–30% of cases.[5] From time to time, despite appropriate therapy, inflammation continues, and the chronic lesions become thickened, vascularized, and firm, giving rise to the name 'ligneous,' meaning woody.

Early in the course of the disease, patients may complain of chronic tearing, mild discomfort, and redness. As the lesions grow, almost all patients complain of pain and photophobia. Severe cases result in almost constant discomfort, making it difficult for patients to carry out activities of daily living. The more severe lesions may extend beyond the lid margin (Fig. 24.3). Bilateral involvement occurs in up to 51% of patients, with the duration of the disease reportedly ranging from a few months to 44 years.[5]

SYSTEMIC FEATURES

Fever or infections of the upper respiratory tract, urinary tract, or female genital tract, may either precede or concomitantly occur with ligneous conjunctivitis, or might even act as a trigger for the development of membranes.[5]

Orophayrnx

The second most frequently affect site is the mouth, with 34% of patients suffering from this in the largest series of patients with severe type 1 plasminogen deficiency.[6] Painless nodular ulcerations or gingival hyperplasia occurs, often resulting in the loss of dental integrity.[12] Similar membranous lesions may occur in the middle and tympanic membrane, causing chronic otitis media and fluctuating hearing loss.[5]

Respiratory Tract

Less frequently, ligneous lesions may develop in the larynx, vocal cords, and tracheobronchial tree. This may cause voice change (dysphonia), recurrent pneumonia, and potentially life-threatening airway obstruction. Recurrent tracheobronchial obstruction by ligneous masses is difficult to manage, and is associated with a poor prognosis.[5]

Genitourinary Tract

Ligneous lesions occurring in the female genital tract have most commonly been reported affecting the cervix, causing ligneous cervicitis.[20] Lesions may also involve the vagina, fallopian tubes, ovary, and endometrium. Dysmenorrhea is the most common presenting symptom, and infertility may occur.[20]

Membranous plaques have been reported in the renal collecting system of two siblings with ligneous

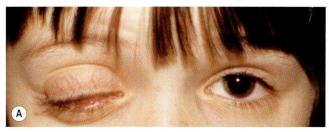
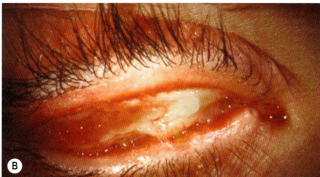

Figure 24.3 Ligneous conjunctivitis in an 8-year-old girl. (**A**) The ligneous lesions involve the entire palpebral and bulbar conjunctiva of the right eye. (**B**) Note the limbal lesions have grown to completely obscure the cornea. (Reproduced from Krachmer et al. Cornea. 3rd ed. Mosby: Elsevier; 2010. Figure 55.2.)

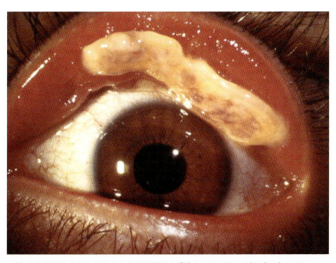

Figure 24.2 Ligneous conjunctivitis of the superior palpebral conjunctiva. Note the white, avascular lesion at the perimeter and the vascularized base. (Reproduced from Krachmer et al. Cornea. 3rd ed. Mosby: Elsevier; 2010. Figure 55.1.)

conjunctivitis.[9] However, involvement of the renal tract appears to be a rare event in patients with ligneous conjunctivitis.[5]

Juvenile Colloid Milium

This is a rare skin condition characterized by the development of small, yellow-brown, translucent papules, typically in sun-exposed areas of the skin.[5] In most cases, it is reported to occur after severe sunburn or chronic sun exposure, and tends to occur prior to puberty. It has been described to be associated with ligneous conjunctivitis.[5]

Congenital Occlusive Hydrocephalus

At least 16 children with ligneous conjunctivitis have been reported to also suffer from congenital occlusive hydrocephalus.[5] Of these, seven have documented plasminogen deficiency.

Management

Plasminogen substitution is presently being investigated as the primary treatment for ligneous conjunctivitis.[3,7,10,21,22] Mingers et al. first proposed the theory of plasminogen deficiency and attempted supplementing plasminogen.[3] Higher doses of intravenous lysine-conjugated plasminogen (1000 units/day, continuous infusion for 2 weeks) have been used successfully in an infant with ligneous conjunctivitis, followed by 2000-unit second daily bolus injections for 2 weeks, and then 1000-unit daily bolus injections long term.[21] Topical plasminogen preparations extracted from fresh frozen plasma, have successfully been employed in the treatment of ligneous conjunctivitis: three patients remained free of recurrences for over 12 months, with topical administration as frequently as every 2 hours.[7] Another patient with hourly plasminogen drop administration had resolution of pseudomembranes in 3 weeks: after tapering, the disease reoccurred and was again quieted with re-administration of plasminogen drops. Chronic low-dose maintenance treatment with topical plasminogen was thought necessary for this patient.[22]

A combination of systemic or subconjunctival fresh frozen plasma (FFP) and topical FFP have shown success in three patients.[23–25] Using FFP bypasses, the need for plasminogen concentrate alone, which has a very short half-life and is difficult to have readily available. No reoccurrence of disease was noted 12 months after pseudomembrane excision in the first two studies, and after 10 months of follow-ups in the third study. A Japanese study successfully treated a 71-year-old and her elder sister with ligneous conjunctivitis, after ocular surgery with a combination of a direct thrombin inhibitor, topical Argatroban, and topical plasma obtained from their healthy family members.[26]

Based on the early observations of the presence of granulation tissue and inflammatory cells in ligneous tissue, topical medical regimens geared toward these non-specific findings were developed. Topical therapy, including topical hyaluronidase, alpha-chymotrypsin, sodium cromoglycate, antibiotics, corticosteroids, and fibrinolysin, have met with limited success.[5] Heparin has been reported to have partial success in controlling ligneous conjunctivitis.[27,28] De Cock et al.[27] treated 17 patients with ligneous conjunctivitis with local excision and immediate, perioperative topical treatment, with intensive heparin and corticosteroids, and in 12 patients additional alpha-chymotrypsin. Overall, 13 of the 17 patients were successfully controlled with this regimen.[27] Cyclosporine had been the most promising element in the therapeutic armamentarium before plasminogen.[15,29] Recently, oral contraceptives have been noted to show a marked increase in plasminogen levels, due to hormonal up-regulation of plasminogen synthesis. In two patients, Sartori et al. showed treatment to be associated with a rise in plasminogen levels and improvement in clinical findings with resolution of disease in one patient.[30] This therapy may be useful in selected female patients with hypoplasminogenemia. Finally, an anecdotal report by Lee and Himmel described successful resolution of a recurrent case of ligneous conjunctivitis with allogeneic serum tears from a family member, confirmed to have normal plasminogen levels.[31] This source of plasminogen may be useful if fresh frozen plasma is not readily available, only after the family member has been cleared of potential blood-borne infectious disease transmission.

Because trauma to the conjunctiva is likely to be an etiologic factor in ligneous conjunctivitis, conjunctival surgery must be performed only with the utmost care. The authors recommend against performing conjunctival autograft for ligneous conjunctivitis. Barabino and Rolando performed amniotic membrane transplantation for conjunctival reconstruction of ligneous conjunctivitis.[32] Following surgery, the patient was given a 6-month course of heparin eye drops (5000 U/mL) with dexamethasone and tobramycin for 2 weeks postoperatively. The patient had small recurrences at 8 months, necessitating regrafting of the amniotic membrane. At 36 months post-procedure, the patient was disease free. The authors would advise pretreating any patient with plasminogen therapy prior to surgery, with slow postoperative tapering. Otherwise, cryosurgery, electrocoagulation, and surgical resection of ligneous lesions, typically result in rapid recurrence of the lesions within days to weeks.

Based on the literature and the authors' clinical experience, the authors recommend the following approach with these patients. All patients should receive a thorough, dilated ocular examination. Otolaryngology and anesthesia are consulted to evaluate the patient's respiratory tract, not only to search for concomitant disease but also because many patients need to be debrided under anesthesia, and any tracheal or laryngeal abnormalities must be discovered before induction. Systemic and topical plasminogen (if available) or FFP treatment is started, as described above, to help soften the pseudomembrane and facilitate removal. The next step would be a complete excisional biopsy of all ocular ligneous lesions. General anesthesia may be used in adults with significant disease and in all children. In advanced disease, excision will require extensive surgery to dissect the substantia propria of the conjunctiva. Eversion of the eyelid is mandatory. Significant bleeding should be expected, and topical epinephrine and cautery might be helpful. Failure to completely remove the lesion results in rapid recurrence because the retained lesion acts as a physical barrier to topical medical treatment.

Immediately after surgery, the patient is continued on systemic and topical FFP and started on a corticosteroid

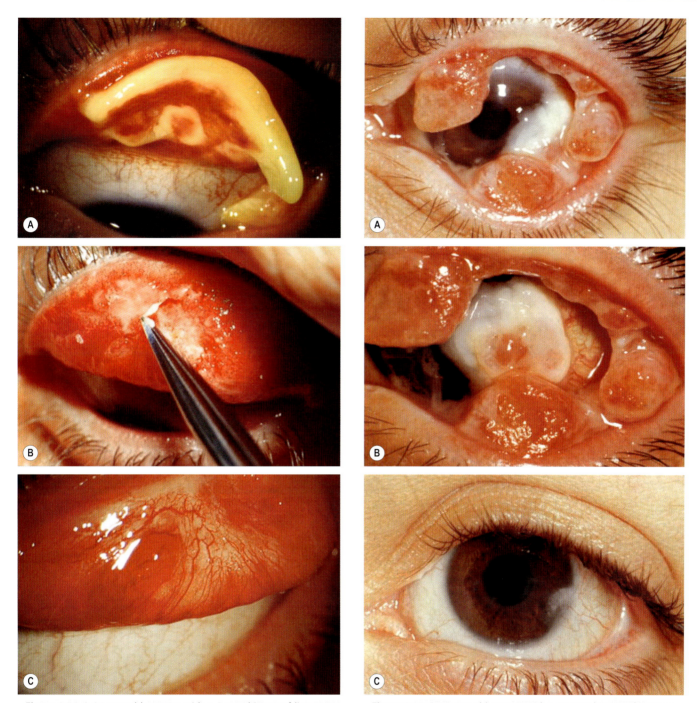

Figure 24.4 A 24-year-old woman with a 3-year history of ligneous conjunctivitis, who had failed prior topical and systemic therapy. (**A**) Note the extensive ligneous lesion of the superior palpebral conjunctiva and the additional lesion of the inferior palpebral conjunctiva of the left eye. (**B**) Postoperative day 1 after excisional biopsy; the early ligneous membrane is being peeled with a jeweler's forceps before administration of topical cyclosporine. (**C**) Nine months after initiation of topical cyclosporine therapy. Note the complete resolution of ligneous conjunctivitis; subepithelial fibrosis can be seen. (Reproduced from Krachmer et al. Cornea. 3rd ed. Mosby: Elsevier; 2010. Figure 55.3.)

Figure 24.5 A 20-year-old woman with a 10-year history of ligneous conjunctivitis of the left eye. (**A**) Extensive vascularized ligneous lesions of the superior and inferior palpebral conjunctiva. (**B**) Note the fleshy ligneous lesion at the 3 o'clock meridian extending over the cornea. (**C**) The same patient showing complete resolution after 9 months of topical cyclosporine and serial excisional biopsies. (Reproduced from Krachmer et al. Cornea. 3rd ed. Mosby: Elsevier; 2010. Figure 55.4.)

and broad-spectrum antibiotic, four times daily with topical cyclosporine A 2% twice daily. These medications must be given after surgery, as early recurrence is the hallmark of this disorder.

Early in the postoperative period, patients must be seen at least once a day. A small but significant amount of recurrence will be seen daily in every patient, and every recurrent lesion must be debrided daily with a jeweler's forceps (Fig. 24.4). If abnormal tissue is allowed to collect for even 1 to 2 days, it will act as a barrier and prevent the topical medications from reaching the basal tissue, which is the origin of the ligneous membranes. Pediatric patients are restrained for their daily examinations, and their parents are taught to debride the lesions with cotton-tipped applicators while they are applying the eye drops.

Within the first few weeks of therapy, the rate and severity of recurrences lessen and the topical medications can be tapered slowly. Some lesions progress despite this aggressive topical therapy. Patients with these lesions must be brought back to the operating room for repeat excisional biopsy. After this surgical procedure, the patient must be placed back on the initial topical regimen, described previously. Results with repeated excisions and aggressive topical management have been satisfactory (Fig. 24.5). As we continue to refine plasminogen therapy, more light is being shed on the pathophysiology of this disease. Overall, the development of systemic and topical plasminogen preparations, as a treatment of ligneous conjunctivitis, carries a new promise for patients with ligneous conjunctivitis.

References

1. Bouisson M. Ophthalmie sur-aigue avec formation de pseudomembranes à la surface de la conjonctive. Ann Ocul 1847;17:100–4.
2. Borel MG. Un nouveau syndrome palpebral. Bull Soc Fr Ophthalmol 1933;46:168–80.
3. Mingers AM, Heimburger N, Zeitler P, et al. Homozygous type I plasminogen deficiency. Semin Thromb Hemost 1997;23:259–69.
4. Tait RC, Walker ID, Conkie JA, et al. Isolated familial plasminogen deficiency may not be a risk factor for thrombosis. Thromb Haemost 1996;76:1004–8.
5. Schuster V, Seregard S. Ligneous conjunctivitis. Surv Ophthalmol 2003;48:369–88.
6. Tefs K, Gueorguieva M, Klammt J, et al. Molecular and clinical spectrum of type I plasminogen deficiency: a series of 50 patients. Blood 2006;108:3021–6.
7. Watts P, Suresh P, Mezer E, et al. Effective treatment of ligneous conjunctivitis with topical plasminogen. Am J Ophthalmol 2002;133:451–5.
8. Ramsby ML, Donshik PC, Makowski GS. Ligneous conjunctivitis: biochemical evidence for hypofibrinolysis. Inflammation 2000;24:45–71.
9. Schuster V, Seidenspinner S, Zeitler P, et al. Compound-heterozygous mutations in the plasminogen gene predispose to the development of ligneous conjunctivitis. Blood 1999;93:3457–66.
10. Mingers AM, Philapitsch A, Schwarz HP, et al. Polymorphonuclear elastase in patients with homozygous type I plasminogen deficiency and ligneous conjunctivitis. Semin Thromb Hemost 1998;24:605–12.
11. Schuster V, Seidenspinner S, Muller C, et al. Prenatal diagnosis in a family with severe type I plasminogen deficiency, ligneous conjunctivitis and congenital hydrocephalus. Prenat Diagn 1999;19:483–7.
12. Mehta R, Shapiro AD. Plasminogen deficiency. Haemophilia 2008;14:1261–8.
13. Chambers JD, Blodi FC, Golden B, et al. Ligneous conjunctivitis. Trans Am Acad Ophthalmol Otolaryngol 1969;73:996–1004.
14. Newcomer V, Klein A. Ligneous conjunctivitis. Arch Dermatol 1977;113:511–2.
15. Rubin BI, Holland EJ, de Smet MD, et al. Response of reactivated ligneous conjunctivitis to topical cyclosporine. Am J Ophthalmol 1991;112:95–6.
16. Schwartz GS, Holland EJ. Induction of ligneous conjunctivitis by conjunctival surgery. Am J Ophthalmol 1995;120:253–4.
17. Rao SK, Biswas J, Rajagopal R, et al. Ligneous conjunctivitis: a clinicopathologic study of 3 cases. Int Ophthalmol 1998;22:201–6.
18. Melikian HE. Treatment of ligneous conjunctivitis. Ann Ophthalmol 1985;17:763–5.
19. Holland EJ, Chan CC, Kuwabara T, et al. Immunohistologic findings and results of treatment with cyclosporine in ligneous conjunctivitis. Am J Ophthalmol 1989;107:160–6.
20. Pantanowitz L. Ligneous conjunctivitis. BJOG 2004;111:635.
21. Schott D, Dempfle CE, Beck P, et al. Therapy with a purified plasminogen concentrate in an infant with ligneous conjunctivitis and homozygous plasminogen deficiency. N Engl J Med 1998;339:1679–166.
22. Heidemann DG, Williams GA, Hartzer M, et al. Treatment of ligneous conjunctivitis with topical plasmin and topical plasminogen. Cornea 2003;22:760–2.
23. Gürlü VP, Demir M, Alimgil ML, et al. Systemic and topical fresh-frozen plasma treatment in a newborn with ligneous conjunctivitis. Cornea 2008;27:501–3.
24. Tabbara KF. Prevention of ligneous conjunctivitis by topical and subconjunctival fresh frozen plasma. Am J Ophthalmol 2004;138:299–300.
25. Pergantou H, Likaki D, Fotopoulou M, et al. Management of ligneous conjunctivitis in a child with plasminogen deficiency. Eur J Pediatr 2011;170:1333–6.
26. Suzuki T, Ikewaki J, Iwata H, et al. The first two Japanese cases of severe type I congenital plasminogen deficiency with ligneous conjunctivitis: successful treatment with direct thrombin inhibitor and fresh plasma. Am J Hematol 2009;84:363–5.
27. De Cock R, Ficker LA, Dart JG, et al. Topical heparin in the treatment of ligneous conjunctivitis. Ophthalmology 1995;102:1654–9.
28. Hiremath M, Elder J, Newall F, et al. Heparin in the long-term management of ligneous conjunctivitis: a case report and review of literature. Blood Coagul Fibrinolysis 2011;22:606–9.
29. Holland EJ, Olsen TW, Ketcham JM, et al. Topical cyclosporin A in the treatment of anterior segment inflammatory disease. Cornea 1993;12:413–9.
30. Sartori TM, Saggiorato G, Pellati D, et al. Contraceptive pills induce an improvement in congenital hypoplasminogenemia in two unrelated patients with ligneous conjunctivitis. Thromb Haemost 2003;90:86–91.
31. Lee WB, Himmel K. Allogeneic serum drops for the treatment of ligneous conjunctivitis. Cornea 2008;28:122–3.
32. Barabino S, Rolando M. Amniotic membrane transplantation in a case of ligneous conjunctivitis. Am J Ophthalmol 2004;137:752–3.

25 Toxic Keratoconjunctivitis

ENRIQUE O. GRAUE-HERNÁNDEZ, ALEJANDRO NAVAS, and
ARTURO RAMÍREZ-MIRANDA

Introduction

The complication of toxic conjunctivitis from topical preparations for the treatment of ophthalmic conditions has long
been recognized. The Ebers papyrus from ancient Egypt
mentions eye remedies including red lead, antimony, lead,
sea salt, iron and sulphur.[1] However, it was not until 1864
that Albrecht von Graefe reported a case of keratoconjunctivitis, following the administration of topical atropine.[2]
In the last few decades, progress in the understanding of
eye diseases' basic mechanisms has increased the number
of therapeutic targets, and the field of ocular pharmacology
has grown accordingly, to provide the physician with many
more topical drugs.[3] Glaucoma therapeutics are of particular importance, since topical therapy may last for decades.[4]
This chapter analyzes the effects of common ophthalmic
treatments on the conjunctiva and cornea.

Pathophysiology

Topical ophthalmic preparations can confuse the diagnosis
of toxic conjunctivitis.[5] Medications often alleviate the
patient's symptoms initially and only at a later time, sometimes years after initiating therapy, will the patient develop
discomfort.[6] Medications can be directly toxic to the conjunctival and corneal epithelium, damaging its structure
and altering its function with or without an inflammatory
response.[7] Some preparations are directly cytotoxic due to
pH, the osmolarity of the solution, or even due to photosensitization.[8] The cellular reaction may reflect the direct effect
of the active compound, the accompanying preservative, or
the breakdown products. Direct toxic effects usually occur
after the first contact and appear after a threshold is
reached.[8] The chronic nature of these substances may lead
to infiltration of the substantia propria, by inflammatory
cells and fibroblasts, eventually generating fibrosis that can
severely disturb the ocular surface.[9]

Topical preparations can also induce damage through
immunological mechanisms. These reactions are classified
into the following categories:

1. Allergic reactions due to type 1 hypersensitivity, triggered by the union of the allergen and initiation of the
   IgE–mast cell axis, leading to degranulation and release
   of inflammatory mediators.[10]
2. Type II–III hypersensitivity, characterized by antibody-
   specific and immune-complex-mediated effects.[11]
3. Type IV or delayed hypersensitivity. This type is associated with marked epithelial and subepithelial edema and
   infiltration by CD4+ lymphocytes and Langerhans
   cells.[12]

Ophthalmic treatments may also be toxic through more
indirect mechanisms. Antimicrobials modify the ocular
external microbiota and may favor bacterial colonization
by selecting resistant strains,[13,14] while corticosteroids
decrease local immune mechanisms. Other indirect effects
on the ocular surface may involve direct cytotoxicity to
goblet cells (preservatives) or decreased tear production
(parasympatholytics and antihistamines).[15] Some preservatives (benzalkonium chloride) may have a detergent effect
on the lipid layer of the tear film, thus, promoting tear
evaporation.[7]

There is no single mechanism responsible for drug intolerance or toxicity, but a combination of these occur simultaneously or in sequence and are accountable for the
patients' symptoms.[16]

Clinical Features

A detailed clinical history is essential for the diagnosis of
toxic conjunctivitis. Patients often neglect communicating
the routine use of over-the-counter eye preparations (artificial tears or vasoconstrictors). The ophthalmologist must
be aware of topical anesthetic abuse or indiscriminate use
of topical antibiotics. Regarding toxicity, it is often valuable
to obtain information on the patients' medication storage
habits and to confirm expiration dates, since patients often
keep previously used treatments for medications use if
symptoms return.

PERIORBITAL SKIN AND EYELIDS

The examination of the ocular adnexa often reveals diagnostic clues. The eyelids and the conjunctiva are contiguous
structures that work in synchrony to stabilize and protect
the ocular surface. Eczema involving the periorbital region
is characteristic of type IV hypersensitivity, specifically if it
appears a few days after the initiation of a new drug (Fig.
25.1). Eczema may rarely simulate seborrheic blepharitis.

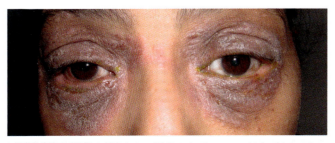

Figure 25.1 Delayed hypersensitivity reaction to topical tobramycin,
72 hours after treatment.

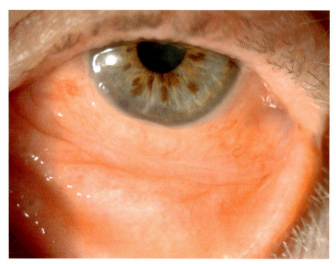

Figure 25.2 Immediate hypersensitivity reaction to topical dorzolamide hydrochloride-timolol maleate ophthalmic solution.

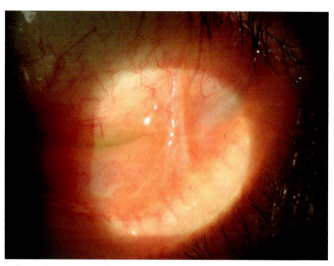

Figure 25.4 Drug induced pemphigoid secondary to timolol maleate 0.5%.

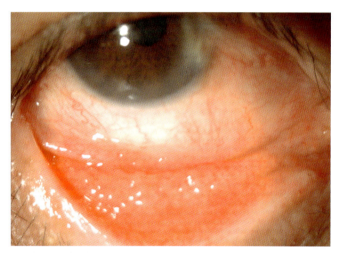

Figure 25.3 Follicular conjunctivitis induced by brimonidine tartrate ophthalmic solution 0.1%.

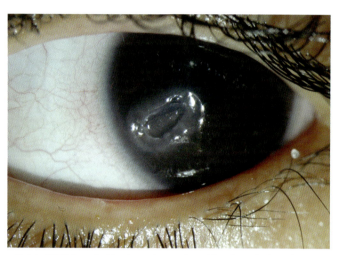

Figure 25.5 Anesthetic abuse (tetracaine chlorydrate) ulcer demonstrating the characteristic inferior-nasal location and rolled edges. Patient was previously diagnosed with recurrent erosion syndrome. (Courtesy of Fernando Peniche MD.)

In turn, pruritus, urticaria and edema of the eyelids are characteristic of Type I hypersensitivity (Fig. 25.2). It is important to examine the lacrimal punctum for patency as some drugs may cause fibrosis and obliteration.[10]

CONJUNCTIVA

Hyperemia, chemosis, and a clear mucoid discharge are characteristic of an allergic reaction. Pruritus is a strong clinical sign of allergy. Follicles are not seen in pure allergy and they should point to toxicity if supported by clinical history (Fig. 25.3). In these cases, the hyperemia and chemosis are more subtle and difficult to assess. Subconjunctival fibrosis, fornix foreshortening, punctal occlusion and symblepharon formation, should direct the clinician toward drug-induced pemphigoid or pseudopemphigoid (Fig. 25.4).[17]

CORNEA

The scope and severity of corneal lesions in toxic keratoconjunctivitis may vary greatly, from very mild punctate epitheliopathy to overt corneal ulceration and necrosis. Toxicity is discovered when epitheliopathy predominates in the inferior-nasal quadrant, where there is maximal contact time between the drug and ocular surface (Fig. 25.5). That is the usual location of corneal ulcers due to anesthetic abuse, which resembles neurotrophic keratitis, in its clinical appearance with rolled edges. Comet's-impact crater keratitis, intense ciliary flush, and papillary response have also been described in this pathology.[5] The corneal epithelium can be opaque and edematous and a hurricane keratopathy can be observed. In the setting of keratoplasty, the latter can be a sign of drug toxicity. Pseudodendrites are also a common feature of drug-induced keratopathy.[2]

Diagnostic Investigations

Many tests have been devised to evaluate the toxic effects of ophthalmic preparations on the ocular surface. However, most of them are not practical or not widely available and are difficult to perform in the clinical setting.

CONJUNCTIVAL BIOPSY

Conjunctival biopsies are reserved for confirmation or exclusion of autoimmune diseases and are usually reserved for the diagnosis of cicatrizing conjunctivitis. These biopsies are not well accepted by the patient unless they are absolutely necessary. Regarding findings of toxic damage, previous studies have shown that squamous metaplasia of the conjunctival epithelium and subconjunctival inflammation and fibrosis are present in patients after long-term glaucoma treatment. Pseudopemghigoid may demonstrate findings identical to idiopathic pemphigoid.[18]

CONJUNCTIVAL SCRAPING

The presence of eosinophils and basophils points to an allergic reaction but it is relatively non-specific, since these cells can also be found in toxic conjunctivitis. In the clinic, they are most often used to rule out infectious disease and allergy.

IMPRESSION CYTOLOGY

Impression cytology can be performed under topical anesthesia and provides a homogenous cell layer for histological studies, with an almost intact architecture and preserved cell junctions. Epithelial cells, goblet cells and inflammatory cells can be differentiated with immunostaining protocols and can even be used for flow cytometry analysis, which permits the measurement of membrane and cytoplasmic inflammatory markers. Some studies have demonstrated that HLA-DR class II antigen and IL-6, IL-8, and IL-10, are strongly expressed in the conjunctival epithelium of patients with history of long-term glaucoma treatment.[19]

Tear samples can be used to measure levels of IgE or inflammatory cytokines, although given their complex processing, they are rarely used except for research purposes. When positive, skin tests and conjunctival allergen challenge are of great clinical value, but negative findings do not rule out allergy.[20]

TOXICITY OF COMMON OPHTHALMIC PREPARATIONS

Preservatives

Multi-dose eye drops contain antimicrobial preservatives. Many substances have been used for this purpose, including benzalkonium chloride, chlorhexidine, chlorbutanol thimerosal, paraben esters, and mercuric salts. Preservatives are probably the most common cause of toxic conjunctivitis. In a study comprising over 9500 patients, signs and symptoms were more frequent in patients taking preserved medications, compared with those using preservative-free eye drops.[21,22]

Benzalkonium chloride (BAK) is a quaternary ammonium hapten highly hydrosoluble with surfactant properties. In concentrations ranging from 0.005% to 0.03%, the drug is generally well tolerated. However, it can cause epithelial toxicity and at higher concentrations can even cause irreversible corneal edema. Thimersoal is an organomercurial derivative used in concentrations varying from 0.001% to 0.004%. It is a common cause of hypersensitivity reactions and follicular conjunctivitis, the reported incidence being as high as 8%. Chlorbutanol is an alcohol that increases lipid solubility and its antimicrobial activity is based on its ability to cross the bacterial lipid layer. It is widely used in many pharmaceuticals and cosmetic products. In concentrations of 0.5% it is normally well tolerated and has been found to be less toxic than BAK or thimerosal.[7,23]

Antivirals, Antibiotics, and Antifungals

Topical antibiotics constitute the main treatment for bacterial conjunctivitis and keratitis. Fortunately, the most allergenic known antibiotic, penicillin, is not used to treat ocular infection. The most used antibiotics are topical aminoglycosides and fluoroquinolones, followed by sulfonamides, macrolides, and chloramphenicol.

Aminoglycosides, such as gentamicin and tobramycin, the latter being the least irritating, can produce conjunctival and corneal hypersensitivity, pruritus and hyperemia.[24] The toxic effects of topical fluoroquinolones, even of the first generations, are less common than those generated by aminoglycosides. The most common corneal finding is a white crystalline precipitate after the use of ciprofloxacin.[13] The current adoption of the fourth-generation fluoroquinolones has resulted in much less toxicity than the aminoglycosides; however, epithelial toxicity, due to the preservative BAK present in the topical preparation of gatifloxacin, can occur. Sulfonamides are the third most commonly used topical antibiotics; and may produce a mild allergic reaction. The most devastating complication associated with this antibiotic is the induction of Stevens–Johnson syndrome or toxic epidermal necrolysis.[14,25] Photosensitization after topical sulfisoxazole ointment use has been reported to cause sunburn of the lid margin.

Antifungals used either in topical commercial preparations or in dilutions prepared from the intravenous forms may impair epithelial healing. Natamycin, the most commonly used topical anti-fungal agent, is generally non-irritating.[26]

All antivirals may cause toxic keratoconjunctivitis to some degree. On the cornea, IDU produces punctate epitheliopathy, epithelial edema, and cornea; erosions. In the conjunctiva, it causes follicular response, subconjunctival scarring and may occlude the puncta. These same effects but to a lesser degree[27] can be caused by trifluorothymidine and vidarabine.

Anesthetics

The indiscriminate use of topical anesthetics is a well known cause of toxic keratoconjunctivitis. Diagnosis is simple when the offending agent is identified, but can be very difficult if the patient hides its misuse. Proparacaine tetracaine, lidocaine, cornecaine, and benoxinate, have all been associated with this entity. The most frequent manifestation is superficial keratopathy, which can be detected even after a single instillation. More severe cases can evolve to corneal ulceration and stromal necrosis. Toxic lesions are due to decreased blinking reflexes, tear film instability with loss of epithelial microvilli, and corneal desiccation. These substances interfere with cell metabolism and cell membrane permeability, alter the function of cytoskeletal proteins, and decrease the rate of epithelial wound healin.[28]

Glaucoma Medications

Patients with glaucoma frequently require topical treatment for decades. Like all ophthalmic medications, any antiglaucoma drop may initiate a sudden allergic response. These events may occur in about 5% of the cases, are usually easy to diagnose, and respond quickly after discontinuation of the offending drug.[4] However, patients may develop a late-onset reaction, appearing months or even decades after treatment. In such cases, local irritation is the rule with foreign body sensation, conjunctival hyperemia, and staining of the conjunctiva with fluorescein and rose bengal.[29] Severe cases may induce subconjunctival fibrosis and a pseudopemphigoid syndrome. Furthermore, long-term therapy may induce subclinical inflammation and increased postoperative fibrosis; hence, the long-term use of topical antiglaucoma drugs is considered as an important risk factor for the failure of filtration surgery failure.[30] Nurturing of the ocular surface and reduction of inflammation before surgery should be achieved whenever possible.[6,17]

Many of the toxic effects on disturbing the ocular surface can be linked to preservatives, such as BAK. However, specific glaucoma medications can be associated with certain clinical manifestations. Pilocarpine and beta-blockers have been associated with follicular conjunctivitis and drug-induced pemphigoid; the latter has also been found to produce pseudodendrites and corneal hypoesthesia. Both epinephrine and dipivefrin can also cause a follicular reaction. The former is associated with pigmented adenochrome deposits in the conjunctiva. Alfa-2-adrenergic agonists may produce an acute allergic blepharoconjunctivitis in up to 30% of the cases.[31]

Others Toxic Agents

Almost all topical treatments used in ophthalmology, given enough time and frequency of use, can be associated with toxicity. Nevertheless, the clinician must be aware that substances other than approved medications may be in contact with the ocular surface. Such is the case of mascara, eyeliner, hair gel, hair sprays, skin preparations, and virtually any substance with direct or indirect contact with the body surface. In many regions of the world, patients still use home-prepared remedies to alleviate common eye complaints, and are often reluctant to disclose their use.[32,33]

Therapeutic Considerations

On encountering a toxic agent, discontinuation of the offending substance is the primary therapeutic strategy. Treatment will depend on the time of exposure and severity of the ocular surface disease. Attempts should be made to stop medications or to substitute them with preservative-free formulations when possible. Contact lenses should be used cautiously, since they can act as a toxic reservoir. For mild disease, a preservative free artificial tear can be used for symptomatic relief. A topical steroid may be beneficial for more symptomatic patients. More severe pathology, such as persistent epithelial defects may require tarsorrhaphy, amniotic membrane grafting, or conjunctival flaps.[34] Keratoplasty may be warranted for corneal ulcerations with impending perforation or necrosis.[35]

References

1. Magnus H. Ophthalmology of the ancients. In: Wayenborgh J, editor. Hirschberg history of ophthalmology, vol. 4. 1st ed. Oostende: Wayenborgh; 1998:4–12.
2. Wilson 2nd FM. Adverse external ocular effects of topical ophthalmic therapy: an epidemiologic, laboratory, and clinical study. Trans Am Ophthalmol Soc 1983;81:854–965.
3. Baudouin C. Detrimental effect of preservatives in eyedrops: implications for the treatment of glaucoma. Acta Ophthalmol 2008; 86:716–26.
4. Baudouin C, Riancho L, Warnet JM, et al. In vitro studies of antiglaucomatous prostaglandin analogues: travoprost with and without benzalkonium chloride and preserved latanoprost. Invest Ophthalmol Vis Sci 2007;48:4123–8.
5. Schwab IR, Abbott RL. Toxic ulcerative keratopathy. An unrecognized problem. Ophthalmology 1989;96:1187–93.
6. Baudouin C, Liang H, Hamard P, et al. The ocular surface of glaucoma patients treated over the long term expresses inflammatory markers related to both T-helper 1 and T-helper 2 pathways. Ophthalmology 2008;115:109–15.
7. Chen W, Li Z, Hu J, et al. Corneal alternations induced by topical application of benzalkonium chloride in rabbit. PLoS One 2011; 6:e26103.
8. Wilson 2nd FM. Adverse external ocular effects of topical ophthalmic medications. Surv Ophthalmol 1979;24:57–88.
9. Thorne JE, Anhalt GJ, Jabs DA. Mucous membrane pemphigoid and pseudopemphigoid. Ophthalmology 2004;111:45–52.
10. Guglielmetti S, Dart JK, Calder V. Atopic keratoconjunctivitis and atopic dermatitis. Curr Opin Allergy Clin Immunol 2010;10: 478–85.
11. Kirzhner M, Jakobiec FA. Ocular cicatricial pemphigoid: a review of clinical features, immunopathology, differential diagnosis, and current management. Semin Ophthalmol 2011;26:270–7.
12. Cone RE, Chattopadhyay S, O'Rourke J. Control of delayed-type hypersensitivity by ocular- induced CD8+ regulatory t cells. Chem Immunol Allergy 2008;94:138–49.
13. Cutarelli PE, Lass JH, Lazarus HM, et al. Topical fluoroquinolones: antimicrobial activity and in vitro corneal epithelial toxicity. Curr Eye Res 1991;10:557–63.
14. Fine HF, Kim E, Eichenbaum KD, et al. Toxic epidermal necrolysis induced by sulfonamide eyedrops. Cornea 2008;27:1068–9.
15. Fraunfelder FW. Corneal toxicity from topical ocular and systemic medications. Cornea 2006;25:1133–8.
16. Dart J. Corneal toxicity: the epithelium and stroma in iatrogenic and factitious disease. Eye (Lond) 2003;17:886–92.
17. Baudouin C, Pisella PJ, Fillacier K, et al. Ocular surface inflammatory changes induced by topical antiglaucoma drugs: human and animal studies. Ophthalmology 1999;106:556–63.
18. Egbert PR, Lauber S, Maurice DM. A simple conjunctival biopsy. Am J Ophthalmol 1977;84:798–801.
19. Barbaro V, Ferrari S, Fasolo A, et al. Evaluation of ocular surface disorders: a new diagnostic tool based on impression cytology and confocal laser scanning microscopy. Br J Ophthalmol 2010;94:926–32.
20. Van D Meid KR, Su SP, Ward KW, et al. Correlation of tear inflammatory cytokines and matrix metalloproteinases with four dry eye diagnostic tests. Invest Ophthalmol Vis Sci 2012;54:1512–8.
21. Jaenen N, Baudouin C, Pouliquen P, et al. Ocular symptoms and signs with preserved and preservative-free glaucoma medications. Eur J Ophthalmol 2007;17:341–9.
22. Baudouin C, Labbe A, Liang H, et al. Preservatives in eyedrops: the good, the bad and the ugly. Prog Retin Eye Res 2010;29:312–34.
23. Beasley R, Burgess C, Holt S. Call for worldwide withdrawal of benzalkonium chloride from nebulizer solutions. J Allergy Clin Immunol 2001;107:222–3.
24. Lass JH, Mack RJ, Imperia PS, et al. An in vitro analysis of aminoglycoside corneal epithelial toxicity. Curr Eye Res 1989;8:299–304.
25. Gottschalk HR, Stone OJ. Stevens–Johnson syndrome from ophthalmic sulfonamide. Arch Dermatol 1976;112:513–4.

26. Foster CS, Lass JH, Moran-Wallace K, et al. Ocular toxicity of topical antifungal agents. Arch Ophthalmol 1981;99:1081–4.
27. Foster CS, Pavan-Langston D. Corneal wound healing and antiviral medication. Arch Ophthalmol 1977;95:2062–7.
28. Yagci A, Bozkurt B, Egrilmez S, et al. Topical anesthetic abuse keratopathy: a commonly overlooked health care problem. Cornea 2011; 30:571–5.
29. Baudouin C, Hamard P, Liang H, et al. Conjunctival epithelial cell expression of interleukins and inflammatory markers in glaucoma patients treated over the long term. Ophthalmology 2004; 111:2186–92.
30. Pflugfelder SC, Baudouin C. Challenges in the clinical measurement of ocular surface disease in glaucoma patients. Clin Ophthalmol 2011;5:1575–83.
31. Noecker RJ, Herrygers LA, Anwaruddin R. Corneal and conjunctival changes caused by commonly used glaucoma medications. Cornea 2004;23:490–6.
32. Satterfield D, Mannis MJ. Episodic bilateral corneal edema caused by hair groom gel. Am J Ophthalmol 1992;113:107–8.
33. Goto T, Zheng X, Gibbon L, et al. Cosmetic product migration onto the ocular surface: exacerbation of migration after eyedrop instillation. Cornea 2010;29:400–3.
34. Altinok AA, Balikoglu M, Sen E, et al. Nonpreserved amniotic membrane transplantation for bilateral toxic keratopathy caused by topical anesthetic abuse: a case report. J Med Case Reports 2010;4:262.
35. Rocha G, Brunette I, Le Francois M. Severe toxic keratopathy secondary to topical anesthetic abuse. Can J Ophthalmol 1995;30: 198–202.

26 *Corneal Epithelial Adhesion Disorders*

ABRAHAM SOLOMON

Introduction

The normal corneal epithelium maintains its adhesion to the underlying basement membrane, through complex adhesion structures, which are composed = of hemidesmosomes, basement membrane components, and structural proteins. Following trauma to the corneal epithelium, new structures are formed as part of the wound healing process. A defect in the appropriate formation of these structures results in inadequate epithelial–stromal attachments, and may lead to localized adhesion problems of the corneal epithelium, manifesting in a distinctive clinical entity entitled *recurrent corneal erosion (RCE) syndrome*.

Corneal epithelial adhesions problems have many etiologies and are collectively referred to as recurrent corneal erosion syndrome. This disorder is characterized by episodes of spontaneous erosions of the corneal epithelium. These episodes are unpredictable and acute, with symptoms ranging from a mild ocular foreign body sensation, to abrupt sharp pain, usually occurring in the middle of the night or upon awakening. The duration of symptoms may last from minutes to hours. This recurrent disorder can last from a few weeks to several years, creating significant disability and suffering for the patient. It poses a significant therapeutic challenge, since there is no definitive treatment to date. Various treatment strategies have been developed over the years, ranging from various topical medications, which are aimed at prevention of these attacks, to surgical procedures which try to create a new stroma–basement membrane–epithelial environment.

Pathophysiology

NORMAL ANATOMY OF THE EPITHELIAL ADHESION COMPLEX

There are two major adherence mechanisms for corneal epithelial cells to adhere to basement membrane. One mechanism is through direct molecular interaction of receptors with ligands located in the extracellular matrix. Three major families of such molecular interactions have been identified. These include the N-CAM family, the cadherin family, and the integrins, which are a family of integral membrane proteins interacting with an extracellular matrix ligand at cell–matrix interfaces.[1]

The second mechanism of cell–matrix adhesion is through adhesive junctions, called hemidesmosomes (Fig. 26.1).[2] The hemidesmosomes are located on the basal membranes of the epithelial cells. On the external side of

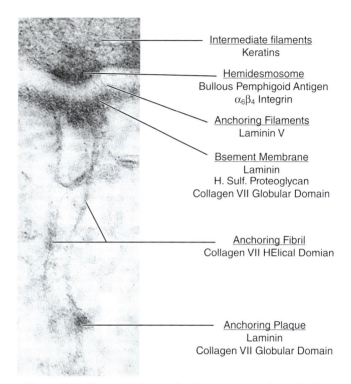

Intermediate filaments
Keratins

Hemidesmosome
Bullous Pemphigoid Antigen
$\alpha_6\beta_4$ Integrin

Anchoring Filaments
Laminin V

Bsement Membrane
Laminin
H. Sulf. Proteoglycan
Collagen VII Globular Domain

Anchoring Fibril
Collagen VII HElical Domian

Anchoring Plaque
Laminin
Collagen VII Globular Domain

Figure 26.1 Electron micrograph demonstrating the adhesion complex of the corneal epithelium. The linked structures of the complex and their known molecular components are identified. 165 000×. (From Albert & Jacobiec's Principles and Practice of Ophthalmology, vol. 1. 3rd ed. Saunders Elseviers; 2009. p. 427.)

the cell membrane at the hemidesmosome, an electron-dense line parallels the membrane and, from it, anchoring filaments extend through the lamina lucida to the lamina densa of the basement membrane (Fig. 26.1). Opposite the lamina densa, anchoring fibrils insert from the stromal side. These fibrils form an intertwining network in the anterior stroma. Distal from their insertions in the basement membrane, anchoring fibrils insert into anchoring plaques, which appear structurally as small segments of basement membrane (Fig. 26.1). Collectively, all these structurally linked components, including intermediate filaments, hemidesmosomes, anchoring filaments, anchoring fibrils and anchoring plaques, are termed the *adhesion complex*.[3]

EPITHELIAL CELL ADHESIONS IN RECURRENT CORNEAL EROSIONS

Immediately after the removal of the corneal epithelium, the denuded stroma in the area of the epithelial defect is coated with fibronectin. This provides a platform for the adjacent viable epithelial cells to slide and migrate to cover the denuded area, and to proliferate to form the superficial cells. The basal cells form adhesion complexes with the underlying structure.

As basal cells of the corneal epithelium begin to migrate to cover a wound, they lose their hemidesmosomes.[4] Re-establishment of the tight adhesion of the corneal epithelium is associated with re-formation of hemidesmosomes and components of the adhesion complex.[5] An interim adhesion junction, termed 'focal adhesion,' is constructed along the cell–matrix interface of epithelial cells during migration, as evident by a dramatic increase in protein synthesis during migration to cover a wound.[6]

The status of the basement membrane at the time of initial injury can influence the outcome of epithelial healing. When the basement membrane is involved in the damage, epithelial cell migration and its adherence to the underlying stroma is delayed up to a few weeks. If the basement membrane remains intact, epithelial cells migrate over the old membrane and form adhesion complexes in a few days.

Ultrastructural studies of the cornea in RCE have demonstrated defective junctional complexes following epithelial trauma, resulting in delayed adhesion of epithelial cells to underlying structures (Fig. 26.2).[5,7] These adhesion complex defects are characterized primarily by the focal absence of the basement membrane and of the hemidesmosomes. The basement membrane may appear multilayered and folded between epithelial cells. In addition, some of the basal corneal epithelial cells appear pale and swollen.[7,8] Areas of healthy epithelium contain intraepithelial pseudocysts, with collections of cellular and amorphous debris.[7] This cellular debris is probably the result of entrapment of the epithelium by aberrant basement membrane. The abnormal adhesion complexes between the basal epithelial cells and the basement membrane, may lead to focal areas of elevation of the epithelium and the accumulation of underlying cellular debris (Fig. 26.2). This leads to formation of abnormal basement membrane, with further focal detachments of the basal epithelium and accumulation of cellular debris, leading to a vicious cycle of aberrant epithelial adhesion and recurrent erosions.

The timing of the erosion corresponds with an abrupt opening of the lids, which is why these episodes occur at night time or while awakening from sleep in the morning. During sleep and lid closure, there is no air between the lids and the tear film, and the surface tension of the tears creates sealing of the lid margins. Abrupt opening the lids creates a shearing force, which is greater than the force of adherence of the epithelium to its basement membrane, and this may result in epithelial avulsion.[9]

MEIBOMIAN GLAND DISEASE AND INFLAMMATORY MEDIATORS

A higher incidence of severe meibomian gland disease (MGD) and acne rosacea was noted in non-traumatic RCE.[10] These patients had inspissation of the meibomian glands, reduced tear film break-up time, conjunctival injection, and facial manifestations of acne rosacea, including facial erythema, flushes, papules, and pustules. The location of the

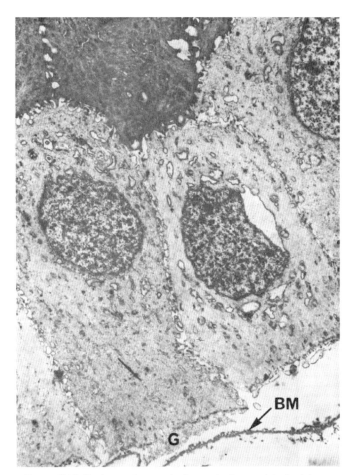

Figure 26.2 Electron micrograph demonstrating a detached basement membrane (BM) with almost complete absence of hemidesmosomes. Cell membranes are poorly demarcated and interrupted. Cellular debris (G) accumulates between the cells and the basement membrane. (From Tripathi RC, Bron AJ. Ultrastructural study of non-traumatic recurrent corneal erosion. Br J Ophthalmol 1972;56:73, Figure 5, page 79.)

corneal erosions was at the inferior cornea, which was explained by a longer contact with the tear film, containing its inflammatory mediators, typical of MGD.[10]

MGD is associated with higher levels of inflammatory cytokines and matrix-degrading enzymes in the tear film, which may potentially disturb the normal healing process, by interfering with the formation of normal hemidesmosomes and adhesion complexes. Increased bacterial lipase has been demonstrated in patients with MGD, which is responsible for the production of free fatty acids, which can interfere with the assembly of the adhesion complexes.[11,12] In addition, inflammatory cytokines and matrix-degrading enzymes, such as interleukin-1 and MMP-9 were found to be elevated in the tears of patients with MGD,[13] further contributing to the damaged healing patterns of the corneal epithelium in RCE.

Elevated levels of MMP-2 and MMP-9 have been observed in the tear fluid of patients with RCE. These matrix-degrading enzymes were found to be up-regulated in human epithelia affected by recurrent erosion. These enzymes are concentrated in basal epithelial cells where they may play an important role in degradation of the epithelial anchoring system and result in recurrent epithelial slippage and erosion.[14]

Etiology

Recurrent corneal erosions are the clinical end result of multiple disorders of the corneal epithelium and basement membrane. Although most of the patients with unilateral RCE will present after a history of acute trauma to the cornea with sloughing or erosion of the corneal epithelium (Fig. 26.3), careful consideration must be given to a wide spectrum of causes, specifically in patients with a bilateral disease, having no prior injury to the cornea.

The etiology of RCE may be classified into primary and secondary disorders (Box 26.1).[9] Primary disorders include genetic disorders, chiefly the corneal dystrophies that involve the epithelium, basement membrane or anterior stroma. Primary disorders are usually bilateral, symmetrical, and may occur in multiple locations in the cornea. The most common of these etiologies is the map-dot finger print dystrophy (Figs 26.4, 26.5). RCE is a common

manifestation in lattice dystrophy, which involves the anterior stroma (Fig. 26.6).[15]

The secondary basement membrane disorders leading to RCE are more common. They are usually acquired disorders, appear in one eye, and are often limited to a single location in the cornea. Of these, minor trauma to the corneal epithelium is the most common cause for RCE.

Box 26.1 Etiology of RCE

Primary

Genetically related basement membrane abnormalities (dystrophies)

Anterior epithelial basement membrane dystrophy
- Map-dot-fingerprint dystrophy
- Cogan's dystrophy
Bowman's layer
- Reis-Bückler's dystrophy
  - Type I: marked visual loss early in life
  - Type II: visual loss late in life

Stromal dystrophy
Lattice dystrophy (RCE common)
Macular dystrophy
Granular dystrophy (RCE rare)

Secondary

Acquired basement membrane abnormalitie
Traumatic epithelial abrasions
Salzmann's nodular degeneration
Band keratopathy
Herpetic infection
Following bacterial ulcers
Meibomian gland dysfunction
Keratoconjunctivitis sicca
Diabetes mellitus
Epidermolysis bullosa
Following refractive surgery

After Ramamurthi S, Rahman MQ, Dutton GN, et al. Pathogenesis, clinical features and management of recurrent corneal erosions. Eye (Lond) 2006;20:635–644.

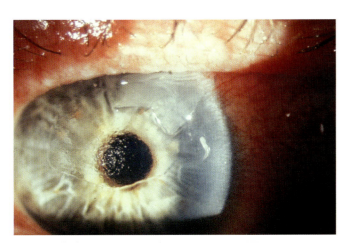

Figure 26.3 Trauma to the corneal epithelium is usually the most common cause of unilateral recurrent corneal erosions. (Courtesy Peter Laibson, MD.)

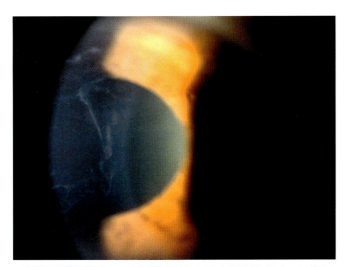

Figure 26.4 Map-like changes in epithelial basement membrane dystrophy. (Courtesy Peter Laibson, MD.)

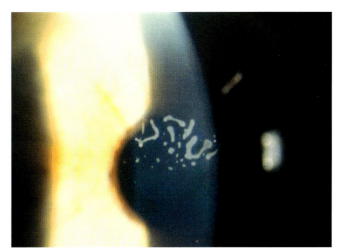

Figure 26.5 Epithelial microcysts which appear as dots in epithelial basement membrane dystrophy (map-dot fingerprint dystrophy). (Courtesy Peter Laibson, MD.)

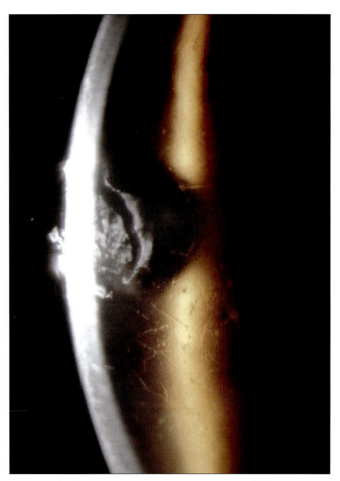

Figure 26.6 Recurrent corneal erosion in a patient with lattice dystrophy. (From Krachmer JH, Mannis JM, Holland EJ. Cornea. 3rd ed. Mosby; 2011. p. 831, Figure 72.13.)

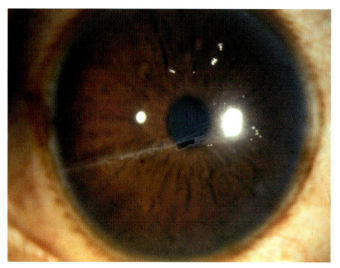

Figure 26.7 A linear erosion in the corneal epithelium, caused by the edge of a paper, may predispose to recurrent corneal erosions. (Courtesy Peter Laibson, MD.)

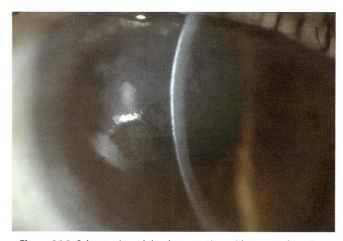

Figure 26.8 Salzmann's nodular degeneration with a corneal erosion. (Courtesy Abraham Solomon, MD.)

Trauma to the epithelium can be caused by a fingernail, plant material, sharp domestic objects, or the edge of a piece of paper (Fig. 26.7).[16] Salzmann's nodular degeneration is another common acquired disorder that may be associated with recurrent erosions (Fig. 26.8).

Rarely, cases may occur spontaneously without any obvious predisposing factor.

Clinical Manifestations

Sharp pain, tearing, photophobia and redness that occur abruptly upon awakening, when opening the lids, or during sleep, mainly due to rapid eye movements, are the hallmark of RCE. The combination of a previous history of minor trauma to the involved eye, episodes of pain on awakening, and a rough irregular area of healing epithelium, is diagnostic of RCE.

Two main forms of erosion have been identified: microform and macroform. The microform erosions are small epithelial breaks, while the macroform erosion is larger and surrounded with a loosely adherent epithelium. Typically, the microform erosions are less severe, occur more frequently, sometimes every night or morning, occur spontaneously and are associated with epithelial basement membrane dystrophy (EBMD). The macroform erosions are associated with a traumatic etiology, and persist for several days.[17]

Although little is known about the epidemiology of RCE, it is thought to be a relatively common problem in specialized cornea services. The incidence of RCE was reported to be 1 : 150 cases following trauma.[9]

Careful slit lamp examination is needed to find the subtle signs of this syndrome, since the epithelium in many cases had already healed. The delicate signs of basement membrane dystrophy (Fig. 26.9), the sites of a previous erosion, or clusters of small epithelial microcysts, may be seen with either a broad slit beam or with retroillumination (Fig. 26.10). Examination of the cornea after pupil dilation, against the red reflex, may disclose subtle changes in the corneal epithelium. Gentle pressure applied to the cornea through the eyelid may demonstrate wrinkling of loosely adherent epithelium. In many cases, no signs are found, and then the patient should be instructed to return immediately after the next episode of pain, without allowing time for the epithelium to heal and cover the erosion. This will facilitate proper diagnosis and correct location of the lesion for the purpose of treatment.

During the acute attack or during the first few days following the attack, the affected corneal epithelium can

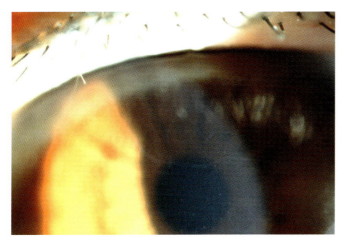

Figure 26.9 Mild changes of epithelial basement membrane dystrophy can be seen at the upper part of the cornea in a patient with RCE. (Source: Abraham Solomon, MD.)

present as a loosely adherent and elevated epithelium, or as epithelial microcysts, or as corneal epithelial defects.[17,18] Stromal infiltrates and opacities may also develop at the site of the erosions.[19] The location of most of the corneal erosions is in the lower half of the cornea.[16] The midline below the horizontal meridian is usually the last area to re-epithelialize, and the closure lines at this area are predisposed to frequent breakdown. In addition, this is the area of maximal exposure, since it opposes the line of lids closure.

A possible complication of RCE is infectious keratitis, occurring as a result of prolonged bandage contact lens use and topical steroids.[9]

When no obvious signs of RCE are evident in the slit lamp examination, the presence of impaired epithelial adhesion is detected by use of a dry cellulose sponge, which is gently rubbed over the area of suspected epithelial erosions. If the intact epithelial sheet is moveable by the sponge, then the lack of adequate epithelial–stromal adhesion must be suspected.[20]

The duration of symptoms may vary, and the frequency and number of attacks are also extremely variable. The frequency of recurrence may range from a minor recurrence every morning to a major recurrence every several months. Recurrences typically last from 1 to 4 hours in the microform condition and 1 to 21 days in the macroform erosions.[17] A more recent study in a large cohort of RCE

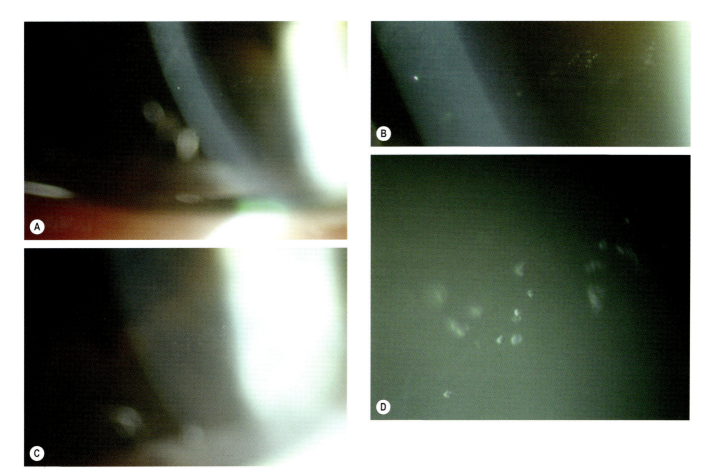

Figure 26.10 Epithelial microcysts in a patient with previous attacks of RCE. The significance of careful evaluation from different angles and magnifications is shown. (**A**) A cluster of epithelial microscysts is seen with retroillumination. (**B**) Same as figure (**A**), under a higher magnification. (**C**) The same cluster of epithelial microcysts is seen with a broad slit beam. (**D**) Same as figure (**C**), under a higher magnification. (Courtesy Abraham Solomon, MD.)

patients demonstrated that after 4 years of follow-up, 59% of all patients were still symptomatic, and most of them complained of symptoms occurring upon waking in the mornings.[21] The median frequency of the attacks was every 60 days; however, 24% of symptomatic patients suffered with an attack at least every week, and 51% of the symptomatic patients suffered an attack at least every month.

Comparing patients with a traumatic etiology with patients who had RCE secondary to EBMD, patients with EBMD were significantly more likely to be symptomatic: 75% of patients with EBMD were symptomatic compared with 46% of patients with traumatic etiology.[21]

Management

The management of RCE is challenging, and to date, not one single therapy was found to be definitive and sufficiently effective. Over the years, multiple treatment strategies were developed, including topical conservative treatments, such as hypertonic lubricants, soft bandage contact lenses, and various aggressive surgical modalities, such as anterior stromal puncture and photorefractive keratectomy, which aim at creating a new basement membrane–epithelial interface (Box 26.2).

The primary goals of management of RCE during the acute attacks include pain relief and promotion of fast and prolonged epithelialization. Stabilization of the healed epithelium and prevention of subsequent erosion episodes are the long-term goals of RCE management. These goals are not easily achieved, and the chronic course of resistant cases of RCE may be frustrating for both patient and physician.

MEDICAL MANAGEMENT

Topical Lubricants and Hyperosmotic Agents

Most patients with an acute episode of RCE can be managed initially with patching and a topical antibiotic ointment.[16,17] To prevent recurrences, the most widely used therapies include topical lubrication and hypertonic saline.[10,16,17,22] Topical lubrication can be administered as drops, gels or ointment. The bedtime application of an ointment will

---

Box 26.2   Management of RCE

Medical treatment for RCE
  Slow eye movements on awakening, gradual lid opening
  Patching, cycloplegia, topical lubrication
  Hyperosmotic agents (5% Sodium Chloride)
  Temporary soft bandage contact lens
  Care of associated lid pathology
  Autologous serum
  MMP inhibitors (oral tetracycline/doxycycline)
Surgical treatment for RCE
  Epithelial debridement
  Anterior stromal puncture (insulin needle or Nd:YAG laser)
  Phototherapeutic keratectomy (PTK)
  Diamond burr superficial keratectomy

After Ramamurthi S, Rahman MQ, Dutton GN, et al. Pathogenesis, clinical features and management of recurrent corneal erosions. Eye (Lond) 2006;20(6):635–644.

---

reduce the amount of friction between the tarsal conjunctiva and the corneal epithelium overnight, during the rapid eye movements (REM), and will protect the corneal epithelium from the shearing action of the eyelids upon awakening, which is the major trigger of recurrence.

Hyperosmotic agents are also routinely used in RCE. During sleep there is a relative hypotonicity of the tear film as a result of decreased tear fluid evaporation. The reduced tear osmolarity at night will cause a shift of water from the tear film into the cornea, resulting in a relative corneal epithelial edema and decreased epithelial adhesion. Hypertonic (5%) sodium chloride, either drops or ointment, will promote epithelial adherence by increasing the tear osmolarity, thereby, decreasing epithelial edema and promoting epithelial adherence. These agents should be continued for a few months after the last attack, as it takes a few months for the adhesion complexes to build up.

Most patients will do well with these conservative treatments, which are effective in relieving the pain and promoting the initial epithelial growth.[22] However, these modalities will not reduce the likelihood of recurrences.[16]

Useful advice for patients is to instruct them to move their eyes slowly to the left and right before opening them, and to gradually retract the lower lid, to facilitate gradual separation between the tarsal conjunctiva and the corneal epithelium. This slower separation of the cornea from the tarsal conjunctiva will prevent the shearing force created on the corneal epithelium during abrupt lid opening, and will prevent the erosion.

Therapeutic Bandage Contact Lenses

Therapeutic bandage contact lenses promote epithelial migration and regeneration of the basement membrane by protecting the corneal epithelium from the friction created by the upper tarsal conjunctiva.[23] To be effective, a bandage contact lens should be worn for a few weeks to several months,[16] replacing it every 2 weeks. This may enable the formation of stable adhesion complexes between the corneal epithelium and the basement membrane.

These contact lenses should be used under close supervision, since long-term continuous use of contact lenses may predispose to bacterial keratitis and neovascularization.[16,24] However, the introduction of the silicon hydrogel extended-wear contact lenses, in recent years, has significantly increased the safety of long-term use of bandage contact lenses.[25,26]

Autologous Serum

Autologous serum has been used effectively in RCE, significantly reducing the incidence of recurrence.[27,28] It is composed of substances that are essential for epithelial healing, such as vitamin A, epidermal growth factor, transforming growth factor β and fibronectin. Fibronectin promotes epithelial cell migration and participates in the adhesion process.[29] The lipids in the serum may act as a substitute for the lipids produced by the meibomian glands. When appropriately prepared and used, autologous serum is safe and no adverse effects have been reported with its use.[28]

Managing Lid Disease

Meibomian gland disease (MGD) and chronic blepharitis are associated with RCE.[10] The tear film in MGD may have increased levels of bacterial lipases, fatty acids, interleukins and MMPs, which can interfere with corneal epithelial healing. Therefore, the usual therapeutic measures employed in the treatment of MGD should be used in RCE as well. These include lid hygiene and oral tetracyclines. Oral tetracyclines were shown to be beneficial in reducing episodes of RCE by reducing the free fatty acids in the tear film of MGD, by inactivating the MMPs, and by reducing the number of colony forming units from lid cultures.[10,30] Low doses of oral tetracyclines should be continued for a few months.

The corneal epithelium produces matrix-degrading enzymes, such as MMP-2 and MMP-9. These enzymes have roles in the wound healing process, and are part of the inflammatory activity in many ocular surface disorders. Increased production of these enzymes, specifically MMP-2, was demonstrated in RCE.[14] Therefore, MMPs may be responsible for the degradation of anchoring molecules in the adhesion complexes of the basement membrane during epithelial healing. This is the basis for the use of inhibitors of MMP in the treatment of resistant RCE.[31] Indeed, a combination of oral doxycycline and topical steroids was successfully used in recalcitrant cases of RCE.[31] Both topical steroids and oral doxycycline were reported to decrease the frequency of RCE in a randomized, controlled clinical trial.[30] In addition, doxycycline and corticosteroids have significant anti-inflammatory properties. Doxycycline decreases the synthesis and bioactivity of interleukin-1, produced by cultured human epithelial cells.[32] The combination of steroids and doxycycline can inhibit the inflammatory cytokines and MMPs and promote rapid resolution and prevent further recurrence in RCE.[31]

SURGICAL MANAGEMENT

When the various medical treatment options fail, surgical therapy can be highly effective. Over the years, a series of surgical procedures have been described for RCE, including diamond burr polishing of Bowman's membrane, anterior stromal puncture with an insulin needle or with YAG laser, and excimer laser phototherapeutic keratectomy (PTK). As these procedures result in high success rates and carry low risks, it is advisable not to defer the surgical options if the medical treatment is not effective.

Debridement of Loose Epithelium

Epithelial debridement is probably indicated when a large area of the epithelium is loose and mobile with lid movements. Debridement of this large area of loose epithelium is necessary for pain relief, and can promote healing from the healthy adherent edges of the intact epithelium. Epithelial debridement may be performed under topical anesthesia with the slit lamp, by removing the loose epithelium with a sterile sponge. A therapeutic bandage contact lens should be placed if the epithelial defect is large. Topical antibiotics and cyclopentolate drops may be added. Epithelial debridement alone cannot reduce the recurrences of epithelial erosions.[16,17,22]

Anterior Stromal Puncture

Anterior stromal puncture is a highly effective and widely used office technique, involving the use of a straight 25-gauge needle to make multiple shallow penetrations through the epithelium into anterior corneal stroma, thus, improving epithelial adhesion. It is theorized that this procedure incites reactive fibrosis and scarring, and production of extra cellular matrix proteins, that are responsible for proper adhesion of the epithelium to its substrate.[33] The procedure is performed with topical anesthesia with a bent 25 gauge (0.1–0.3 mm turned end) needle attached to a 3-mL syringe. Topical nonsteroidal drops, such as ketorolac or diclofenac should be instilled prior to the procedure to reduce postoperative pain. Fluorescein can be instilled topically before the treatment to better define the affected area (Fig. 26.11). The angled tip of the needle is kept perpendicular to the surface of the cornea, and multiple superficial punctures are placed approximately 0.5 mm apart in the affected area (Fig. 26.11). Treatment is extended to 1–2 mm into the normal epithelium bordering the lesion, because the loose epithelium usually extends beyond the visible limits of the erosion. Treatment within the pupil area should be minimized if possible. Since anterior stromal puncture may result in subepithelial scars (Fig. 26.12),

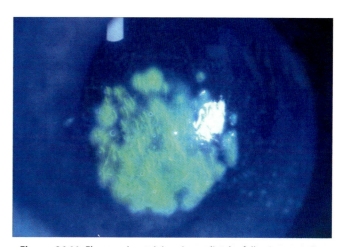

Figure 26.11 Fluorescein staining immediately following anterior stromal puncture. (Courtesy Peter Laibson, MD.)

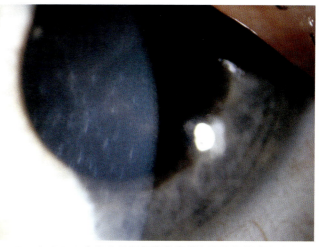

Figure 26.12 Subepithelial scarring after anterior stromal puncture. (Courtesy Peter Laibson, MD.)

its use is not advisable if the erosion directly involves the visual axis, since a central scar may result in glare and a reduction in visual acuity. Immediately after the treatment, a bandage contact lens is placed and antibiotics are given for 1 week.[18,22]

Success rates of up to 80% have been reported in recalcitrant RCE.[18] Treatment failure is associated with a too small treatment area, and erosions then develop outside of the treated area. A second, larger treatment can often resolve the erosions in patients in whom the initial procedure was unsuccessful.

Anterior stromal puncture can also be performed with a short-pulsed Nd:YAG laser.[34] Energy levels ranging of 1.8–2.2 mJ can be used. The advantage of laser puncture over needle puncture is that the laser puncture is more reproducible, shallow, and translucent.

Phototherapeutic Keratectomy (PTK)

Studies have shown that partial ablation of Bowman's layer, with the excimer laser, provides a smooth bed for migrating epithelium, and results in new hemidesmosomal adhesion complexes.[35,36] Human studies have shown that the basal epithelial layer forms hemidesmosomes and new basement membrane within 2 weeks of laser photoablation.[37] Thus, new hemidesmosomes, anchoring fibrils, and epithelial basement membrane are synthesized rapidly and in increasing amounts after PTK. In addition, removing the basement membrane allows the epithelium to come into direct contact with stromal elements, stimulating the synthesis of new anchoring fibrils and hemidesmosomes.[38]

The safety and efficacy of PTK for RCE have been well established.[38,39] The advantages of PTK are removal of corneal tissue with extreme precision, without damage to the non-ablated area, and simultaneous treatment of wider areas. The aim is to remove a 6.0-mm diameter of thick anterior stromal layer. The defective epithelium is removed with a cellulose sponge and a 7.0–8.0-mm diameter flat beam is programmed to ablate a 6.0-mm diameter layer of the anterior stroma. The eye is usually padded after cycloplegic and antibiotic drops. Bandage contact lenses may be needed during the postoperative period. The success rate of PTK is between 60% and 100%.[40,41] PTK results in a higher rate of success for RCE following trauma than corneal dystrophies.[40,41]

The main disadvantags of PTK are the postoperative discomfort and the hyperopic shift caused by the central flattening of the cornea. More advanced PTK treatments, based on flying spot beam profiles, are associated with fewer undesirable refractive changes, compared to those with older, broader beam lasers.

Diamond Burr Superficial Keratectomy

Epithelial debridement and diamond burr polishing of Bowman's membrane is another, less commonly used option in the treatment of RCE. This procedure includes the debridement of loose sheets of epithelium from the cornea, using a combination of peeling with forceps and gentle wiping with a cellulose sponge. If the erosion is within the visual axis, the entire corneal surface is polished with a fine diamond burr, using multiple circular movements to prevent an irregular surface. The limbal epithelium is left intact in the 1–2-mm circumferential periphery. Treatment is limited to the anterior part of Bowman's layer. A bandage contact lens is applied and antibiotics are given following the treatment.

The results of diamond burr are comparable to those of PTK.[42] A subtle granular subepithelial deposit is initially noticed. The haze clears in up to 3 months postoperatively. A study on cases with RCE and anterior basement membrane dystrophy showed significantly less haze after diamond burr polishing compared to PTK. Diamond burr polishing is a simple, less expensive procedure with a smaller incidence of haze and fewer recurrences compared to PTK. In addition, it can be used to treat RCE involving the visual axis.

Conclusion

Epithelial adhesion disorders are common problems encountered by most cornea specialists. Recurrent corneal erosions occur most commonly after mild trauma to the corneal epithelium, but may also result from various inherited dystrophies of the corneal epithelium, basement membrane and anterior stroma. RCE is symptomatic with episodes of pain upon awakening, and can cause considerable impairment of the quality of life. Careful slit lamp examination is needed to find subtle changes associated with either mild trauma or EBMD. The majority of cases are mild and respond to simple, conservative medical treatment, such as lubricants and hyperosmotic agents. However, a minority of patients will develop a more persistent course of RCE and will require surgical intervention, including anterior stromal puncture or PTK. Tailoring the proper treatment strategy to each patient is the key to a successful control of these disorders.

References

1. Hynes RO. Integrins: a family of cell surface receptors. Cell 1987; 48:549–54.
2. Gipson IK. Adhesive mechanisms of the corneal epithelium. Acta Ophthalmol Suppl 1992;202:13–7.
3. Gipson IK, Spurr-Michaud SJ, Tisdale AS. Anchoring fibrils form a complex network in human and rabbit cornea. Invest Ophthalmol Vis Sci 1987;28:212–20.
4. Buck RC. Hemidesmosomes of normal and regenerating mouse corneal epithelium. Virchows Arch B Cell Pathol Incl Mol Pathol 1982;41(1-2):1–16.
5. Khodadoust AA, Silverstein AM, Kenyon KR, et al. Adhesion of regenerating corneal epithelium. The role of basement membrane. Am J Ophthalmol 1968;65:339–48.
6. Zieske JD, Bukusoglu G, Gipson IK. Enhancement of vinculin synthesis by migrating stratified squamous epithelium. J Cell Biol 1989; 109:571–6.
7. Rodrigues MM, Fine BS, Laibson PR, et al. Disorders of the corneal epithelium: a clinicopathologic study of dot, geographic, and fingerprint patterns. Arch Ophthalmol 1974;92:475–82.
8. Tripathi RC, Bron AJ. Ultrastructural study of non-traumatic recurrent corneal erosion. Br J Ophthalmol 1972;56:73–85.
9. Ramamurthi S, Rahman MQ, Dutton GN, et al. Pathogenesis, clinical features and management of recurrent corneal erosions. Eye 2006; 20:635–44.
10. Hope-Ross MW, Chell PB, Kervick GN, et al. Recurrent corneal erosion: clinical features. Eye 1994;8(Pt 4):373–7.
11. Dougherty JM, McCulley JP. Bacterial lipases and chronic blepharitis. Invest Ophthalmol Vis Sci 1986;27:486–91.
12. Dougherty JM, McCulley JP. Analysis of the free fatty acid component of meibomian secretions in chronic blepharitis. Invest Ophthalmol Vis Sci 1986;27:52–6.

13. Afonso AA, Sobrin L, Monroy DC, et al. Tear fluid gelatinase B activity correlates with IL-1alpha concentration and fluorescein clearance in ocular rosacea. Invest Ophthalmol Vis Sci 1999;40:2506–12.

14. Garrana RM, Zieske JD, Assouline M, et al. Matrix metalloproteinases in epithelia from human recurrent corneal erosion. Invest Ophthalmol Vis Sci 1999;40:1266–70.

15. Zechner EM, Croxatto JO, Malbran ES. Superficial involvement in lattice corneal dystrophy. Ophthalmologica 1986;193:193–9.

16. Hykin PG, Foss AE, Pavesio C, et al. The natural history and management of recurrent corneal erosion: a prospective randomised trial. Eye 1994;8(Pt1):35–40.

17. Brown N, Bron A. Recurrent erosion of the cornea. Br J Ophthalmol 1976;60:84–96.

18. Rubinfeld RS, Laibson PR, Cohen EJ, et al. Anterior stromal puncture for recurrent erosion: further experience and new instrumentation. Ophthalmic Surg 1990;21:318–26.

19. Ionides AC, Tuft SJ, Ferguson VM, et al. Corneal infiltration after recurrent corneal epithelial erosion. Br J Ophthalmol 1997;81:537–40.

20. Kenyon KR, Paz H, Greiner JV, et al. Corneal epithelial adhesion abnormalities associated with LASIK. Ophthalmology 2004;111:11–7.

21. Heyworth P, Morlet N, Rayner S, et al. Natural history of recurrent erosion syndrome – a 4-year review of 117 patients. Br J Ophthalmol 1998;82:26–8.

22. Reidy JJ, Paulus MP, Gona S. Recurrent erosions of the cornea: epidemiology and treatment. Cornea 2000;19:767–71.

23. Donnenfeld ED, Selkin BA, Perry HD, et al. Controlled evaluation of a bandage contact lens and a topical nonsteroidal anti-inflammatory drug in treating traumatic corneal abrasions. Ophthalmology 1995;102:979–84.

24. Kent HD, Cohen EJ, Laibson PR, et al. Microbial keratitis and corneal ulceration associated with therapeutic soft contact lenses. CLAO J 1990;16:49–52.

25. Blackmore SJ. The use of contact lenses in the treatment of persistent epithelial defects. Cont Lens Anterior Eye 2010;33:239–44.

26. Mely R. Therapeutic and cosmetic indications of lotrafilcon a silicone hydrogel extended-wear lenses. Ophthalmologica 2004;218(Suppl. 1):29–38.

27. Ziakas NG, Boboridis KG, Terzidou C, et al. Long-term follow up of autologous serum treatment for recurrent corneal erosions. Clin Experiment Ophthalmol 2010;38:683–7.

28. del Castillo JM, de la Casa JM, Sardina RC, et al. Treatment of recurrent corneal erosions using autologous serum. Cornea 2002;21:781–3.

29. Fujikawa LS, Foster CS, Harrist TJ, et al. Fibronectin in healing rabbit corneal wounds. Lab Invest 1981;45:120–9.

30. Hope-Ross MW, Chell PB, Kervick GN, et al. Oral tetracycline in the treatment of recurrent corneal erosions. Eye 1994;8(Pt 4):384–8.

31. Dursun D, Kim MC, Solomon A, et al. Treatment of recalcitrant recurrent corneal erosions with inhibitors of matrix metalloproteinase-9, doxycycline and corticosteroids. Am J Ophthalmol 2001;132:8–13.

32. Solomon A, Rosenblatt M, Li DQ, et al. Doxycycline inhibition of interleukin-1 in the corneal epithelium. Invest Ophthalmol Vis Sci 2000;41:2544–57.

33. Katsev DA, Kincaid MC, Fouraker BD, et al. Recurrent corneal erosion: pathology of corneal puncture. Cornea 1991;10:418–23.

34. Geggel HS. Successful treatment of recurrent corneal erosion with Nd:YAG anterior stromal puncture. Am J Ophthalmol 1990;110:404–7.

35. Aitken DA, Beirouty ZA, Lee WR. Ultrastructural study of the corneal epithelium in the recurrent erosion syndrome. Br J Ophthalmol 1995;79:282–9.

36. Marshall J, Trokel SL, Rothery S, et al. Long-term healing of the central cornea after photorefractive keratectomy using an excimer laser. Ophthalmology 1988;95:1411–21.

37. Lohmann CP, Gartry DS, Muir MK, et al. Corneal haze after excimer laser refractive surgery: objective measurements and functional implications. Eur J Ophthalmol 1991;1:173–80.

38. O'Brart DP, Muir MG, Marshall J. Phototherapeutic keratectomy for recurrent corneal erosions. Eye 1994;8(Pt 4):378–83.

39. Cavanaugh TB, Lind DM, Cutarelli PE, et al. Phototherapeutic keratectomy for recurrent erosion syndrome in anterior basement membrane dystrophy. Ophthalmology 1999;106:971–6.

40. Dausch D, Landesz M, Klein R, et al. Phototherapeutic keratectomy in recurrent corneal epithelial erosion. Refract Corneal Surg 1993;9:419–24.

41. Fagerholm P, Fitzsimmons TD, Orndahl M, et al. Phototherapeutic keratectomy: long-term results in 166 eyes. Refract Corneal Surg 1993;9(Suppl. 2):S76–S81.

42. Soong HK, Farjo Q, Meyer RF, et al. Diamond burr superficial keratectomy for recurrent corneal erosions. Br J Ophthalmol 2002;86:296–8.

27 *Neurotrophic Keratopathy*

SATHISH SRINIVASAN and DOUGLAS A.M. LYALL

Introduction

The cornea is one of the most richly innervated organs. Corneal innervation not only provides sensation but is integral in the maintenance of the structure and function of the cornea. Normal innervation helps the cornea to regulate epithelial integrity, proliferation and wound healing. Neurotrophic keratopathy (NK) is a degenerative condition of the cornea, characterized by lack of or decreased corneal sensation. This results in increased susceptibility of the corneal surface to injury and compromised healing. In severe cases this can lead to corneal ulceration, stromal melt and perforation. The cornea is supplied by the long ciliary nerve, derived via the nasociliary nerve from the ophthalmic branch of the trigeminal nerve. Any ocular, localized or systemic condition affecting the nerve function along this course can create corneal anesthesia, resulting in NK (Box 27.1).[1] Management of NK can be formidable, with the aim of therapy being prevention of disease progression, preservation of globe integrity and promotion of ocular surface repair.

Pathogenesis

Most of the corneal nerves are derived from the ophthalmic division of the trigeminal nerve, via the anterior ciliary nerves and to a lesser degree from the maxillary nerve. The limbus and the peripheral cornea also receive autonomic sympathetic innervation from the superior cervical ganglion.[2]

Nerves enter the cornea in the middle third of the stroma and run forward anteriorly in a radial fashion towards the center where they lose their myelin sheath approximately 1 mm from the corneal limbus, giving rise to branches that innervate the anterior and mid-stromal layers. In the interface between Bowman's layer and the anterior stroma, the stromal nerves form the subepithelial nerve plexus. They perforate Bowman's layer and form the sub-basal epithelial nerve plexus, providing innervation to the basal epithelial cell layer, to terminate finally within the superficial epithelial layers (Fig. 27.1).[3] Thin branches of the subepithelial plexus ascend and penetrate Bowman's layer, bending almost at a right angle to form the sub-basal nerve plexus at the basal epithelial cell layer (Fig. 27.2).[4]

In vivo confocal microscopy has emerged as a powerful tool to image the corneal cellular structure, including the corneal nerves (Fig. 27.3). The density of the sub-basal plexus varies depending on the method of examination and method of analysis. However, when compared to normal controls, the density of the plexus is reduced in NK and

several predisposing disease states, including diabetes mellitus and viral keratitis (Fig. 27.4 and Fig. 27.5).[5]

Alteration in the density of sub-basal nerves has been shown to alter the concentration of several neuromediators and growth factors on the ocular surface.[6,7] These neuromediators contribute to the homeostatic cycle that maintains a healthy ocular epithelial surface, in addition to

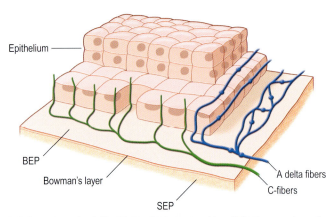

Figure 27.1 Three-dimensional representation of the innervation of the human cornea. BEP, basal epithelial plexus; SEP, subepithelial plexus. (Modified from Guthoff RF, Wienss H, Hahnel C, et al. Epithelial innervation of human cornea: a three-dimensional study using confocal laser scanning fluorescence microscopy. Cornea 2005;24:608–13.)

altering tear production rate. These include substance P, calcitronin gene-related peptide, neuropeptide Y, vasoactive intestinal peptide, galanin, methionine-enkephalin and acetylcholamine.[6–8]

Deficiencies in such mediators have been shown to reduce mitosis rates in epithelial cells, leading to epithelial thinning and surface breakdown. Limbal stem cells fail to replace central epithelium, leading to a persistent epithelial defect. There is also a reduction in microvilli on the epithelial surface, resulting in poor tear adherence to the cornea.[1] Tear composition is also altered by a reduction in goblet cell density within the conjunctival epithelium.[9]

Nerve growth factors (NGF) are a family of circulating mediators that are known to be essential for development and maintenance of both sympathetic and sensory nerves. NGF has also been shown to play a role in the production of acetylcholine and substance P.[10] The cornea and conjunctiva are known to possess specific NGF receptors and it is likely that it plays a multifactorial role in maintaining normal corneal nerve density and preservation of the epithelium.[11] NGF and neuromediators have been the target for several therapeutic agents for neurotrophic keratopathy.

Clinical Presentation

Neurotrophic keratopathy (NK) can present with varied clinical signs. Groos divided the clinical sings into three stages (Box 27.2).[12] Stage 1, the least severe, is characterized by punctate keratopathy, altered tear viscosity with shorter tear break time, peripheral corneal vascularization and punctate staining of the palpebral conjunctiva. Stage 2 is characterized by a compromised corneal epithelial surface, with the defect often bordered by edematous and loose epithelium that forms a smooth edge. Compromise of the epithelium can also lead to stromal edema and visible folds in Descemet's membrane (Fig. 27.6 – Fig. 27.8). Stage 3, the most severe form, is characterized by stromal melting and eventually corneal perforation (Fig. 27.9).

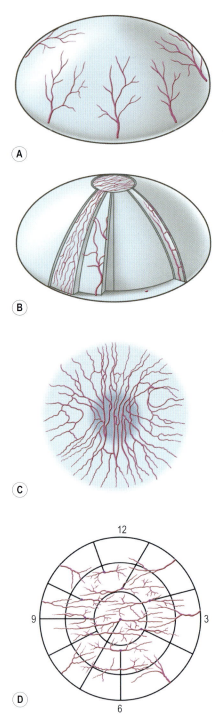

Figure 27.2 Schematic distribution of the corneal nerves. (Reproduced from Muller LJ, Vrensen GF, Pels L, et al. Architecture of human corneal nerves. Invest Ophthalmol Vis Sci 1997;38:985–94.)

Assessment

HISTORY

A systemic and drug history will reveal disease such as diabetes or stroke, or medications that may predispose to NK. A social history may identify patients with vitamin A deficiency, as patients with alcohol excess may be prone to self-neglect and dietary deficiency. Systemic inquiry may

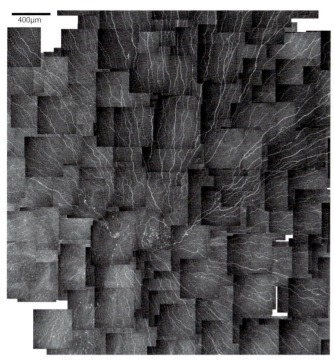

Figure 27.3 A montage of laser scanning in vivo confocal microscopy images depicting the architecture of the human corneal sub-basal nerve plexus. (Image courtesy of Dipika Patel & Charles McGhee.)

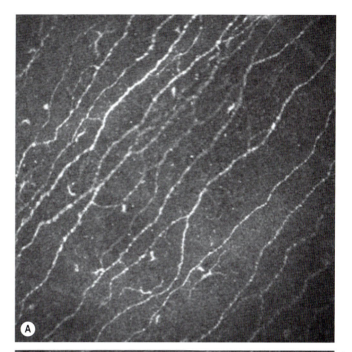
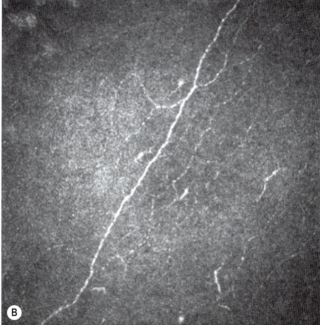

Figure 27.4 (**A**) Confocal microscopy images of corneal nerves in Bowman's layer from a healthy subject. (**B**) Confocal microscopy images of corneal nerves in Bowman's layer from a diabetic patient with severe neuropathy. Note the marked reduction in the density of corneal nerves. (Courtesy of Mitra Tavakoli, PhD.)

Box 27.2 Clinical Stages of Neurotrophic Keratopathy

Stage 1

Punctate corneal epithelium (Gaule spots)
Superficial vascularization
Stromal scarring
Decreased tear break-up time
Increased tear mucus viscosity
Epithelial hyperplasia and irregularity
Hyperplastic precorneal membrane
Staining of palpebral conjunctiva with rose bengal

Stage 2

Epithelial defect, usually in superior half of cornea
Smooth and rolled epithelial defect edges
Surrounding rim of loose epithelium
Stromal edema
Anterior chamber inflammation

Stage 3

Corneal ulcer
Stromal melting
Perforation

(From Groos Jr E. Neurotrophic keratitis. In: Cornea: Fundamentals of Cornea and External Disease. St Loius: Mosby; 1997.)

also reveal previous head trauma, cranial surgery or pathology, such as intracranial neoplasia (acoustic neuroma) that may have led to trigeminal nerve dysfunction. An anesthetic cornea may be the first presentation of an intracranial lesion or abnormality that requires a complete neurological assessment. In addition, past ocular conditions, such as previous herpetic keratitis, trauma, contact lens use, laser refractive eye surgery and topical anesthetic abuse should be documented.

EXAMINATION

Systemic examination should be guided by the history and may warrant referral to an internist for further assessment. Cranial nerve examination should be performed to identify any other potentially relevant neurological deficit.

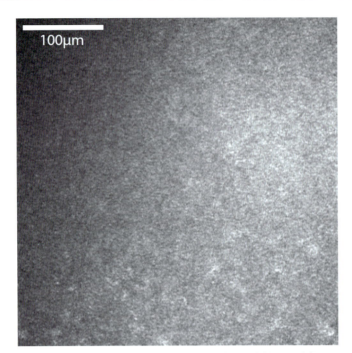

Figure 27.5 Bowman's layer in herpes zoster keratitis. Bowman's layer appears bare, with absent sub-basal nerves when imaged by laser scanning in vivo confocal microscopy in a patient with a history of multiple episodes of herpes zoster disciform keratitis. (Image courtesy of Dipika Patel & Charles McGhee.)

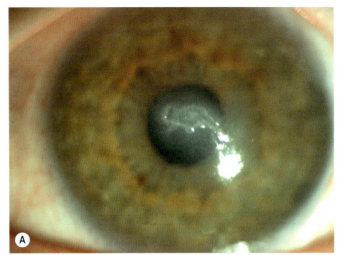

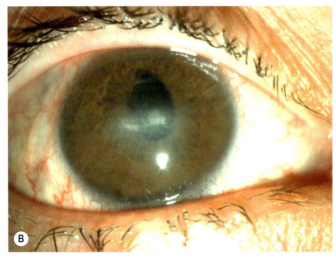

Figure 27.6 Clinical photograph of a 25-year-old-type 1 diabetic with severe diabetic neuropathy. Note the central persistent epithelial defect with raised borders and surrounding epithelial haze

Correctly identifying dysfunction of cranial nerves two to eight, including other divisions of the trigeminal nerve, may help to localize the site of any underlying pathology causing corneal anesthesia. Such pathology may warrant imaging of either the brain or orbit to localize potential lesions. Suspicion of an underlying systemic disease may warrant further blood tests, such as serum glucose to investigate diabetes and serum vitamin levels to investigate hypovitaminosis A.

Orbital and adnexal examination is required to assess the protection offered to the ocular surface by the eyelids. Overexposure of the cornea can lead to a dry ocular surface that may accelerate breakdown of the corneal epithelium. Previous thyroid eye disease may cause proptosis and a potential for associated eyelid retraction. The eyelid may also be unable to close adequately as a result of previous surgery, trauma or a seventh cranial nerve palsy. The presence of blepharitis may also contribute to ocular surface inflammation. Therefore, careful inspection of the lid margin, including the meibomian glands, should be performed as part of routine assessment.

The blink rate should also be assessed, as a reduction can result in a failure to evenly distribute tears over the ocular surface. This can lead to secondary dryness and exposure. There is a reduction in conjunctival goblet cell density and mucin production in neurotrophic keratopathy, resulting in tear instability. There might also be a reduction in tear production as a result of a lack of reflex tearing from corneal irritation.[9] A Schirmer test should be performed as part of the work-up. Corneal sensitivity can be measured with a Cochet – Bonnet esthesiometer. A difference in corneal sensitivity in different quadrants of the cornea might indicate a local cause for anesthesia, such as viral keratitis. An

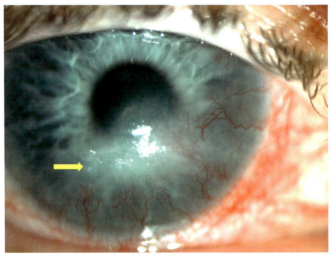

Figure 27.7 Clinical photograph of a 40-year-old with severe neurotrophic keratitis following herpes zoster ophthalmicus. Note the persistent epithelial defect (*arrow*), epithelial and stromal haze, and stromal vascularization.

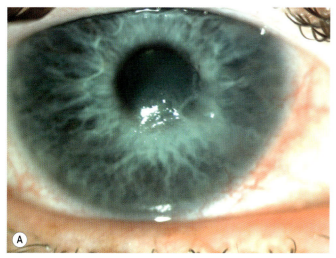

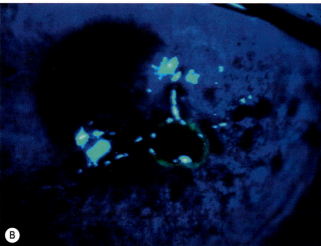

Figure 27.8 (**A**) Clinical photograph of a 40-year-old with neurotrophic keratitis secondary to herpes zoster ophthalmicus. Note the epithelial defect with surrounding epithelial haze. (**B**) Fluorescein staining of a patient highlighting the persistent epithelial defect with neurotrophic keratopathy from herpes zoster keratitis.

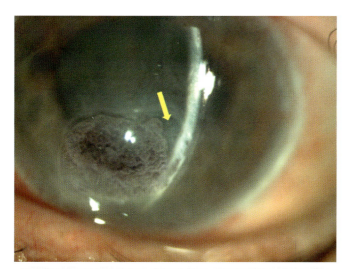

Figure 27.9 Clinical photograph of a 70-year-old with neurotrophic keratitis secondary to herpes zoster ophthalmicus that perforated. Note the cyanoacrylate glue and the underlying persistent epithelial defect (*arrow*).

alternative to an esthesiometer is the use of a wisp of a sterile cotton-tipped applicator.

Slit lamp biomicroscopy of the cornea should include assessment of any epithelial defect. The visualization of ocular surface damage can be assisted by the use of vital dyes, including fluorescein, rose bengal or lissamine green. A corneal examination may also reveal an ocular cause of anesthesia, such as stromal scars from previous keratitis, evidence of previous corneal refractive laser surgery or previously asymptomatic corneal dystrophies. Secondary bacterial infection also requires prompt assessment and treatment. Further investigation in the form of corneal or conjunctival sampling should be performed if a secondary infection is suspected.

A complete ocular examination should also be performed. Inspection of the conjunctiva may reveal Bitot spots, which are associated with hypovitaminosis A. Anterior chamber activity may be related to uveitis associated with chronic inflammatory disease, that may have lead to corneal anesthesia. A dilated fundus examination is required to allow inspection of the optic disc. There might be either optic disc pallor or swelling if corneal anesthesia is secondary to an underlying neurological pathology. Dilated fundus examination may also reveal evidence of diabetic retinopathy or previous laser or cryotherapy to the retina in the vicinity of the posterior ciliary nerves.

Differential Diagnosis

Neurotrophic keratopathy may have a similar clinical appearance to other ocular surface disorders at each clinical stage. History is often helpful in directing the diagnosis towards neurotrophic keratopathy and the presence of an anesthetic cornea on clinical assessment is a critical sign. The presence of a surface punctate keratopathy in early neurotrophic keratopathy may lead to the incorrect diagnosis of dry eye, exposure keratopathy, surface irritation from topical therapy, or limbal stem cell deficiency. Symptoms of ocular pain or discomfort would not normally be reported in neurotrophic keratopathy and their presence might support these other diagnoses. Limbal stem cell deficiency could also be differentiated from corneal neovascularization by impression cytology, which would distinguish corneal from conjunctival epithelium.[13]

In the later stages of neurotrophic keratopathy, the differential diagnosis would include an infective or inflammatory corneal ulcer, a traumatic epithelial defect, toxic ulcer or recurrent corneal erosion (RCE). Microbiological studies would identify any potential infective cause, the presence of systemic autoimmune disease would raise the suspicion of an inflammatory ulcer, history of topical therapy would be necessary for a toxic-related corneal ulcer and a history of trauma, even a mild injury, would be suggestive of a traumatic epithelial defect or RCE.

Treatment

The primary aim of treatment is to protect the corneal surface and to promote epithelial regrowth. The specific measures taken are dependent on the stage of the disease at the time of presentation and severity of anesthesia. In stage 1 disease, topical lubricants can be used to protect the corneal epithelium. To minimize ocular surface irritation from long-term use, preservative-free topical preparations should be considered for both lubricants and other topical preparations, if used for pre-existing ocular co-morbidity.[8] Ideally, other topical medications should be discontinued if possible. A review of concurrent topical and systemic medications should be undertaken to minimize the use of therapies that might predispose to neurotrophic keratopathy. In order to increase tears on the ocular surface, punctal plugs may be considered.[1] Eyelid hygiene and treatment of blepharitis optimizes meibomian gland function and reduces the risk of secondary infection. Oral doxycycline can be prescribed to treat blepharitis and reduce tear concentrations of matrix metalloproteinases (MMPs). MMPs have been implicated as a contributing factor of the surface epithelium failing to heal in RCE syndrome.[14] The use of a bandage contact lens as a temporary measure to protect the corneal surface has previously been proposed. However, this may introduce infection and be a risk factor for secondary infective keratitis.[15] Any exposure of the corneal surface, secondary to either an eyelid defect or lid malposition, should be addressed by surgical correction.

In more advanced disease when an epithelial defect occurs, the above conservative measures should also be administered. All topical treatment for other ocular conditions should be discontinued, as there is significant risk of stromal lysis and globe perforation. Topical collagenase inhibitors may be considered. A lateral tarsorrhaphy can be performed to reduce the palpebral aperture and corneal exposure.[16] A measure that may be considered as an alternative to tarsorrhaphy, is inducing a temporary ptosis by injection of botulinum toxin A into the levator muscle.[17]

While the mainstay of topical therapy is lubrication, there are several adjunctive topical therapies available to promote both corneal epithelial and nerve regrowth. Treatment with autologous serum eye drops has been shown to promote epithelial regeneration and increase nerve density in the sub-basal plexus.[18] Umbilical cord serum eye drops have also been shown to promote healing in a similar manner.[19] Both preparations have been found to have significantly higher concentrations of neuromediators that play a role in corneal epithelial healing than human tears.[19] Use of adjunctive therapy may be performed in combination with punctal plugging or a bandage contact lens. Preparations of individual neuromediators have also been studied as a treatment of neurotrophic keratopathy. This includes substance P in combination with insulin-like growth factor-1, epidermal growth factors, fibronectin and NGF.[20–22] NGF has been found in one prospective study of 45 eyes with either stage 2 or 3 neurotrophic disease to promote persistent epithelial defect resolution, an associated improvement in visual acuity and an increase in corneal sensitivity long after cessation of treatment.[20] A persisting epithelial defect only recurred in three patients who had had trigeminal nerve resection and this resolved with a further course of NGF therapy.

The presence of other ocular surface conditions in the setting of neurotrophic keratopathy requires prompt treatment. Secondary bacterial keratitis requires microbiological sampling and intensive preservative-free antimicrobial therapy. In cases where ocular inflammation is part of the underlying etiology, the use of mild topical steroids may be advocated to dampen the inflammatory process. However, such treatment requires close observation, as there is a significant risk of precipitating stromal lysis and perforation. Nonsteroidal anti-inflammatory topical therapies have not been shown to have a positive effect on the course of the disease, and there use may be a relative contraindication, due to the potential of corneal melting as a side effect from their anesthetic properties.

In cases of unilateral neurotrophic keratopathy, surgical replacement of the dysfunctional nerve in the form of corneal neurotization has been described.[23] Branches of the contralateral supraorbital and supratrochlear nerves originating from the contralateral supraorbital foramen are isolated, tunneled over the bridge of the nose to the lid crease before being directed through the lid, conjunctiva, Tenon's space, and attached at the limbus of the anesthetic cornea.

In stage 3 disease, the cornea is at significant risk of perforation. Immediate intervention is required to halt stromal lysis. In such cases, preservation of the globe integrity rather than preservation of vision takes precedent. In addition to the above measures to protect the corneal surface, either an amniotic membrane graft or conjunctival pedicle graft may be considered.[24,25] In the presence of small perforations, corneal glue may be used followed by insertion of a bandage contact lens.[26] In larger perforations, both lamellar keratoplasty and penetrating keratoplasty have been reported.[1] Lamellar keratoplasty must only be performed if it is deemed that enough endothelium is preserved so to avoid decompensation. However, as cases of neurotrophic keratitis are characterized by altered innervation and there is invariably limbal neovascularization, performing keratoplasty is associated with a high failure rate and recurrence of an epithelial defect. The use of a Boston keratoprosthesis (Kpro) has also been suggested as an alternative to keratoplasty in the treatment of an anesthetic cornea, but the risk of device extrusion from keratolysis and inflammatory factors must be considered prior to Kpro surgery.[27]

Conclusion

Neurotrophic keratopathy remains a challenging clinical entity for the practicing eye care professional. Even with prompt and aggressive therapy, significant visual loss and globe perforation can occur. Patients should be aware of the need for regular assessment, as significant disease progression can recur in the absence of any noticeable symptoms. Any surgical intervention carries a high failure rate, due to the lack of normal corneal innervation and healing mechanisms. Adjuncts to preservative-free lubrication, particularly nerve growth factor, appear to offer promise as a means to restore normal epithelial healing, resolve persistent epithelial defects, improve corneal sensation, and maintain globe integrity. Such treatments hold promise for the future therapeutic agents.

References

1. Bonini S, Rama P, Olzi D, et al. Neurotrophic keratitis. Eye (Lond) 2003;17:989–95.

2. Marfurt CF, Murphy CJ, Florczak JL. Morphology and neurochemistry of canine corneal innervation. Invest Ophthalmol Vis Sci 2001; 42:2242–51.

3. Guthoff RF, Wienss H, Hahnel C, et al. Epithelial innervations of human cornea: a three-dimensional study using confocal laser scanning fluorescence microscopy. Cornea 2005;24:608–13.

4. Muller LJ, Vrensen GF, Pels L, et al. Architecture of human corneal nerves. Invest Ophthalmol Vis Sci 1997;38:985–94.

5. Hamrah P, Cruzat A, Dastjerdi MH, et al. Corneal sensation and sub-basal nerve alterations in patients with herpes simplex keratitis: an in vivo confocal microscopy study. Ophthalmology 2010;117:1930–6.

6. Garcia-Hirschfeld J, Lopez-Briones LG, Belmonte C. Neurotrophic influences on corneal epithelial cells. Exp Eye Res 1994;59: 597–605.

7. Nishida T. Neurotrophic mediators and corneal wound healing. Ocul Surf 2005;3:194–202.

8. Lambiase A, Rama P, Aloe L, et al. Management of neurotrophic keratopathy. Curr Opin Ophthalmol 1999;10:270–6.

9. Heigle TJ, Pflugfelder SC. Aqueous tear production in patients with neurotrophic keratitis. Cornea 1996;15:135–8.

10. Donnerer J, Amann R, Schuligoi R, et al. Complete recovery by nerve growth factor of neuropeptide content and function in capsaicin-impaired sensory neurons. Brain Res 1996;741:103–8.

11. Lambiase A, Bonini S, Micera A, et al. Expression of nerve growth factor receptors on the ocular surface in healthy subjects and during manifestation of inflammatory diseases. Invest Ophthalmol Vis Sci 1998;39:1272–5.

12. Groos Jr E. Neurotrophic keratitis. In: Cornea: Fundamentals of cornea and external disease. St Loius: Mosby; 1997.

13. Elder MJ, Hiscott P, Dart JK. Intermediate filament expression by normal and diseased human corneal epithelium. Hum Pathol 1997; 28:1348–54.

14. Ramamurthi S, Rahman MQ, Dutton GN, et al. Pathogenesis, clinical features and management of recurrent corneal erosions. Eye 2006; 20:635–44.

15. Kent HD, Cohen EJ, Laibson PR, et al. Microbial keratitis and corneal ulceration associated with therapeutic soft contact lenses. CLAO J 1990;16:49–52.

16. Cosar CB, Cohen EJ, Rapuano CJ, et al. Tarsorrhaphy: clinical experience from a cornea practice. Cornea 2001;20:787–91.

17. Naik MN, Gangopadhyay N, Fernandes M, et al. Anterior chemodenervation of levator palpebrae superioris with botulinum toxin type-A (Botox) to induce temporary ptosis for corneal protection. Eye 2008; 22:1132–6.

18. Rao K, Leveque C, Pflugfelder SC. Corneal nerve regeneration in neurotrophic keratopathy following autologous plasma therapy. Br J Ophthalmol 2010;94:584–91.

19. Yoon KC, You IC, Im SK, et al. Application of umbilical cord serum eyedrops for the treatment of neurotrophic keratitis. Ophthalmology 2007;114:1637–42.

20. Bonini S, Lambiase A, Rama P, et al. Topical treatment with nerve growth factor for neurotrophic keratitis. Ophthalmology 2000;107: 1347–51.

21. Daniele S, Gilbard JP, Schepens CL. Treatment of persistent epithelial defects in neurotrophic keratitis with epidermal growth factor: a preliminary open study. Graefes Arch Clin Exp Ophthalmol 1992; 230:314–7.

22. Nishida T, Yanai R. Advances in treatment for neurotrophic keratopathy. Curr Opin Ophthalmol 2009;20:276–81.

23. Terzis JK, Dryer MM, Bodner BI. Corneal neurotization: a novel solution to neurotrophic keratopathy. Plast Reconstr Surg 2009;123: 112–20.

24. Alino AM, Perry HD, Kanellopoulos AJ, et al. Conjunctival flaps. Ophthalmology 1998;105:1120–3.

25. Park JH, Jeoung JW, Wee WR, et al. Clinical efficacy of amniotic membrane transplantation in the treatment of various ocular surface diseases. Cont Lens Anterior Eye 2008;31:73–80.

26. Sharma A, Kaur R, Kumar S, et al. Fibrin glue versus N-butyl-2-cyanoacrylate in corneal perforations. Ophthalmology 2003;110: 291–8.

27. Pavan-Langston D, Dohlman CH. Boston keratoprosthesis treatment of herpes zoster neurotrophic keratopathy. Ophthalmology 2008; 115(Suppl. 2):S21–3.

28 *Filamentary Keratitis*

WOODFORD S. VAN METER, DOUGLAS KATZ, and BYRON G. COOK

Introduction

Filamentary keratitis is a condition in which mucoid filaments are attached to the anterior corneal surface and cause a foreign body sensation in the patient (Fig. 28.1). Filamentary keratitis is associated with dry eyes, superficial punctate keratopathy, ptosis, and tear film stasis. Patients affected with filamentary keratitis are often highly symptomatic; the filaments may cause a persistent foreign body sensation, photophobia, and redness, that can range from moderate to severe in intensity. Filamentary keratitis is associated with a wide range of conditions in which the ocular surface is abnormal. Treatment can be acute or chronic, and severe cases may require multiple therapeutic modalities.

Etiology

The filaments adherent to the corneal epithelium in filamentary keratitis are gelatinous and refractile in appearance and can vary from 0.5 mm sessile adhesions, to 10 mm strings;[1] filaments are generally attached to the basement membrane of the corneal epithelium at one end, with the other end freely moveable. Movement of the lids causes the filament to elongate and coil, which is thought to produce patient discomfort. Filamentary keratitis is associated with underlying basement membrane abnormalities, most of which are related to hypertonic tear film states. A list of conditions that are associated with filamentary keratitis can be seen in Box 28.1.[2–18]

A relative deficiency in the aqueous component of the tear film is usually present in filamentary keratitis, which produces a relative increase in the mucinous component. The ratio of mucus to aqueous is usually increased because of a decrease in aqueous tear production, but can also occur from mucus production[19] or abnormal mucus accumulation. Abnormalities of the ocular surface result in defects in the corneal epithelium that allow for anchoring of filaments. Ptosis may lead to a reduction in oxygenation of the corneal epithelium, as well as poor tear distribution underneath the lid, which can predispose to or exacerbate filament formation.[2] Reactive ptosis from discomfort only serves to worsen the problem.

Box 28.1   Conditions Associated with Filamentary Keratitis

Aqueous tear deficiency and exposure syndromes
  Keratoconjunctivitis sicca[1,28]
  Meibomian gland dysfunction[15]
  Seventh-nerve palsy[1]
  Neurotrophic keratopathy[1]
  Radiation keratopathy
  Atopic/vernal keratoconjunctivitis[1]
  Acute viral keratoconjunctivitis[1]
  Lacrimal gland agenesis[5]
Occlusion syndromes
  Blepharoptosis[1,2,8]
  Chronic patching[2]
  Large-angle strabismus[7]
  Floppy-eyelid syndrome[15]
  Contact lens overwear[3]
  Profound CNS damage[4]
  Reactive ptosis[2]
Post-surgical syndromes
  Status post penetrating keratoplasty[9,12]
  Status post extracapsular cataract extraction[6]
  Status post limbal stem cell transplantation[10]
  Status post strabismus surgery[11]
Manifestations of systemic disease
  Sjögren's syndrome[1,28]
  Superior limbic keratoconjunctivitis[18]
  Diabetes mellitus[16]
  Sarcoidosis
  Psoriasis[1]
  Stevens-Johnson syndrome
  Graft-versus-host disease
  Systemic lupus erythematosus
  Hereditary hemorrhagic telangiectasis[14]
Medication-related
  Topical medications
  Anticholinergic medications[13]
  Cetuximab (EGFR antibody)[17]
Ocular surface abnormalities
  Ocular cicatricial pemphigoid
  Aniridia[1]
  Trachoma

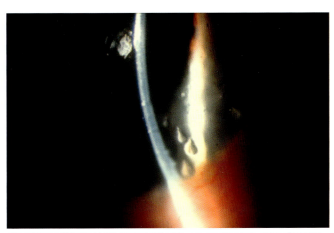

Figure 28.1 Filaments are composed of chains of epithelial cells and mucus attached to the corneal epithelial surface and can cause a foreign body sensation on blinking. (Courtesy Mark J. Mannis.)

The disorder most frequently associated with filamentary keratitis is dry eye disease. The increase in the mucus-to-aqueous ratio in the tear film may be brought about by either reduced aqueous tear secretion or increased tear film stasis, both of which effectively increase tear film osmolarity. Mucus serves as a disposal system for exfoliated epithelial cells.[20] For example, changes in the composition of the mucinous layer, in which mucus becomes more viscous, enhance the adherence of mucus to irregularities in the corneal epithelium. One example of this change occurs when the normally predominant sialomucin is replaced by more viscous sulfomucin in certain disease states.[19] Adherence of mucus to the epithelium is more likely with the latter. The combination of epithelial damage, such as that seen in dry eyes or stasis conditions, combined with an increase in mucus viscosity, can increase the potential for filaments to form on the cornea. Aqueous tear insufficiency decreases lubrication and increases the viscosity of the mucin layer, thereby leading to increased sloughing of epithelial cells, epithelial defects, and viscous mucus – the basic constituents of the corneal filament.

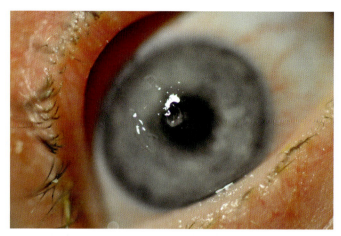

Figure 28.2 Filaments which are attached to the epithelial surface of the cornea are associated with dry eyes and stasis conditions of the precorneal tear film. (Courtesy Mike Hanson.)

Diagnosis

SUBJECTIVE

Patients with filamentary keratitis usually complain of a foreign body sensation. This irritation is exacerbated by blinking and usually present throughout the day. Patients may not be symptomatic with their eyes closed. Patients with severe filamentary keratitis may also complain of photophobia, blepharospasm, and tearing.

OBJECTIVE

Filaments can vary in size from 0.5 mm to 10 mm in length. On biomicroscopy they appear as small, gray, mucoid threads that firmly adhere to the cornea (Fig. 28.2). Occasionally, blinking may dislodge large filaments. Small filaments can cause discomfort commenserate with larger filaments because of the underlying foreign body sensation, caused by the lids tugging on the filaments during blinking. Filaments stain with rose bengal, lissamine green and fluorescein; however, care should be taken during examination not to confuse frank epithelial defects, where a filament may have been dislodged, from sessile filaments that pool with fluorescein and may mimic small corneal abrasions.

The location of the filaments may provide a clue as to the cause of the filamentary keratitis.[1] Filaments associated with dry eye or exposure keratopathy are frequently found in the interpalpebral space. Filaments associated with ptosis, prolonged lid closure, or superior limbic keratoconjunctivitis are frequently found superiorly. Filaments related to ocular surgery are often found in the vicinity of the surgical trauma. For example, following corneal transplantation, filaments can be seen near sutures at the graft–host junction (Fig. 28.3). After cataract surgery, they may be overlying or alongside the corneal incision. Surgery-specific factors, such as the disruption of proper tear flow, pooling, toxicity from medications, and local trauma, may predispose to filament formation.

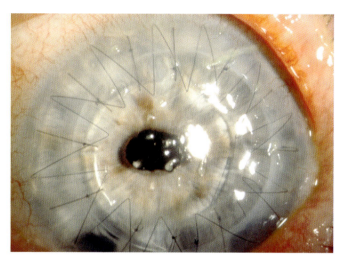

Figure 28.3 Filamentary keratitis can occur on the graft following penetrating keratoplasty in patients with dry eyes or tear film stasis. (Courtesy Mark J. Manni.s)

Histopathology

Traditional teaching has centered on the premise that the filament is composed of mucus and degenerated epithelial cells, and is adherent to the corneal epithelium at the base. However, debate still exists over the exact structure of the filament because observations of the filament on a microscopic level have been heterogeneous in approach and conclusion. Wright used standard histochemical stains to suggest that filaments form when mucus in the tear film attaches to receptors on the corneal surface.[21] Subsequent proliferation of a filament occurs as mucus accumulates cellular and other degenerative material. In contrast, Zaidman et al. used electron microscopy to report that scattered groups of inflammatory cells and fibroblasts are present below the basement membrane of the corneal epithelium where filaments are attached.[22] The authors hypothesized that an underlying pathological process damages the basement epithelium, which leads to focal areas of basement membrane detachment from the underlying Bowman's layer. This raised epithelium subsequently becomes a nidus for mucus and degenerated cells.[22] Tabery confirmed these findings with in vivo photographs, showing aggregations of mucus and cell debris adherent to the corneal surface, adjacent to focal excrescences of the basement membrane.[23] Recently, based on observations made with light microscope and immunohistochemical analysis of 13 cases of filamentary keratitis, Tanioka et al. proposed an alternate theory. They observed that corneal epithelial cells form the core of the filament and an admixture of multiple surface mucins, DNA material, and degenerated conjunctival epithelial cells become wound around the core to produce a braided shape.[24] They theorize that blinking then transmits stress to the base of the filament, which in turn incites an inflammatory response below the corneal epithelial basement membrane.

Treatment

Filamentary keratitis can be an acute or chronic condition. Some acute conditions resolve spontaneously, but more often than not, treatment is chronic. Because of the multifactorial cause of filamentary keratitis and variability in patient discomfort, treatment of filamentary keratitis can be frustrating for both the patient and the treating physician.

Initially, improving the ocular surface by treating any underlying dry eye and blepharitis is undertaken. The underlying causes of filament formation, such as keratoconjunctivitis sicca, contact lens over wear, medication toxicity, or ptosis, should initially be identified and treated. For example, resolution of filamentary keratitis in a patient with blepharoptosis has been reported following blepharoptosis surgery.[8] Because surgical correction of ptosis may lead to increased corneal exposure and subsequent exacerbation of filamentary keratitis, the exact etiology of the condition should be clearly identified prior to electing for surgical intervention.

MEDICAL

The first line of treatment is administration of topical tear film substitutes throughout the day and ointments or higher viscosity tears at bedtime. Ideally, non-preserved tears are used. Lower viscosity tears may be helpful, improving the tear film osmolarity, but more viscous tear substitutes can also provide substantial relief from microscopic corneal abrasions, and so different tear substitutes should be tried and individualized to the patient. There are many different tear formulations available and any of them may be beneficial in a given patient. Chronic treatment of dry eye with topical cyclosporine can be considered. Oral tetracycline derivatives, omega-3 fatty acid supplementation, topical azithromycin, and lid hygiene, may be beneficial to help control meibomian gland dysfunction.

Hamilton and Wood reported a 95% success rate using 5% sodium chloride ophthalmic solution administered four times daily.[25] This regimen reportedly works directly at the level of the corneal epithelium by reducing edema of the epithelium and obviating the focal detachments. While our experience with this modality is not quite as dramatic, it certainly can be useful in some patients.

N-acetylcysteine has similarly been used topically for treatment.[26] N-acetylcysteine is a mucolytic agent that decreases the viscosity of mucus in the precorneal tear film. The ocular solution is not commercially available and must be compounded without preservatives from the commercially available respiratory preparation (20% solution) to create a 5% to 20% solution. However, the discomfort of the drops and the expense and difficulty of obtaining N-acetylcysteine in a preservative-free status, minimizes the usefulness of this treatment.

A bandage contact lens is frequently successful in treating cases of filamentary keratitis that do not respond to ocular lubrication.[27] The contact lens protects the corneal epithelium from the shearing forces of the lids and may help to eliminate or reduce reactive ptosis that often occurs and exacerbates the condition in these patients. High Dk soft contact lenses should be used and are well tolerated with frequent topical artificial tears and a prophylactic topical antibiotic. Patients should be closely monitored because of the inherent risks of contact lens wear in dry eye patients with a suboptimal ocular surface.

Treatment may also target inflammation. Marsh and Pflugfelder demonstrated in a retrospective case series 100% efficacy of topical methylprednisolone for resolution of filamentary keratitis, in the setting of Sjögrens's syndrome and symptomatic keratoconjunctivitis sicca.[28] In their study, satisfactory control of symptoms and filaments was achieved with only short bursts of therapy in most cases.[28] Administration of topical nonsteroidal anti-inflammatory drugs (NSAIDs) has also been shown to reduce patient discomfort and accelerate resolution of severe cases.[29,30] The toxicity of NSAIDs on the damaged epithelium in a dry eye patient should be carefully weighed along with their beneficial effect in evaluating the pros and cons of this therapy.

SURGICAL

Debridement of filaments may be helpful initially in treating severe cases, but is rarely permanently successful without adjunctive therapy. Filaments may be removed at the slit lamp microscope with topical anesthesia and tying forceps. Care should be taken to remove the entire filament, yet not disrupt the epithelium at the base of the filament. A prophylactic topical antibiotic should be prescribed for several days following mechanical debridement of filaments. Likewise, a pressure patch with lubricating ointment or a bandage contact lens can be used to minimize patient discomfort in severe cases.

Punctal occlusion may be helpful in increasing the aqueous tear component in some cases. Temporary punctal plugs should be utilized, before permanent punctal occlusion is attempted, because in many cases, temporary improvement in tear film volume can cause resolution of filamentary keratitis, without the need for permanent punctal occlusion. It is important to treat any underlying meibomian gland dysfunction so as to minimize the retention of mucus in the tear film from punctal occlusion.

Conclusion

Filamentary keratitis is generally an easy diagnosis to make but often challenging to resolve. It is associated with a wide variety of corneal and systemic conditions. While the presentation is variable, the distinctive-appearing, gray, mucoid threads attached to the surface of the corneal epithelium noted on biomicroscopy are typical. The threads, which move on blinking, cause a foreign body sensation for the patient. The cornerstone of treatment consists of eliminating the offending cause, increasing lubrication, bandage contact lenses, and supplementing the precorneal tear film. Adjunctive topical medications, such as hypertonic saline, N-acetylcysteine, corticosteroids and NSAIDs, may offer a therapeutic benefit in selected cases. Cases refractory to treatment can be frustrating for both patient and physician; however, treatment should be continued to keep the disease from progressing and to protect the corneal epithelium from additional insult due to dryness or trauma.

References

1. Davidson RS, Mannis MJ. Filamentary keratitis. In: Krachmer JH, Mannis MJ, Holland EJ, editors. Cornea. Vol 1. 3rd ed. Philadelphia: Elsevier/Mosby; 2011. p. 1093–6.
2. Baum JL. The Castroviejo Lecture. Prolonged eyelid closure is a risk to the cornea. Cornea 1997;16:602–11.
3. Dada VK. Contact lens induced filamentary keratitis. Am J Optom Physiol Opt 1975;52:545–6.
4. Davis WG, Drewry RD, Wood TO. Filamentary keratitis and stromal neovascularization associated with brain-stem injury. Am J Ophthalmol 1980;9 0:489–91.
5. Demetriades AM, Seitzman GD. Isolated unilateral congenital lacrimal gland agenesis presenting as filamentary keratopathy in a child. Cornea 2009;28:87–8.
6. Dodds HT, Laibson PR. Filamentary keratitis following cataract extraction. Arch Ophthalmol 1972;88:609–12.
7. Good WV, Whitcher JP. Filamentary keratitis caused by corneal occlusion in large-angle strabismus. Ophthalmic Surg 1992;23:66.
8. Kakizaki H, Zako M, Mito H, et al. Filamentary keratitis improved by blepharoptosis surgery: two cases. Acta Ophthalmol Scand 2003; 81:669–71.
9. Mannis MJ, Zadnik K, Miller MR, et al. Preoperative risk factors for surface disease after penetrating keratoplasty. Cornea 1997;16: 7–11.
10. Miri A, Said DG, Dua HS. Donor site complications in autolimbal and living-related allolimbal transplantation. Ophthalmology 2011; 118:1265–71.
11. Pons ME, Rosenberg SE. Filamentary keratitis occurring after strabismus surgery. Journal of AAPOS 2004;8:190–1.
12. Rotkis WM, Chandler JW, Forstot SL. Filamentary keratitis following penetrating keratoplasty. Ophthalmology 1982;89:946–9.
13. Seedor JA, Lamberts D, Bergmann RB, et al. Filamentary keratitis associated with diphenhydramine hydrochloride (Benadryl). Am J Ophthalmol 1986;101:376–7.
14. Wolper J, Laibson PR. Hereditary hemorrhagic telangiectasis (Rendu–Osler–Weber disease) with filamentary keratitis. Arch Ophthalmol 1969,81:272–7.
15. Diller R, Sant S. A case report and review of filamentary keratitis. Optometry 2005;76:30–6.
16. Holly FJ. Biophysical aspects of epithelial adhesion to stroma. Invest Ophthalmol Vis Sci 1978;17:552–7.
17. Kawakami H, Sugioka K, Yonesaka K, et al. Human epidermal growth factor eyedrops for cetuximab-related filamentary keratitis. J Clin Oncol 2011;29:e678–9.
18. Cher I. Blink-related microtrauma: when the ocular surface harms itself. Clin Exp Ophthalmol 2003;31:183–90.
19. Wright P, Mackie IA. Mucus in the healthy and diseased eye. Trans Ophthalmol Soc UK 1977;97:1–7.
20. Adams AD. The morphology of human conjunctival mucus. Arch Ophthalmol 1979;97:730–4.
21. Wright P. Filamentary keratitis. Trans Ophthalmol Soc UK 1975; 95:260–6.
22. Zaidman GW, Geeraets R, Paylor RR, et al. The histopathology of filamentary keratitis. Arch Ophthalmol 1985;103:1178–81.
23. Tabery HM. Filamentary keratopathy: a non-contact photomicrographic in vivo study in the human cornea. Eur J Ophthalmol 2003; 13:599–605.
24. Tanioka H, Yokoi N, Komuro A, et al. Investigation of the corneal filament in filamentary keratitis. Invest Ophthalmol Vis Sci 2009;50: 3696–702.
25. Hamilton W, Wood TO. Filamentary keratitis. Am J Ophthalmol 1982;93:466–9.
26. Absolon MJ, Brown CA. Acetylcysteine in kerato-conjunctivitis sicca. Br J Ophthalmol 1968;52:310–6.
27. Bloomfield SE, Gasset AR, Forstot SL, et al. Treatment of filamentary keratitis with the soft contact lens. Am J Ophthalmol 1973;76: 978–80.
28. Marsh P, Pflugfelder SC. Topical nonpreserved methylprednisolone therapy for keratoconjunctivitis sicca in Sjögren syndrome. Ophthalmology 1999;106:811–6.
29. Avisar R, Robinson A, Appel I, et al. Diclofenac sodium, 0.1% (Voltaren Ophtha), versus sodium chloride, 5%, in the treatment of filamentary keratitis. Cornea 2000;19:145–7.
30. Grinbaum A, Yassur I, Avni I. The beneficial effect of diclofenac sodium in the treatment of filamentary keratitis. Arch Ophthalmol 2001;119:926–7.

LIMBAL STEM CELL DISEASE

29 Chemical and Thermal Injuries to the Ocular Surface

CHARLES N.J. MCGHEE, ALEXANDRA Z. CRAWFORD, and DIPIKA V. PATEL

Introduction

Chemical or thermal injury to the eye constitutes an ophthalmic emergency, due to the potential for permanent visual impairment and the threat to the structural integrity of the eye. The prognosis for severe injury is typically poor and may result in widespread damage to the ocular surface epithelium, cornea and anterior segment.[2] However, in recent years, the prognosis of severe ocular burns has improved, with advances in the understanding of the physiology of the cornea and the resultant development of enhanced medical and surgical treatments. The final visual prognosis is influenced by the nature of the chemical insult, the extent of ocular damage, and the timing and efficacy of treatment.

Epidemiology

Chemical or thermal burns represent 7.7% to 18% of cases of ocular trauma.[1,3] Responsible chemicals are numerous and include cleaning agents, fertilizers, refrigerants, cement, preservatives and fireworks.[2] Alkali injuries occur more frequently than acid injuries, as a result of their more ubiquitous presence in household and industrial products.[2] Ocular burns caused by detergents and thermal agents are less common.[2,4,5]

Fortunately, the majority of chemical injuries are classified as mild[2,5,6] and the estimated incidence of severe chemical injuries in the United Kingdom is approximately 0.02 per 100 000. Injured parties are characteristically young and male[5-8] and exposure most commonly occurs in a variety of agricultural, industrial and domestic settings, or less commonly in association with a criminal assault.[2,5,8] Unfortunately, studies report an increasing number of patients presenting with chemical eye injuries resulting from assault.[6]

OCULAR CHEMICAL INJURY

Etiology of Chemical Injury: Causative Agents

ALKALIS

More than 25,000 chemical products with the potential to cause chemical eye injuries have been identified, many of which may be classified as acids or bases, oxidizing or reducing agents, or corrosives. The most frequently implicated chemical agents are acids and bases. The severity of the injury is related to the nature, concentration, quantity and pH of the chemical involved, and the duration and surface area of exposure.[3] In particular, a history of a high-velocity (explosive) chemical or thermal injury should always raise suspicion of an associated intraocular foreign body.

Wet and dry cement, ammonia, lye, potassium hydroxide, magnesium hydroxide, and lime, constitute the most common causes of alkali injury to the eye.[2,5,8] The severity of an alkali injury is governed by the pH, rather than the properties of the cation.[2] Therefore, the most severe injuries are typically caused by ammonia and lye[8] which are both capable of rapid penetration into the eye. The damage inflicted by lime injuries is reduced by the formation of calcium soaps that precipitate and hinder further penetration.[2] Firework injuries deserve special mention as the presence of magnesium hydroxide results in a combined chemical and thermal injury. The most important agents causing alkali and acid injuries to the eye are summarized in Table 29.1.

ACIDS

The most common causes of acid burns are sulphuric, sulphurous, hydrofluoric, acetic, chromic, and hydrochloric acids.[2] The strength of an acid depends on its ability to lose a proton; strong acids ionize completely in an aqueous solution. However, the most severe acid injuries are caused by hydrofluoric acid, as a result of its unique properties. In addition to the action of the dissociated proton, which is the primary mechanism of damage by other acids, hydrofluoric acid has a unique dissolving action which allows it to quickly penetrate into deeper tissues.[2] Moreover, hydrofluoric acid chelates all calcium and magnesium from cells, thereby halting cellular biochemical activity.

Although alkalis typically cause the most serious chemical injuries, the presence of an acid injury does not preclude an equally devastating ocular injury as very strong acids penetrate just as rapidly as alkalis. Indeed, studies have shown no clinically significant differences in clinical course and prognosis between severe acid and alkali burns.[9]

Pathophysiology

STRUCTURAL AND BIOCHEMICAL ALTERATIONS

The severity of an ocular chemical injury is influenced by the ability of the chemical to penetrate the eye. Alkalis characteristically penetrate the eye more rapidly than acids.[2,3,10]

Table 29.1   Common Causes of Alkali and Acid Injuries[2]

Common Acids/Alkalis	pH of 0.1 M Solution	Sources/Uses	Comments
Sulphuric (H_2SO_4)	1.2	Battery acid, industrial cleaners	Diprotic acid
Sulphurous (H_2SO_3)	1.5	Fruit and vegetable preservatives, bleach, refrigerants	Good penetration
Hydrofluoric (HF)	2.1	Mineral refining and production, glass polishing and frosting, gasoline alkylation.	Severe injury due to rapid penetration and chelation of calcium and magnesium ion
Acetic (CH_3COOH)	2.9	Vinegar	Classified as a weak acid but corrosive in concentrated form
Hydrochloric (HCL)	1.1	Gastric acid, household cleaning, plastics production	Stable on storage
Chromic (H_2CrO_4)	1	Chrome plating	Diprotic acid
Ammonium hydroxide (NH_3)	11.1	Fertilizers, refrigerants, cleaning agents.	Rapid penetration
Sodium Hydroxide (NaOH) – Lye	13	Caustic soda, drain cleaner, manufacture of pulp, paper, textiles and soaps.	Rapid penetration
Potassium hydroxide (KOH)	12	Caustic potash	Dissolution in water strongly exothermic. Corrosive
Magnesium Hydroxide Mg $(OH)_2$	10.5	Fireworks	Combined chemical and thermal injury
Calcium hydroxide ($Ca(OH)_2$) – Lime	12.4	Cement, plaster, whitewash, industrial cleaners	Often found in composite mixtures. Poor penetration. Retained particulate matter provides sump for on-going toxicity.

(Adapted from Wagoner MD. Chemical injuries of the eye: current concepts in pathophysiology and therapy. Surv Ophthalmol 1997;41:275–313.)

The hydroxyl ion (OH) saponifies plasma membranes, resulting in cell disruption and death, while the cation is responsible for the penetration of the specific alkali.[2,3,10] Stronger alkalis are associated with more rapid penetration and the penetration rate increases in ascending order from calcium hydroxide, potassium hydroxide, sodium hydroxide to ammonium hydroxide.[10] Changes in aqueous humor pH are observed within a few seconds of contact with ammonium hydroxide, and within 3–5 minutes after sodium hydroxide injury.[10,11] Ultimately, irreversible tissue damage occurs when the pH rises above 11.5.[2,10]

In alkali injuries, cations react with the carboxyl (COOH) groups of stromal collagen and glycosaminoglycans.[2,10] Hydration of glycosaminoglycans results in loss of clarity of the stroma, whereas, hydration of collagen fibrils causes distortion of the trabecular meshwork and the release of prostaglandins, these sequelae combine to produce elevations in intraocular pressure.[10]

In general, as previously noted, acids penetrate the corneal stroma much less readily than alkalis.[2,3,10,12] The hydrogen ion mediates damage due to pH alteration, while the anion causes precipitation and denaturation of proteins in the corneal epithelium and anterior stroma.[10] Precipitation of the epithelial proteins affords a degree of protection by providing a physical barrier against further ingress.[2,3,10,12] However, in the event that an acid succeeds in penetrating the stroma, the damage to ocular structures is similar to that observed in alkali injury.[2] Alterations include precipitation of extracellular glycosaminoglycans and corneal opacification, distortion of the trabecular meshwork, changes in anterior chamber pH, damage to anterior chamber structures, and reduced aqueous ascorbate levels.[2,10] Vascular damage results in ischemic injury.

Both acids and bases may mediate osmolar damage to the delicate physiology of the cornea.[2] Chemical insults to the eye may initiate large changes in osmolarity, and the resultant osmolar stress gives rise to cellular dysfunction and destruction. The limited buffering capacity of the cornea affords little protection against a variety of chemical and toxic insults. In the event that the buffering capacity is overwhelmed, there is an immediate cessation of biochemical activity, such as protein synthesis.[13]

INJURY, REPAIR AND DIFFERENTIATION

Ocular Surface

Following corneal epithelial injury, recovery is dependent on the centripetal migration of cells from the most proximal region of viable epithelium.[14] The extent of the injury dictates the source of regenerating epithelium; epithelial defects involving a portion, or the entirety of the cornea are replenished by adjacent corneal epithelium and limbus, respectively. However, in the event of complete corneal and limbal epithelial loss, the conjunctiva is the only source of regenerating epithelium. The source of regenerating epithelium influences the rate of re-epithelialisation and the ultimate phenotype of the restored epithelium.[2]

A variety of factors may retard the rate of re-epithelisation following chemical injury, including a robust and persistent inflammatory response, and structural damage to the epithelial basement membrane.[2] Non-healing corneal epithelial wounds pose a significant risk as they expose the cornea to potential microbial infection.

Stroma

Severe chemical injuries deplete stromal keratocyte populations, and initiate collagenolytic processes which degrade collagen fibrils.[2] These processes undermine the structural integrity of the corneal stroma, and may culminate in corneal ulceration and perforation. Keratocytes play a critical role in the maintenance and regeneration of the corneal stroma. Following corneal injury, keratocytes migrate into areas of damaged stroma from adjacent tissue. Keratocytes are responsible for collagen synthesis, and collagen production is maximal between days 7 and 56, with a peak at day 21 post injury.[2] Collagen synthesis requires ascorbate and thus, may be significantly impaired by the scorbutic state induced in the cornea following severe chemical injury.[15,16]

INFLAMMATION

Chemical injury to the eye is associated with a dramatic release of pro-inflammatory mediators and the infiltration of inflammatory cells into injured tissue. Regulation of this inflammatory response is crucial, as a robust and prolonged inflammatory response may have a detrimental effect on wound healing.

Severe chemical injuries are characterized by two waves of inflammation; the first wave occurs in the first 24 hours and the second wave begins at approximately 7 days and peaks 2 to 3 weeks post injury. The intensity of the first wave may be critical for the recruitment of the second wave.[2] The second wave of inflammation coincides with the period of maximal corneal degradation and repair, and may facilitate the sterile enzymatic digestion of the corneal stroma. Sterile ulceration is associated with the infiltration of polymorphonuclear leukocytes, and conversely, the exclusion of inflammatory cells from the corneal stroma is associated with cessation of sterile ulceration.[2]

SEQUELAE

A summary of potential ophthalmic sequelae of chemical burns is provided in Table 29.2. Figure 29.1 highlights some of the complications of chemical burns.

Emergency Treatment

IRRIGATION

Emergency management is oriented towards prompt irrigation and the removal of residual chemical debris from the eye. The objectives are to minimize the ingress of the chemical agent into the anterior chamber, and to remove a potential reservoir for ongoing injury. The most important intervention is immediate copious irrigation at the scene of the incident.[17,18] Irrigation should be continued until pH neutralization is achieved. Animal models have demonstrated that external irrigation for 90 minutes reduces the pH by 1.5 units.[11] In a non-controlled human study involving 66 eyes, immediate copious irrigation resulted in less severe injury, compared with eyes which were not irrigated.[17] Although there may be an advantage in the use of amphoteric buffering solutions,[10] urgency may necessitate the use of any available neutral irrigation fluid.

Where possible, topical anesthetic drops should be applied to reduce pain and blepharospasm, thereby enhancing irrigation. Care should be taken to remove all particulate matter, and this mandates eyelid eversion (double eversion may be necessary) and cleaning of the fornices. In some

Table 29.2 Potential Ophthalmic Sequelae of Chemical Burns

Lids	Posterior displacement of meibomian orifices
	Trichiasis
	Ectropion
	Entropion
	Lagophthalmos
Ocular surface	Dry eye
	Loss of goblet cells
	Damage to lacrimal system
	Corneal melt
	Corneal opacity/scarring
	Corneal neovascularization
	Intraocular inflammation
	Limbal stem cell deficiency
	Recurrent corneal erosions
	Non healing epithelial defects
	Symblepharon/ankyloblepharon
	Microbial keratitis
Elevated intraocular pressure	Secondary glaucoma
Intraocular structures	Iris ischemia
	Fixed dilated pupil
	Ciliary body shut down with secondary hypotony
	Cataract
	Retinal detachment
	Phthisis

severe cases, a general anesthetic or sedation may be necessary to effectively remove particulate matter.

AQUEOUS HUMOR REPLACEMENT

External irrigation is of limited value in eliminating chemicals once they have reached the intraocular chambers. Animal models of alkali injuries have shown that paracentesis lowers the aqueous humor pH by 1.5 pH units. Subsequent anterior chamber reformation, with buffered phosphate solution, lowers the aqueous humor pH by a further 1.5 pH units.[11] However, the value of paracentesis and irrigation of the anterior chamber following a severe chemical injury remains controversial.[2] Nonetheless, it may be reasonable to consider aqueous humor replacement in patients with severe injuries presenting within the first 2 hours post exposure.

Classification

Early assessment should include careful documentation of the extent and severity of limbal, corneal and bulbar and palpebral conjunctival involvement, as it provides an important reference tool in subsequent evaluation and treatment design. Photographic documentation is recommended where possible.

Classification schemes for grading the severity of the initial injury are useful in guiding treatment and provide an estimation of prognosis. The Roper–Hall classification system[19] (Table 29.3) was introduced in the mid-1960s and is the most established and commonly applied system. It provides prognostic guidelines based on the degree of corneal haze and the amount of perilimbal ischemia.

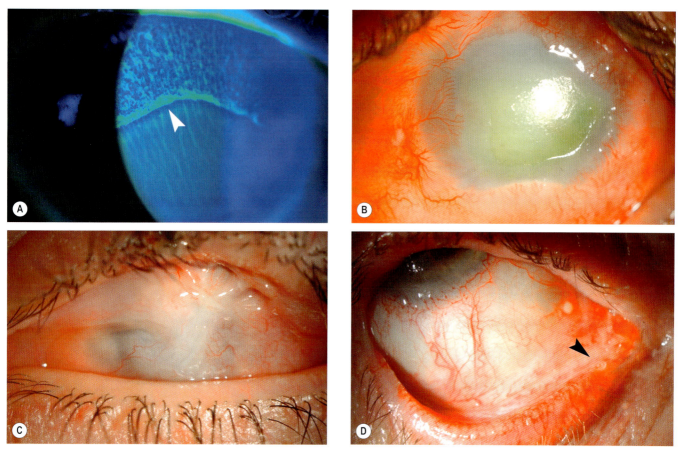

Figure 29.1 Complications of ocular chemical burns. (**A**) An epithelial ridge (*arrowhead*) with conjunctivalization of the cornea indicative of limbal stem cell deficiency. (**B**) Limbal stem cell deficiency exhibiting corneal neovascularization, subepithelial scarring and a non-healing epithelial defect. (**C**) Extensive symblepharon and corneal scarring. (**D**) Shortening of the inferior fornix with effacement of the caruncle, and a silicone plug in the punctum (*arrowhead*). (Courtesy of McGhee/Crawford/Patel.)

Table 29.3 Roper–Hall Classification 1965[19]

Grade	Prognosis	Corneal Appearance	Limbal Ischemia
I	Good	Epithelial damage	None
II	Good	Haze but iris details visible	<1/3
III	Guarded	Total epithelial loss with haze that obscures iris detail	1/3 to 1/2
IV	Poor	Cornea opaque with iris and pupil obscured	>1/2

(From Roper-Hall MJ. Thermal and chemical burns. Trans Ophthalmol Soc UK 1965;85:631–53.)

Table 29.4 Dua Classification 2001[34]

Grade	Prognosis	Clock hours of Limbal Involvement	Conjunctival Involvement	Analog Scale*
I	Very good	0	0%	0/0%
II	Good	≤3	<30%	0.1–3/1–29.9%
III	Good	>3–6	>30–50%	3.1–6%/31–50%
IV	Good to guarded	>6–9	>50–75%	6.1–9/51–75%
V	Guarded to poor	>9 – <12	75–<100%	9.1–11.9/75.1–99.9%
VI	Very poor	12	100%	12/100%

*The analog scale records accurately the limbal involvement in clock hours of affected limbus/percentage of conjunctival involvement. While calculating percentage of conjunctival involvement, only involvement of bulbar conjunctiva, up to and including the conjunctival fornices is considered.

(From Dua HS, King AJ, Joseph A. A new classification of ocular surface burns. Br J Ophthalmol 2001;85:1379–83.)

However, the years following the introduction of the Roper–Hall classifications have seen changes in the understanding and management of ocular surface burns. An enhanced understanding of the role of the limbus in wound healing has been of particular importance. In order to reflect these changes, Dua proposed a new classification scheme in 2001 (Table 29.4) based upon clock hours of limbal involvement (as opposed to ischemia), as well as the percentage of conjunctival involvement. In a recent study, Gupta et al.[20] concluded that the Dua classification had superior prognostic

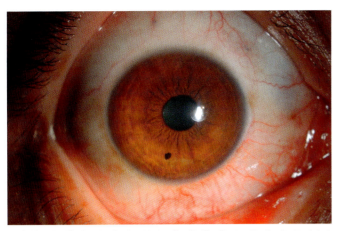

Figure 29.2 Mild chemical injury demonstrating a clear cornea with inferior limbal inflammation. (Kindly provided by Dr Chi-Ying Chou MBChB, University of Auckland Department of Ophthalmology, New Zealand.)

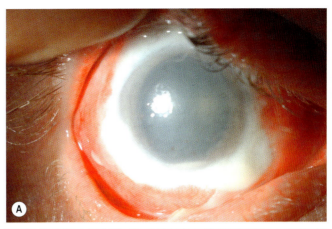

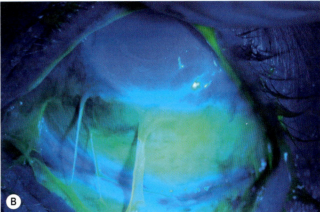

Figure 29.4 Severe chemical injury. (**A**, **B**) A 33-year-old patient presenting with severe bilateral hydrochloric acid injury. (Courtesy of McGhee/Crawford/Patel.)

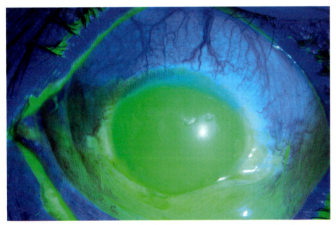

Figure 29.3 Moderate chemical injury. Total corneal epithelial loss with less than 6 clock hours of limbal involvement highlighted by fluorescein staining. (Courtesy of McGhee/Crawford/Patel.)

value over the Roper–Hall classification scheme in the context of severe ocular burns.

Examples of mild, moderate and severe chemical burns are highlighted in Figures 29.2, 29.3, and 29.4, respectively.

Medical Treatment

A retrospective study of patients with alkali burns revealed that intensive therapy with a combination of topical corticosteroids, antibiotics, ascorbate and citrate, atropine, and oral vitamin C, was most effective in the treatment of patients with Roper–Hall grade III injuries, with reference to time to re-epithelialization and visual acuity.[21] Conversely, intensive therapy delayed re-epithelialization in the context of grade I and II injuries, presumably as a result of drug toxicity and inhibition of re-epithelialization by corticosteroid.

A suggested treatment flow chart is provided in Figure 29.5.

PRESERVATIVE-FREE ANTIBIOTICS

Epithelial defects warrant the use of a topical antibiotic for antimicrobial prophylaxis. A variety of topical antibiotics have been employed or advocated in the literature in drop or ointment form, including: chloramphenicol,[6,21,22] tetracycline[2] and ofloxacin.[23] The choice of antibiotic must be considered with reference to the likelihood of microbial contamination at the time of injury, balanced with the potential for antibiotic or preservative-induced epithelial toxicity, which may hinder epithelial repair. Commercially available, non-preserved, antibiotic eye drops include chloramphenicol, moxifloxacin and ofloxacin. The presence of an unclean injury or microbial keratitis may necessitate the use of fortified antibiotics, such as tobramycin and cefazolin. However, these antibiotics must be used judiciously as they have a low therapeutic : toxic ratio.

TOPICAL CORTICOSTEROIDS

There is continuing controversy regarding the use and timing of topical corticosteroids in the treatment of chemical burns. While corticosteroids have the advantageous effects of inflammatory cell suppression and collagenase inhibition, they also suppress keratocyte migration and collagen production, and therefore, may cause corneal thinning. Indeed, an early animal study by Donshik et al.[24]

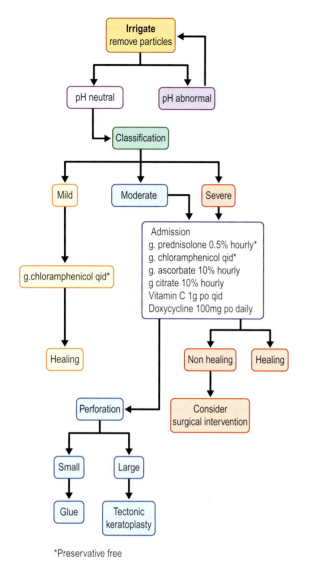

*Preservative free

Figure 29.5 Chemical burns treatment flow chart. (Courtesy of McGhee/Crawford/Patel.)

observed that the prolonged use of topical corticosteroids was associated with an increase in the incidence and severity of corneal ulceration.

Sterile ulceration occurs when there is an imbalance between collagen synthesis and proteolytic degradation. Consequently, the risk of sterile ulceration in the first week following a chemical injury is relatively modest but increases as the corneal repair process becomes established around day 14 post injury.[2] Experimental models have demonstrated that the use of corticosteroids in the first 10 days post injury does not appear to have an adverse effect on outcome.[24] Interestingly, more recent studies have suggested that the corneal ulceration observed in the Donshik et al. study with longer duration topical corticosteroid,[24] may have actually been a product of the prolonged scorbutic state of the aqueous humor, rather than a direct action of topical steroids per se.[22] Consequently, Davis et al.[22] and Brodovsky et al.[21] concluded that the prolonged use of topical steroids is not associated with corneoscleral melting, when used in conjunction with topical ascorbate.

ASCORBATE

Following a chemical injury, ascorbate levels in the aqueous humor may fall as a result of damage to the ciliary body epithelium.[2,15] This scorbutic state has the potential to compromise stromal repair because ascorbate is a key co-factor in collagen synthesis.[15] Topical or systemic supplementation of depleted aqueous ascorbate levels has been demonstrated to reduce the incidence of corneal thinning and ulceration, following experimental alkali injuries if an aqueous humor concentration of 15 mg/dL can be achieved.[25] Supplementation can be achieved through the hourly topical application of 10% sodium citrate eye drops and/or 1000 mg of oral ascorbic acid, given four times a day.

In severe injuries, topical administration is superior to systemic administration, presumably as a result of the reduced capacity of the ciliary body epithelium to concentrate ascorbate into the aqueous humor.[25] Early supplementation is absolutely critical as ascorbate has no demonstrable effect on the progression of established ulceration.[2]

CITRATE

Citrate chelates extracellular calcium and diminishes the activity of polymorphonuclear leukocytes by reducing membrane and intracellular calcium levels.[2] In the early and late phases following chemical injury, it has been shown to reduce neutrophil infiltration by 63% and 92%, respectively.[26] Citrate also has an inhibitory effect on collagenase.

In contrast to ascorbate, citrate is effective in both preventing and retarding the progression of corneal ulcers.[16] The topical route is superior to the systemic route and a 10% solution of citrate eye drops may be administered hourly.

Both citrate and ascorbate have been demonstrated to reduce corneal ulceration, albeit by different mechanisms. The combined effect of citrate and ascorbate has a therapeutic advantage over citrate treatment alone.[16] Citrate has a greater effect than ascorbate on more severely injured eyes because of its inhibitory action on the inflammatory response.[16] Severe chemical injuries may deplete collagen-producing fibroblast populations in the corneal stroma, thereby limiting the beneficial effect of ascorbate.[16]

CYCLOPLEGIC AGENTS

A cycloplegic agent, such as cyclopentolate 1% or atropine 1%, will reduce pain and minimize the risk of posterior synechiae. However, phenylephrine hydrochloride and other adrenergic drugs should be avoided, as their vasoconstrictor action may exacerbate limbal ischemia.

PRESERVATIVE-FREE LUBRICANTS

Chemical burns may result in tear film abnormalities, resulting from damage to conjunctival goblet cells. Severe injuries may also directly damage the lacrimal system. Therefore, frequent preservative-free tear substitutes may assist in promoting healing and re-epithelialization, both by washing out debris and inflammatory cells, and by hydrating the ocular surface.[3] Temporary or permanent punctal occlusion may also augment the function of tear substitutes.

ANTIHYPERTENSIVES

Alterations of the trabecular meshwork and the release of inflammatory mediators may impair aqueous outflow, resulting in elevated intraocular pressure.[2] In this context, suppression of aqueous humor production is the treatment of choice. In the absence of contraindications, short-term oral administration of acetazolamide may be preferable to minimize epithelial toxicity from preservatives in topical agents.[27]

TETRACYCLINES

The efficacy of tetracyclines in reducing collagenase activity and corneal ulceration has been demonstrated in experimental alkali injuries.[2,3] This action is independent of their antimicrobial properties and is thought to occur through the chelation of zinc; an element indispensable to the activity of matrix metalloproteinases.[2,3] Tetracyclines also inhibit the activity of polymorphonuclear leucocytes.[2,3]

ANTIVASCULAR ENDOTHELIAL GROWTH FACTOR (VEGF)

In murine models of ocular chemical burn, local bevacizumab has been shown to exhibit both anti-inflammatory and antineovascular properties.[28] Experimental studies have demonstrated that the neovascularization cascade develops early, with significantly increased levels of VEGF expression, detectable as little as 6 hours after an alkali burn.[28] Consequently, early initiation of treatment may be superior to delayed treatment. However, the use of anti-VEGF on corneal neovascularization in chemical burns has not been evaluated in humans. Theoretically, anti-VEGF agents could actually aggravate scleral ischemia and necrosis, and, therefore, anti-VEGF therapy in acute chemical burns must currently be viewed with caution.[28]

SERUM EYE DROPS

Both peripheral blood serum and umbilical cord serum have been shown to be effective in the treatment of a variety of ocular surface diseases owing to the presence of various growth factors. A recent study revealed that umbilical cord serum therapy is more effective than autologous serum eye drops or artificial tears in ocular surface restoration after chemical burns in patients with Dua classification grade III, IV and V injuries.[23] Presumably this reflects the higher concentration of growth factors in umbilical cord serum, compared with peripheral blood serum.

Early Surgical Intervention

In the acute phase, a general anesthetic may be required to effectively remove foreign material and debride the conjunctiva and fornices of necrotic tissue. As previously mentioned, anterior chamber paracentesis and aqueous exchange may be considered; however, there are no large studies reporting this practice in humans.

The prevention of symblepharon formation should be considered in all burns involving the conjunctiva.[29] Strategies to maintain the fornices include breaking symblepharon, by repeatedly using a glass rod, inserting a symblepharon ring and lining the eyelid and palpebral conjunctiva with amniotic membrane or a sutured plastic drape.[3] However, the success of these techniques will be limited in the setting of a severe injury.

TENON'S ADVANCEMENT

The presence of a severe ocular burn with total loss of limbal vasculature places the eye at immediate risk of anterior segment necrosis. A Tenon's advancement may be effective in reestablishing limbal circulation and curbing the progression towards necrosis and aseptic ulceration.[3] This procedure consists of advancing a viable Tenon's sheet from the orbital region to the level of the limbus in order to cover the ischemic or ulcerating sclera with healthy vascularized tissue.[27] While it may not prevent subsequent limbal stem cell deficiency, this technique is useful in preventing scleral perforation.

Intermediate Surgical Intervention

Intermediate surgical intervention is directed toward encouraging re-epithelialization, controlling inflammation, and protecting and maintaining the ocular surface. Persistent epithelial defects, with the attendant risk of microbial and sterile ulceration, may develop if the corneal epithelium fails to regenerate. Various strategies may be employed to promote epithelialization, including botulinum toxin-induced ptosis, surgical tarsorrhaphy, or an amniotic membrane graft.[29] These procedures may also be useful in reducing ocular pain. Bandage contact lenses are not commonly used as they are frequently not tolerated by patients and they may increase the risk of infection in inflamed or dry eyes.

AMNIOTIC MEMBRANE TRANSPLANT

Amniotic membrane transplantation (AMT) can be considered an early or intermediate surgical procedure to promote epithelialization and suppress inflammation in order to prevent or diminish scarring-induced sequelae in the late phase.[30] AMT fosters epithelial healing by acting as a basement membrane rich in growth factors, such as transforming growth factors β1 (TGF-β1) and β2 (TGF-β2), hepatocyte growth factor (HGF) and epithelial growth factor (EGF).[27] The action of growth factors in concert with other cytokines is thought to stimulate epithelialization and inhibit fibrosis.[27] Amniotic membrane also functions as a barrier against the influx of immune cells as it exhibits anti-angiogenic properties and tempers the immune response.[27]

A study by Gupta et al.[20] suggests that AMT in conjunction with medical therapy results in improved outcomes, compared with medical treatment alone, in patients with Dua classification grade IV injuries. However, there was no demonstrable improvement with AMT in patients with grade VI burns. These observations are in agreement with the earlier work of Meller and colleagues[30] who concluded that AMT was ineffective in preventing the development of limbal stem cell deficiency in severe chemical burns (Roper–Hall grade IV). In such cases, AMT should be performed in conjunction with a limbal stem cell transplant (LSCT). However, LSCT should not be performed in eyes with significant inflammation, as the success rate is very low. The delay for LSCT is especially important when the source of the stem cells is the fellow eye or a living relative. AMT may help prevent corneal perforation in severe cases and may provide a more favorable platform for future restorative procedures.[27] However, the presence of a robust inflammatory process may rapidly dissolve the AMT, necessitating a number of repeat surgeries. (Refer to Chapter 37 for further details regarding AMT.)

TENONPLASTY FLAPS

Tenonplasty is an alternative method of promoting corneal epithelialization and preventing ulceration following severe injuries. This technique involves rotating a vascularized pedicle of Tenon's capsule over the cornea.[29]

CONJUNCTIVAL FLAPS

Simple conjunctival flaps should generally be avoided in relation to corneal complications as they cause excessive vascularization and are not effective in sealing leaks. Moreover, they can complicate future ocular surface reconstruction procedures.

TISSUE GLUE

In the event of corneal thinning with threatened or actual perforation, the application of tissue glue offers a means of preserving the integrity of the globe. Tissue glue is usually accompanied by the application of a soft bandage contact lens, which enhances comfort and reduces the risk of glue dislodgement.[2] In addition to providing tectonic support, tissue glue can stop further melting by excluding inflammatory cells and their mediators.[29]

Tissue adhesives provide a means of delaying penetrating keratoplasty and, thereby, modifying the risk of graft rejection, which is extremely high in the acute phase. However, a tectonic keratoplasty may be unavoidable for large perforations. Neither tissue glue nor tectonic keratoplasty in isolation ameliorate underlying ocular surface deficiency and aberrant repair mechanisms – in particular, they do not address any avascular limbal zone. Consequently, these temporizing procedures do not prevent progressive vascularization, and scarring is, therefore, inevitable in the absence of adjunctive treatment.[2]

Intermediate/Late Surgical Interventions

Intermediate/late surgical interventions are targeted towards optimizing the ocular surface environment in order to provide more favorable conditions for subsequent ocular surface reconstruction.[29] Strategies which enhance the prognosis of ocular surface reconstruction include reconstruction of the fornices and correction of eyelid malposition. Surgery may also be necessary to eliminate corneal exposure.

CONJUNCTIVAL TRANSPLANTATION

Conjunctival transplantation is a means of restoring the conjunctival fornices after they have been morphologically altered by cicatricial fibrosis.[3] The advantage of a conjunctival transplant over other mucosal sources is that it provides compatible tissue with a basement membrane, in addition to mucus cells.[3] However, conjunctival grafts are only available if the contralateral eye remains undamaged. The procedure involves taking a sample of upper bulbar conjunctiva from the contralateral eye but this must not compromise the limbus or conjunctiva, thus, limiting the size of donor graft.

BUCCAL AND NASAL MUCOSA TRANSPLANTATION

Buccal mucosa grafts can be used to treat symblepharon, trichiasis, distichiasis, entropion or a keratinized zone of the conjunctiva of the palpebral margin.[3] The graft is usually obtained from the posterior aspect of the upper or lower lip. The advantage of nasal mucosal grafts resides in the ability to obtain large-sized grafts, and the transplantation of intraepithelial mucus cells.[3] The sample is taken from the septum and the lower or medium turbinates.

Late Surgical Interventions

LIMBAL STEM CELL TRANSPLANT

Limbal compromise results in ocular surface abnormalities characterized by chronic epithelial defects, stromal inflammation, and corneal conjunctivalization and neovascularization.[2,31] Surgical options to reconstruct the ocular surface pivot around limbal stem cell transplantation which offers the possibility of restoring the corneal epithelial phenotype.[29] Limbal autografts are the treatment of choice as there is no risk of rejection. However, they are only available in unilateral limbal deficiencies where there is a healthy contralateral donor eye. Typically, two 60–90-degree segments encompassing peripheral cornea, conjunctiva and limbus are harvested from the superior and inferior cornea of the donor eye.[29] The graft must not encircle more than 180 degrees in order to avoid limbal deficiency in the donor eye.[3] The abnormal epithelium of the recipient eye is removed and the two donor segments are sutured to the superior and inferior cornea of the host eye.[29] Additional protection is afforded by an amniotic membrane onlay graft, a therapeutic contact lens or temporary tarsorrhaphy.

Alternatively, in vitro amplification techniques can be used to minimize the size of the limbal biopsy taken from the healthy donor eye (Fig. 29.6).[31] A small 2-mm biopsy is taken from the limbus of the unaffected eye and cultured in the laboratory on a carrier such as amniotic membrane or fibrin sheet. Once a confluent epithelial layer is obtained, the tissue is grafted onto the affected eye. The relative

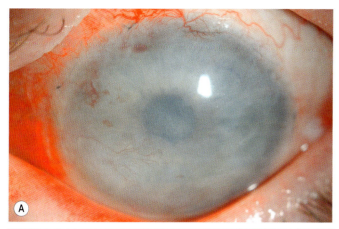

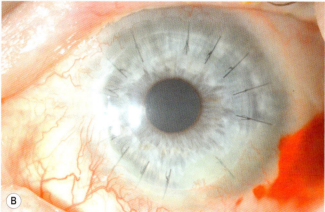

Figure 29.6 Ex vivo cultivated limbal epithelial stem cell transplant. (**A**) Day 1 postoperatively. (**B**) Two years postoperatively. (Courtesy of McGhee/Crawford/Patel.)

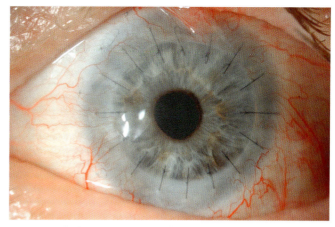

Figure 29.7 Penetrating keratoplasty in a patient with a previous firework injury, note superior symblepharon. (Courtesy of McGhee/Crawford/Patel.)

success of in vitro amplification techniques appears to be similar to that of conjunctival limbal autograft.[29]

Limbal allografts address bilateral limbal deficiencies and may be harvested from eye bank eyes or living donors. However, limbal allografts are accompanied by a significant risk of rejection and, therefore, require long-term systemic immunosuppression.[3]

The process of limbal stem cell transplantation is discussed in greater detail in Part V of this book.

CORNEAL TRANSPLANTATION

Penetrating Keratoplasty

The choice of corneal transplantation procedures in chemical burns must always be considered in relation to the status of the adjacent limbus. Ultimately, long-term corneal graft clarity is untenable in the absence of a stable ocular surface. When severe, widespread corneal injury occurs, large diameter (11–12 mm) penetrating keratoplasties may confer two advantages: enhanced tectonic support, and the passage of corneal limbal stem cells from the donor globe.[3] However, the success of large-diameter grafts is undermined by the significant risk of rejection. Consequently, a normal-diameter (≤8.00 mm) graft preceded, or accompanied by a limbal stem cell transplant, is the preferred treatment where extensive corneal and limbal damage coincide (Fig. 29.7).

In general, chemical burns are associated with a high risk of subsequent corneal graft rejection, largely due to the presence of corneal neovascularization. The prognosis for successful penetrating keratoplasty correlates with the severity and sequelae of the original chemical insult.[2] The likelihood of success is remote in the setting of intraocular abnormalities, such as glaucoma, hypotony, anterior chamber membrane formation, and retinal detachment.[2] Preliminary rehabilitation of the ocular surface is vital to the success of penetrating keratoplasty.

Deep Anterior Lamellar Keratoplasty

Deep anterior lamellar keratoplasty may be considered where the injury has spared Descemet's membrane and the corneal endothelium. The risk of allograft rejection is reduced compared with penetrating keratoplasty.

The End-Stage Eye

KERATOPROSTHESIS

Artificial corneas represent the last treatment avenue in patients with severely damaged eyes who are unsuitable for penetrating keratoplasty. Keratoprosthesis offers the potential for visual recovery, and early studies suggest favorable retention rates.[12] Complications of keratoprosthesis placement include infection, corneal melt, glaucoma and the formation of a retroprosthetic membrane.[12] Keratoprosthesis is discussed in greater detail in Chapters 49 to 53.

EVISCERATION OR ENUCLEATION

Evisceration or enucleation may be required in the context of a painful blind eye, in which all treatment options have been exhausted.

Glaucoma Surgery

Secondary glaucoma recalcitrant to maximal medical therapy requires surgical treatment. However, filtration surgery is complicated by extensive scarring of the perilimbal and bulbar conjunctiva, combined with foreshortening of the fornices. Cyclodiode ablation of the ciliary body may be considered as a last resort in the event of intractable glaucoma. However, the results are unpredictable and may initiate a terminal spiral of hypotony and eventual phthisis.

OCULAR THERMAL BURNS

Facial burns are a frequent component of thermal trauma and ocular involvement is estimated to affect between 7.5% and 27% of patients admitted to burn units.[4] Fortunately, thermal burns are not commonly associated with severe ocular sequelae, courtesy of inherent protective mechanisms, such as the blink reflex, Bell's phenomenon, and reflex shielding movements of the head and arms.[3] The loss of an eye primarily from thermal trauma is uncommon and the risk of permanent visual impairment can be minimized with timely and effective treatment.[4] Involvement of the eyelids and lid margins is the most frequent ophthalmic manifestation, and ocular complications are more commonly secondary to lid pathology than the result of direct thermal damage to the eye.[4] However, ocular trauma may occur in the absence of eyelid injury and all patients who have been exposed to fumes, heat and smoke warrant comprehensive ophthalmic evaluation. Figure 29.8 shows two examples of a combined chemical and thermal injury from a firework.

The majority of ocular thermal burns can be divided into flame and contact burns; flame burns are secondary to fire, and contact burns are the result of direct exposure to a hot object.

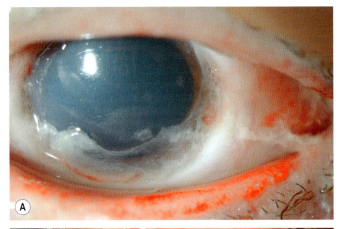

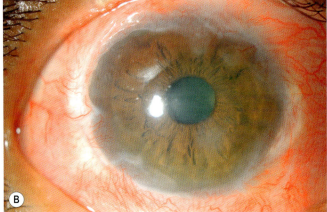

Figure 29.8 (A, B) Two eyes of two individuals with firework injuries that resulted in combined thermal and chemical damage. (**A**, Severe acute; **B**, 3 months post injury.) (Courtesy of McGhee/Crawford/Patel.)

Pathophysiology

The severity of a thermal ocular injury is a function of the thermal dose and the surface area of contact. A thermal dose can be defined by a time-temperature relationship. Goldblatt et al.[32] explored the limits of thermal tolerance of rabbit corneas, by applying well-defined heat doses (temperature × time) and examining the gross and histological effects on the tissue. They determined that a heat dose of 45°C resulted in no perceptible damage to the cornea when applied for 15 minutes, and produced only mild transient stromal edema when applied for 45 minutes. Higher thermal doses produced a spectrum of damage, with total destruction of cellular elements, massive edema and stromal disorganization at a temperature of 59°C for 45 minutes. This degree of thermal insult resulted in severe degeneration of all structures and total necrosis at 1 week.

Clinical Evaluation

Patients with suspected ocular thermal trauma should undergo early ophthalmic evaluation to assess the extent of the injury and exclude the possibility of an intraocular or intraorbital foreign body.[4,12] The frequency of ophthalmic review must balance the risk of ocular sequelae with the

risk of contaminating a susceptible burns victim. Early assessment is preferable, as subsequent conjunctival and lid edema may preclude a comprehensive examination. A critical issue is to establish the integrity of the ocular surface. Most ocular thermal injuries result in superficial burns to the cornea or conjunctiva. Superficial burns may produce a spectrum of damage limited to the corneal epithelium, ranging from minor punctate changes, to widespread loss of epithelium. Deeper injuries generate a characteristic ground-glass appearance which may result in stromal scarring. The resultant eschar eventually sloughs off, leaving a thin corneal tissue that is susceptible to ectatic changes.[4] Severe injuries may instigate a catastrophic process of corneal necrosis and eventual perforation.

The extent and depth of eyelid and facial burns should be assessed and carefully documented, as most ocular sequelae are secondary to the development of eyelid deformities, such as lagophthalmos and entropion.[3,4,12,33] The loss of eyebrow hairs and eyelashes is usually associated with a deep partial-thickness or full-thickness burn.[4] Initial assessment should note the presence or absence of Bell's phenomenon and corneal sensation in order to appraise the risk of corneal ulceration from corneal exposure. An absent Bell's phenomenon in the presence of lagophthalmos warrants daily ophthalmic review. Lagophthalmos from contracture of the eyelids may begin within 2 weeks post injury.

Patients with extensive burns are at risk of orbital compartment syndrome as a result of profound capillary leak into the enclosed space of the orbit.[4] Elevated intraorbital pressure may result in ischemic optic neuropathy secondary to elevated intraocular pressure. In the presence of orbital compartment syndrome, an urgent lateral canthotomy and inferior cantholysis is indicated.

Clinical Management

Initial management involves careful removal of debris with irrigation and sterile cotton swabs. Early prophylactic ocular lubrication is recommended, as patients may have reduced tear production, blink reflex, and eyelid mobility or excursion.[4] Ointments are considered to be more effective than drops. The presence of an epithelial defect necessitates the addition of prophylactic topical antibiotics to the lubrication regimen.[3] Preservative-free chloramphenicol can be used in the presence of punctate staining, and a frank epithelial defect can be treated with preservative-free ofloxacin drops. In general, topical corticosteroids should be avoided due to the risk of secondary infection.

Singed or scorched lashes should be removed to prevent char from falling into the eye. The management of scorched lashes has largely been neglected in the literature and the relative merits of trimming eyelashes compared with epilating have not been evaluated. One study advocated trimming lashes with scissor blades coated with an ophthalmic ointment in order to prevent cut lashes from falling into the conjunctival sac.[4] In the cases where cicatricial entropion may occur, epilation is the preferred option. Management of eyelid and facial burns should be conducted in close collaboration with oculoplastic or plastic surgery services.[12] Tarsorrhaphy is recommended in the context of a non-healing epithelial defect, secondary to lagophthalmos and a poor Bell's phenomenon.

In contrast to ocular chemical injuries, the efficacy of citrate and ascorbate in the context of ocular thermal injuries has not been scientifically assessed. Consequently, a lack of consensus is found in the literature. Some articles recommend the addition of citrate and ascorbate to treatment protocols,[12,33] whereas others exclude their use.[3,4]

In the event of corneal necrosis and perforation, surgical interventions such as lamellar keratoplasty, penetrating keratoplasty or a limbal stem cell transplant procedure may be employed.[12] The principles of surgical management are similar to those of ocular chemical burns.

OCULAR RADIATION BURNS

Both ultraviolet (UV) and infrared rays have the ability to cause radiant injury to the eyes. Burns from UV rays are the most frequent.[3] The sources of emission are various and include strongly reflected sunlight and welding lights. Ultraviolet rays are almost totally absorbed by the cornea, where they produce epithelial disturbances and stromal edema. Within 12 hours after exposure, UV burns manifest with pain, blepharospasm and tearing. Ocular examination reveals the presence of punctate epithelial erosions and conjunctival hyperemia. They typically heal within 48 hours and can be treated symptomatically with topical lubricants.

Burns from infrared rays are uncommon and may be caused by events, such as explosions and solar eclipses. Although corneal damage mediated by infrared light, it is usually limited to a superficial punctate keratitis, prolonged infrared light may also induce cataract or chorioretinitis.

Conclusion

Severe ocular chemical and thermal injuries are uncommon but may result in profound visual impairment and may compromise globe integrity. The physical, psychological and emotional consequences for injured individuals, often young men, are considerable. Although alkalis tend to cause more severe injuries, strong acids may be equally as destructive as strong alkalis. Prompt and copious irrigation remains the single most important intervention. Subsequent therapy is oriented towards addressing secondary complications, maintaining the integrity of the globe, and optimizing the prognosis of reconstructive procedures. Classification of severity is important in providing an estimation of prognosis and in guiding treatment. Although recent advances have improved the outcomes of severe chemical burns, they continue to present a medical and surgical challenge.

References

1. Pfister RR. Chemical injuries of the eye. Ophthalmology 1983; 90:1246–53.
2. Wagoner MD. Chemical injuries of the eye: current concepts in pathophysiology and therapy. Surv Ophthalmol 1997;41: 275–313.
3. Merle H, Gérard M, Schrage N. Ocular burns. J Fr Ophtalmol 2008; 31:723–34.
4. Malhotra R, Sheikh I, Dheansa B. The management of eyelid burns. Surv Ophthalmol 2009;54:356–71.
5. Morgan SJ. Chemical burns of the eye: causes and management. Br J Ophthalmol 1987;71:854–7.
6. Beare JD. Eye injuries from assault with chemicals. Br J Ophthalmol 1990;74:514–8.
7. Hong J, Qiu T, Wei A, et al. Clinical characteristics and visual outcome of severe ocular chemical injuries in Shanghai. Ophthalmology 2010;117:2268–72.
8. Kuckelkorn R, Makropoulos W, Kottek A, et al. Retrospective study of severe alkali burns of the eyes. Klin Monatsbl Augenheilkd 1993; 203:397–402.
9. Kuckelkorn R, Kottek A, Reim M. Intraocular complications after severe chemical burns–incidence and surgical treatment. Klin Monatsbl Augenheilkd 1994;205:86–92.
10. Kuckelkorn R, Schrage N, Keller G, et al. Emergency treatment of chemical and thermal eye burns. Acta Ophthalmol Scand 2002; 80:4–10.
11. Paterson CA, Pfister RR, Levinson RA. Aqueous humor pH changes after experimental alkali burns. Am J Ophthalmol 1975;79: 414–9.
12. Fish R, Davidson RS. Management of ocular thermal and chemical injuries, including amniotic membrane therapy. Curr Opin Ophthalmol 2010;21:317–21.
13. Schrage N. Chemical ocular burns. New York: Springer; 2010.
14. Dua HS, Azuara-Blanco A. Limbal stem cells of the corneal epithelium. Surv Ophthalmol 2000;44:415–25.
15. Levinson RA, Paterson CA, Pfister RR. Ascorbic acid prevents corneal ulceration and perforation following experimental alkali burns. Invest Ophthalmol 1976;15:986–93.
16. Pfister RR, Haddox JL, Yuille-Barr D. The combined effect of citrate/ascorbate treatment in alkali-injured rabbit eyes. Cornea 1991; 10:100–4.

17. Ikeda N, Hayasaka S, Hayasaka Y, et al. Alkali burns of the eye: effect of immediate copious irrigation with tap water on their severity. Ophthalmologica 2006;220:225–8.

18. Burns FR, Paterson CA. Prompt irrigation of chemical eye injuries may avert severe damage. Occup Health Saf 1989;58:33–6.

19. Roper-Hall MJ. Thermal and chemical burns. Trans Ophthalmol Soc UK 1965;85:631–53.

20. Gupta N, Kalaivani M, Tandon R. Comparison of prognostic value of Roper Hall and Dua classification systems in acute ocular burns. Br J Ophthalmol 2011;95:194–8.

21. Brodovsky SC, McCarty CA, Snibson G, et al. Management of alkali burns: an 11-year retrospective review. Ophthalmology 2000;107: 1829–35.

22. Davis AR, Ali QK, Aclimandos WA, et al. Topical steroid use in the treatment of ocular alkali burns. Br J Ophthalmol 1997;81:732–4.

23. Sharma N, Goel M, Velpandian T, et al. Evaluation of umbilical cord serum therapy in acute ocular chemical burns. Invest Ophthalmol Vis Sci 2011;52:1087–92.

24. Donshik PC, Berman MB, Dohlman CH, et al. Effect of topical corticosteroids on ulceration in alkali-burned corneas. Arch Ophthalmol 1978;96:2117–20.

25. Pfister RR, Paterson CA, Spiers JW, et al. The efficacy of ascorbate treatment after severe experimental alkali burns depends upon the route of administration. Invest Ophthalmol Vis Sci 1980;19: 1526–9.

26. Pfister RR, Nicolaro ML, Paterson CA. Sodium citrate reduces the incidence of corneal ulcerations and perforations in extreme alkali-burned eyes–acetylcysteine and ascorbate have no favorable effect. Invest Ophthalmol Vis Sci 1981;21:486–90.

27. Gicquel JJ. Management of ocular surface chemical burns. Br J Ophthalmol 2011;95:159–61.

28. Hosseini H, Nowroozzadeh MH, Salouti R, et al. Anti-VEGF Therapy with bevacizumab for anterior segment eye disease. Cornea 2012; 31:322–34.

29. Tuft SJ, Shortt AJ. Surgical rehabilitation following severe ocular burns. Eye 2009;23:1966–71.

30. Meller D, Pires RT, Mack RJ, et al. Amniotic membrane transplantation for acute chemical or thermal burns. Ophthalmology 2000; 107:980–9.

31. Crawford AZ, McGhee CNJ. Management of limbal stem cell deficiency in severe ocular chemical burns. Clin Exp Ophthalmol 2012; 40:227–9.

32. Goldblatt WS, Finger PT, Perry HD, et al. Hyperthermic treatment of rabbit corneas. Invest Ophthalmol Vis Sci 1989;30:1778–83.

33. Czyz CN, Kalwerisky K, Stacey AW, et al. Initial treatment of ocular exposure and associated complications in severe periorbital thermal injuries. J Trauma 2011;71:1455–9.

34. Dua HS, King AJ, Joseph A. A new classification of ocular surface burns. Br J Ophthalmol 2001;85:1379–83.

30 Erythema Multiforme, Stevens–Johnson Syndrome and Toxic Epidermal Necrolysis

ANDREA Y. ANG, FLORENTINO E. PALMON, and EDWARD J. HOLLAND

Introduction

Erythema multiforme (EM), Stevens–Johnson syndrome (SJS), and toxic epidermal necrolysis (TEN) are considered as a spectrum of epidermal bullous diseases involving the skin and mucous membranes, usually triggered by drugs or infection. Although rare diseases, they are important since they cause high mortality and morbidity, with ocular involvement often being the most serious long-term sequela. Initial management involves early recognition, prompt hospitalization, and immediate cessation of the offending agent. During the acute self-limited course of the illness, management is primarily supportive in providing fluid management and prevention of sepsis. During the acute stage, it is important to manage the ocular surface inflammation aggressively with supportive treatment, so as to minimize the development of cicatricial changes that lead to chronic ocular surface disease.

History

In 1866, the Austrian dermatologist Ferdinand von Hebra first described erythema multiforme as a self-limited cutaneous disease characterized by multiform skin lesions.[1] In association with the erythematous skin lesions, his findings included a severe stomatitis and purulent conjunctivitis. In 1922, two American pediatricians, Stevens and Johnson, described two boys with a more severe mucocutaneous disease with ophthalmologic manifestations, naming the disease eruptive fever with stomatitis and ophthalmia.[2] This nomenclature was not adopted. However, since that time, erythema multiforme major has been most commonly referred to as Stevens–Johnson syndrome. In 1950, Thomas suggested the division of erythema multiforme into two forms: minor (von Hebra) and major (SJS).[3] In 1956, Lyell introduced the term toxic epidermal necrolysis, a condition characterized by more extensive skin loss in conjunction with mucous membrane involvement.[4]

Classification

There was confusion in the nomenclature and diagnostic criteria for the erythema multiforme spectrum of diseases until an international classification was adopted in 1993.[5] Traditionally, erythema multiforme was divided into minor

Table 30.1 Diagnostic Criteria for Bullous Skin Diseases

ERYTHEMA MULTIFORME MINOR
- <20% body area involvement
- Target (iris) lesions (typical or atypical)
- Individual lesions <3 cm in diameter
- No or minimal mucous membrane involvement
- Biopsy specimen compatible with EM minor

STEVENS–JOHNSON SYNDROME (ERYTHEMA MULTIFORME MAJOR)
- <20% of body area involved in first 48 hours
- >10% of body area involvement
- Target (iris) lesions (typical or atypical)
- Individual lesions <3 cm in diameter (lesions may coalesce)
- Mucous membrane involvement (at least 2 areas)
- Fever
- Biopsy specimen compatible with EM major

TOXIC EPIDERMAL NECROLYSIS
- Bullae and/or erosions over 20% of body area
- Bullae develop on erythematous base
- Occurs on non-sun-exposed skin
- Skin peels off in >3-cm sheets
- Mucous membrane involvement frequent
- Tender skin within 48 hours of onset of rash
- Fever
- Biopsy specimen compatible with TEN

(Adapted from Chan HL, Stern RS, Arndt KA, et al. The incidence of erythema multiforme, Stevens–Johnson syndrome, and toxic epidermal necrolysis. A population-based study with particular reference to reactions caused by drugs among outpatients. Arch Dermatol 1990;126:43–7.)

and major forms, with the minor form only involving skin, with no or minimal mucous membrane involvement and not involving the eye. Table 30.1 outlines the diagnostic criteria for bullous skin diseases.[6] Although the terms EM major and SJS are often used interchangeably, international collaborators have now differentiated them by their etiology and pattern of cutaneous lesions.[7] The major etiologic factor for EM major (or bullous EM) is herpes simplex virus (HSV), compared to drug-induced SJS. An international consensus collaboration further classified the overlap between SJS and TEN. They defined five categories based on the pattern of skin lesions and extent of epidermal detachment as shown in Table 30.2.[5]

Incidence

Although EM/SJS/TEN are rare conditions, they are important because they cause high mortality and morbidity. Chan (USA) reported an overall incidence of these diseases

Table 30.2　Proposed Classification of Cases in the Spectrum of Severe Bullous EM

Classification	Bullous EM	SJS	Overlap SJS–TEN	TEN with spots	TEN without spots
Detachment	<10%	<10%	10–30%	>30%	>10%
Typical targets	Yes				
Atypical targets	Raised	Flat	Flat	Flat	
Spots		Yes	Yes	Yes	
Distribution	Localized (acral)	Widespread	Widespread	Widespread	Widespread

EM, erythema multiforme; SJS, Stevens–Johnson syndrome; TEN, toxic epidermal necrolysis.
(Adapted from Bastuji-Garin. Clinical classification of cases of toxic epidermal necrolysis, Stevens–Johnson syndrome, and erythema multiforme. Arch Dermatol 1993;129:92–6.)

Table 30.3　Etiologies of Stevens–Johnson Syndrome

Etiologic agent	Most frequently described
Drugs	Sulfas, NSAIDs, antiepileptics, barbiturates, allopurinol, tetracyclines, antiparasitics
Viral	HIV, herpes simplex, Epstein–Barr, influenza, coxsackie, lymphogranuloma venereum, variola
Bacterial	Mycoplasma pneumonia, typhoid, tularemia, diphtheria, group A streptococci
Fungal	Dermatophytosis, histoplasmosis, coccidiomycosis
Protozoal	Trichomoniasis, plasmodium

NSAIDs, nonsteroidal anti-inflammatory drugs; HIV, human immunodeficiency virus.
(Adapted from Hazin R, Ibrahimi OA, Hazin MI, Kimyai-asadi A. Stevens–Johnson syndrome: Pathogenesis, diagnosis, and management. Ann Med 2008;40:129–38.)

at 4.2 per million person-years (TEN 0.5 per million person-years),[6] and Rzany (Germany) reported an overall incidence of 1.89 per million person-years.[8] Schöpf (Germany) reported an incidence of SJS at 1.1 per million person-years and incidence of TEN at 0.93 per million person-years.[9] Roujeau (France) reported an incidence of TEN at 1.2 to 1.3 per million person-years.[10] The reported mortality rate is 1% for EM, 1% to 7% for SJS, and 30% to 45% for TEN.[9–11] Both the incidence and the mortality appear to be higher in immunocompromised patients with these risks correlated with weaker immune function.[12] EM is more common in males, whereas TEN is more common in women, with a ratio ranging from 1.5:1 to 2.0:1.[9–11] Although these conditions can occur at any age, EM and SJS tends to occur in younger patients in their second to third decades, whereas TEN occurs in older patients in their fifth to seventh decades.[9–11]

Etiology

Drugs and infections are the most common inciting causes of disease, as shown in Table 30.3. Drug-related reactions typically begin within 3 weeks of initiation of therapy. In cases of re-exposure to the drug, the reaction may begin within hours of restarting the therapy.[6] TEN is usually drug-related. Drugs are an important cause of SJS, but infections, or a combination of infections and drugs has also been implicated. Infections, especially viral, are the most common cause of EM. In large epidemiology studies,

drugs accounted for 89% to 95.5% of cases of TEN,[9,10] 54% to 64% of cases of SJS,[9,11] and 18% for EM major.[11] In the international prospective SCAR (severe cutaneous adverse reactions) study, recent or recurrent herpes was the principal risk factor for EM major (etiologic fractions of 29% and 17%, respectively) and had a role in SJS (etiologic fractions of 6% and 10%) but not in overlap cases or TEN.[11] *Mycoplasma pneumoniae* has also been associated with EM Major in several studies.[11,13]

In the SCAR study, the use of antibacterial sulfonamides, anticonvulsants, oxicam nonsteroidal anti-inflammatory drugs (NSAIDs), allopurinol, chlormezanone, and corticosteroids were associated with large increases in the risk of SJS or TEN.[14] However, it is important to note that these reactions are rare, since for each of these drugs the excess risk did not exceed five cases per million users per week. Among drugs usually used for months or years, the increased risk was confined largely to the first 2 months of treatment. Table 30.4 lists drugs that have been associated with these diseases.

Pathogenesis

The exact pathophysiologic mechanism of EM/SJS/TEN remains unknown. Prevailing evidence indicates an immune-mediated response, in particular those mediated by memory cytotoxic T cells, to drugs and infections. Histologically, keratinocyte death occurs from extensive apoptosis.[15] The proposed initiating mechanism involves the interaction between Fas and Fas ligand (FasL), which is either membrane bound on keratinocytes or soluble.[16] Activation of the Fas signaling cascade leads to widespread keratinocyte apoptosis and subsequent epithelial necrosis. It has been suggested that soluble FasL is secreted by peripheral blood mononuclear cells and is elevated in EM and TEN patients.[17] Other studies have also linked perforin, a pore-making monomeric granule released from natural killer T lymphocytes, which is thought to initiate the keratinolysis seen early in the development of SJS.[18] Granulysin has also been implicated as a key mediator for disseminated keratinocyte death in SJS/TEN. Granulysin levels are much higher in patients with SJS/TEN, compared to healthy controls, and also correlate with clinical severity.[19]

Genetic factors may also play a role in the development of erythema multiforme disorders. Slow acetylators and those taking medications, such as azoles, protease inhibitors, serotonin-specific reuptake inhibitors, and quinolones

Table 30.4 Drugs Associated with EM/SJS/TEN

Antimicrobials	Metals
Sulfonamides	Arsenic
Sulfones	Bromides
Penicillins	Mercury
Cephalosporins	Gold
Griseofulvin	Iodides
Rifampicin	Lithium
Tetracyclines	**Miscellaneous Agents**
Ethambutol	
Isoniazid	Adrenocorticotropin
Streptomycin	Alkylating agents
Thiacetazone	Allopurinol
Vancomycin	Atropine
Chloramphenicol	Bismuths
Chloroquine	Cimetidine
Ciprofloxacin	Chlorpropamide
Clindamycin	Codeine
Quinine	Cyclophosphamide
Fluconazole	Clofibrate
Lincomycin	Danazol
Nystatin	Dipyridamole
Nonsteroidal Anti-inflammatory Drugs	Estrogens
	Ethanol
Salicyclates	Methaqualone
Fenbufen	Nitrogen mustard
Ibuprofen	Pentazocine
Sulindac	Phenolphthalein
Pyrazolone derivatives	Progesterone
Isoxicam	Vaccinating agents
Anticonvulsants	Ethosuximide
	Glucagon
Barbiturates	Glucocorticoids
Carbamazepines	Hydroxyurea
Hydantoin derivatives	Methotrexate
Trimethadione	Methylthiouracil
Lamotrigine	Indapamide
Central Nervous System Drugs	Methenamine
	Nalidixic acid
Mianserin	Novobiocin
Phenothiazines	Theophylline
Trazodone	Vitamin A
Cardiovascular Drugs	Tolbutamide
	Dorzolamide
Captopril	Nevirapine
Acetazolamide	Tipranavir
Enalapril	Darunavir
Iopamidol	Etravirine
Propranolol	Enfuvirtide
Quinidine	Raltegravir
Furosemide	Maroviroc
Hydralazine	
Minoxidil	
Thiazide diuretics	
Diltiazem	
Verapamil	

(Adapted from Palmon et al. Cornea. 3rd ed. Elsevier 2011. p. 604.)

are at increased risk of developing SJS. The reduced rate of acetylation causes the accumulation of reactive metabolites that induce cell-mediated cytotoxic reactions against the epidermis, resulting in keratinocyte apoptosis.[12]

In studies in Western populations,[14,20] antibiotics, particularly sulfonamides, are the most common drug trigger. In the largest Asian study by Chang et al.,[13] anticonvulsants, particularly carbamazepine, and allopurinol were the most common drug triggers. A study by Chung et al.[21] found a strong association in Han Chinese between the human leukocyte antigen (HLA) B*1502 and SJS induced by carbamazepine. Another study showed that HLA-B*5801 is highly associated with allopurinol-induced SJS/TEN.[22] These associations suggest the importance of pharmacogenetic mechanisms on the risk of developing SJS/TEN.

Histopathology

The initial diagnosis of EM/SJS/TEN is based on clinical presentation; however, skin biopsies should be taken for both routine histopathology and direct immunofluorescence in order to distinguish these conditions from autoimmune blistering disorders. The typical histopathology of EM/SJS/TEN is characterized by vacuolization of epidermal cells and necrosis of keratinocytes within the epidermis, along with dermoepidermal detachment and perivascular lymphocytic infiltration.[23] The dermal infiltrate is more pronounced in EM major, compared to SJS or TEN.[24] In TEN, subepidermal blistering associated with full-thickness epidermal necrosis occurs.

Clinical Findings

INITIAL PRESENTATION

Typically, EM/SJS/TEN begins with a systemic prodrome of vague upper respiratory tract symptoms and fever, headache, and malaise within 1 to 3 weeks of the precipitating factor. Within 1 to 3 days of the prodrome, there is rapid onset of the typical mucocutaneous lesions that may continue to erupt for up to 4 weeks. The disease is self-limited and typically lasts 4 to 6 weeks.

SYSTEMIC FEATURES

Mucous membrane involvement occurs in more than 90% of affected patients, and the absence of such lesions should cast doubt on the diagnosis. There is no correlation between the extent and severity of mucous membrane erosions and the extent of epidermal detachment.[5,8] Painful erosions of the mucous membrane may affect the lip, oral cavity, conjunctiva, nasal cavity, urethra, vagina, gastrointestinal tract, and respiratory tract. Mucous membrane ulceration can result in both short-term dysfunction and morbidity, and lead to long-term complications, due to fibrosis and stricture formation. In the study by Chang et al.[13] the most common sites of mucosal involvement were the mouth (72%), eye(s) (60%), genitalia (37%), and anus (8%). Mucous membrane erosions sometimes persist for months after the reparation of the epidermis and may leave atrophic scars.

EM/SJS/TEN skin lesions have characteristic patterns and are described in Table 30.2 and shown in Figure 30.1.[11] The rash of EM is predominantly on the extremities, including the dorsal aspect of the hands and feet, and on the extensor surface of the forearms, legs, palms and soles.[11] Typical target lesions are < 3 cm in diameter, with a regular round shape, well-defined border, and at least three different zones, i.e. two concentric rings around a central disc (Fig. 30.1A). Raised atypical targets are round, edematous,

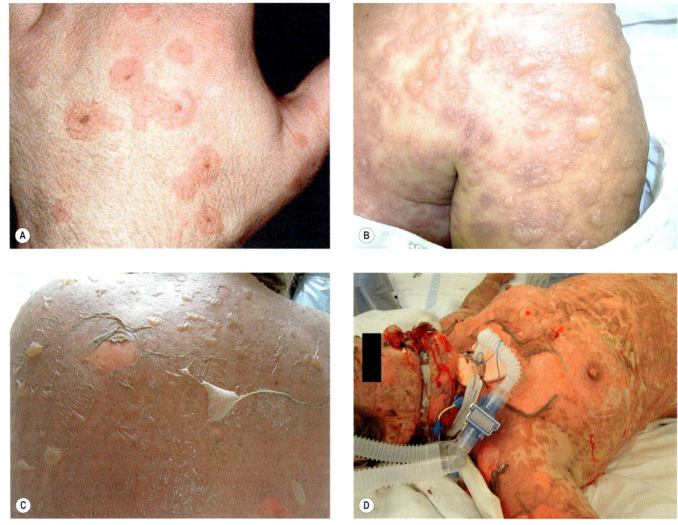

Figure 30.1 Characteristic skin lesions of EM/SJS/TEN. (**A**) Erythema multiforme: typical targets. (**B**) Stevens–Johnson syndrome: erythematous or purpuric macules with irregular shape and size, and blisters. (**C**) and (**D**) Toxic epidermal necrolysis: widespread detachment of >30% of body surface area. (**A**, Reproduced from Werchniak, AE, Schwarzenberger, K. Poison ivy: An underreported cause of erythema multiforme, J Am Acad Dermatol 2004;51(Suppl. 5):S159–60. **B**, Reproduced from Weinberger, CH, Bhardwaj, SS, Bohjanen, KA. Toxic epidermal necrolysis secondary to emergency contraceptive pills, J Am Acad Dermatol 2009;60:708–9. **C** & **D**, Reproduced from Downey, A, Jackson, C, Harun, N, et al. Toxic epidermal necrolysis: Review of pathogenesis and management, J Am Acad Dermatol 2012;66:995–1003.)

palpable lesions, reminiscent of EM but with only two zones and/or a poorly defined border.

The rash in SJS consists of flat atypical target lesions and erythematous macules that then develop central necrosis to form vesicles, bullae, and areas of denudation on the face, trunk, and extremities. Flat atypical targets are round, non-palpable lesions reminiscent of EM but with only two zones and/or a poorly defined border. Macules are non-palpable, erythematous or purpuric spots with irregular shape and size, and often confluent. Blisters often occur on all or part of the macule (Fig. 30.1B).

In TEN, the cutaneous lesions begin suddenly with burning and painful red skin, often symmetrically distributed on the face and chest that rapidly extends over the skin surface, including the trunk and proximal extremities. The maximal extension of the lesions is obtained in 3 to 4 days, and sometimes in a few hours.[5,8] The hallmark of TEN is a widespread necrosis and detachment of full-thickness epidermis (Figs 30.1C and 30.1D). A positive Nikolsky's sign may be present, where there is detachment of the full-thickness epidermis when light lateral pressure is applied with the examining finger. Re-epithelialization of the epidermis begins about 1 week after onset of the skin lesions, and most of the skin surface is re-epithelialized in 2 to 3 weeks.

Death usually results from sepsis or multi-organ failure. In the Power et al.[20] and Chang et al.[13] studies, the most frequent causes of mortality were overwhelming sepsis, respiratory failure, and renal failure. The SCORTEN (TEN-specific severity of illness score) scale[25,26] was developed as a tool to predict the severity of the disease and risk of mortality, with prognostic factors, including age, amount of body surface area involved, heart rate, and renal function (Table 30.5).

Table 30.5 SCORTEN Scale: Prognostic Factors for SJS and TEN

Variable	Value
Age	>40 years
Malignancy	Yes
Body surface area detached	>10%
Heart rate	>120 per minute
Serum urea	>10 mmol/L
Serum glucose	>14 mmol/L
Serum bicarbonate	<20 mmol/L

One point is assigned for each positive variable. A patient's mortality is predicted by the total number of points: 0–1 points=3.2%; 2 points=12.1%, 3 points=35.3%, 4 points=58.3%, ≥5 points=90.0%. (Adapted from Guegan S, Bastuji-Garin S, Poszepczynska-Guigne E, et al. Performance of the SCORTEN during the first five days of hospitalization to predict the prognosis of epidermal necrolysis. J Invest Dermatol 2006;126:272–6.)

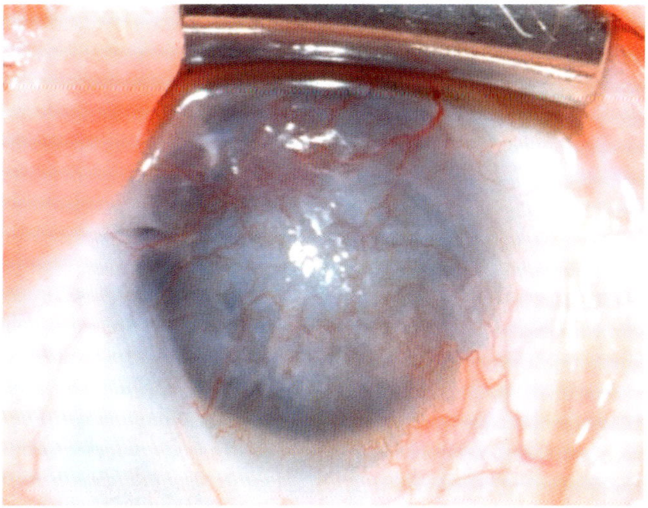

Figure 30.2 Preoperative photo of an SJS patient with total ocular surface failure. There is conjunctivalization and keratinization centrally.

OCULAR FEATURES

Incidence

Acute ocular complications develop in over half (i.e. 50% to 81%) of patients hospitalized for SJS and TEN, and 25% of these exhibit severe involvement.[13,20] Chronic ocular sequelae occur in up to 35% patients with blinding corneal damage being the most severe long-term complication for survivors.[27] In the Power et al. study,[20] ocular involvement was seen in 9% of patients with EM, 50% of patients with TEN, and 69% of patients with SJS. Similarly, in the Chang et al. study,[13] ocular involvement was more frequent in TEN (66.7%) and SJS (81.3%) than in those with EM (22.7%).

Acute Ocular Features

The acute stage may involve the entire ocular surface, including the eyelids, conjunctiva, and cornea. Initially, the eyelids may be swollen and erythematous, with crusting and ulceration of the lid margin and tarsal conjunctiva. A non-specific conjunctivitis usually occurs at the same time or may precede the onset of the skin lesions, and its severity usually parallels that of the skin lesions.[20] More severe involvement can result in pseudomembranous or membranous conjunctivitis. Secondary purulent bacterial conjunctivitis may occur. Conjunctival vesicles are rare. The acute inflammation may rapidly produce scarring, causing symblepharon and ankyloblepharon formation, and fornix foreshortening. In the acute stage, corneal epithelial defects may occur and these may be uncommonly complicated by corneal infiltrates and rarely by corneal perforation. Acute uveitis is uncommon but can occur. The initial eye findings usually last only 2 to 3 weeks.[28]

Power et al.[20] classified severity of ocular involvement as mild, moderate, or severe. Mild involvement was defined as complications requiring routine eye care with full resolution prior to hospital discharge: lid edema, and conjunctival injection and chemosis. Moderate involvement included specific ocular complications that required specific treatment with near complete resolution of active disease upon discharge: conjunctival membrane formation, corneal epithelial loss <30%, evidence of corneal ulceration or corneal infiltrates. Severe complications included sight-threatening disease, ongoing ocular inflammation with reduced vision, and the need for specific ongoing care after discharge: conjunctival fornix foreshortening, symblepharon formation, and ongoing active corneal disease at the time of discharge. Chang et al.[13] used the same classification system and they both found that ocular involvement was not only more frequent but also more severe in SJS and TEN, compared to EM. Power et al. also found that the use of systemic corticosteroids had no effect on the incidence or the severity of ocular manifestations.

Chronic Ocular Features

Chronic ocular features include cicatrizing changes of the conjunctiva and eyelids, severe dry eye, and ocular surface failure. Corneal damage is the most severe long-term complication for survivors of SJS and TEN. These late features may not only result from severe ocular inflammation during the acute phase, but may also be a result of later recurrent episodes of conjunctival inflammation, and perpetuated by the severe dry eye and eyelid pathologies.[29,30]

Conjunctival inflammation and scarring may cause foreshortening of the fornices, symblepharon, ankyloblepharon, distichiasis, trichiasis, entropion or ectropion. Disorders of the lid–lash complex may cause microtrauma and perpetuate chronic inflammation through the mechanical rubbing of lashes against the ocular surface.[30] Ectropion or lagophthalmos can cause exposure keratopathy and further exacerbate the extremely dry ocular surface. Severe dry eye results from conjunctival goblet cell destruction, fornix foreshortening and destruction of the aqueous-secreting glands of Wolfring and Krause, lacrimal gland ductule scarring, and meibomian gland dysfunction.

Corneal involvement includes chronic epitheliopathy, persistent epithelial defects, fibrovascular pannus formation, stromal scarring and neovascularization, conjunctivalization, and in severe cases keratinization of the surface (Fig. 30.2). Keratinization also occurs on the posterior lid margin and tarsal conjunctiva, further abrading the ocular surface. Ocular surface failure may appear early as a consequence of the acute stage of disease, or can manifest several years later.[30] Destruction of the limbus during the acute phase of the disease may cause partial limbal stem cell deficiency (LSCD), but leave enough transient amplifying cells to maintain a normal corneal epithelium for some time. Further destruction of the remaining stem cells by chronic inflammation may cause late stem cell failure.

Recurrent Disease

Most people do not take the inciting drug again; however, in the Chang et al. study,[13] recurrences of EM/SJS/TEN occurred in six cases (2.4%) from 3 months to 6 years after the first attack. All initial and recurrent attacks were attributed to drugs, of which three recurrences occurred because the cause of the initial episode had not been recognized. Therefore, great care should be taken to document all medications associated with an episode of EM/SJS/TEN, and patients need to be acutely aware of the inciting medications to avoid future exposure. In other studies, most recurrences were attributable to herpes simplex virus infections. Of the 552 patients in the SCAR study,[11] 51 (9%) were recurrent. Recurrence rates were higher in EM (30%), compared to SJS (3%) and TEN (3%), due to the association of EM with herpes simplex virus. Prevention by oral antiviral drugs should be considered in cases of recurrent EM, due to herpes simplex virus.[31] Recurrence episodes of conjunctival inflammation not associated with external factors may occur.[29,32]

Differential Diagnosis

The differential diagnosis of the dermatological manifestations of EM/SJS/TEN is broad, due to the varying presentations of the skin lesions and unknown etiology in some cases. The most common diagnoses mistaken for these disorders are staphylococcal scalded skin syndrome, toxic shock syndrome, exfoliative dermatitis, autoimmune bullous diseases, and chemical/thermal burns.[12] It is critical to distinguish SJS and TEN from staphylococcal scalded skin syndrome and toxic shock syndrome, which are both bacterial in nature and require immediate appropriate antibiotic therapy to arrest release of the exotoxins responsible for the disease.

The chronic ocular findings of SJS most closely resemble those of ocular cicatricial pemphigoid, however, with less extensive symblepharon formation. The differential diagnosis also includes other diseases that produce cicatrizing changes of the eyelids and conjunctiva: atopic or toxic keratoconjunctivitis, severe infectious keratoconjunctivitis, ocular rosacea, linear IgA disease, chemical burns, avitaminosis A, and trachoma. Careful history taking should elucidate the diagnosis; however, conjunctival biopsy may be necessary in some cases. Immunofluorescence microscopy of the involved mucosa in ocular cicatricial pemphigoid will show linear immune deposits along the basement membrane.

Management

SYSTEMIC

Effective management of EM/SJS/TEN involves prompt recognition of the disease, and identification and immediate cessation of all potential offending agents. Immediate cessation of the involved medication reduces mortality and improves prognosis.[33] Comprehensive treatment requires a multidisciplinary approach with specialized nursing and medical care to address the complex, systemic response to the disease. Supportive care involves a similar therapeutic protocol as used in burns management: warming of the environment, minimizing transepidermal fluid loss, treatment of electrolyte imbalances, administration of high-calorie nutrition and intravenous fluids, and prevention of sepsis.[12] For more extensive cutaneous involvement, early referral to a burns unit reduces the risk of infection, mortality, and length of hospitalization significantly.[34,35] The largest trial showed a mortality of 29.8% after transfer to a burns unit with 7 days versus 51.4% ($p<0.05$) after 7 days in TEN patients.[35] Although sepsis is a major source of mortality, prophylactic systemic antibiotics are not recommended and should be reserved for culture-proven sepsis.[12]

Skin lesions should be treated with antimicrobial materials, such as copper sulfate, silver nitrate or sulfadiazine cream (which contains sulfonamide and may cross-react with sulfonamide antibiotics) to improve barrier function and to prevent infection.[36] Biologic dressings, such as cadaver or porcine skin have also been used.[36] Nanocrystalline silver dressings, which serve as an antimicrobial agent and is released for up to 7 to 14 days, have been shown to be beneficial and reduce the frequency of painful dressing changes.[37]

No treatment modality has been established as the gold standard for patients with EM/SJS/TEN. Given the immune-mediated background of these diseases, treatment with immunosuppressive medication should be expected to be beneficial; however, its use has met with intense debate over the years. Corticosteroids, while beneficial in many other acute inflammatory disorders, are controversial in EM/SJS/TEN. Other immunosuppressants, such as intravenous immunoglobulin (IVIG), cyclosporine, cyclophosphamide, thalidomide, infliximab, azathioprine, methotrexate, and plasmapheresis have also been tried in small case series.[36] However, the efficacy of these agents in the treatment of EM/SJS/TEN has not been demonstrated by any controlled clinical trial.

Several studies have shown that corticosteroid use is detrimental in the treatment of SJS or TEN, resulting in increased mortality and morbidity, most commonly infection and gastrointestinal bleeding.[34,38,39] Systemic steroids may also mask early signs of sepsis, impair wound healing, and prolong recovery. However, a large retrospective review of 281 patients enrolled in EuroSCAR (case-control study of mortality risk factors in SJS/TEN patients) found that neither corticosteroids, nor IVIG showed any significant effect on mortality, compared to supportive care alone.[40] Studies have shown that IVIG arrests Fas-mediated keratinolysis in vitro,[41] which provides a pathophysiologic explanation of why it has been shown to be beneficial, with rapid cessation of skin lesions and decreased mortality, in several small case series.[42] However, other studies have found a higher mortality and a longer hospitalization,[43] or no benefit in outcomes with IVIG.[40]

OCULAR – ACUTE

The key to preventing long-term sequelae is early involvement of the ophthalmologist, particularly when efforts may be concentrated on life-threatening issues and hidden ocular involvement can be missed. In addition, eye examination is often difficult in the setting of an intensive care unit and in children. The aim during the acute stage is to prevent cicatricial complications of the ocular surface from developing: if the ocular surface inflammation and ulceration is not expeditiously managed, the ensuing wound healing usually results in scarring. It is important to evert the eyelids if possible, to examine for epithelial defects or ulcers involving the tarsi and fornices which may otherwise remain hidden.

Good ocular surface hygiene should be maintained by frequent lid soaks and conjunctival irrigation to remove accumulated mucous discharge. Prophylactic topical antibiotics should be used to prevent secondary infection, and the ocular surface kept well lubricated with frequent preservative-free artificial tears. Topical steroids should be used judiciously to decrease ocular inflammation; however, patients need to be monitored closely for secondary bacterial infection. Early efforts to prevent symblepharon and ankyloblepharon formation involve daily symblepharolysis with a glass rod or the use of a symblepharon ring to maintain the fornices.

If corneal epithelial defects develop, progressive stromal lysis should be prevented by the use of topical and systemic anticollagenases and frequent lubrication. Careful use of topical steroids should be employed in an effort to balance their anti-inflammatory effects with their risk of accelerated stromal lysis. If microbial keratitis is suspected, microscopy and cultures should be obtained, and fortified antibiotics started. Corneal perforation or impending corneal perforation may be managed with a lamellar or penetrating keratoplasty. An impending perforation may also be managed with a conjunctival flap, or cyanoacrylate glue and bandage contact lens.

There have been several case series reporting success with the use amniotic membrane (AMT) during the acute phase of SJS/TEN.[44–46] AMT is the innermost layer of the placental membrane, consisting of a thick basement membrane and an avascular stroma. It exerts anti-inflammatory and antiscarring actions and is used to facilitate wound healing, including persistent corneal epithelial defects, acute chemical or thermal burns, or recurrent pterygiums.[46] In SJS/TEN, cryopreserved AMT is sutured to cover the entire ocular surface from lid margin to lid margin as a temporary biological bandage as shown in Figure 30.3.[45,47] The eyelashes are trimmed, and the edge of the piece of AMT is sutured to the external eyelid skin 1–2 mm from the lash line using an 8-0 nylon running suture.[44–46] The AMT is oriented stromal surface in contact with conjunctiva. It is spread to cover tarsal conjunctiva and fornix, then reflected to cover bulbar conjunctiva using muscle hooks. The AMT is anchored to skin using double-armed 6-0

prolene sutures passed through the eyelids and secured over the skin with a bolster. The AMT is fixed to the episclera with a continuous 10-0 nylon suture near the limbus. Either a symblepharon ring or Kontour bandage contact lens is used to separate eyelid from eyeball. Prokera™, a symblepharon ring with a sheet of AMT clipped to it, has also been used but has been found to provide inadequate coverage of the forniceal and palpebral conjunctiva and lid margins.[44,45] If Prokera™ is used, it is recommended that one must also use separate AMT to cover the eyelid margin and palpebral conjunctiva. Gregory[44] reported successfully treating 10 patients with AMT, with all patients having epithelial sloughing involving large areas of the ocular surface. They were treated within 10 days of onset of symptoms, and the AMT repeated every 10 to 14 days if inflammation and sloughing persisted. Dry eye severity and ocular surface and eyelid scarring was mild to moderate in all patients.

OCULAR – CHRONIC

The goals of treatment in the chronic stages of EM/SJS/TEN are:

1. Management of dry eye
2. Restoration of eyelid function
3. Restoration of ocular surface.

Management of Dry Eye

The extent of compromise of tear function preoperatively is inversely correlated with the success rate of ocular surface reconstruction procedures.[48] Frequent non-preserved artificial tears should be used to treat the keratoconjunctivitis sicca that results from loss of goblet cells and scarring of the lacrimal ductules. Autologous serum eye drops (ASE) have been recommended as a useful alternative treatment in severe dry eye.[49] Topical transretinoic acid is commercially available and been shown to improve clinical features of dry eye in correlation with the degree of squamous metaplasia in patients with severe dry eye disorders.[50] Chronic conjunctival inflammation will perpetuate the dry eye state and should be managed with topical steroids and cyclosporine. Punctal occlusion to retain the tear film, and medial or lateral tarsorrhaphies to prevent exposure of the tear film to evaporation may also be helpful. The severe dry eye state can result in persistent corneal epithelial defects, and cause the patient to be in a constant state of photophobia and irritation. This may be improved with long-term bandage contact lenses. One study of 39 patients (67 eyes) fitted with scleral lenses for SJS/TEN found a significant improvement in visual acuity and ocular surface symptoms.[51] Similarly, PROSE (prosthetic replacement of the ocular ecosystem) scleral lenses may be used to manage chronic ocular surface disease.

Management of Lid Disease

Abnormal eyelid anatomy may perpetuate corneal complications[30] and should be addressed prior to any ocular surface reconstructive procedure. Trichiasis is a recurrent problem in these patients and may be managed by various techniques, including epilation, electrolysis, argon laser

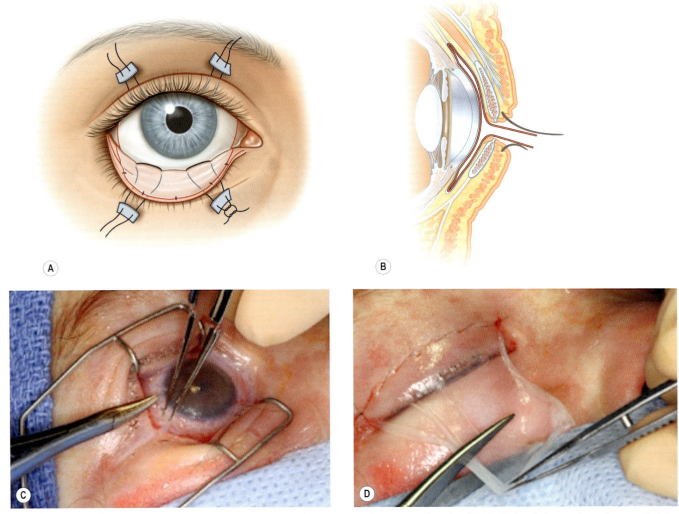

Figure 30.3 Schematic drawing showing the surgical technique of amniotic membrane transplantation (AMT). (**A**) Amniotic membrane is secured with two double-armed horizontal mattress sutures tied over the skin with bolsters and interrupted sutures to the lid margin. (**B**) Side view of AMT showing how AM covers the entire ocular surface from the upper lid margin to the lower lid margin. (**C** and **D**) Sheets of AMT are secured to cover the eyelid margin, and tarsal and bulbar conjunctiva. (**A** & **B**, Reproduced with permission from Meller D, Pires RT, Mack RJ, et al. Amniotic membrane transplantation for acute chemical or thermal burns. Ophthalmology 2000;107:980–9. **C** & **D**, Reproduced with permission from Shammas MC, Lai EC, Sarkar JS, et al. Management of acute Stevens-Johnson syndrome and toxic epidermal necrolysis utilizing amniotic membrane and topical corticosteroids. Am J Ophthal 2010;149:202–13.)

treatment, and cryotherapy. Symblepharon and fornix foreshortening may be addressed by symblepharolysis and conjunctival recession, with the placement of mucous membrane grafts, such as hard palate, nasal or buccal mucosa, or amniotic membrane. Symblepharon may also be addressed at the time of keratolimbal allograft. Cicatricial entropion or ectropion may be corrected by a variety of surgical methods, including placement of a skin or mucous membrane graft.

Ocular Surface Reconstruction

EM/SJS/TEN patients with LSCD have the worst prognosis for ocular surface reconstruction surgery, due to chronic ocular surface inflammation (stage c ocular surface disease),[52] extremely dry eye, and other cicatricial complications. It is important to manage the ocular inflammation preoperatively and to wait until the inflammation is minimized before proceeding with surgery. If surgery is performed during active inflammation, there is an increased risk of delayed epithelial healing, corneal melts, and immune rejection postoperatively. A lateral and/or medial tarsorrhaphy should be strongly considered at the time of ocular surface reconstruction surgery.

EM/SJS/TEN is a bilateral disease, so a conjunctival limbal autograft from the fellow eye is not an option. The two remaining options are ocular surface stem cell transplantation (OSST) from an allograft donor with or without an optical keratoplasty, or keratoprosthesis (KPro) surgery with either a Boston KPro or osteo-odonto-keratoprosthesis (OOKP). We do not advocate Boston Type 1 KPro surgery as the primary ocular surface reconstructive procedure in these patients, and the prognosis for Boston Type 1 KPro surgery in EM/SJS/TEN patients is worse than for other disorders.[53] Due to the severe dry eye there is a high

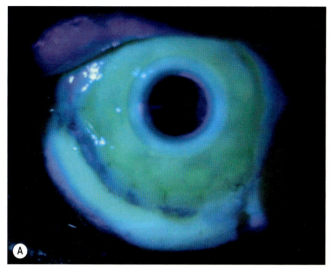

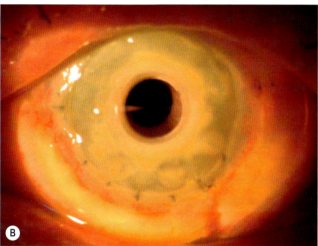

Figure 30.4 SJS patient with KPro complicated by fungal keratitis. (**A**) Fluorescein staining demonstrates a epithelial defect. (**B**) A white infiltrate can be seen 360 degrees under the optic edge.

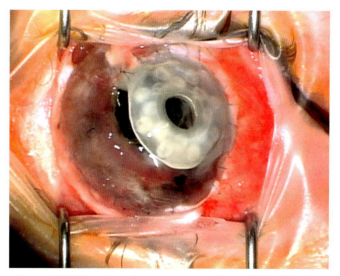

Figure 30.5 SJS patient (same eye as in Figure 30.2) with KPro extrusion.

risk of corneal melting, infectious keratitis, endophthalmitis, and KPro extrusion. Figure 30.4 shows fungal keratitis and Figure 30.5 shows KPro extrusion in a patient with SJS who had undergone Boston type 1 KPro surgery.

We recommend firstly performing OSST surgery to reestablish the corneal epithelium and possibly the deficient conjunctival goblet cells (as discussed below). Once a healthy corneal epithelium has become stabilized after OSST, a penetrating keratoplasty (PK) or deep anterior lamellar keratoplasty (DALK) may be performed if there is significant stromal scarring. A KPro may be considered over a PK or DALK if there is a past history of recurrent endothelial failure from previous PKs, or if the surface fails after OSST surgery.

Allograft transplantation can be from a cadaver-donor keratolimbal allograft (KLAL) or living-related conjunctival limbal allograft (lr-CLAL), or a combination of both lr-CLAL/KLAL (the Cincinnati procedure).[54] A further option is transplantation of ex vivo cultured stem cells. Systemic immunosuppression is required in allograft transplantation to prevent immune rejection of the richly vascularized and antigenic limbal stem cells. SJS-related ocular surface

disease carries a worse prognosis compared to other indications for these procedures, such as aniridia or contact lens-induced keratitis.[55–57] Aside from the chronic inflammation and cicatricial eyelid pathology, one of the major reasons for ocular surface failure is the severe dry eye and mucin deficiency seen in these patients. It has been suggested that combining lr-CLAL and KLAL is beneficial in replacing not only deficient limbal stem cells, but also conjunctival goblet cells.[54] Figure 30.6 shows the preoperative photographs of severe ocular surface failure in a patient with SJS, and the postoperative appearance after combined lr-CLAL/KLAL and penetrating keratoplasty.

In eyes with severe keratinization an osteo-odonto-keratoprosthesis (OOKP)[58] or a Boston type 2 keratoprosthesis[59] may be more suitable. However, these procedures are highly complex and performed only in a few centers around the world.

Conclusion

Erythema multiforme (EM), Stevens–Johnson syndrome (SJS), and toxic epidermal necrolysis (TEN) are rare conditions usually caused by drugs or infections. SJS and TEN are more commonly associated with ocular involvement, and the acute conjunctival inflammation leads to subsequent chronic cicatricial changes in the ocular surface which are usually the most devastating long-term sequelae in these patients. In the acute phase, systemic corticosteroids have gone out of favor, due to the increased risk of infection and associated higher mortality, and intravenous immunoglobulins are being investigated as a promising alternative. Amniotic membrane has been shown to be successful in protecting the ocular surface in the acute phase, alongside topical antibiotics and steroid drops, and regular symblepharolysis. Reconstruction of the ocular surface is challenging in these patients, and aggressive management of the severe dry eye and cicatrizing eyelid pathology is necessary to optimize chances of success.

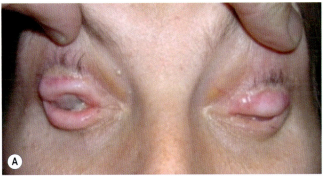

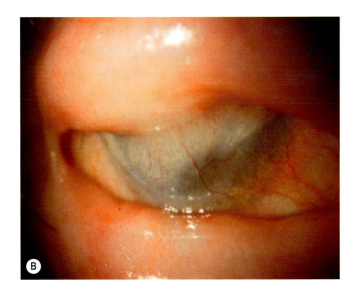

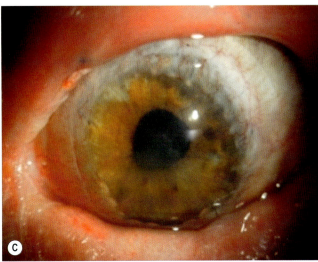

Figure 30.6 (**A**) Preoperative appearance of a patient with SJS showing marked cicatricial ectropion and ocular surface failure. (**B**) Total ocular surface failure and symblepharon of the right eye of the same patient. (**C**) Postoperative appearance of the same patient after lr-CLAL/KLAL and penetrating keratoplasty.

References

1. Hebra F. On diseases of the skin, including the exanthemata. Translated and edited by CH Fagge. London: New Sydenham Society; 1866.
2. Stevens AM, Johnson FC. A new eruptive fever associated with stomatitis and ophthalmia: report of two cases in children. Am J Dis Child 1922;24:526–33.
3. Thomas BA. The so-called Stevens–Johnson syndrome. Br Med J 1950;1:1393–7.
4. Lyell A. Toxic epidermal necrolysis: an eruption resembling scalding of the skin. Br J Dermatol 1956;68:355–61.
5. Bastuji-Garin S, Rzany B, Stern RS, et al. Clinical classification of cases of toxic epidermal necrolysis, Stevens–Johnson syndrome, and erythema multiforme. Arch Dermatol 1993;129:92–6.
6. Chan HL, Stern RS, Arndt KA, et al. The incidence of erythema multiforme, Stevens–Johnson syndrome, and toxic epidermal necrolysis. A population-based study with particular reference to reactions caused by drugs among outpatients. Arch Dermatol 1990;126: 43–47.
7. Assier H, Bastuji-Garin S, Revuz J, et al. Erythema multiforme with mucous membrane involvement and Stevens–Johnson syndrome are clinical different disorders with distinct causes. Arch Dermatol 1995;131:539–43.
8. Rzany B, Mockenhaupt M, Baur S, et al. Epidemiology of erythema exudativum multiforme majus, Stevens–Johnson syndrome, and toxic epidermal necrolysis in Germany (1990–1992): structure and results of a population-based registry. J Clin Epidemiol 1996;49:769–73.
9. Schöpf E, Stühmer A, Rzany B, et al. Toxic epidermal necrolysis and Stevens–Johnson syndrome. An epidemiologic study from West Germany. Arch Dermatol 1991;127:839–42.
10. Roujeau JC, Guillaume JC, Fabre JP, et al. Toxic epidermal necrolysis (Lyell syndrome). Incidence and drug etiology in France, 1981–1985. Arch Dermatol 1990;126:37–42.
11. Auquier-Dunant A, Mockenhaupt M, Naldi L, et al; SCAR Study Group. Severe cutaneous adverse reactions. Correlations between clinical patterns and causes of erythema multiforme majus, Stevens–Johnson syndrome, and toxic epidermal necrolysis: results of an international prospective study. Arch Dermatol 2002;138:1019–24.
12. Hazin R, Ibrahimi OA, Hazin MI, et al. Stevens–Johnson syndrome: Pathogenesis, diagnosis, and management. Ann Med 2008;40: 129–38.
13. Chang YS, Huang FC, Tseng SH, et al. Erythema multiforme, Stevens–Johnson syndrome, and toxic epidermal necrolysis. Acute ocular manifestations, causes, and management. Cornea 2007;26:123–9.
14. Roujeau JC, Kelly JP, Naldi L, et al. Medication use and the risk of Stevens–Johnson syndrome or toxic epidermal necrolysis. N Engl J Med 1995;333:1600–7.
15. Paul C, Wolkenstein P, Adle H, et al. Apoptosis as a mechanism of keratinocyte death in toxic epidermal necrolysis. Br J Dermatol 1996;134:710–4.
16. French LE. Toxic epidermal necrolysis and Stevens–Johnson syndrome: our current understanding. Allergol Int 2006;55:9–16.
17. Abe R, Shimizu T, Shibaki A, et al. Toxic epidermal necrolysis and Stevens–Johnson syndrome are induced by soluble Fas ligand. Am J Pathol 2003;162:1515–20.
18. Inachi S, Mizutani H, Shimizu M. Epidermal apoptotic cell death in erythema multiforme and Stevens–Johnson syndrome. Contribution of perforin-positive cell infiltration. Arch Dermatol 1997;133: 845–9.
19. Chung WH, Hung SI, Yang JY, et al. Granulysin is a key mediator for disseminated keratinocyte death in Stevens-Johnson syndrome and toxic epidermal necrolysis. Nat Med 2008;14:1343–13450.
20. Power WJ, Ghoraishi M, Merayo-Lloves J, et al. Analysis of the acute ophthalmic manifestations of the erythema multiforme/Stevens–Johnson syndrome/toxic epidermal necrolysis disease spectrum. Ophthalmology 1995;102:1669–72.

21. Chung WH, Hung SI, Hong HS, et al. Medical genetics: a marker for Stevens–Johnson syndrome. Nature 2004;428–86.

22. Hung SI, Chung WH Liou LB, et al. HLA-B*5801 allele as a genetic marker for severe cutaneous adverse reactions caused by allopurinol. Proc Natl Acad Sci USA 2005;102:4134–9.

23. Paquet P, Pierard GE. Erythema multiforme and toxic epidermal necrolysis: a comparative study. Am J Dermatopathol 1997;19: 127–32.

24. Rzany B, Hering O, Mockenhaupt M, et al. Histopathological and epidemiological characteristics of patients with erythema exudativum multiforme major, Stevens–Johnson syndrome and toxic epidermal necrolysis. Br J Dermato 1996;135:6–11.

25. Guegan S, Bastuji-Garin S, Poszepczynska-Guigne E, et al. Performance of the SCORTEN during the first five days of hospitalization to predict the prognosis of epidermal necrolysis. J Invest Dermatol 2006;126:272–6.

26. Bastuji-Garin S, Fouchard N, Bertocchi M, et al. SCORTEN: a severity-of-illness score for toxic epidermal necrolysis. J Invest Dermatol 2000;115:149–53.

27. Arstikais MJ. Ocular aftermath of Stevens–Johnson syndrome. Arch Ophthalmol 1973;90:376–9.

28. Tauber J. Autoimmune diseases affecting the ocular surface. In: Holland EJ, Mannis MJ, editors. Ocular surface disease: medical and surgical management. New York: Springer-Verlag; 2002.

29. De Rojas MV, Dart JK, Saw VP. The natural history of Stevens–Johnson syndrome: patterns of chronic ocular disease and the role of systemic immunosuppressive therapy. Br J Ophthalmol 2007; 91:1048–53

30. Di Pascuale MA, Espana EM, Liu DT, et al. Correlation of corneal complications with eyelid cicatricial pathologies in patients with Stevens–Johnson syndrome and toxic epidermal necrolysis syndrome. Ophthalmology 2005;112:904–12.

31. Tatnall FM, Schofield JK, Leigh IM. A double-blind placebo-controlled trial of continuous acyclovir therapy in recurrent erythema multiforme. Br J Dermatol 1995;132:267–70.

32. Foster CS, Fong LP, Azar D, et al. Episodic conjunctival inflammation after Stevens–Johnson syndrome. Ophthalmology 1988;95: 453–62.

33. Garcia-Doval I, LeCleach L, Bocquet H, et al. Toxic epidermal necrolysis and Stevens–Johnson syndrome: does early withdrawal of causative drugs decrease the risk of death? Arch Dermatol 2000;136: 323–7.

34. Kelemen JJ, Cioffi WG, McManus WF, et al. Burns center care for patients with toxic epidermal necrolysis. J Am Coll Surg 1995; 180:273–8.

35. Palmiere TL, Greenhalgh DG, Saffle JR, et al. A multicenter review of toxic epidermal necrolysis treated in U.S. burn centers at the end of the twentieth century. J Burn Care Rehabil 2002;23:87–96.

36. Gerull R, Nelle M, Schaible T. Toxic epidermal necrolysis and Stevens–Johnson syndrome; a review. Crit Care Med 2011;39: 1521–32.

37. Dalli RL, Kumar R, Kennedy P, et al. Toxic epidermal necrolysis/Stevens–Johnson syndrome: current trends in management. ANZ J Surg 2007;77:671–6.

38. Halebian PH, Corder VJ, Madden MR, et al. Improved burn center survival of patients with toxic epidermal necrolysis managed without corticosteroids. Ann Surg 1986;204:503–12.

39. Rasmussen JE. Erythema multiforme in children. Response to treatment with systemic corticosteroids. Br J Dermatol 1976;95:181–6.

40. Schneck J, Fagot FP, Sekula P, et al. Effects of treatments on the mortality of Stevens–Johnson syndrome and toxic epidermal necrolysis: a retrospective study on patients included in the prospective EuroSCAR study. J Am Acad Dermatol 2008;58:33–40.

41. Viard I, Wehrli P, Bullani R, et al. Inhibition of toxic epidermal necrolysis by blockade of CD95 with human intravenous immunoglobulin. Science 1998;282:490–3.

42. Prins C, Kerdel FA, Padilla RS, et al. Treatment of toxic epidermal necrolysis with high-dose intravenous immunoglobulins: a multicenter retrospective analysis of 48 consecutive cases. Arch Dermatol 2003;139:26–32.

43. Brown KM, Silver GM, Halerz M, et al. Toxic epidermal necrolysis: does immunoglobulin make a difference? J Burn Care Rehabil 2004;25: 81–8.

44. Gregory DG. Treatment of acute Stevens–Johnson syndrome and toxic epidermal necrolysis using amniotic membrane: a review of 10 consecutive cases. Ophthalmology 2011;118:908–14.

45. Shammas MC, Lai EC, Sarkar JS, et al. Management of acute Stevens–Johnson syndrome and toxic epidermal necrolysis utilizing amniotic membrane and topical corticosteroids. Am J Ophthalmol 2010; 149:202–13.

46. Shay ES, Kheirkhah A, Liang L, et al. Amniotic membrane transplantation as a new therapy for the acute ocular manifestations of Stevens–Johnson syndrome and toxic epidermal necrolysis. Surv Ophthal 2009;54:686–96.

47. Meller D, Pires RT, Mack RJ, et al. Amniotic membrane transplantation for acute chemical or thermal burns. Ophthalmology 2000; 107:980–9.

48. Shimazaki J, Shimmura S, Fujishima H, et al. Association of preoperative tear function with surgical outcome in severe Stevens–Johnson syndrome. Ophthalmology 2000;107:1518–23.

49. Management and Therapy Subcommittee members of the International Dry Eye Work Shop. Management and therapy of dry eye disease: Report of the Management and Therapy Subcommittee of the International Dry Eye Work Shop (2007). Ocul Surf 2007;5: 163–78.

50. Tseng SCG. Topical tretinoin treatment for severe dry-eye disorders. J Am Acad Dermatol 1986;15(4 Pt 2):860–6.

51. Tougeron-Brousseau B, Delcampe A, Gueudry J, et al. Vision-related function after scleral lens fitting in ocular complications of Stevens–Johnson syndrome and toxic epidermal necrolysis. Am J Ophthalmol 2009;148:852–9.

52. Schwartz GS, Gomes JAP, Holland EJ. Preoperative staging of disease severity. In: Holland EJ, Mannis MJ, editors. Ocular surface disease: medical and surgical management. New York: Springer-Verlag; 2002.

53. Yaghouti F, Nouri M, Abad JC, et al. Keratoprosthesis: preoperative prognostic categories. Cornea 2001;20:19–23.

54. Biber JM, Skeens HM, Neff KD, et al. The Cincinnati procedure: technique and outcomes of combined living-related conjunctival limbal allografts and keratolimbal allografts in severe ocular surface failure. Cornea 2011;30:765–71.

55. Solomon A, Ellis P, Anderson DF, et al. Long-term outcome of keratolimbal allograft with or without penetrating keratoplasty for total limbal stem cell deficiency. Ophthalmology 2002;109:1159–66.

56. Samson CM, Nduaguba C, Baltatzis S, et al. Limbal stem cell transplantation in chronic inflammatory eye disease. Ophthalmology 2002;109:862–8.

57. Shimazaki J, Higa K, Morito F, et al. Factors influencing outcomes in cultivated limbal epithelial transplantation for chronic cicatricial ocular surface disorders. Am J Ophthalmol 2007;143:945–53.

58. Liu C, Okera S, Tandon R, et al. Visual rehabilitation in end-stage inflammatory ocular surface disease with the osteo-odonto-keratoprosthesis: results from the UK. Br J Ophthalmol 2008; 92:1211–7.

59. Pujari S, Siddique SS, Dohlman CH, et al. The Boston keratoprosthesis type II: the Massachusetts Eye and Ear Infirmary experience. Cornea 2011;30:1298–303.

31 *Mucous Membrane Pemphigoid*

TAIS HITOMI WAKAMATSU and JOSE ALVARO PEREIRA GOMES

Introduction

Mucous membrane pemphigoid (MMP), previously known as cicatricial pemphigoid, is a systemic cicatrizing autoimmune disease characterized by chronic blistering of mucous membranes, including ocular, oral, genital, nasopharyngeal, anogenital, and laryngeal mucosa, with ocular (60.1–80%) and oral (90.2%) involvement the most common.[1] The disease causes subepithelial damage and excessive scar tissue formation, which can be life threatening if the trachea or esophagus is involved, or sight threatening if the eyes are involved. Cutaneous involvement is seen in approximately 20% of the patients and usually affects the head, neck, and upper trunk.[2]

Ocular MMP, also known as ocular cicatricial pemphigoid (OCP), is seen as a progressive cicatrizing conjunctivitis, which, if left untreated, bears the risk of symblepharon, ocular surface diseases, corneal ulceration and neovascularization, and ankyloblepharon, causing visual impairment or blindness. It generally presents a chronic course, characterized by periods of activity subsequent to quiescent phases. In large series, approximately 80% of the patients with MMP have ocular involvement,[3] and blindness has been reported to occur in 27%.[4]

The diagnosis of this disease is made difficult because of its early presenting symptoms that can be subtle and non-specific. The signs of MMP often go unrecognized until the resulting erosions and scarring are established. As a chronic and progressive disorder with sequelae that are irreversible and often debilitating, early diagnosis is critical.

Epidemiology

The incidence of MMP is approximately one new case per million inhabitants per year. MMP is considered a potentially fatal autoimmune disease with a mortality usually secondary to aero-digestive tract stricture formation, quoted as 0.028 per 100 000 in the United States during 1992–2002.[5]

OCP is a relatively rare disease with an estimated incidence of 1 in 15 000 to 1 in 60 000 ophthalmic patients.[6] However, these studies do not report the true epidemiologic incidence of this disease because the reported cases are usually not in their earliest stages.[3] Typical presentation involves a patient in the sixth or seventh decade of life, although it is recognized that OCP can begin at least as early as the third decade of life.[7] In a study involving 130 patients, Foster et al. described that the average age was 64 years with a range of 20 years to 87 years. Females are affected two to three times as frequently as males. It has no racial or geographic predilection.[3]

Pathogenesis

Ocular cicatricial pemphigoid (OCP) is an autoimmune chronic cicatrizing conjunctivitis (CCC) associated with linear deposition of IgG and IgA aoutoantibodies directed against autoantigens at the conjunctival epithelial basement membrane zone (BMZ)[3] that sets in motion a complex series of events. Bhol et al. concluded that a 205-kilodalton (KDa) protein molecule is the putative target antigen for OCP.[8] Among others, the target antigen identified by the sera of patients with OCP is located in the basal epithelial cell hemidesmosome cytoplasmic domain of β4 subunit of the α6β4 integrin heterodimer.[9] Autoantibodies are thought to cause scarring of the conjunctiva via activation of complement, neutrophils and proinflammatory cytokines. In addition, immunohistochemical study of the conjunctiva from patients with active OCP revealed significantly more T-helper-inducer cells (CD4+) and Langerhans cells in the epithelium and active T cells, fibroblasts and macrophages in the substantia propria compared to the control group.[10] Staining for transforming growth factor-beta (TGF-β) is also significantly increased.

The subacute phase of the disease is histologically similar to acute disease. The chronic phase is characterized by an infiltration with T lymphocytes, HLA-DR-expressing cells and macrophages which are mildly increased in number. The epithelium may become thickened, metaplastic and may keratinize at any phase.

Fibrosis results from the stimulation of fibroblasts, often by fibrogenic growth factors as TGF-β, PDGF, TNF and IL-1.[11] When quiescent fibroblasts are stimulated to proliferate by these modulators, there is transient expression of proto-oncogenes, including c-fos, c-myc and c-myb. These are a series of genes that are transducers of external growth factors and probably trigger the activation of genes that are required for proliferation.

Several human leukocyte antigens (HLAs), including HLA-DR4 and HLA-DQw3 were first reported to be associated with increased susceptibility to the OCP.[12] Furthermore, a prevalence of HLA-DQB1*0301 was first described in patients with pure ocular mucous membrane pemphigoid.[13] This allele, however, was later found to be associated with all clinical sites of involvement and possibly to be linked to antibasement membrane IgG production. Interestingly, these studies also suggested a role for this allele in disease severity. Environmental triggers, such as microbial infection or drug exposure may stimulate the genetically susceptible individuals and induce the development of the disease.

Diagnosis

CLINICAL FEATURES

The natural history of OCP begins with unilateral chronic conjunctivitis that becomes bilateral after a variable period. In relapsing-remitting OCP, symptoms and signs typically evolve over a period of several weeks, stabilize, and then often extend over many years with periods of activity followed by quiescent phases every few months. Diagnosis of this disease in its early stages is difficult and most cases are not recognized as OCP until they reach the advanced stage.

Early in the disease, signs of subepithelial fibrosis appear in the inferior and superior tarsal conjunctiva and consist of fine white lines that are often perivascular. Ocular symptoms are variable and consist of foreign body sensation, burning sensation, discharge, and hyperemia. They are not always correlated to disease severity, and progressive fibrosis can occur even in asymptomatic patients. Subsequently, the fibrosis progresses and leads to fornix foreshortening, symblepharon formation, entropion, trichiasis, and, in the terminal stage, ankyloblepharon. Conjunctival fibrosis also can cause severe dry eye syndrome because of the destruction of goblet cells and obliteration of lacrimal gland ductules. Corneal lesions are frequent in this setting and may be complicated by bacterial and fungal superinfection and lead to corneal perforation and xerosis.

To assess the progression of the fibrotic process and treatment efficacy, it is important to quantify fibrosis and conjunctival inflammation. The classification of Foster et al. (Fig. 31.1) uses as an index the degree of inferior fornix foreshortening and the number and extension of symblephara.[14] Subepithelial fibrosis is characteristic of stage I of OCP, with stage II showing fornix foreshortening. Symblepharon formation is the hallmark of stage III. Stage IV,

I. Chronic conjunctivitis, sub-epithelial fibrosis

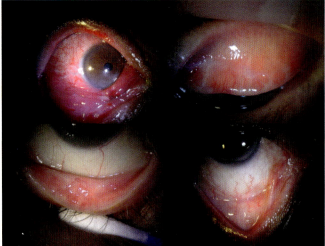

II. Inferior fornix foreshortening

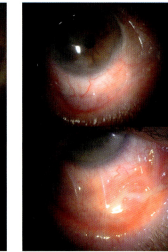

III. Symblepharon, corneal vasc., trichiasis

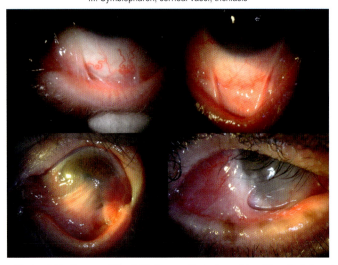

IV. Ankyloblepharon, surface keratinization

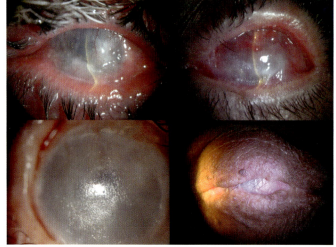

Figure 31.1 Stages of the OCP disease. Stage I consists of tarsal white subepithelial stria and fibrosis formation. In stage II, in addition to the subepithelial fibrosis, a fornix shortening is visible. In stage III, symblepharon is detected, most easily seen with lower lid retracted and patient gazing upwards. In stage IV, total ankyloblepharon and surface keratinization are observed.

end-stage disease, is characterized by ankyloblepharon and surface keratinization. Mondino's classification quantifies inferior fornix depth loss.[15] Stage II is a reduction of 25–50%; stage III, 50–75%; stage IV, more than 75%. Normal depth is approximately 11 mm.

LABORATORIAL FEATURES

Immunopathological techniques may be helpful in characterizing the underlying pathogenetic processes in mucous membrane pemphigoid. Conjunctival biopsies using the immunofluorescent or immunoperoxidase technique provide the only definitive evidence of OCP. Direct and indirect immunofluorescence are sensitive but non-specific indicators for OCP, because findings are often indistinguishable from those seen in patients with other subepithelial blistering diseases.

Immunochemical techniques, including immunoblotting, immunoprecipitation and enzyme-linked immunosorbent assay (ELISA), have simplified the diagnostic process and have identified novel protein targets recognized by autoantibodies in different subgroups of mucous membrane pemphigoid.

Direct Immunopathology

Direct methods of immunofluorescence microscopy or immunohistochemistry examinations on perilesional mucosa biopsies detect continuous deposits of any one or combination of the following in the epithelial BMZ: IgG, IgA, and/or C3 (Fig. 31.2). Direct immunofluorescence (DIF) evidence has been recommended as a mandatory requirement for the diagnosis of MMP.[16] However, conjunctival DIF is positive in only 20–83% of cases of ocular MMP,[17] and the results can be initially positive then subsequently negative, and vice versa, during the course of the disease, apparently unrelated to disease activity or treatment.

Indirect Immunofluorescence

Indirect immunofluorescence testing of patients' serum using chemically separated normal human epithelial substrate is a sensitive method for detecting circulating

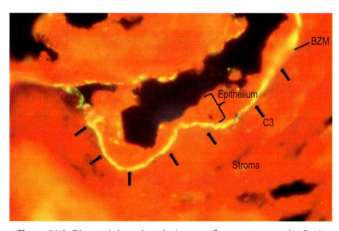

Figure 31.2 Diagnosis based on the immunofluorescence results. Positive conjunctival direct immunofluorescence in a patient with OCP. Note the linear deposition of complement C3 in the BZM of the conjunctiva. (magnification ×400).

autoantibodies to epithelial BMZ components in affected patients. Current assays that identify circulating autoantibodies have a limited role in serological diagnosis, since sensitivity is determined by substrate used; even the best available substrate yielded only a 52% positive result.[18]

More sensitive assays include the radioimmunoassay[19] and immunoblot assay (IBA),[8] and an ELISA assay for detection of such circulating autoantibodies is currently being developed.

Histopathological Examination.

Findings from routine light microscopy studies of lesional tissues stained with hematoxylin and eosin typically demonstrate subepithelial blisters with or without a significant leukocyte infiltrate.

Differential Diagnosis

The differential diagnosis of MMP includes other immunobullous diseases, erythema multiforme, lupus erythematosus, lichen planus, and lichenoid drug eruptions. Similar to OCP, many disorders may cause subepithelial fibrosis with or without inflammation (Box 31.1).[20] OCP may represent the sequela of a prior bout of Stevens–Johnson syndrome, occurring a few months to as much as 30 years previously. Drug-induced cicatrizing or inflammatory conjunctivitis, also known as ocular pseudopemphigoid, can arise from long-term use of certain ophthalmologic preparations (antiviral and glaucoma medications) or biologic drugs (epidermal growth factor receptor tyrosine kinase inhibitors).

Management

The course of ocular disease is variable, and determining disease activity and progression represents a major challenge. Patients are often diagnosed in advanced stages of disease when the signs and symptoms of disease are severe and mandate aggressive therapy.

Management strategies are aimed at early diagnosis together with the prevention of both life- and sight-threatening complications through the removal of factors that precipitate inflammation, dry eye, basement membrane abnormalities, eyelids abnormalities and limbal stem cell deficiency.

Treatment

INFLAMMATION

Inflammation resulting from systemic immune imbalance requires treatment with systemic immunosuppressive agents. Previous studies showed that almost 75% of the patients require systemic immunosuppression[21] and 46% require continuing systemic treatment to avoid disease reactivation. There is no evidence that topical therapy alters the natural history of the disease.[3]

The immunosuppressive therapeutic approach should take into consideration the severity and the progression of

Box 31.1 Differential Diagnosis of Cicatrizing Conjunctivitis

1A. Static or Very Slowly Progressive Conjunctival Scarring

1. Trauma
   Physical, chemical, thermal, radiation injury, artefacta
2. Infection
   Trachoma, membranous streptococcal and adenoviral conjunctivitis
   Corynebacterium diphtheria, chronic mucocutaneous candidiasis
3. Allergic eye disease
   Atopic keratoconjunctivitis
4. Drug-induced conjunctival cicatrization†
5. Mucocutaneous disorders
   Stevens–Johnson syndrome and toxic epidermal necrolysis†
   Graft-versus-host disease
6. Immunobullous disorders
   Linear IgA disease,† epidermolysis bullosa acquisita†
   Dermatitis herpetiformis, bullous pemphigoid
   Pemphigus vulgaris
   Discoid and systemic lupus erythematosus*
7. Systemic disease
   Rosacea, Sjögren's syndrome, inflammatory bowel disease, sarcoidosis, scleroderma, immune complex diseases, ectodermal dysplasia, porphyria cutanea tarda, erythroderma ichthyosiform congenital

1B. Progressive Conjunctival Scaring

1. Neoplasia
   Squamous cell carcinoma, sebaceous cell carcinoma, lymphoma
2. Mucous membrane pemphigoid (MMP)
   a. MMP with ocular involvement
   b. Ocular MMP associated with other disorders
      Linear IgA disease
      Epidermolysis bullosa acquisita
      Paraneoplastic MMP
      Drug-induced ocular MMP
      Stevens–Johnson syndrome
3. Other mucocutaneous & immunobullous disorders
   a. Mucocutaneous disorders
      Lichen planus
   b. Immunobullous disorders
      Paraneoplastic pemphigus

*Rare cases can develop progressive scarring.
†A subset of patients with these diseases may develop autoantibody-positive progressive conjunctival scarring similar to MMP.
(In: Ocul Surf 2008;6:128–42. Ocular mucous membrane pemphigoid: diagnosis and management strategies. Saw VP, Dart JK.)

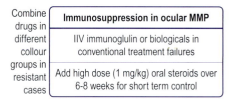
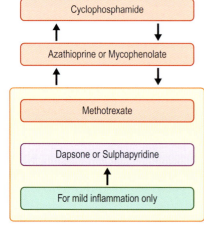

Figure 31.3 Stepladder immunosuppressive therapy for ocular MMP. For severe disease, commence with cyclophosphamide and plan introduction of less toxic drugs and withdrawal of cyclophosphamide once the disease is under control. For mild disease, use dapsone (or sulfapyridine if dapsone is not tolerated) or methotrexate and step up to azathioprine or mycophenolate. If treatment fails with this, then progress to cyclophosphamide. Oral prednisolone for 6 weeks is usually combined with cyclophosphamide, while awaiting the commencement of immunosuppressive effect. Combinations of a sulpha-based agent (dapsone or sulphapyridine) with a myelosuppressive agent (cyclophosphamide, azathioprine, mycophenolate) and prednisolone are also effective.

the disease, the patient's age, health and anticipated tolerance of treatment-related side effects, and the response to treatment (Fig. 31.3). For patients with severe disease or rapid progression of disease, the initial treatment should be with cyclophosphamide (1–2 mg/kg/day) and prednisone (1–1.5 mg/kg/day)[22] for 6–8 weeks, and sometimes in conjunction with intravenous pulses of methylprednisolone (500 mg–1 g, up to three doses over 3 days). Because cyclophosphamide is associated with an increased risk of bladder carcinoma, the safe duration of treatment with this agent is limited to 12–18 months. Cyclophosphamide can also be administered intravenously if patients cannot tolerate the oral form. When the disease is controlled, prednisone administration should be slowly tapered while maintaining the immunosuppressive regimen for a longer period. In a preliminary study, intravenous immunoglobulin has been reported to be a safe and effective therapy for recalcitrant ocular disease[23] or as an alternative to conventional immunosuppression. Monoclonal antibody therapies are potential treatments for severe refractory MMP.

For moderate disease, patients should be treated with azathioprine (1–2 mg/kg/day) or mycophenolate mofetil (500 mg–1 g/day). Nicotinamide and tetracycline have also been reported as an effective therapy in mild to moderate case, with 50% of patients responding to the treatment. For patients with mild disease, initial treatment with dapsone (diaminodiphenylsulfone; 50–200 mg/day) for 12 weeks or sulphapyridine (500 mg one or two times/day, given as sulfasalazine 500 mg one or two times/day when sulphapyridine is unavailable) should be initiated.

Topical ocular immunomodulation treatment can be used for improving symptoms and for adding additional control of the conjunctival inflammation. This local treatment can be done with topical corticosteroids (e.g. fluoromethalone or prednisolone 0.5%), 0.05–2% cyclosporine, tacrolimus or pimecrolimus.

DRY EYE

Dry eyes in OCP patients may be caused by lacrimal gland duct obstruction, cicatricial meibomian gland dysfunction and/or poor lid apposition. Tear deficiency is a major cause of symptoms, although loss of vision is usually due to surface failure before the onset of aqueous tear deficiency. Surface failure and stem cell deficiency occur late in the progression of the disease. Management of the dry eye must be integrated with the management of the other components of both the ocular surface disease and inflammation.

Treatment of dry eye starts with the use of lubricants. The use of lubricants without preservatives avoids toxicity. Autologous serum drops improve the ocular surface due to their effect as a physiological tear replacement as serum contains many of the components of tears, including growth factors, vitamins, and albumin.

The lacrimal puncta are often occluded spontaneously as part of the disease. In case they are not closed, occlusion is helpful and its use has been associated with objective and subjective improvement. The wearing of moisture chamber spectacles helps to alleviate ocular discomfort associated with dry eye, increasing the periocular humidity in patients wearing such spectacles. Contact lenses, either large limbal-diameter rigid gas-permeable or gas-permeable scleral lenses, are useful for treating dry eye and improving vision in some patients.

Several potential topical or systemic pharmacologic agents may stimulate aqueous secretion, mucous secretion, or both. The topical agents currently under investigation are diquafosol, rebamipide, gefarnate, ecabet sodium and 15(S)-HETE. Two orally administrated cholinergic agonists, pilocarpine and cevilemine, have been evaluated in clinical trials and were found to significantly improve symptoms of dryness and aqueous tear production. Salivary gland transplantation may also constitute an option for the treatment of severe dry eye secondary to OCP. This may be considered a step prior to limbal stem cell and corneal transplantation.[24]

EYELID ABNORMALITIES

Trichiasis is a common and potentially sight-threatening complication of ocular cicatricial pemphigoid (OCP) and is the major risk factor for microbial keratitis. It may also cause punctate epitheliopathy, corneal abrasions, conjunctival metaplasia, provoke additional conjunctival inflammation, and increase ocular surface symptoms. It is usually secondary to cicatricial entropion and may involve either the upper or lower lid. Trichiasis can be treated with several methods: laser thermoablation, lid split through the gray line and anterior lamellar reposition, excision with oral mucous membrane or amniotic membrane transplantation or cryotherapy. Another option of protection against the trauma provoked by the eyelashes in contact to the conjunctiva and cornea is a scleral contact lens.[25]

BASENMENT MEMBRANE ABNORMALITIES

The complex autoimmune disorder with multiple components of the immune system participating in the OCP results in an inflamed conjunctiva at the BZM level with formation of bullae and scarring. Chronic conjunctivitis is the common cause of many complications of this disease. In order to establish control of the inflammation and maintain a stable conjunctiva, decreasing the symblepharon formation in patients with OCP, several studies have been performed using amniotic membrane transplantation (Fig. 31.4). It has unique properties that improve the pain, confer anti-inflammatory, antiadhesive and antiangiogenic effects, has the ability to stimulate re-epithelialization and lacks immunogenicity. Previous studies demonstrated that amniotic membrane can be used as an initial step in attempting to reconstruct the ocular surface in patients with advanced OCP.[26]

LIMBAL STEM CELL DEFICIENCY

Progressive conjunctival scarring results in loss of goblet cells and keratinization of the ocular surface epithelia with

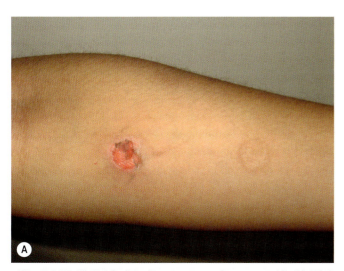
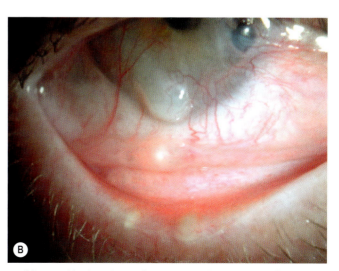

Figure 31.4 Clinical findings in mucous membrane pemphigoid. (**A**) Cutaneous blisters with ulceration and cicatrization. (**B**) Formation of bullae in the corneal epithelium.

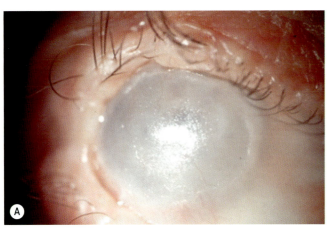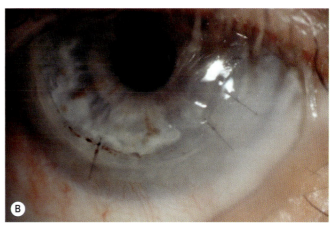

Figure 31.5 Ocular surface reconstruction. (**A**) Total surface keratinization. (**B**) After immunosuppressive therapy, limbal transplantation and penetrating keratoplasty. Note the decrease of keratinization and the transparency of the cornea.

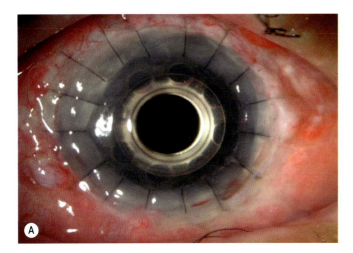

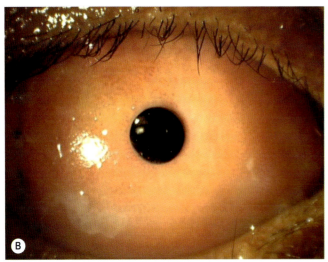

Figure 31.6 Keratoprosthesis for end stage of OCP. (**A**) Boston type I keratoprosthesis. (**B**) Osteo-odonto-keratoprosthesis. (Courtesy of Donald Tan.)

complete corneal opacification. Prolonged inflammation, which is associated with conjunctivalization of the cornea, destroys corneal stem cells and is the main reason for the failure of penetrating keratoplasty in these cases. Furthermore, the long-term success of a limbal allograft is at risk because of ongoing inflammation.

Tsubota et al. reported successful visual improvement in 9/9 eyes with use of limbal allografts and amniotic membrane transplantation in conjunction with systemic immunosuppression with dapsone and cyclosporine. Penetrating keratoplasty was also performed in 5 of the 9 eyes.[26] Other reports of the outcomes of surface reconstructive surgery that used living-related limbal allografts[27] or cultivated epithelial stem cells[28] describe results for only two or three OCP eyes. Once ocular surface inflammation and progression have been controlled, attention can be turned to other means of improving vision (Fig. 31.5).

When ocular surface reconstruction and penetrating keratoplasty fail, keratoprosthesis (KPro) surgery may provide the only potential means of restoring vision in patients with progressive OCP (Fig. 31.6). However, transcorneal KPros, such as the Boston type I device have shown limited results in the long-term follow-up of advanced OCP patients with severe dry eye. This device carries a guarded prognosis in OCP due to the high risk of corneal melting and device extrusion. Boston type II KPros or the osteo-odonto-keratoprosthesis (OOKP) devices appear to be better options for these cases of OCP in comparison to the Boston type 1 device.[29]

References

1. Thorne JE, Anhalt GJ, Jabs DA. Mucous membrane pemphigoid and pseudopemphigoid. Ophthalmology 2004;111:45–52.
2. Williams GP, Radford C, Nightingale P, et al. Evaluation of early and late presentation of patients with ocular mucous membrane pemphigoid to two major tertiary referral hospitals in the United Kingdom. Eye (Lond) 2011;25:1207–18.
3. Foster CS. Cicatricial pemphigoid. Trans Am Ophthalmol Soc 1986;84:527–663.
4. Hardy KM, Perry HO, Pingree GC, et al. Benign mucous membrane pemphigoid. Arch Dermatol 1971;104:467–75.
5. Risser J, Lewis K, Weinstock MA. Mortality of bullous skin disorders from 1979 through 2002 in the United States. Arch Dermatol 2009;145:1005–8.

6. Lever WF, Talbott JH. Pemphigus: a historical study. Arch Dermatol Syph 1942;46:800.

7. Kharfi M, Khaled A, Anane R, et al. Early onset childhood cicatricial pemphigoid: a case report and review of the literature. Pediatr Dermatol 2010;27:119–24.

8. Bhol K, Mohimen A, Neumann R, et al. Differences in the anti-basement membrane zone antibodies in ocular and pseudo-ocular cicatricial pemphigoid. Curr Eye Res 1996;15:521–32.

9. Bhol KC, Dans MJ, Simmons RK, et al. The autoantibodies to alpha 6 beta 4 integrin of patients affected by ocular cicatricial pemphigoid recognize predominantly epitopes within the large cytoplasmic domain of human beta 4. J Immunol 2000;165:2824–9.

10. Rice BA, Foster CS. Immunopathology of cicatricial pemphigoid affecting the conjunctiva. Ophthalmology 1990;97:1476–83.

11. Muller R, Bravo R, Burckhardt J, et al. Induction of c-fos gene and protein by growth factors precedes activation of c-myc. Nature 1984;312:716–20.

12. Zaltas MM, Ahmed R, Foster CS. Association of HLA-DR4 with ocular cicatricial pemphigoid. Curr Eye Res 1989;8:189–93.

13. Ahmed AR, Foster S, Zaltas M, et al. Association of DQw7 (DQB1*0301) with ocular cicatricial pemphigoid. Proc Natl Acad Sci UA 1991; 88:11579–82.

14. Foster CS, Wilson LA, Ekins MB. Immunosuppressive therapy for progressive ocular cicatricial pemphigoid. Ophthalmology 1982; 89:340–53.

15. Mondino BJ, Ross AN, Rabin BS, et al. Autoimmune phenomena in ocular cicatricial pemphigoid. Am J Ophthalmol 1977;83:443–50.

16. Chan LS, Ahmed AR, Anhalt GJ, et al. The first international consensus on mucous membrane pemphigoid: definition, diagnostic criteria, pathogenic factors, medical treatment, and prognostic indicators. Arch Dermatol 2002;138:370–9.

17. Tauber J, Jabbur N, Foster CS. Improved detection of disease progression in ocular cicatricial pemphigoid. Cornea 1992;11:446–51.

18. Power WJ, Neves RA, Rodriguez A, et al. Increasing the diagnostic yield of conjunctival biopsy in patients with suspected ocular cicatricial pemphigoid. Ophthalmology 1995;102:1158–63.

19. Ahmed AR, Khan KN, Wells P, et al. Preliminary serological studies comparing immunofluorescence assay with radioimmunoassay. Curr Eye Res 1989;8:1011–9.

20. Saw VP, Dart JK. Ocular mucous membrane pemphigoid: diagnosis and management strategies. Ocul Surf 2008;6:128–42.

21. Elder MJ, Bernauer W, Leonard J, et al. Progression of disease in ocular cicatricial pemphigoid. Br J Ophthalmol 1996;80:292–6.

22. Elder MJ, Lightman S, Dart JK. Role of cyclophosphamide and high dose steroid in ocular cicatricial pemphigoid. Br J Ophthalmol 1995; 79:264–6.

23. Sami N, Letko E, Androudi S, et al. Intravenous immunoglobulin therapy in patients with ocular-cicatricial pemphigoid: a long-term follow-up. Ophthalmology 2004;111:1380–2.

24. Sant' Anna AE, Hazarbassanov RM, de Freitas D, et al. Minor salivary glands and labial mucous membrane graft in the treatment of severe symblepharon and dry eye in patients with Stevens–Johnson syndrome. Br J Ophthalmol 2011;96:234–9.

25. Siqueira AC, Santos MS, Farias CC, et al. [Scleral contact lens for ocular rehabilitation in patients with Stevens-Johnson syndrome]. Arq Bras Oftalmol 2010;73:428–32.

26. Tsubota K, Satake Y, Ohyama M, et al. Surgical reconstruction of the ocular surface in advanced ocular cicatricial pemphigoid and Stevens–Johnson syndrome. Am J Ophthalmol 1996;122:38–52.

27. Santos MS, Gomes JA, Hofling-Lima AL, et al. Survival analysis of conjunctival limbal grafts and amniotic membrane transplantation in eyes with total limbal stem cell deficiency. Am J Ophthalmol 2005; 140:223–30.

28. Nishida K, Yamato M, Hayashida Y, et al. Corneal reconstruction with tissue-engineered cell sheets composed of autologous oral mucosal epithelium. N Engl J Med 2004;351:1187–96.

29. Dohlman CH, Terada H. Keratoprosthesis in pemphigoid and Stevens–Johnson syndrome. Adv Exp Med Biol 1998;438:1021–5.

32 *Congenital Stem Cell Deficiency*

HEATHER M. SKEENS

Stem cells are present in all self-renewing tissues.[1] Multiple studies have demonstrated that the stem cells for the corneal surface are located at the limbus. Davanger and Evensen[2] were the first to speculate that the cells involved in the process of normal corneal epithelial renewal are located at the limbus when they observed that pigmented cells from the area of the limbus were moving centrally in the cornea. The pattern of movement they observed from the peripheral to the central cornea suggested a centripetal migration of corneal epithelial cells; we now know that the process of corneal epithelial cell renewal is very elaborate and involves a migration of epithelial cells from the periphery of the cornea to the central cornea where the older cells are then shed.[3] Around the same time, a separate study observed that the basal cells of the limbal area are less differentiated than those cells that are found in other areas of the cornea epithelium. This observation was made by following the patterns of expression of a cornea-specific 64K keratin protein present in all corneal epithelial cells, except the limbal basal cells.[4] The absence of expression of this protein in the limbal basal cells led Schermer and coworkers to speculate that corneal epithelial stem cells must be located in the less differentiated limbus.[4] Additional studies demonstrated that the cells in the less differentiated limbus display another property in that they exhibit a long cell cycle consistent with the long cell cycles characteristic of other stem cell populations.[5] The incorporation of tritiated thymidine for long time intervals into the limbal basal cells demonstrated this concept.[5] Finally, Ebato and associates[6] reported that human ocular limbal epithelial cells grew better in culture and had a higher rate of mitotic activity than peripheral corneal epithelial cells.

The importance of sustaining a healthy limbal stem cell population is evident in the appearance and function of the ocular surface when a deficiency of stem cells exists. A deficiency of the limbal stem cell population leads to a very unstable ocular surface. The cornea becomes conjunctivalized and vascularized, and the patient experiences repeated epithelial defects and ulcerations of the cornea. Vision becomes limited, due to the loss of transparency of the cornea. Patients with decreased vision from other causes, such as macular abnormalities, glaucoma, and cataract, will experience further vision loss from this keratopathy.

The most common causes of limbal stem cell deficiency (LSCD) are secondary in nature and include chemical and thermal burns, Stevens–Johnson syndrome and ocular cicatricial pemphigoid, multiple surgeries, topical medications, including antimetabolite use, neoplasias, and contact-lens induced LSCD.[7–10] Congenital stem cell deficiency is less common and includes such conditions as congenital aniridia, some ectodermal dysplasias and sclerocornea.

Aniridia

Classic congenital aniridia is a bilateral, panocular disorder presenting with decreased best-corrected visual acuity, foveal hypoplasia, and nystagmus.[11] Abnormalities in the cornea, anterior chamber angle, iris, lens, optic nerve, macula, and retina have all been reported.[11] Glaucoma and cataract may occur. The prevalence is between $1:64\,000$ and $1:100\,000$.[11] About two-thirds of cases of aniridia arise via familial inheritance and one-third of cases arise sporadically.[11] A *PAX6* gene mutation has been identified as the underlying cause of aniridia in the vast majority of patients, although some genetic heterogeneity has recently been identified.[12]

ANIRIDIC KERATOPATHY

While 'aniridia' was traditionally named for the near complete absence of the iris, foveal hypoplasia is most often responsible for the initial poor visual acuity in affected patients. However, many of these patients are susceptible to further visual loss from a progressive aniridic keratopathy (AK).[13] This keratopathy, due to a congenital deficiency of the limbal stem cells, progresses to involve the total cornea, and eventually may lead to severe corneal stromal scarring and complete conjunctivalization of the ocular surface.[13]

Deficiency of the limbal stem cells in aniridia has been proven. Tseng[14] proposed an initial model of LSCD in AK, and this model was further elucidated in a separate study by Nishida et al.[15] through the process of impression cytology. Aniridic patients in the Nishida study demonstrated a clinical absence of the limbal palisades of Vogt, and the presence of conjunctival goblet cells on the cornea, implying either a primary absence of the limbal stem cells or abnormal limbal stem cells in aniridia.

Although the term 'aniridic keratopathy' was not coined at the time, clinicians began to recognize corneal changes in their aniridic patients well over a hundred years ago. As early as 1893, corneal opacities were mentioned in aniridia, and casual references were made to corneal haze, peripheral dystrophy, and corneal clouding.[16] In 1979, Mackman and colleagues[16] grouped the corneal changes in AK into four stages. In their stage 0, the aniridic cornea is clinically normal. In their stage 1A, the cornea displays abnormal epithelium and vascularization in the 6- and 12-o'clock meridians, which progresses to 360-degree corneal involvement in stage 1B. In stage 2 AK, there is central corneal involvement with stromal scarring as well. However, the changes seen in AK present in more clinically distinct stages and it may be more helpful to the clinician to separate these out even further.

Holland has proposed the following classification of AK, which more accurately details the cornea changes (unpublished results). AK occurs in five stages, with each stage progressing to the next unless the LSCD is corrected (Figs 32.1–32.7). In stage 1, a peripheral corneal epitheliopathy exists. Patients may display increased fluorescein uptake in the area of the peripheral cornea and exhibit a characteristic of LSCD known as late-staining. Clinically abnormal epithelium is evident in the periphery of the cornea. Stage 2 AK occurs when the peripheral epitheliopathy moves

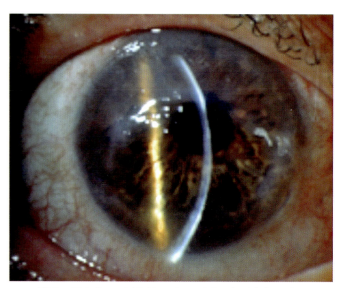

Figure 32.3 Stage 2 AK. Note the peripheral epitheliopathy.

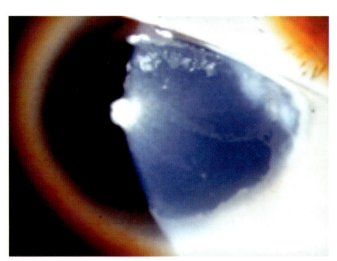

Figure 32.1 Stages 1 and 2 aniridic keratopathy (AK). Note the peripheral epitheliopathy inferiorly (Holland stage 1) which expands to involve the pericentral cornea superiorly (Holland stage 2). The central cornea is quickly becoming involved (Holland stage 3).

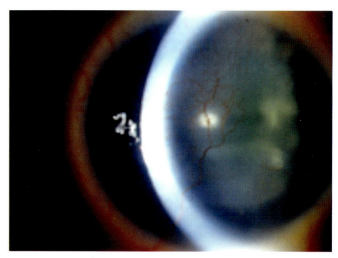

Figure 32.4 Stage 3 AK. Note the total epitheliopathy and neovascularization (NV). As noted in the text, NV can occur in any stage of AK and is not helpful in identifying the stage.

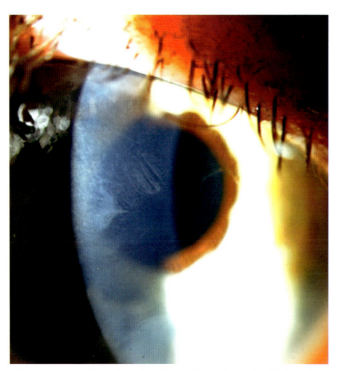

Figure 32.2 Holland stage 2 AK. Note the peripheral epitheliopathy that is extending to the pericentral cornea. Also note the presence of ectropion uveae. This patient has variant aniridia.

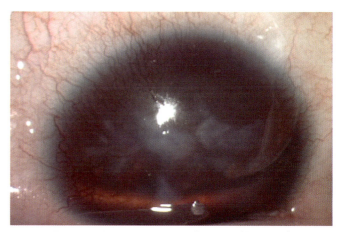

Figure 32.5 Stage 4 AK. Note the total epitheliopathy along with subepithelial fibrous tissue.

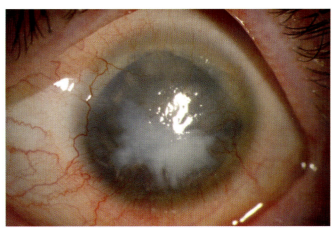

Figure 32.6 Stage 5 AK. There is total epitheliopathy along with sub-epithelial and stromal scar tissue.

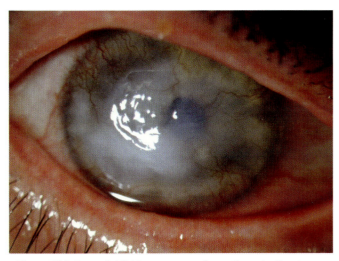

Figure 32.7 Stage 5 AK. The presence of scar tissue in the stroma denotes the stage.

centrally, involving the pericentral cornea. In stage 3 AK, the epitheliopathy involves the central cornea. At any stage, neovascularization may be seen and is non-specific for AK and not helpful in identifying the stage of AK a patient may be exhibiting. In stage 4 AK, the cornea displays complete epitheliopathy and subepithelial fibrosis. Total epitheliopathy is required before the process of subepithelial fibrosis (SEF) can occur. Without further treatment, stage 5 AK ensues, and in this stage the cornea exhibits total epitheliopathy and deeper scarring now involving the stroma. Clinically, it is important to recognize and diagnose AK before SEF and deep scarring of the cornea ensues (prior to stage 4), as the patient will require both correction of the LSCD and a cornea transplant beyond this point.

The PAX6 gene plays an important role for the ocular surface in all individuals, not just aniridics. Studies have demonstrated PAX6 expression in the limbal stem cells.[17] PAX6 has also been demonstrated in embryonic, as well as mature corneal and conjunctival tissues, and it may play a role in the maintenance and proliferation of the limbal stem cells.[17] As mentioned, the underlying genetic defect in aniridia involves a mutation in the PAX6 gene, although other genes are now being identified. In aniridia, one copy of the PAX6 gene expresses the mutation while the second copy of the gene is normal. Patients who are born with two mutated copies of the PAX6 gene do not live.[18]

The mutated PAX6 gene has implications for the aniridic patient. The normal centripetal migration of corneal epithelial cells from the area of the limbus to the central cornea is impaired in aniridia secondary to the mutated PAX6 gene.[11] PAX6 also regulates the expression of cytokeratins 3 and 12, which are critical for normal cell-to-cell binding, and in anchoring cells to their underlying basal lamina. In aniridia, the epithelium is more fragmented secondary to the reduced expression of cytokeratins as a result of the mutated PAX6 gene.[11] Furthermore, the expression of adhesion molecules desmogleine, B-catenin, and gamma-catenin, is decreased in the aniridic because these too are controlled by the PAX6 gene.[11] The absence of these adhesion molecules gives rise to spaces between the corneal epithelial cells.[11] Finally, PAX6 regulates the development of cell surface proteins that are required for the normal migration of cells in response to injury, and in aniridia these proteins are absent.[11] Cells cannot migrate in response to injury. The PAX6 gene also controls the production of matrix metalloproteinase 9 (MMP 9), a protein required for wound healing which is as a result, abnormal in aniridia. The end result is that aniridics have a fragile corneal surface that is not able to properly heal itself, and patients experience repeated epithelial defects and ulcerations.

While other genes are being discovered, the vast majority of patients with classic congenital aniridia are found to be heterozygous for a mutation in the PAX6 gene. Interestingly, only two of six patients with a congenital aniridia variant (variant aniridia; see below) in a study by Skeens et al.[18] had definitive PAX6 mutations and one had a potentially disease-causing variant. Although the precise reason for this is unclear, one possibility is that patients with a milder, variant aniridic keratopathy phenotype may have sequence changes in regulatory or intronic regions of the PAX6 gene. In fact, distinct cis-acting DNA modules have been shown to specifically direct PAX6 expression in ocular surface tissues and lens during development.[19] Alternatively, there may be genetic heterogeneity for this phenotype. Although, the molecular techniques in the aforementioned study were not designed to identify large genomic deletions or rearrangements of the PAX6 gene, most patients with such deletions have a classic congenital aniridia phenotype, and the authors of this study felt that this was unlikely to be a cause of disease in their patients. Also of note is that, as mentioned, while the vast majority of aniridia is caused by a PAX6 gene mutation, there are isolated patients who may have mutations in other genes leading to the development of aniridia.

VARIANT ANIRIDIA

Early reports of classic congenital aniridia emphasized the severe abnormalities of the iris on clinical examination as essential in making the diagnosis of this condition.[20] Because of this terminology, many ophthalmologists now think to diagnose aniridia only in patients who display a near complete absence of the iris (Fig. 32.8). The term 'aniridia' is actually a misnomer. In 1994, Pearce first reported on the variability that may occur in the structural changes in the iris in aniridia.[20] He cited the case reports of other authors who had not described complete absence of the iris, but instead reported atypical colobomas, stromal hypoplasia, full-thickness iris holes, and radial stromal defects in patients who had the additional ophthalmic findings consistent with what we define as classic congenital aniridia (poor visual acuity, fovea hypoplasia, nystagmus, cataract, and glaucoma).[20] Hence to be diagnosed with 'aniridia,' a patient may have not only a near complete absence of the iris, but may present with any of these structural defects of the iris instead (Fig. 32.9).[20] In fact, the abnormalities in each ocular structure affected in classic congenital aniridia may present along a wide spectrum. For example, not all patients develop cataracts and glaucoma,

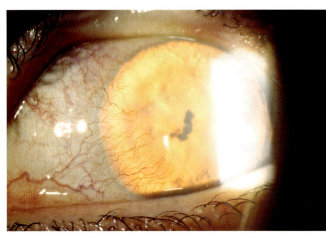

Figure 32.8 A patient with classic congenital aniridia with almost complete absence of the iris. Although the iris looks entirely absent in this photograph, a stump can always be found.

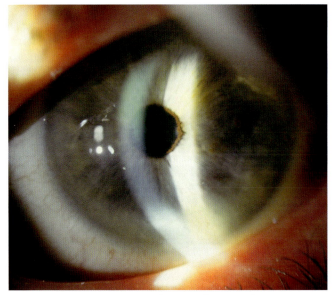

Figure 32.9 This patient has variant aniridia. Note the presence of ectropion uveae along with the cornea nodule.

and patients may present with varying degrees of foveal hypoplasia, visual acuity, and nystagmus. While the process is bilateral, it can be asymmetric in its severity and progression. As previously discussed, Skeens et al. described a subset of patients referred for undiagnosed cornea pathology who presented with signs and symptoms of aniridic keratopathy.[18] Because iris findings were generally mild and because nystagmus or other findings of classic aniridia, including foveal hypoplasia, were mild or not present, the diagnosis of aniridic keratopathy was not previously entertained by the referring physicians. Nonetheless, it was demonstrated that a subset of these patients had defined mutations in *PAX6* (see above) and all patients responded well to keratolimbal allograft.

Other authors have confirmed the same findings. In 1986, Kivlin et al. coined the term 'dominantly inherited keratitis' to represent a group of patients presenting with a dominantly inherited fibrovascular replacement of Bowman's layer, associated with inflammation and vascularization of the cornea.[21] Abnormalities of the iris were not reported, but their patients underwent penetrating keratoplasty of the cornea with a quick recurrence in the grafts of all original findings. Pearce et al. challenged 'dominantly inherited keratitis' as a possible 'aniridia variant' when they reported the same cornea changes as Kivlin's in 15 affected family members of a four-generation family who also had associated macular hypoplasia and iris abnormalities that included stromal atrophy and ectropion uveae.[22] Some of their patients also underwent penetrating keratoplasty with a recurrence of the cornea findings in the grafts. The authors also noted that the patients had more subtle degrees of macular hypoplasia, with visual acuities as good as 20/25 to 20/30, and iris abnormalities which included radial defects, ectropion uveae, iris coloboma, and absent crypts and collarettes. Pearce thus declared a wider picture of familial aniridia to include those patients with the less severe changes in iris structure, little to no nystagmus, and improved visual acuities.[22] He suggested we reconsider the diagnosis of 'aniridia without aniridia.'[22] A *PAX6* gene mutation was identified as the underlying cause of 'autosomal dominant keratitis.'[23]

Patients with a complete or partial absence of the iris will present to their ophthalmologists as infants because the pediatrician usually recognizes the abnormal anterior segment. These patients will be monitored closely for the development of glaucoma and cataract. Patients with 'variant aniridia' will usually not present until a later age because the visual acuity can be close to normal and nystagmus is absent. These patients usually present to their ophthalmologists as young adults complaining of decreasing visual acuity and sensitivity to light that arises from the development of AK. The keratopathy is misdiagnosed because the variability in iris anomalies and the subtle degree of foveal hypoplasia are not recognized as being a result of classic aniridia.

Clinically, it is important to recognize the subtle iris anomalies that may be associated with the other findings seen in classic aniridia because patients need to be followed as such. The most devastating consequence would be undetected glaucoma. Patients with congenital aniridia without glaucoma usually undergo intraocular pressure measurement every 6 months to screen for glaucoma. Glaucoma can develop at any point in the life of an aniridic. We may see it in infants arising from angle closure as a developmental anomaly in the angle of the iris, but more commonly as the patient ages, open-angle glaucoma may arise from a yet completely undetermined mechanism. An alteration in the trabecular meshwork mechanics has been identified as a result of the genetic mutation.

Foveal hypoplasia may be identified clinically by the absence of a foveal light reflex, the absence of the normal darker pigmentation seen in the fovea, and/or the presence of vessels crossing the fovea. Foveal hypoplasia has also recently been elucidated using optical coherence tomography (OCT).[24]

Patients may undergo keratolimbal allograft with success following their clinical diagnosis (Fig. 32.10). All grafts in the study cited by Skeens et al. were successful,[18] and the patients in that study currently maintain a stable ocular surface. It is important to identify that the corneal changes in these patients are associated with AK because without limbal stem cell transplantation, routine penetrating keratoplasty is destined to fail.

Of all the ocular findings in both classic and variant aniridia, the progression of aniridic keratopathy will be the presenting clinical feature among patients with a complaint of a decrease in their vision from baseline. Clinicians should consider this diagnosis even when the iris displays only subtle changes, the fovea is mildly affected, and no nystagmus is present.

Treatment of the keratopathy of classic congenital or variant aniridia is of great value in patients whose vision has been reduced by the corneal changes. Cornea transplant (PK or deep anterior lamellar keratoplasty – DALK) alone will fail because without correction of the primary limbal stem cell deficiency, the findings of AK will develop in the transplanted tissue.[25] Since the underlying corneal abnormality arises in the limbal stem cells, replacement of the limbal stem cells is required for proper treatment of AK. As previously mentioned, it is also important to treat the

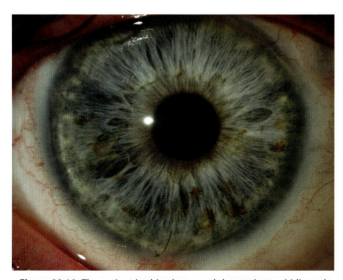

Figure 32.10 The patient in this photograph has variant aniridia and has undergone keratolimbal allograft placement (KLAL). Note the grossly normal iris. Upon close inspection, stromal atrophy of the iris is recognized.

LSCD prior to the development of stage 4 and 5 AK, as described by Holland, so that further cornea transplant will not also be required following limbal stem cell replacement.

TREATMENT OF ANIRIDIC KERATOPATHY

The surgical details of the various methods of stem cell transplantation will be discussed thoroughly throughout this textbook. Briefly, the procedure of keratolimbal allograft (KLAL) is the following. The recipient eye is prepared first. A 360-degree limbal peritomy is performed, and the conjunctiva is resected posteriorly 2 to 3 mm from the limbus with Westcott scissors. Light cautery is used to maintain hemostasis. Excess Tenon's tissue is excised with a Westcott scissors. Any abnormal corneal epithelium and fibrovascular pannus are removed by superficial dissection with a No. 64 Beaver or crescent blade.

Cadaveric donor tissue is used for the stem cell transplantation in a KLAL. Two corneas are requested from the eye bank and the indication for surgery is listed as KLAL. Each donor tissue is placed endothelial side up in the standard fashion of cutting a corneal button in preparation for penetrating keratoplasty. The central cornea of each corneoscleral rim is excised with a 7.5-mm trephine on an Iowa trephine press. The remaining corneoscleral rims are cut into equal halves and scissors are used to dissect the excess peripheral scleral tissue. The posterior one-half to two-thirds of each hemisection is removed by lamellar dissection using a crescent blade. The four pieces are placed in storage media until secured onto the eye. The cadaveric donor lenticles are placed in ring fashion around the limbus in the same anatomical orientation with the limbal edge at the recipient limbus. 10-0 nylon sutures and/or tissue glue are used to secure the lenticles. Once concluded, subconjunctival steroid and antibiotic are administered and the eye is patched for 4 hours, at which time the patch is removed and topical medications are started.

Holland and coauthors[25] reported on the success of KLAL in 31 eyes of 23 patients with classic congenital aniridia. Seventy-four percent of patients achieved a stable ocular surface. Visual acuity improved in the patients from 20/1000 to 20/165. Ninety percent of patients in the study who received systemic immunosuppression maintained a stable ocular surface whereas only 40% of patients not receiving systemic immunosuppression maintained a stable ocular surface. KLAL was determined to be an effective treatment for AK with patients receiving systemic immunosuppression more likely to maintain a healthy ocular surface than those who did not.

The safety of systemic immunosuppression in patients receiving ocular surface stem cell transplants has been reviewed. Holland and coauthors[26] reported on the effects of systemic immunosuppression in 136 patients who underwent stem cell transplantation for varying diagnosis between 1997 and 2007. The most common systemic immunosuppression regimen consisted of tacrolimus, mycophenolate mofetil, and a short course of oral prednisone. The mean duration of use of systemic immunosuppression was 42.1 months. Only two patients experienced severe adverse events and 19 patients experienced minor adverse events, with 47.6% of those 19 having previous systemic co-morbidities. The authors concluded that the prevention of graft rejection post ocular surface transplant is critical and should be approached with the same rigor as in solid organ transplantation. With proper long-term follow-up by the transplant surgeon and close monitoring of physical health while taking immunosuppression, ocular surface transplant patients experience minimal irreversible toxicity.

Another approach to ocular surface stem cell transplantation in these patients involves the use of HLA-matched living related conjunctival tissue, termed a living related conjunctival limbal allograft (lr-CLAL). The advantage to this approach is that the patient may not need to be systemically immunosuppressed or may require a shorter term of immunosuppression because the tissue is matched for donor compatibility. Scocco et al.[27] reported on 39 eyes of 32 patients with bilateral surface disorders and LSCD who underwent HLA-matched lr-CLAL. The donor limbus was obtained from a sibling or a parent after an appropriate class I and II HLA match. Vision improved in 46.2% of patients, ambulatory vision was achieved in 48.7%, and a stable corneal surface was achieved in 84.6% of the eyes. They concluded that HLA-matched lr-CLAL could be an adequate method of treatment for bilateral surface disorders. While none of the patients in their study had aniridia, three had ectodermal dysplasia, another congenital stem cell deficiency disorder discussed later in this chapter.

In congenital stem cell deficiency, the patient will require 360-degree replacement of the limbal tissues. A third alternative in patients with congenital stem cell deficiency involves the combination of lr-CLAL and KLAL. Biber et al.[28] have reported on the success of 'The Cincinnati Procedure.' In this technique, 50% of the recipient limbus is replaced by HLA-matched lr-CLAL, and the remainder is replaced by non-matched KLAL. Again, the advantage to this technique is a decreased duration of systemic immunosuppression use.

Finally, the Boston keratoprosthesis is a suitable alternative to limbal stem cell transplantation in patients with congenital stem cell deficiency (Figs 32.11, 32.12). Akpek et al.[29] evaluated the long-term outcomes of keratoprosthesis as an alternative surgical procedure in the management of AK. Sixteen eyes of 15 patients in their study underwent a Boston type I keratoprosthesis procedure. Device retention rate, intraoperative and postoperative complications, and preoperative and postoperative visual acuity were reviewed. The patients were followed for an average of 17 months. All devices were retained throughout the follow-up period with only one device requiring repair, but not exchange. The visual acuity improved in all patients with the exception of one. The authors concluded that the keratoprosthesis provides significant vision benefits in this group of patients.

Ectodermal Dysplasia

Over 150 separate forms of ectodermal dysplasia exist.[30] Ectrodactyly-ectodermal dysplasia-clefting syndrome (EEC) is one form of ectodermal dysplasia. EEC consists of ectrodactyly (lobster-claw deformity) of the hands and feet, ectodermal dysplasia, and cleft lip and palate. The EEC syndrome,

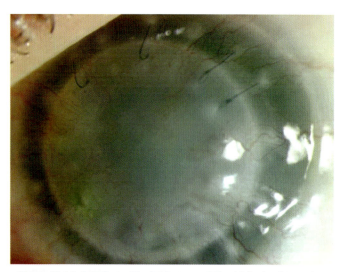

Figure 32.11 A patient with classic congenital aniridia that has undergone both limbal stem cell transplant and PK. The PK has failed and the patient now has an opacified cornea.

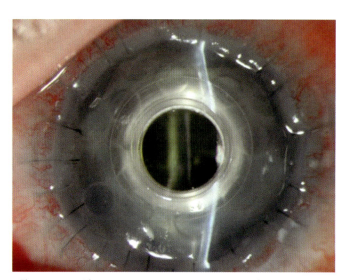

Figure 32.12 The same patient as in Figure 32.11 after undergoing keratoprosthesis placement.

an acronym coined by Rüdiger et al. in 1970,[31] was first recognized as a distinct clinical entity by Cockayne in 1936.[32] He drew attention to the dacryocystitis that commonly affects these patients, and found that it was associated with atresia of the lacrimal ducts. Since that description in 1936, several other reports have appeared in the literature detailing the ocular findings in the EEC syndrome. Many ocular structures are derived from surface ectoderm, so it is not surprising that the abnormal ocular findings in EEC may consist of absent meibomian glands, lacrimal drainage abnormalities, and a progressive keratopathy.[33] Interestingly, the crystalline lens, a surface ectoderm-derived structure, is not affected.[33]

Limbal stem cell failure is the cause of the progressive keratopathy that develops in the EEC syndrome. Iorio et al.[34] reviewed 23 patients affected by the EEC syndrome to assess the pathogenic basis of their visual morbidity. While all patients had ocular involvement, and the commonest involvement was anomaly of the meibomian glands and lacrimal drainage system, the major cause of visual morbidity was progressive LSCD that occurred in 61% of patients. LSCD was related to advancing age and caused a progressive keratopathy resulting in a dense corneal pannus.[34] Clinical examination of the limbal palisades of Vogt along with impression cytology by the authors did confirm the presence of LSCD. The authors also confirmed that heterozygous mutations in the p63 gene are responsible for the limbal stem cell failure.[34] Approximately 40 different pathogenic p63 mutations have been identified in EEC syndrome.[34] Patients develop corneal conjunctivalization, cornea ulceration, and corneal neovascularization as a result of the LSCD that develops secondary to the mutations.[34] Mutational analysis of p63 was performed in this study by polymerase chain reaction-based bidirectional Sanger sequencing.[34] The p63 gene is essential in epithelial development for the regenerative proliferation of epithelial cells.[34] The p63 gene also distinguishes human keratinocyte stem cells from their transient amplifying cell (TAC) progeny, and is expressed by the basal cells of the limbal epithelium but not by the transient amplifying cells covering the corneal surface.[34] Briefly, the normal process of a stem cell involves an asymmetric cell division so that one of the daughter cells remains a stem cell while the other becomes a TAC.[35] The TAC then differentiates into a postmitotic cell (PMC) and finally into a terminally differentiated cell (TDC).[35] The TAC and PMC have no ability to divide.

Saw et al.[36] reported on a subgroup of ectodermal dysplasia patients presenting with severe cicatrizing conjunctivitis and sharing clinical and immunopathological features of ocular mucous membrane pemphigoid (MMP). Six patients with ectodermal dysplasia (four with EEC and two with hypohidrotic ectodermal dysplasia) demonstrated circulating and mucosa-deposited antibasement membrane zone antibodies. Clinically severe ocular surface inflammation (OSI) was controlled with systemic immunosuppression in 83% of patients. Patients with MMP develop severe cicatrizing conjunctivitis and LSCD as a result of uncontrolled OSI.[37] The need to control OSI in these patients in order to prevent cornea conjunctivalization and vascularization with loss of vision is evident in MMP, as should it be in patients with ectodermal dysplasia presenting with severe inflammation of the ocular surface.

Case reports of penetrating keratoplasty in patients with EEC syndrome and keratopathy cite unsuccessful results, which is not surprising given that limbal stem cell failure has been identified as the cause of the corneal abnormalities. Mader and Stulting[38] reported the outcome of PK in two related patients with EEC syndrome who underwent surgery after a spontaneous corneal perforation. One patient developed microbial keratitis postoperatively, and the second developed recurrent vascularization, peripheral scarring, and recurrent epithelial erosions. Baum and Bull[39] reported on a 5-year-old child with EEC syndrome who underwent PK, but 1 month postoperatively only 1 to 2 mm of the donor button had re-epithelialized and the corneal graft subsequently opacified and failed. Replacement of the abnormal limbus in these patients with stem cells prior to PK is beneficial. Daya and Ilari[40] reported on the success of HLA matched lr-CLAL in two eyes with ectodermal

dysplasia and one additional with EEC syndrome. Keratoprosthesis placement could be an alternative to limbal stem cell transplant in these patients; however, no reports exist to date on this treatment.

Not all forms of ectodermal dysplasia display corneal involvement. Keratitis–ichthyosis–deafness, or KID, syndrome, also called Senter's syndrome, is an ectodermal dysplasia that does, however, have corneal involvement with presumed limbal stem cell deficiency. In 1915, Burns described a patient with progressive corneal inflammatory disease, diffuse hyperkeratotic erythroderma, and neurosensory hearing loss.[41] The acronym 'KID' was coined by Skinner et al.[42] to represent the triad of keratitis, ichthyosis, and deafness. KID syndrome consists of congenital neurosensory hearing loss, ectodermal dysplasia, and progressive corneal vascularization and conjunctivalization.[43] Chronic bacterial and mycotic infections, an increased risk of squamous cell carcinoma, liver disease, and mental retardation have all been associated in some patients as well.[43] Gicquel et al.[44] reported on LSCD as a major pathologic factor in this syndrome.

Hereditary hypohidrotic ectodermal dysplasia may be a variant of the KID syndrome. Patients present with decreased sweating, generalized hypotrichosis, and dental abnormalities, as well as ectodermal dysplasia. Corneal vascularization and conjunctivalization have been reported.[45] Bowman's membrane is replaced with a fibrovascular pannus with inflammatory cells present.[45] The corneal epithelium demonstrates acanthosis and dyskeratosis.[45]

Autoimmune Polyglandular Endocrinopathy–Candidiasis–Ectodermal Dysplasia (APECED)

Keratitis early in life associated with multiple endocrine deficiency (failure of the parathyroid glands, adrenal cortex, gonads, pancreatic beta cells, gastric parietal cells, thyroid gland, and hepatitis), chronic mucocutaneous candidiasis, dystrophy of dental enamel and nails, alopecia, and vitiligo, has been coined the APECED syndrome.[46] Also known as autoimmune polyendocrinopathy syndrome type 1, APECED syndrome is a rare autosomal recessive disease, due to a defect in the AIRE (autoimmune regulator) gene.[47] Corneal conjunctivalization and vascularization is characteristic.[47] Impression cytology of the cornea demonstrates goblet cells consistent with conjunctivalization of the cornea.[47] It is uncertain whether this represents a congenital stem cell deficiency or an acquired one. Stem cell grafts from living related donors have been reported in this disorder.[48]

Sclerocornea

Sclerocornea is congenital and usually bilateral. The cornea is often flat with complete opacification and no appreciable limbal area, or only peripheral corneal opacification may exist. Autosomal dominant inheritances, as well as sporadic occurrence have been reported.[49] Sclerocornea is often not an isolated anomaly but is seen in conjunction with Peter's anomaly, microphthalmos, and aniridia. In peripheral sclerocornea, the changes are usually not progressive, suggesting that stem cells are present to maintain central corneal clarity.[50] Demonstration of limbal stem cell deficiency has not been reported, but in the more severe cases with total sclerocornea and no defined limbus, it is likely that a stem cell deficiency is present.

Conclusion

Congenital stem cell deficiency is not the most common type of limbal stem cell deficiency, but it is a very important form to diagnose and treat early. Classic congenital aniridia and variant aniridia, along with some ectodermal dysplasias and sclerocornea, are the diagnoses most often associated with congenital stem cell deficiency. The ocular findings in what has been termed classic congenital aniridia present along a spectrum. Varying levels of visual acuity development arise from different degrees of foveal hypoplasia. Some patients develop cataract and glaucoma while others do not. Aniridic keratopathy also may present along a spectrum, with stages of progression, and patients may present in any stage of AK. Briefly, a peripheral corneal epitheliopathy advancing to the pericentral and then central cornea will be followed by a total corneal epitheliopathy with subepithelial fibrosis, and finally a total epitheliopathy with deeper stromal scarring. Some patients progress quickly to stromal scarring, while others advance very slowly and may live most of their lives with only peripheral cornea involvement. The reason for this is unclear.

Limbal stem cell deficiency is the cause for the progressive keratopathy that develops in the EEC syndrome. And while demonstration of LSCD has not been reported in sclerocornea, in the more severe cases with total sclerocornea and no defined limbus, it is likely that a stem cell deficiency is present.

It is important to make these diagnoses clinically and treat the stem cell deficiency before the patient develops irreversible cornea scarring, necessitating a cornea transplant in addition.

References

1. Holland EJ. Epithelial transplantation for the management of severe ocular surface disease. Trans Am Ophthalmol Soc 1996;94:677–743.
2. Davanger M, Evensen A. Role of the pericorneal papillary structure in renewal of corneal epithelium. Nature 1971;229:560–1.
3. Lim M, Goldstein MH, Tuli S, et al. Growth factor, cytokine, and protease interactions during cornea wound healing. Ocul Surf 2003;1:53–65.
4. Schermer S, Galvin S, Sun TT. Differentiation-related expression of a major 64K corneal keratin in vivo and in culture suggests limbal location of corneal epithelial stem cells. J Cell Biol 1986;103:49–62.
5. Cotsarelis G, Dong G, Sun TT, et al. Differential response of limbal and corneal epithelial to phorbol myristate acetate (TPA). Invest Ophthalmol Vis Sci 1987;28(suppl. 1):1.
6. Ebato B, Friend J, Thoft RA. Comparison of limbal and peripheral human corneal epithelium in tissue culture. Invest Ophthalmol Vis Sci 1988;29:1533–7.
7. Margo CE. Congenital aniridia: a histopaphologic study of the anterior segment in children. J Pediatr Ophahalmol Strabismus 1983;20:192–8.
8. Nelson LB, Spaeth GL, Nowinski T, et al. Aniridia: a review. Surv Ophthalmol 1984;28:621–42.
9. Tugal-Tutkun I, Akova YA, Foster CS. Penetrating keratoplasty in cicatrizing conjunctival diseases. Ophthalmology 1995;102:576–85.
10. Jenkins C, Tuft S, Liu C, et al. Limbal transplantation in the management of chronic contact-lens associated epitheliopathy. Eye 1993;7:629–33.
11. Lee H, Khan R, O'Keefe M. Aniridia: Current pathology and management. Acta Ophthalmologica 2008;86:708–15.
12. Ito Y, Footz T, Berry F, et al. Severe molecular defects of a novel FOXC1 W152G mutation result in aniridia. Invest Ophthalmol Vis Sci 2009;50:3573–9.
13. Mayer KL, Nordlund ML, Schwartz GS, et al. Keratopathy in congenital aniridia. Ocul Surf 2003;1:74–9.
14. Tseng SCG. Concept and application of limbal stem cells. Eye 1989;3:141–57.
15. Nishida K, Kinoshita S, Ohashi Y, et al. Ocular surface abnormalities in aniridia. Am J Ophthalmol 1995;120:368–75.
16. Mackman G, Brightbill FS, Optiz JM. Corneal changes in aniridia. Am J Ophthalmol 1979;87:497–502.
17. Karoma BM, Yang JM, Sundin OH. The Pax-6 homeobox gene is expressed throughout the corneal and conjunctival epithelia. Invest Ophthalmol Vis Sci 1997;38:108–20.
18. Skeens HM, Brooks BP, Holland EJ. Congenital aniridia variant: minimally abnormal irides with severe limbal stem cell deficiency. Ophthalmology 2011;118:1260–4.
19. Kammandel B, Chowdhury K, Stoykova A, et al. Distinct cis-essential modules direct the time-space pattern of the Pax6 gene activity. Dev Biol 1999;205:79–97.
20. Pearce WG. Variability of iris defects in autosomal dominant aniridia. Can J Ophthalmol 1994;29:25–9.
21. Kivlin JD, Apple DJ, Olson RJ, et al. Dominant inherited keratitis. Arch Ophthalmol 1986;104:1621–3.
22. Pearce WG, Mielke BW, Hassard DT, et al. Autosomal dominant keratitis: a possible aniridia variant. Can J Ophthalmol 1995;30:131–7.
23. Mirzayans F, Pearce WG, MacDonald IM, et al. Mutation of the PAX6 gene in patients with autosomal dominant keratitis. Am J Hum Genet 1995;57:539–48.
24. Holstrom G, Eriksson U, Hellgren K, et al. Optical coherence tomography is helpful in the diagnosis of foveal hypoplasia. Acta Ophthalmol 2010;88:439–42.
25. Holland EJ, Djalilian AR, Schwartz GS. Management of aniridic keratopathy with keratolimbal allograft: a limbal stem cell transplantation technique. Ophthalmology 2003;110:125–30.
26. Holland EJ, Mogilishetty G, Skeens HM, et al Systemic immunosuppression in ocular surface stem cell transplantation: results of a 10-year experience. Cornea 2012;31:655–61.
27. Scocco C, Kwitko S, Rymer S, et al. HLA-matched living-related conjunctival limbal allograft for bilateral ocular surface disorders: long-term results. Arq Bras Oftalmol 2008;71:781–7.
28. Biber JM, Skeens HM, Neff KD, et al. The Cincinnati procedure: technique and outcomes of combined living-related conjunctival limbal allografts and keratolimbal allografts in severe ocular surface failure. Cornea 2011;30:765–71.
29. Arpek EK, Harissi-Dagher M, Petrarca R, et al. Outcomes of Boston keratoprosthesis in aniridia: a retrospective multicenter study. Am J Ophthalmol 2007;144:227–31.
30. Freire-Maia N, Pinheiro M. Ectodermal dysplasias: a review of the conditions described after 1984 with an overall analysis of all the conditions belonging to this nosologic group. Rev Brasil Genet 1988;10:403–14.
31. Rüdiger RA, Haase W, Passarge E. Association of ectrodactyly, ectodermal dysplasia, and cleft lip-palate. Am J Dis Child 1970;120:160–3.
32. Cockayne EA. Cleft palate–lip, hare lip, dacryocystitis and cleft hand and foot. Biometrika 1936;28:60–63.
33. Mcnab A, Potts M, Welham R. The EEC syndrome and its ocular manifestations. Br J Ophthalmol 1989;73:261–4.
34. Di Iorio E, Kaye S, Ponzin D, et al. Limbal stem cell deficiency and ocular phenotype in ectrodactyly-ectodermal dysplasia-clefting syndrome caused by p63 mutations. Ophthalmology 2010;119:74–83.
35. Leblond CP. The life history of cells in renewing systems. Am J Anat 1981;160:114–58.
36. Saw VP, Dart JK, Sitaru C, et al. Cicatrising conjunctivitis with anti-basement membrane autoantibodies in ectodermal dysplasia. Br J Ophthalmol 2008;92:1403–10.
37. Thorne JE, Anhalt G, Jabs D. Mucous membrane pemphigoid and pseudopemphigoid. Ophthalmology 2004;111:45–52.

38. Mader TH, Stulting RD. Penetrating keratoplasty in ectodermal dysplasia. Am J Ophthalmol 1990;110:319–20.

39. Baum JL, Bull MJ. Ocular manifestations of the ectrodactyly, ectodermal dysplasia, cleft lip-palate syndrome. Am J Ophthalmol 1974; 78:211–6.

40. Daya SM, Ilari L. Living related conjunctival limbal allograft for the treatment of stem cell deficiency. Ophthalmology 2001;108: 126–34.

41. Burns FS. A case of generalized congenital keratoderma, with unusual involvement of the eyes, ears, and nasal and buccal mucous membranes. J Cutan Dis 1915;33:255–60.

42. Skinner BA, Greist MC, Norins AL. The keratitis, ichthyosis, and deafness (KID) syndrome. Arch Dermatol 1981;117: 285–9.

43. Messmer EM, Kenyon KR, Rittinger O, et al. Ocular manifestations of Keratitis-Ichthyosis-Deafness (KID) syndrome. Ophthalmology 2005; 112:e1–e6.

44. Gicquel JJ, Lami MC, Catier A, et al. Limbal stem cell deficiency associated with KID syndrome, about a case [in French]. J Fr Ophtalmol 2002;25:1061–4.

45. Wilson FM, Grayson M, Pieroni D. Corneal changes in ectodermal dysplasia. Am J Ophthalmol 1973;75:17–27.

46. Ahonen P, Myllarniemi S, Sipila I, et al. Clinical variation of autoimmune polyendocrinopathy-candidiasis-ectodermal dystrophy (APECED) in a series of 68 patients. N Engl J Med 1990; 322:1829–36.

47. Rajendram R, Deane JA, Barnes M, et al. Rapid onset childhood cataracts leading to the diagnosis of Autoimmune Polyendocrinopathy-Candidiasis-Ectodermal Dystrophy. Am J Ophthalmol 2003;136: 951–2.

48. Tseng SCG, Meller D, Pires RTF, et al. Corneal surface reconstruction by limbal epithelial cells ex vivo expanded in amniotic membrane. Investigative Ophthalmol Vis Sci 2000;41:S756 Abst No 4016.

49. Elliott JH, Feman SS, O'Day DM, et al. Hereditary sclerocornea. Arch Ophthalmol 1985;103:676–9.

50. Waizenegger UR, Kohnen T, Weidle EG, et al. Kongenitale familiar cornea plana mit Ptosis, peripherer Sklerokornea und Bindehaut-Xerose. Klin Monatsbl Augenheilk 1995;206:111–6.

33 Iatrogenic Causes of Limbal Stem Cell Deficiency

VICTOR L. PEREZ and JESSICA CHOW

Introduction

Proper functioning of limbal stem cells is crucial to the maintenance of a stable and healthy ocular surface. Limbal stem cells provide a renewal source of corneal epithelial cells and act as a barrier to the extension of conjunctival epithelial cells onto the corneal surface. Limbal stem cell deficiency (LSCD) results in breakdown of the corneal epithelium and poor wound healing, eventually leading to conjunctivalization and opacification of the cornea.[1] Symptoms of LSCD include redness, irritation, photophobia, and decreased vision. Early findings on slit lamp examination include corneal neovascularization, pannus, and loss of the palisades of Vogt. As the condition progresses, punctate epithelial keratopathy and frank epithelial defects may develop. Due to decreased wound healing, these epithelial defects may become persistent, which can lead to stromal scarring, ulceration, and perforation. Conjunctivalization of the cornea may occur, where the corneal epithelium is replaced with a conjunctival epithelial phenotype.[2] Staining of the conjunctivalized epithelium with fluorescein may occur. If conjunctival stem cells, which are thought to reside in the fornices, are also compromised, the entire ocular surface may become keratinized.[3,4]

Causes of limbal stem cell deficiency include both inherited and acquired etiologies. Aniridia is a condition in which anterior segment dysgenesis results in a decreased number of limbal stem cells. Aniridic individuals are born with a normal ocular surface. However, as the patient ages, limbal stem cell dysfunction manifests as corneal epitheliopathy which begins in the peripheral cornea and progresses to involve the central cornea, leading to corneal ulceration, scarring and decreased vision. Other congenital causes of LSCD include Peters anomaly and ectodermal dyplasia.[1] Autoimmune disorders can also result in limbal stem cell deficiency (Fig. 33.1). Typically, these conditions cause chronic inflammation of the conjunctiva with secondary involvement of the limbus. Stevens–Johnson syndrome, toxic epidermal necrolysis, and ocular cicatricial pemphigoid are all diseases in which chronic conjunctival and limbal inflammation diminishes the stem cell population. Limbal lesions, such as conjunctival or corneal intraepithelial neoplasia (CIN) are also associated with limbal stem cell deficiency.[5] Stem cell deficiency is thought to result from replacement of normal stem cells with neoplastic cells. Pterygia have also been associated with LSCD, presumably, due to chronic limbal inflammation.[6] Direct trauma to the limbus by alkali, acid, or thermal injury is another common cause of LSCD.[3] Other acquired causes of LSCD include infectious causes, such as herpesviruses and trachoma.

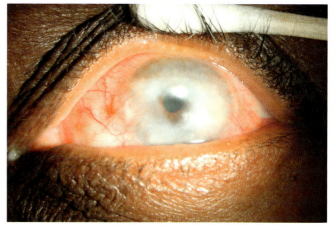

Figure 33.1 Autoimmune LSCD associated with immune complex deposition causing diffuse corneal opacification and pannus formation. (Courtesy Victor L. Perez, MD.)

Recent reports of mustard gas-induced LSCD have also been described.[7]

The categories above represent the most common causes of LSCD as reported in the literature. However, another group of patients develop LSCD secondary to iatrogenic etiologies, defined as directly resulting from intervention or treatment by a physician or surgeon. Many of these cases are multifactorial, and while they are treated with the same methods as those used for classically described causes of stem cell deficiency, awareness of induced etiologies may be useful for both the early recognition and prevention of LSCD in these patients. This chapter will review examples of iatrogenic causes of LSCD (Box 33.1).

Multiple Ocular Surgery-Induced Iatrogenic Stem Cell Deficiency

Limbal stem cell deficiency can occur as a result of multiple ocular surgeries (Fig. 33.2). Puangsricharern and Tseng classified limbal stem cell deficiency etiologies into two groups, resulting from either hypofunction or aplasia of stem cells.[6] In the latter category, patients had a clear history of limbal stem cell destruction by chemical/thermal burns, Stevens–Johnson syndrome, severe microbial keratitis, contact lens-induced keratopathy, and a previously undescribed group of patients had undergone multiple surgeries or cryotherapies to the limbal region. Patients had clinical signs of LSCD, including corneal vascularization and irregular corneal epithelium, as well as impression

Box 33.1   Etiologies of Limbal Stem Cell Deficiency

Inherited
Aniridia
Peters anomaly
Ectodermal dysplasia
Autoimmune
Stevens–Johnson syndrome
Toxic epidermal necrolysis
Ocular cicatricial pemphigoid
Neoplastic
Conjunctival intraepithelial neoplasia
Corneal intraepithelial neoplasia
Pterygium
Trauma
Chemical burn
Thermal injury
Mustard gas
Infection
Trachoma
Herpes virides
Iatrogenic
Multiple ocular surgeries
Contact lens-induced
Cryotherapy
Medication toxicity – mitomycin C, 5-fluorouracil
Radiation therapy
Chemotherapy
Phototherapeutic keratectomy
Multiple intravitreal injections

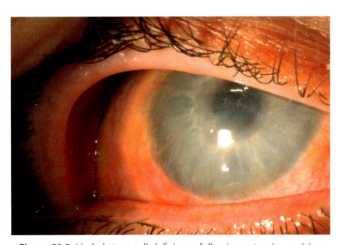

Figure 33.2 Limbal stem cell deficiency following extensive excision of conjunctival melanoma with cryotherapy. (Courtesy Carol Karp, MD.)

cytology demonstrating goblet cell-containing conjunctival epithelial cells on the corneal surface.[6]

In 1998, Schwartz and Holland described a group of patients with limbal stem cell disease not secondary to a known diagnosis, which they termed 'iatrogenic limbal stem cell deficiency.'[8,9] The patients were similar to the above group in Puangsricharern's study who had undergone 'multiple surgeries or cryotherapies of the limbal region.' Schwartz's study comprised 14 eyes of 12 patients. All eyes had a history of prior ocular surgery involving the corneoscleral limbus, as well as concurrent external disease, including pterygium, keratoconjunctivitis sicca,

rosacea, herpes simplex keratitis, or corneal edema. Eleven eyes had received long-term topical medications. In all eyes, the superior quadrants that corresponded to the areas of prior limbal surgery were affected by corneal scarring and neovascularization. Many of the eyes had undergone multiple ocular surgeries. Nine eyes had undergone prior ICCE, three had ECCE, and nine had penetrating keratoplasties.

All eyes exhibited a chronic, progressive epitheliopathy that began in the peripheral cornea and extended centrally, in a pattern consistent with limbal stem cell deficiency. The epitheliopathy was initially sectoral and located in an area of previous limbal surgery, in contrast to classically described causes of LSCD which involve the entire limbus. The authors noted that the epitheliopathy did not resolve with therapy for dry eye management or with cessation of topical medications, implying a permanent alteration in the stability of the ocular surface. They hypothesized that direct surgical trauma to the limbus resulted in localized stem cell deficiency, resulting in increased susceptibility to further damage from both external disease and toxicity from long-term topical medications. All patients had presumed multifactorial LSCD secondary to prior corneoscleral limbal surgery combined with topical medications.[8]

Sridhar et al. reported three cases of impression cytology-proven LSCD following limbal surgeries.[10] One patient had undergone multiple pterygium surgeries, while the other two had undergone therapeutic penetrating keratoplasties. In all cases, limbal stem cell deficiency was confirmed by detection of goblet cells on the surface of the cornea by impression cytology. Surgical trauma to the limbus was the predisposing factor for the development of LSCD in all three cases, while use of topical medications in cases of therapeutic penetrating keratoplasty was felt to be a contributing factor.

Glaucoma Surgery and Iatrogenic Limbal Stem Cell Deficiency

The development of limbal stem cell deficiency in patients who have undergone glaucoma procedures is multifactorial and, due to a combination of mechanical insult from surgery and toxic injury from antimetabolite and chronic topical medication use.[8,11] Antimetabolites, such as 5-fluorouracil and mitomycin C that are used in conjunction with glaucoma surgery are well known to cause corneal toxicity.[11–13] 5-fluorouracil (5-FU), a cell-cycle-specific antimetabolite, inhibits fibroblast proliferation and is used to prevent scarring and closure of the filtration sites in glaucoma procedures. In the acute phase, the cornea exhibits epithelial toxicity and sloughing following the administration of 5-FU, is likely due to its antimetabolite effect on corneal epithelial progenitor cells. With prolonged and recurrent use of 5-FU, damage to the slower-cycling limbal stem cells can result in corneal conjunctivalization and persistent epithelial breakdown.[13] In 2000, Pires et al. reported two cases of iatrogenic limbal stem cell deficiency in post-trabeculectomy patients who had each received over 105 mg 5-FU injections in the postoperative period. Limbal stem cell deficiency was confirmed by impression cytology. One patient with partial limbal stem cell deficiency recovered well after amniotic membrane transplantation while the other, who exhibited total limbal stem cell deficiency, required limbal stem cell transplantation to stabilize the ocular surface.[13]

Mitomycin C (MMC), a potent DNA cross-linker, is an antimetabolite that targets dividing cells. MMC is usually applied during glaucoma surgery by soaking the drug in sponges and placing them in contact with the conjunctiva near the filtration site. However, this technique can lead to wound leak, due to delayed conjunctival healing.[12,14] Sauder and Jonas reported a case series of seven patients who underwent trabeculectomy with a modified technique, in which mitomycin C was administered subconjunctivally prior to opening of the conjunctiva. In this series, three patients developed signs and symptoms of limbal stem cell deficiency, including avascularity of over 50% of the limbal circumference, dry eye, corneal epithelial irregularities, and corneal opacities. The other four patients did not show similar sequelae, but, of note, were each followed for less than 14 months, compared to the three patients with MMC-related complications that were followed for at least 2 years. The authors concluded that subconjunctival MMC in conjunction with trabeculectomy could result in delayed postoperative complications, including late limbal stem cell deficiency, and should therefore be avoided.[14]

Contact Lens-Induced Iatrogenic Limbal Stem Cell Deficiency

Contact lens-induced keratopathy has long been recognized as a cause of ocular surface disease, due to limbal stem cell deficiency. In 1984, Bloomfield et al. described mild cases of LSCD in contact lens wearers as contact lens-induced keratoconjunctivitis.[15] Patients exhibited papillary hypertrophy of the superior tarsus, superior limbal hypertrophy, and superior punctate staining. Severe cases of contact lens-related LSCD, which were classified as contact lens-induced keratopathy, demonstrated superficial punctate keratitis, epithelial irregularities, and a superior 'V'-shaped vascularized pannus of the cornea in the region of stem cell deficiency.[15]

Several theories for the development of contact lens-induced keratopathy have been proposed. Bloomfield proposed that mechanical rubbing from poorly fitting contact lenses can damage the limbus and result in limbal stem cell compromise.[15] Chronic irritation to the limbal region can cause perilimbal capillaries to grow between the corneal epithelium and Bowman's membrane, forming a pannus. These capillaries are accompanied by fibroblasts which produce collagen and dissolve Bowman's membrane, producing a superficial corneal scar and irregular astigmatism. Mechanical pressure from blinking of the upper lid may contribute to superior pannus formation.[16] Pannus may also occur from chronic tight lens syndrome[17] or from long-term hypoxia from low oxygen permeable soft contact lenses. Signs of tight lens syndrome include corneal edema, punctate epithelial erosions, iritis, and lack of lens movement upon blink. An imprint in the anterior conjunctiva can sometimes be seen upon lens removal.[18]

In one study, contact lens-induced keratopathy comprised 15% of LSCD cases.[19] Another large retrospective study of over 500 soft contact lens wearers identified risk factors for asymptomatic corneal conjunctivalization.[20] These patients were predominantly female, myopic, and had been wearing daily disposable soft contact lenses for more than 10 hours per day for 6 or more years. The authors suggested that early diagnosis of the condition, reduced length of contact lens wear, suspension of contact lens use, or refitting with either high oxygen permeability soft or RGP contact lenses, would be useful in decreasing the prevalence of contact lens-related LSCD.[20]

Toxicity from contact lens solutions can also damage limbal stem cells. Thimerosal is an organic mercurial that was commonly used as an antimicrobial preservative in contact lens disinfecting solutions in the 1980s. Jenkins et al. described chronic corneal epitheliopathy with a history of thimerosal exposure in soft contact lens wearers.[16] All patients exhibited corneal changes characterized by epithelial haze and superficial stromal vascularization with significantly decreased visual acuity. In vitro cell studies have shown the cytotoxic effects of thimerosal, which include inhibition of mitotic activity in human corneal epithelial cells, loss of cell membrane integrity, and initiation of mitochondria-mediated and caspase-3-dependent apoptosis in human neurons and fibroblasts.[21] Thimerosal toxicity has been reported to cause total limbal stem cell failure with secondary corneal vascularization and opacification.[22]

A recent study by Jeng et al. investigated the management of focal limbal stem cell deficiency secondary to long-term contact lens use (Fig. 33.3).[23] Nine out of ten patients were women, and superior involvement was present in all eighteen eyes. LSCD was diagnosed based on clinical findings, including the appearance of irregular corneal epithelium seen as dull opaque-appearing tissue of variable thickness originating from the limbus; impression cytology was not available to confirm the diagnosis. Most of the eyes responded to conservative therapy with cessation of contact lens use and administration of artificial tears with corticosteroids; however, one eye underwent conjunctival autograft and another eye underwent amniotic membrane transplantation for more aggressive disease, both with successful visual outcomes.[23]

Iatrogenic Limbal Stem Cell Deficiency Associated with Ocular Surface Tumor Therapy

Ocular surface neoplasias in and of themselves are associated with limbal stem cell deficiency, presumably to the replacement of healthy stem cells with dysfunctional neoplastic cells.[5] The treatment of ocular surface neoplasias, including conjunctival intraepithelial neoplasia (CIN), atypical primary acquired melanosis (PAM), and conjunctival melanoma may involve wide surgical excision with cryotherapy to the conjunctiva and limbus, the application of topical adjuvant medications, such as mitomycin C and 5-fluorouracil, or radiation therapy, all of which result in additional insult to the limbal stem cell population.

Limbal stem cell deficiency following the treatment of CIN is likely secondary to a combination of inherent stem cell dysfunction from the neoplastic process and multiple

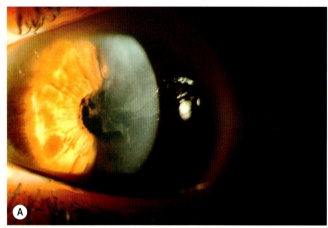

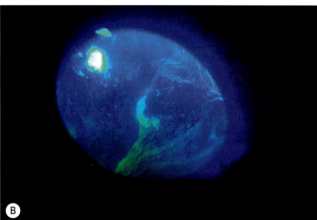

Figure 33.3 (A) Contact lens induced LSCD demonstrating superior wedge-shaped corneal conjunctivalization. (Courtesy Bennie Jeng, MD, reproduced with permission from Wolters Kluwer Health[23] Jeng BH, Halfpenny CP, Meisler DM, Stock EL. Management of focal limbal stem cell deficiency associated with soft contact lens wear. Cornea. 2011;30:18–23.) **(B)** Contact lens-induced LSCD with fluorescein stain demonstrating corneal epithelial irregularity. (Courtesy Bennie Jeng, MD, reproduced with permission from Wolters Kluwer Health[23] Jeng BH, Halfpenny CP, Meisler DM, Stock EL. Management of focal limbal stem cell deficiency associated with soft contact lens wear. Cornea. 2011;30:18–23.)

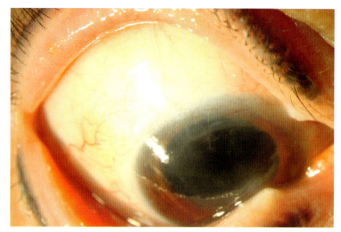

Figure 33.4 Limbal stem cell deficiency following resection of conjunctival melanoma, cryotherapy and treatment with topical mitomycin C. (Courtesy Carol Karp, MD.)

treatment modalities that result in limbal injury. Puangsricharern and Tseng reported LSCD in two patients with CIN who underwent multiple tumor resections and cryotherapies.[6] In one case, additional conjunctival scraping for recurrent tumor was performed several years after the initial resection, and the patient subsequently developed superficial pannus and corneal epithelial irregularity. Impression cytology revealed the presence of goblet cells on the corneal surface, indicating LSCD. The patient's ocular surface stabilized and his visual acuity improved after limbal transplantation from the contralateral eye.[6] A recent study by Asoklis et al. demonstrated two cases of partial limbal stem cell deficiency following the excision of limbal tumors with cryotherapy applied to the resected edge of conjunctiva and to the limbus and amniotic membrane grafting. In both cases, there was an extensive limbal invasion of the tumor involving more than one-fourth of the limbus.[24]

Mitomycin C (MMC) is frequently used in the treatment of ocular surface neoplasias, including CIN, PAM, and

conjunctival melanoma, and can result in limbal stem cell deficiency (Fig. 33.4). Dudney et al. first described a case of LSCD in a patient who was treated for conjunctival–corneal intraepithelial neoplasia with a total of 5 week-long courses of topical mitomycin C 0.04%.[25] The patient subsequently developed superior stromal haze and nonhealing epithelial defects, presumably secondary to limbal stem cell dysfunction, but was lost to follow-up. In a recent study of 21 patients who underwent MMC therapy for PAM with atypia, five patients were noted to develop limbal stem cell deficiency, diagnosed clinically and confirmed by impression cytology.[26] Older age and longer treatment periods were found to be significant risk factors for this complication. Partial resolution of LSCD occurred in three of the patients, as evidenced by normalization of the corneal epithelium and improved visual acuity. Ditta et al. reported LSCD as a complication of long-term MMC therapy in a cohort of patients with conjunctival melanoma. Four out of 15 patients (26.7%) developed clinical signs of stem cell deficiency.[27] Russell et al. performed a 10-year review of topical MMC for ocular surface neoplasia, including primary acquired melanosis (PAM), melanoma, corneal–conjunctival intraepithelial neoplasia (CCIN), squamous cell carcinoma (SCC) and sebaceous gland carcinoma (SGC).[28] The overall rate of long-term complications was higher than previously reported, at 33%. Seven out of 58 patients developed corneal epithelial changes, due to presumed limbal stem cell deficiency (LSCD), but five of these patients also underwent surgical excision with cryotherapy, which likely contributed to the limbal insult. The remaining two patients had MMC as a primary treatment; thus, it is likely that MMC was the cause of this complication.[28]

Radiation Therapy-Induced Iatrogenic Limbal Stem Cell Deficiency

Local radiation therapy is known to cause ocular toxicity and visual loss by affecting multiple ocular structures.

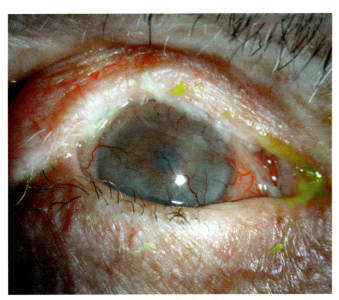

Figure 33.5 External radiation-induced limbal stem cell deficiency after therapy for skin tumor with orbital involvement inducing diffuse corneal neovascularization and pannus years later after therapy. (Courtesy Victor L. Perez, MD.)

Plaque radiotherapy for ocular melanomas can result in radiation retinopathy, neovascular glaucoma, and optic neuropathy.[29] Radiation can also result in cataract, corneal epithelial toxicity and limbal stem cell deficiency (Fig. 33.5).

In 1996, Fujishima et al. reported a case of temporary corneal stem cell dysfunction after radiation therapy for maxillary cancer.[30] The patient received a dose of 61 gy over 44 days, and experienced ocular surface discomfort and vision loss to 20/500. Examination revealed corneal epithelial opacity, and impression cytology demonstrated goblet cells on the cornea. After conservative management with artificial tears and topical antibiotic ointment, the ocular surface improved and 4 months later, visual acuity recovered to 20/40. Repeat impression cytology demonstrated no goblet cells; therefore, the authors concluded that the LSCD had been temporary.

Smith et al. reported a case of permanent LSCD following local radiotherapy for orbital lymphoma in a 31-year-old male patient who received a total of 4600 cGY over 21 sessions.[31] Several years later, the patient demonstrated superficial vascularization of the cornea. Immunostaining of impression cytology specimens demonstrated a conjunctival phenotype over portions of the cornea, indicating delayed limbal stem cell deficiency. LSCD can also occur after proton radiotherapy for ocular surface neoplasias, such as conjunctival melanoma.[32]

Systemic Chemotherapy-Induced Iatrogenic Limbal Stem Cell Deficiency

Limbal stem cell deficiency may arise from the treatment of systemic disease. Ellies et al. reported a case of bilateral corneal epitheliopathy in a patient undergoing systemic chemotherapy for chronic myelocytic leukemia with hydroxyurea.[33] Hydroxyurea is a cytotoxic agent that arrests DNA replication. Impression cytology revealed focal LSCD localized to the temporal and inferior portion of the right cornea by exhibiting conjunctival goblet cells and mucins on the cornea and diffuse squamous metaplasia of the left cornea with partial loss of the limbal area. Cessation of hydroxyurea therapy resulted in significant improvement of the ocular surface in both eyes, although the left eye still required keratolimbal allograft with amniotic membrane transplantation for visual rehabilitation.[33]

Another case of LSCD arising from systemic hydroxyurea use was reported in 2009.[34] The patient, who had sickle cell disease, was placed on hydroxyurea for pulmonary hypertension, and developed pterygium-like peripheral corneal neovascularization in both eyes with progressive pannus. Histopathologic analysis of the conjunctiva revealed pingueculae, loss of goblet cells with scar tissue formation, and corneal neovascularization consistent with limbal stem cell deficiency.[34]

Rare Causes of Iatrogenic Limbal Stem Cell Deficiency

Unusual causes of iatrogenic LSCD have been presented in the literature. Nghiem-Buffet et al. reported one case of stem cell deficiency following phototherapeutic keratectomy (PTK).[35] The patient, who had a history of diabetes mellitus and rosacea, underwent PTK for recurrent epithelial erosions. The procedure consisted of complete epithelial debridement and photoablation of the central 8 mm-diameter area of the cornea. He subsequently developed a vascular pannus and underwent excision of the pannus with limbal autografting from the contralateral eye. The diagnosis of LSCD was confirmed by histologic examination of the pannus demonstrating goblet cells within the corneal epithelium.[35]

Recently, Capella et al. reported a case of LSCD following multiple Avastin injections.[36] The patient, who had a history of idiopathic choroidal polypoidal vasculopathy, underwent five sessions of photodynamic therapy, one transpupillary thermal therapy, and seven injections of intravitreal bevacizumab in the superonasal quadrant. He subsequently developed a superior corneal pannus and central epithelial irregularity at the site of the multiple intravitreal injections. LSCD was confirmed by impression cytology. He underwent limbal autograft from the same eye, which resulted in significant improvement of the epitheliopathy and stabilization of the ocular surface.[36]

It is possible that some iatrogenic causes of LSCD have not yet been identified. UV light exposure has been associated with limbal stem cell deficiency.[37,38] A relatively new and increasingly popular early intervention for keratoconus and post-refractive ectasia is corneal collagen cross-linking, which involves the use of UVA irradiation of the cornea after topical application of the photosensitizer riboflavin. Long-term studies are necessary to assess the potential effects of this procedure on limbal stem cells.

Medical Management/Prevention of Iatrogenic Limbal Stem Cell Deficiency

The treatment of iatrogenic limbal stem cell deficiency may be challenging, and is similar to therapy for other causes of limbal stem cell deficiency. However, the key difference is that in iatrogenic cases, the clinician should be aware of the risk of LSCD, and therefore, can be proactive in prevention, early diagnosis, and management of the condition.

Certain cases of iatrogenic limbal stem cell deficiency may not require therapy. If the patient is only mildly symptomatic and the visual axis is not involved, conservative management with preservative-free artificial tears may be sufficient to achieve patient comfort. If LSCD results from chronic use of topical medications, such as antiglaucoma agents or antibiotics, these medications should be discontinued, if possible, to avoid further toxicity.

Topical corticosteroids may be useful both to minimize patient discomfort and to control the inflammatory component of LSCD. Corticosteroids may help in the regression of corneal neovascularization. Anti-VEGF agents, such as bevacizumab may also prove beneficial in the management of corneal neovascularization secondary to LSCD. In a small interventional case series by Bock et al., four patients with limbal stem cell deficiency and aggressive corneal neovascularization were treated with topical bevacizumab. All patients showed a decrease in neovascularization, although the response was highly variable. None of the patients experienced adverse corneal side effects.[39]

Severe cases of LSCD may require surgical intervention with limbal stem cell transplantation.

Conclusion

Iatrogenic limbal stem cell deficiency comprises a variety of etiologies in which patients develop LSCD as a result of intervention for ocular or systemic medical conditions. It is important to recognize these causes, as they can lead to visually significant sequelae, including corneal scarring and vision loss. Early recognition and preventative measures may help to reduce the rate of iatrogenically induced LSCD in the future.

References

1. Hatch KM, Dana R. The structure and function of the limbal stem cell and the disease states associated with limbal stem cell deficiency. Int Ophthalmol Clin 2009;49:43–52.
2. Lim P, Fuchsluger TA, Jurkunas UV. Limbal stem cell deficiency and corneal neovascularization. Semin Ophthalmol 2009;24:139–48.
3. Dua HS, Saini JS, Azuara-Blanco A, et al. Limbal stem cell deficiency: concept, aetiology, clinical presentation, diagnosis and management. Ind J Ophthalmol 2000;48:83–92.
4. Wei ZG, Wu RL, Lavker RM, et al. In vitro growth and differentiation of rabbit bulbar, fornix, and palpebral conjunctival epithelia. Implications on conjunctival epithelial transdifferentiation and stem cells. Invest Ophthalmol Vis Sci 1993;34:1814–28.
5. Erie JC, Campbell RJ, Liesegang TJ. Conjunctival and corneal intraepithelial and invasive neoplasia. Ophthalmology 1986;93:176–83.
6. Puangsricharern V, Tseng SCG. Cytologic evidence of corneal diseases with limbal stem cell deficiency. Ophthalmology 1995;102:1476–85.
7. Javadi MA, Jafarinasab MR, Feizi S, et al. Management of mustard gas-induced limbal stem cell deficiency and keratitis. Ophthalmology 2011;118:1272–81.
8. Schwartz GS, Holland EJ. Iatrogenic limbal stem cell deficiency. Cornea 1998;17:31–7.
9. Holland EJ, Schwartz GS. Iatrogenic limbal stem cell deficiency. Trans Am Ophthalmol Soc 1997;95:95–107.
10. Sridhar MS, Vemuganti GK, Bansal AK, et al. Impression cytology-proven corneal stem cell deficiency in patients after surgeries involving the limbus. Cornea 2001;20:145–8.
11. Schwartz GS, Holland EJ. Iatrogenic limbal stem cell deficiency: when glaucoma management contributes to corneal disease. J Glauc 2001;10:443–5.
12. Hau S, Barton K. Corneal complications of glaucoma surgery. Curr Opin Ophthalmol 2009;20:131–6.
13. Pires RTF, Chokshi A, Tseng SCG. Amniotic membrane transplantation or conjunctival limbal autograft for limbal stem cell deficiency induced by 5-fluorouracil in glaucoma surgeries. Cornea 2000;19:284–7.
14. Sauder G, Jonas JB. Limbal stem cell deficiency after subconjunctival mitomycin C injection for trabeculectomy. Am J Ophthalmol 2006;141:1129–30.
15. Bloomfield SE, Jakobiec FA, Theodore FH. Contact lens induced keratopathy: a severe complication extending the spectrum of keratoconjunctivitis in contact lens wearers. Ophthalmology 1984;91:290–4.
16. Jenkins C, Tuft S, Liu C, et al. Limbal transplantation in the management of chronic contact-lens-associated epitheliopathy. Eye 1993;7:629–33.
17. Arentsen JJ. Corneal neovascularization in contact lens wearers. Int Ophthalmo Clin 1986;26:15–23.
18. Achong RAC. Limbal stem cell deficiency in a contact lens-related case. Clin Eye Vis Care 1999;11:191–7.
19. Donisi PM, Rama P, Fasolo A, et al. Analysis of limbal stem cell deficiency by corneal impression cytology. Cornea 2003;22:533–8.
20. Martin R. Corneal conjunctivalisation in long-standing contact lens wearers. Clin Exp Optom 2007;90:26–30.
21. Baskin DS, Ngo H, Didenko VV. Thimerosal induces DNA breaks, caspase-3 activation, membrane damage, and cell death in cultured human neurons and fibroblasts. Toxicol Sci 2003;74:361–8.
22. Nguyen DQ, Srinivasan S, Hiscott P, et al. Thimerosal-induced limbal stem cell failure: report of a case and review of the literature. Eye Contact Lens 2007;33:196–8.
23. Jeng BH, Halfpenny CP, Meisler DM, et al. Management of focal limbal stem cell deficiency associated with soft contact lens wear. Cornea 2011;30:18–23.
24. Asoklis RS, Damijonaityte A, Butkiene L, et al. Ocular surface reconstruction using amniotic membrane following excision of conjunctival and limbal tumors. Eur J Ophthalmol 2011;21:552–8.
25. Dudney BW, Malecha MA. Limbal stem cell deficiency following topical mitomycin C treatment of conjunctival-corneal intraepithelial neoplasia. Am J Ophthalmol 2004;137:950–1.
26. Lichtinger A, Pe'er J, Frucht-Pery J, et al. Limbal stem cell deficiency after topical mitomycin C therapy for primary acquired melanosis with atypia. Ophthalmology 2010;117:431–7.
27. Ditta LC, Shildkrot Y, Wilson MW. Outcomes in 15 patients with conjunctival melanoma treated with adjuvant topical mitomycin C: complications and recurrences. Ophthalmology 2011;118:1754–9.
28. Russell HC, Chadha V, Lockington D, et al. Topical mitomycin C chemotherapy in the management of ocular surface neoplasia: a 10-year review of treatment outcomes and complications. Br J Ophthalmol 2010;94:1316–21.
29. Chan MD, Melhus CS, Mignano JE, et al. Analysis of visual toxicity after gamma knife radiosurgery for treatment of choroidal melanoma: identification of multiple targets and mechanisms of toxicity. Am J Clin Oncol 2011;34:517–23.
30. Fujishima H, Shimazaki J, Tsubota K. Temporary corneal stem cell dysfunction after radiation therapy. Br J Ophthalmol 1996;80:911-4. Epub 1996/10/01.
31. Smith GT, Deutsch GP, Cree IA, et al. Permanent corneal limbal stem cell dysfunction following radiotherapy for orbital lymphoma. Eye 2000;14:905–7.
32. Wuestemeyer H, Sauerwein W, Meller D, et al. Proton radiotherapy as an alternative to exenteration in the management of extended conjunctival melanoma. Graefe's Arch Clin Exp Ophthalmol 2006;244:438–46.

33. Ellies P, Anderson DF, Topuhami A, et al. Limbal stem cell deficiency arising from systemic chemotherapy. Br J Ophthalmol 2001;85: 373–4.

34. Ding X, Bishop RJ, Herzlich AA, et al. Limbal stem cell deficiency arising from systemic chemotherapy with hydroxycarbamide. Cornea 2009;28:221–3.

35. Nghiem-Buffet MH, Gatinel D, Jacquot F, et al. Limbal stem cell deficiency following phototherapeutic keratectomy. Cornea 2003; 22:482–4.

36. Capella MJ, Álvarez de Toledo J, de la Paz MF. Limbal stem cell deficiency following multiple intravitreal injections. Archivos de la Sociedad Española de Oftalmología. 2011;86:89–92.

37. Passchier WF, Bosnjakovic BFM. Human exposure to ultraviolet radiation : risks and regulations: proceedings of a seminar held in Amsterdam, 23–25 March 1987. Amsterdam; New York, NY, USA: Excerpta Medica. Sole distributors for the USA and Canada, Elsevier Science Pub. Co. 1987.

38. Zaidi FH, Bloom PA, Corbett MC. Limbal stem cell deficiency: a clinical chameleon. Eye 2003;17:837–9.

39. Bock F, Konig Y, Kruse F, et al. Bevacizumab (Avastin) eye drops inhibit corneal neovascularization. Graefe's Arch Clin Exp Ophthalmol 2008;246:281–4.

PART 4

MANAGEMENT OF SEVERE OCULAR SURFACE DISEASE

34 Medical Management of Ocular Surface Disease

MARIAN MACSAI and GIOCONDA MOJICA

Introduction

As an orchestra is composed of various instrumentalists playing together to form a unified sound, optimal management of the ocular surface entails fine tuning the performance of its collective players (lids, lacrimal gland, cornea, conjunctiva). Recognized as an integrated system working in concert for quality of ocular surface health and vision, the burgeoning field of ocular surface disease (OSD) has witnessed an explosion in the literature. Advances in our understanding of the pathophysiology driving various conditions affecting the health of the ocular surface has helped clinicians develop and broaden medical and surgical therapies, leading to improved outcomes. This chapter will focus primarily on medical treatment, including topical and systemic regimens.

The medical management of OSD is required prior to surgical intervention. In our understanding of OSD, numerous factors are intertwined. Inflammation, anatomical malpositioning, systemic hormonal levels, and changes in the ocular tear film are individual causative factors that play a role in this complex disease. Central to each of these factors is an underlying inflammatory state, as seen in blepharitis, meibomitis, conjunctivitis, and keratitis. The medical management of OSD requires controlling the inflammation and restoring the normal anatomy and tear film to promote healing of the ocular surface. Careful attention to the medical management of the ocular surface is paramount to the outcomes of any surgical intervention and may indeed preclude its necessity.

Topical Treatment

ARTIFICIAL TEARS

Method of Action

The tear layer represents a complex mixture of mucins for increased viscosity, antimicrobial proteins, growth factors, inflammatory suppressors, and electrolytes for proper osmolarity (Fig. 34.1). Artificial tears cannot completely substitute this complex composition of human tears. Their mechanism of action includes adding volume to the tear film while in contact with the ocular surface. In order to remain in contact with the ocular surface, hydrogels are an essential ingredient of artificial tears. Hydrogels are polymers that swell in water and retain moisture to increase viscosity. The mucous adhesive properties of hydrogels prolong the contact time of artificial tears on the eye. The following hydrogels have been used in artificial tears:

hydroxypropyl methylcellulose (HPMC), carboxymethylcellulose (CMC), polyvinyl alcohol (PVA), carbopol, polyvinyl pyrrolidone, polyethylene glycol (PEG), polyvinyl alcohol (PVA), dextran, hyaluronic acid, glycerin, and carbomer 940 (polyacrylic acid). There have been no large scale, masked, comparative clinical trials to evaluate the wide variety of hydrogels available. However, using wavefront sensing and ocular coherence tomography, PEG drops showed significant worsening of visual quality, compared with CMC, PVA, and glycerin-containing artificial tears.[1]

There are many different types of preservatives in artificial tears. Benzalkonium chloride (BAK) and chlorobutanol, which can be toxic when used more than four times a day, are older preservatives. Preservatives, such as GenAqua (Sodium Perborate), Purite (sodium chlorite) and Polyquad (Polyquaternium-1) are less damaging to the ocular surface than BAK.[2,3] Purite degrades to chloride ions and water after instillation. GenAqua is converted to water and oxygen on contact with the tear film.

The presence of 'inactive ingredients' provides unique surface protective properties to artificial tears. For example,

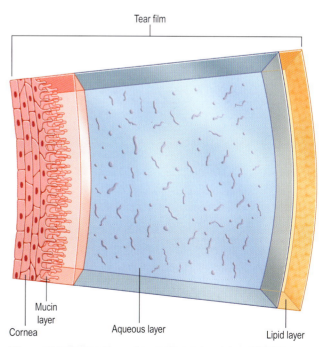

Figure 34.1 Composition of tears. (Reproduced from Allergan. 'Tear film.' Online image. Mydryeyes.com. 2012. 15 August 2012. http://www.mydryeyes.com/what_is_a_healthy_tear_film.cfm.)

compatible solutes may help surface healing by osmoprotection. HP-Guar forms a cross-linked viscoelastic gel when exposed to eye surface (pH 7.5). This gel increases viscosity and bioadhesive properties while promoting the retention of its two demulcents (polyethylene glycol 400 and polypropylene glycol). It has been suggested that HP-guar preferentially binds to the more dry or damaged areas of the surface epithelial cells, providing protection for these cells.[4–6]

Viscous tears have a longer retention time, as they are not easily drained out of the eye through the lacrimal outflow system. Oil-containing eye drops may be added if meibomian gland dysfunction is present. These eye drops will replenish the lipid layer of the tear film and prevent tear evaporation. Moderately hypotonic artificial tears containing PVA, as well as bicarbonate-containing tears have been shown to promote OSD healing in severe dry eyes.[7–10]

Delivery System

Artificial tears are available in multidose preserved formulations, as well as single-use non-preserved formulations.

Dosage

Artificial tears may be dosed on many different schedules, including an as-needed basis. BAK-preserved drops are usually well tolerated when used four times a day or less. If artificial tears are needed more than four times a day then GenAqua or Polyquad preserved tears are better choices, avoiding the toxicity of BAK. In moderate to severe OSD, preservative-free solutions should be used. It is apparent that there is no single artificial tear eye drop that provides the entire surface healing strategies required in OSD (bicarbonate ions, hypotonicity, viscosity, non-preserved). However, understanding of the mechanism of action of the different hydrogels, additives and preservatives in artificial tears will aid the clinician in directing the OSD patient to the optimal tear substitute.

Side Effects

Side effects of artificial tear substitutes may include redness, stinging and ocular irritation, as well as allergy to one of the ingredients. Viscous artificial tears may cause unacceptable blurry vision in some individuals. Higher-viscosity tears can cause eye irritation by crystallization on the lids and lashes.

TOPICAL CORTICOSTEROIDS

Mechanism of Action

Topical corticosteroids are currently the most effective, potent treatment modalities for the medical management of ocular inflammation, an important hallmark of OSD. Although there is no generally accepted explanation for the mechanism of action of ocular corticosteroids, they are thought to act by inducing lipocortins, proteins that inhibit phospholipase A2. It is postulated that these proteins control the biosynthesis of potent inflammatory mediators, including prostaglandins and leukotrienes by inhibiting the release of arachidonic acid, their common precursor. Corticosteroids inhibit the inflammatory response to a variety of inciting agents that may delay wound healing. They inhibit fibrin and collage deposition, capillary dilation, capillary proliferation, leukocyte migration, fibroblast

Table 34.1 Active Ingredients and Available Formulations for Topical Ophthalmic Steroid Preparations

Topical Ocular Steroid	Concentration/Formulation
Prednisolone acetate	0.125, 1.0% suspension
Difluprednate	0.05% emulsion
Prednisolone sodium phosphate	0.125, 0.5 1.0% solution
Dexamethasone alcohol	0.05–0.1% susp, ointment
Fluorometholone acetate	0.1% suspension
Fluorometholone alcohol	0.1% suspension, ointment 0.25% suspension
Rimexolone	0.5–1% suspension
Medrysone alcohol	1.0% suspension
Lotoprednol etabonate	0.2, 0.5% suspension

proliferation, and scar tissue formation associated with the process of inflammation. The two traditional groups of corticosteroids are the ketone steroids (prednisolone, dexamethasone, fluorometholone, medrysone, rimexolone, and difluprednate) and the ester steroids (loteprednol).

Delivery System

Corticosteroids are available in a diverse range of preparations, including solutions, suspensions, emulsions and ointments (Table 34.1). Topical steroids in a suspension, or viscous formulation have increased ocular contact time and can thereby double the corneal and aqueous steroid concentrations, compared with the same drug used as a solution.[11] There is no prospective clinical trial comparing the relative efficacy of generic with branded topical steroids, though studies point to the possible advantage of smaller particle size in branded drops conferring greater efficacy and bioavailability.[12] The relative potency of corticosteroids depends on the molecular structure, concentration, and release from the vehicle. For example, dexamethasone is a very potent steroid, but does not penetrate ocular tissues well. In contrast, prednisolone is less potent and has better ocular penetration. Steroids, such as loteprednol etabonate and fluorometholone are less potent, but have safer side effect profiles. Compared to dexamethasone and prednisolone, loteprednol etabonate and fluorometholone are reported to have lower rates of intraocular pressure (IOP) spikes. A retrospective review of 30 patients with IOP elevation to a mean of 31.1 millimeters of mercury after prednisolone acetate use for keratoplasty reported a 41% reduction in IOP after switching to loteprednol etabonate. Yet in one study, IOP elevations with loteprednol occurred more commonly in females after an average of 2 months of treatment.[13]

Dosage

To our knowledge, no studies have conclusively outlined the optimal steroid concentrations for treating various OSD conditions. Studies have evaluated topical corticosteroid penetration into human aqueous humor (Fig. 34.2).[14] For conditions primarily affecting the ocular surface where intraocular antiinflammatory therapy is not needed, fluorometholone alcohol 0.1%, loteprednol etabonate 0.5% and prednisolone sodium phosphate 0.5% are viable options. When intraocular penetration is indicated, the

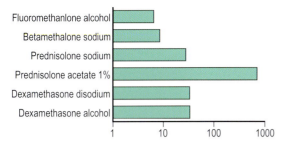

Figure 34.2 Comparison of peak aqueous concentration of topically applied commercially available ophthalmic steroid preparations.

more potent prednisolone acetate, dexamethasone or diflu-prednate emulsion should be considered. In randomized, controlled studies, loteprednol etabonate has demonstrated excellent results in treating external inflammation, such as seasonal allergic conjunctivitis and giant papillary conjunctivitis with a favorable side effect profile.[15,16] Topical corticosteroids with lower aqueous penetration are not as effective as those with higher intraocular penetration in the management of intraocular inflammation.[14] Compared to prednisolone acetate 1%, loteprednol etabonate 0.5% has been found to be less effective in patients with acute anterior uveitis.[17]

Side Effects

Prolonged administration of corticosteroids may result in a rise in IOP with subsequent damage to the optic nerve. In glaucoma patients or patients with a previous steroid response, close monitoring of the IOP is extremely important. Use of corticosteroids may also result in formation or progression of posterior subcapsular cataracts. Additional side effects include delayed wound healing, corneal and scleral thinning or perforation. Prolonged treatment with corticosteroids may suppress the host response and thus increase the susceptibility of secondary ocular infections, including bacterial, viral, fungal, and parasitic infections. In patients whose symptoms worsen with attempted corticosteroid weaning, switching to less potent antiinflammatory therapy is a viable alternative. Due to the well-known complications associated with prolonged corticosteroid therapy, long-term treatment should be reserved for severe, disabling OSD, and such patients must be closely monitored. Compared to dexamethasone, difluprednate, and prednisolone, loteprednol and fluorometholone have lower rates of these complications. Patients with corneal disease that may affect the measurement of IOP need be closely followed for side effects of corticosteroid use, as these measurements may be inaccurate in cases of corneal thinning or edema.

Considered a corticosteroid primarily targeting ocular surface inflammation, fluorometholone alcohol 0.1% may adequately control signs and symptom of dry eyes in patients with keratoconjunctivitis sicca (KCS). In a randomized, controlled trial, fluorometholone alcohol 0.1% used q.i.d. for 30 days demonstrated a beneficial effect on both subjective and objective clinical parameters of moderate-to-severe KCS patients, reportedly without complications.[18] A mild corticosteroid with low intraocular penetration, fluorometholone alcohol 0.1% may have a lower likelihood of increasing intraocular pressure, compared to prednisolone

or dexamethasone.[14] A short-term treatment option for patients with moderate keratoconjunctivitis sicca, topical loteprednol etabonate 0.5% used four times a day for 4 weeks may be beneficial in improving objective clinical parameters with an acceptable benefit–risk ratio. A randomized, masked clinical trial comparing loteprednol to vehicle reported greater improvement in objective variables, including corneal fluorescein staining and conjunctival injection, particularly in a subset of patients with more severe clinical findings of inflammation.[19]

TOPICAL CYCLOSPORINE

Mechanism of Action

Cyclosporine A (CsA) is a fungal-derived peptide that prevents activation and nuclear translocation of transcription factors that are required for inflammatory cytokine production and T-cell activation. Its major clinical effect is disruption of expression of interleukin-2 by helper T cells, thereby preventing T-cell proliferation. Studies have demonstrated that cyclosporine 0.05% can be an effective treatment for management of herpetic stromal keratitis, graft-versus-host disease (GVHD), ocular rosacea, vernal keratoconjunctivitis (VKC), atopic keratoconjunctivitis (AKC), and post-LASIK dry eye.[20]

Delivery System

Available as an FDA-approved treatment for dry eye disease since 2003, cyclosporine 0.05% ophthalmic emulsion has been investigated for management of ocular surface diseases that have an underlying inflammatory etiology. Cyclosporine is not water soluble, and as a result must be mixed in a lipophillic vehicle. Different soluents have variable tolerance in patients. Compounding of cyclosporine drops is possible in cyclodextran, gum cellulose, maize oil and olive oil in concentrations ranging from 0.05% to 2.0%.

Dosage

In severe cases, higher concentration cyclosporine A 2% can provide symptomatic relief. A double-masked, placebo-controlled trial to evaluate the short-term efficacy and safety of topical 2% cyclosporine A in a preservative-free vehicle for patients with severe VKC demonstrated a statistically significant decrease in both signs and symptoms with no observed side effects over the course of the study.[21] For the treatment of patients with steroid-dependent atopic keratoconjunctivitis (AKC), cyclosporine A 2% dissolved in maize oil and dosed four times daily to both eyes appears to be an effective means to improve signs and symptoms, allowing patients to be weaned off topical corticosteroids.[22]

Cyclosporine 0.05% may lead to improved tear film regularity and ocular surface health. In a randomized clinical study of moderate to severe dry eye patients, baseline tear production, as determined by Schirmer testing (with anesthesia), increased to a significantly greater degree in the cyclosporine 0.05% group than in the vehicle group. Also, compared to vehicle, patients treated with cyclosporine 0.05% demonstrated greater improvements in blurred vision that could be explained by the improvement in corneal fluorescein staining.[23] Combination therapy with topical cyclosporine A and topical steroids has been successfully used in treating moderate to severe DES. While cyclosporine does not contribute to the rapid anti-inflammatory effect of corticosteroids, it has a better side effect profile and is safer for long-term use. It is possible to begin treatment of the ocular surface by prescribing both topical steroids and cyclosporine at the same time. The concurrent short-term use of a topical steroid tapered over 1–2 months provides the benefit of faster symptom relief and improvement of ocular signs without accompanying serious complications.[24]

Side Effects

The drug-related side effects of blurred vision, ocular stinging, and conjunctival hyperemia with drop instillation make this medication difficult to tolerate, especially with prolonged use. Other common reactions include discharge, tearing, and foreign body sensation.

AZITHROMYCIN

Mechanism of Action

Azithromycin is a broad-spectrum macrolide antibiotic that contains nitrogen on its macrolide ring. It inhibits bacterial protein synthesis by binding to the 50S ribosomal subunit of susceptible microorganisms. It has high tissue penetration and a prolonged half-life. Macrolide antibiotics, such as azithromycin exhibit antiinflammatory properties. Studies have demonstrated that they can inhibit the production of proinflammatory cytokines and the production of matrix metalloproteinases (MMPs).[25]

Although the specific antiinflammatory mechanism of action remains unknown, the suppression of the nuclear transcription factor nuclear factor kappa B (NF-κB) has been shown to play a role. Furthermore, the concentration of macrolide antibiotics, such as azithromycin within polymophonuclear leukocytes (PMNs) may also modulate their role in infection-mediated inflammation.[26,27] With respect to ocular inflammatory diseases, an in vitro study found azithromycin in DuraSite as effective in suppressing MMPs in the corneal epithelium and endothelium as doxycycline (a tetracycline analog with known antiinflammatory properties, see below) in both human and bovine cells.[28]

Delivery System

Azithromycin is extremely lipophillic, making a stable aqueous preparation difficult. When coupled with a vehicle containing polycarbophil it can be formulated into a stable aqueous preparation. It binds to the mucin-coated surfaces of the eye (including the palpebral conjunctiva), resulting in the formation of a sustained-release gel that prolongs the release and availability of the drug on the ocular surface and enhances the penetration of the drug into the eyelids, conjunctiva, and cornea.[29,30]

Dosage

The recommended dose of azithromycin is one drop twice a day for the first 2 days and then one drop a day for the next 5 days. A single topical dose in healthy individuals demonstrated azithromycin achieved significant tissue concentrations and maintained those levels for up to 24 hours.[31] Peak concentrations of azithromycin of more than 200 μg/g of tissue were achieved in human eyelid tissue as the drug accumulated over the 7 days of therapy. Furthermore, 5 days after discontinuing the medication, tissue concentrations of azithromycin of more than 50 μg/g were still present in the eyelids. Similar results were found for corneal and conjunctival samples.[30]

Side Effects

Eye irritation occurs in approximately 1–2% of patients. Other adverse reactions from topical azithromycin were reported in less than 1% of patients and included ocular reactions (blurred vision, burning, stinging and irritation upon instillation, contact dermatitis, corneal erosion, dry eye, eye pain, itching, ocular discharge, punctate keratitis and visual acuity reduction) and non-ocular reactions (facial swelling, hives, nasal congestion, periocular swelling, rash, sinusitis, urticaria).

TOPICAL VITAMIN A

Mechanism of Action

Vitamin A is essential for maintaining the health of epithelial cells throughout the body. Vitamin A deficiency adversely affects conjunctival and corneal epithelial cells, causing loss of goblet cells and leading to increased epidermal keratinization and squamous metaplasia of the mucous membranes.[32] Vitamin A can exist in three forms: retinol, retinal, and retinoic acid. Many tissues requiring vitamin A store the vitamin as an ester of retinal. Vitamin A is stored as fatty acyl esters of retinol in the lacrimal gland. It is also present as retinol in the tears of rabbits and humans. Its presence in tears provides the rationale for treating OSD with vitamin A.[32]

Delivery System

Topical vitamin A is available as aqueous ophthalmic retinyl palmitate solution 0.05% combined with polysorbate 80 1% (an emulsifier). Vitamin A (All trans retinoic acid) can be formulated as a suspension or an ointment ranging in strength from 0.005% to 0.05%.

Dosage

Topical vitamin A used four times daily has demonstrated improvement in blurred vision, Schirmer scores without anesthesia, and impression cytologic analysis in patients with dry eye.[32] Topical therapy with retinoic acid ointment 0.05% can be an effective treatment of keratinization seen in cicatrizing diseases involving the cornea and conjunctiva. Vitamin A eye drops can be used as adjunct therapy with artificial lubricants for treatment of dry eyes.

Side Effects

Topical vitamin A is known to be an irritant of the ocular surface and its dose should be progressively reduced to the minimal effective dose to treat ocular surface keratinization.[33]

AUTOLOGOUS SERUM

Mechanism of Action

Natural human tears contain essential components for maintaining the ocular surface, such as vitamin A, epidermal growth factor, fibronectin, and other cytokines. Because

Table 34.2 Biochemical Comparison of Serum and Normal, Unstimulated Human Tears

	Serum	Unstimulated Tears
pH	7.4	7.4
Osmolality (SD)	296	298 (10)
EGF (ng/mL)	0.5	0.2–3.0
Vitamin A (mg/mL)	46	0.02
TGF-β	6–33	2–10
Surface IgA (μg/mL) (SD)	2	1190 (904)
Lysozyme (mg/mL) (SD)	6	1.4 (0.2)
Fibronectin (μg/mL)	205	21

these components are also present in serum, the application of autologous serum is thought to offer advantages over artificial tear substitutes that lack these essential components. Compared to pharmaceutical lubricants, autologous serum eye drops more closely mirror the biochemical components of natural tears, containing vitamins, immunoglobulins, and growth factors, some in higher concentrations than natural tears. The pH of natural tears and serum is 7.4 and the osmolarity of tears and serum is approximately equivalent. Certain components are present in higher concentration in serum, compared with natural tears: vitamin A, TGF-β, lysozyme, and fibronectin (Table 34.2).[34] It is possible that serum concentration of certain components may be harmful to the ocular surface, which explains the rationale for using dilute serum.

Delivery System

In previously reported studies, the serum concentration has ranged from 20% to 100%.[35] In order to formulate autologous serum eye drops, blood is drawn from the patient and allowed to coagulate. Autologous serum is separated from other blood components through centrifugation. The separated serum is then re-suspended in balanced salt solution or artificial tears in either a 20% or 50% concentration and frozen in small aliquots. Prior to freezing, the containers should be covered to prevent exposure of the contents to light, as some of the serum components may degrade. The lack of a preservative in the autologous serum requires the necessary aliquot or small amount be defrosted and refrigerated between applications.

Dosage

Protocols reported for preparation and use of autologous serum eye drops exhibit considerable variation. Currently, no data have definitively defined the optimal concentration of autologous serum most appropriate for the treatment OSD. Studies have described the use of serum eye drops for treatment of persistent epithelial defects, severe dry eyes, KCS associated with Sjögren's syndrome and graft-versus-host disease, superior limbal keratoconjunctivitis, and recurrent erosion syndrome.[35–38] In patients with neurotrophic keratopathy, topical autologous serum drops used six to eight times per day, results in improved visual acuity, decreased corneal fluorescein staining, and increased corneal sensitivity that correlated with improvement in corneal nerve morphology as measured with confocal microscopy.[39] Autologous serum has been shown to be superior to conventional treatment with artificial tears in a randomized, crossover study, including patients with severe KCS. After 3 months of 50% autologous serum, patients showed significant improvement in subjective symptoms and impression cytology analysis, corneal staining with rose bengal staining, Schirmer's test without anesthesia, and fluorescein tear clearance test in comparison with those who instilled artificial tears.[40] The use of 50% autologous serum eye drops appears to be an efficacious medical treatment modality for persistent corneal epithelial defects that are recalcitrant to conventional medical therapy.[41]

Side Effects

A potential disadvantage of serum eye drops is the limited stability. The bottles of autologous serum must be kept in the freezer or the refrigerator. Currently, no studies delineate the minimum freezer temperature required for adequate storage. After approximately 30 days, the bottle kept in the refrigerator must be discarded and replaced with a new bottle. Another disadvantage is the risk of blood-borne infection arising for patients and others handling serum. A donor could potentially transmit hepatitis to a recipient or to staff handling the serum. With prolonged use, an initially sterile dropper could become contaminated. Bacterial contamination poses a potential risk either during the production of the serum tears or during prolonged use of the eye drops. The drops are also not typically covered by insurance and must be made by a compounding pharmacy, so continued use can become expensive. Caution should be exercised in prescribing autologous serum eye drops as scleral vasculitis and melting has been reported in a patient with rheumatoid arthritis. Immune complex deposition in the peripheral cornea and subsequent inflammation could be encountered given that antibodies are found in serum. Other possible side effects include discomfort, worsening corneal epitheliopathy, microbial keratitis and conjunctivitis, and eyelid eczema.[34]

TACROLIMUS

Method of Action

Tacrolimus is a macrolide immunosuppressive agent produced by the fermentation of *Streptomyces tsukubaensis*. The method of action of tacrolimus involves the blockage of transcription of cellular communications molecules, including interleukin 2, inhibiting the antigen presenting role of Langerhans cells, and reducing the activation of T cells.[42,43])

Delivery System

Tacrolimus ointment is approved for the treatment of moderate to severe atopic dermatitis. It is available in 0.03% and 0.1% ointment for cutaneous use. Inactive ingredients include mineral oil, paraffin, propylene carbonate, white petrolatum and white wax.

Dosage

Tacrolimus can be compounded into a 0.02% ophthalmic suspension or ointment by a compounding pharmacy. Its use in the eye is considered off-label. There have been no prospective comparative trials of the efficacy of the different strengths. Tacrolimus dermatologic ointment has been reported to control ocular surface inflammation in all three strengths when applied 1–2 times a day in the inferior fornix, without any detectable blood levels. Tacrolimus has been demonstrated to treat intractable allergic conjunctivitis, atopic blepharoconjunctivitis, atopic keratitis, recalcitrant vernal keratoconjunctivitis, and giant papillary conjunctivitis.[44-47] In a retrospective interventional case series, tacrolimus 0.02% placed twice daily in the inferior fornix was effective in severe ocular surface inflammatory diseases.[48] Application of tacrolimus dermatological ointment may present an alternative treatment in advanced ocular surface inflammation without the potential side effects of long-term steroid use.

Side Effects

Reported side effects include redness, stinging, and burning of the eyes. Allergic reaction to the dermatologic formulation has also been reported. Other side effects with doses used for dermatologic conditions may include acne, swollen or infected hair follicles, increased sensitivity of the skin to cold or hot temperatures, lymphadenopathy, skin tingling, flu-like symptoms, skin infections, chickenpox or shingles. Tacrolimus may have a potential to impair local immune surveillance.

Systemic Therapies

SECRETOGOGUES

Mechanism of Action

Derived from a South American shrub *Pilocarpus jaborandi*, pilocarpine is a muscarinic cholinergic parasympathomimetic agonist that binds to muscarinic M3 receptors. In humans, it can cause pharmacologic smooth muscle contraction and exocrine gland stimulation.[49] Cevimeline hydrochloride is an orally administered derivative of acetylcholine that also binds to muscarinic M3 receptors in exocrine glands and stimulates exocrine gland secretion.

Delivery System

Pilocarpine (Salagen tablets, Novartis Pharmaceuticals, Basel, Switzerland) is currently available in 5 and 7.5 mg tablets for oral use. Cevimeline (Evoxac, Daiichi Pharmaceutical Corp, Montvale, NJ) 30 mg tablets are typically taken three times daily; maximum dosage is 90 mg/day.[50]

Dosage

Use of oral secretogogues is beneficial for addressing both the ocular and oral mucosal manifestations of Sjögren's syndrome. Most patients require 20 mg/d of pilocarpine in divided doses for a therapeutic response. According to recommendations in a review article published in JAMA, in cases with residual salivary gland function, oral pilocarpine and cevimeline are the treatment of choice. Recommended doses balancing efficacy and adverse effects are the following: pilocarpine 5 mg q.i.d. and cevimeline 30 mg t.i.d.[51] In a placebo-controlled clinical trial of Sjögren's syndrome patients suffering from xerosis of the eyes and mouth, significant relief in reported ocular symptoms, including decreased use of artificial tears was noted at a dose of 30 mg/day after 12 weeks of therapy.[49] Response to pilocarpine may require 6–12 weeks of therapy.

Side Effects

With oral pilocarpine use, excessive sweating is the most commonly reported side effect, occurring in approximately 40% of patients. Other common reactions include side effects of cholinergic stimulation, such as the following: nausea and vomiting, rhinitis, diarrhea, excessive salivation, salivary gland enlargement, miosis, headache and GI irritation, tremor, and bradycardia. Patients should be closely monitored for severe reactions include arrhythmias, AV block, severe hypotension, and bronchospasm.

Oral Cyclines

TETRACYLINES

Mechanism of Action

Tetracyclines are oral antibiotics originally derived from *Streptomyces aureofaciens*. Their method of action is through inhibition of binding of aminoacyl-tRNA primarily to 70S ribosomes but also to 30S ribosomes. The inhibition leads to a bacteriostatic effect of the tetracyclines, including doxycycline. Additionally, this class of antibiotics also exhibits antiinflammatory properties. The tetracyclines inhibit metalloproteinases, reduce angiogenesis, and reduce apoptosis.

Delivery Systems

The tetracyclines are available in numerous oral compounds, including tetracycline, the semisynthetic doxycycline hyclate, doxycycline monohydrate and minocycline.[52] Tetracycline must be taken on an empty stomach half an hour before, or 2 hours after meals. This is because food prevents absorption of tetracycline into the bloodstream. Minocycline and doxycycline absorption are not affected by food and can be taken at mealtime. All of these tetracyclines must be taken with a full glass of water to prevent esophageal ulceration.

Dosage

Tetracycline is available in 250 and 500 mg tablets; Doxycycline is available in 20, 50, and 100 mg tablets. Minocycline is available in 50 and 100 mg tablets.

Side Effects

In addition to gastrointestinal (GI) concerns, all of the tetracyclines may stain developing teeth in children, induce vaginal or oral candidiasis, and cause dose-related dizziness and photosensitivity. Tetracycline may make the skin more sensitive to sunlight (photosensitivity); this effect depends on the variety of tetracycline and the amount taken. Photosensitization is most likely with doxycycline and least likely with minocycline. Additionally, minocycline may be associated with the development of autoantibodies, including antinuclear antibody (ANA), antineutrophil cytoplasmic antibody (ANCA) and antiphospholipid antibodies with or without associated clinical symptoms. Minocycline may result in dose-related dizziness. It has been reported to cause pseudotumor cerebri and to precipitate arthritis and systemic lupus erythematosus, especially in young women.[53,54]

Tetracyclines as a group in general can be poorly tolerated, due to gastrointestinal upset and require a difficult dosing regimen. Patients can better tolerate doxycyclines, due to their easier dosing regimen. Due to its acidic pH of 2-3, doxycycline hyclate can result in GI upset. Enteric-coated doxycycline hydrate (Doryx) is better tolerated, while doxycycline monohydrate (pH 5-6) is best tolerated with the least amount of gastrointestinal adverse reaction. In the treatment of OSD, doxycycline and minocycline are used at lower doses than those required for the bacteriostatic effect, and are used for a longer treatment period. At the lower doses, these drugs appear to have a greater antiinflammatory effect.

ORAL VITAMIN A

Mechanism of Action

Vitamin A is essential for the differentiation of mucus-secreting epithelium of the eyes, skin, gastrointestinal tract, and genitourinary tract. Loss of mucin and goblet cells in the conjunctiva leads to squamous metaplasia with keratinization of the conjunctiva and cornea. Severe forms of hypovitaminosis A, such as xerosis, corneal ulceration, and keratomalacia, can be seen in countries with a high prevalence of malnutrition.[55] In the developed world, hypovitaminosis A can present in the wake of malnutrition from a variety of causes, such as psychiatric conditions, chronic gastrointestinal and liver disease and bariatric surgery through the disruption of fat-soluble vitamin absorption.[56] It is important to have a high clinical suspicion of hypovitaminosis A, as it can initially be misdiagnosed or overlooked, in part, due to clinical signs being easily represented as simple epithelial erosions seen in keratoconjunctivitis sicca or exposure keratopathy. Without appropriate vitamin A supplementation, ocular surface conditions can be refractory to medical or surgical intervention and lead to progressive blinding disease. With the increasing popularity of bariatric surgery, the risk of vitamin A deficiency is increasing in the developed world. As a result, the ophthalmologist must be mindful of this possible etiology in the differential diagnosis of ocular surface disease.

Delivery System

Prescription-strength vitamin A dosage forms are available from 8,00 up to 250000 units. Various over-the-counter preparations can be obtained in doses lower than prescription-strength. Vitamin A is fat soluble and is therefore only available in capsule form or as an oil liquid supplement.

Dosage

Recommended daily intake and various dosing regimens are highlighted in Table 34.3. The dose of vitamin A is variable, depending on the level of deficiency. Vitamin A levels can be determined by blood test.

Side Effects

With usual doses, no common reactions have been reported. Serious reactions reported with high-dose supplementation include the following: hepatotoxicity, severe nausea and vomiting, mood changes, such as irritability, drowsiness, vertigo, delirium, headache, increased intracranial pressure, papilledema, coma and anorexia.

Table 34.3 Adult Dosing of Oral Vitamin A Supplementation

Dietary Reference Intake	Dosing
Male	3000 units p.o. daily; max: 10000 units/day
Female	2330 units p.o. daily; max: 10000 units/day
Vitamin A deficiency	100000 units p.o. daily × 3 days, then 50000 units p.o. daily × 14 days
Severe vitamin A deficiency with xerophthalmia	500000 units p.o. daily × 3 days, then 50000 units p.o. daily × 14 days, then 10000- 20000 units p.o. daily × 2 mon
Prophylaxis, malabsorption syndromes	10000–50000 units p.o. daily
Retinitis pigmentosa	150000 units p.o.daily
Ichthyosis vulgaris	50000–500000 units p.o. daily
Keratosis follicularis	50000–500000 units p.o. daily

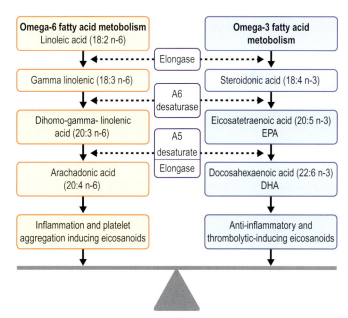

Figure 34.3 Metabolic pathways for omega-3 and omega-6 fatty acids.

NUTRITIONAL SUPPLEMENTS

Mechanism of Action

Dietary modifications and nutritional supplements can promote ocular surface health. An essential part of normal growth and development, essential fatty acids (EFA) cannot be synthesized and must therefore be acquired through dietary intake. Precursors of eicosanoids, omega-3 and omega-6 EFAs are hormones involved in the inflammatory cascade. Four groups of eicosanoids have been identified: leukotrienes, thromboxanes, prostacyclins, and prostaglandins. Omega-3 molecules act as antiinflammatory and anticoagulation mediators. On the converse, omega-6 molecules are proinflammatory and proplatelet aggregator mediators. The overall inflammatory state in the body is influenced by the ratio of omega-6 to omega-3 fatty acids. Omega-3 and omega-6 fatty acids compete for the same enzyme in two distinct pathways that result in antiinflammatory and proinflammatory derivatives, respectively (Fig. 34.3).[57]

Delivery System

Essential fatty acids can be obtained via dietary supplementation. Omega-3 essential fatty acids include docosahexaenoic acid (DHA), alpha linoleic acid (ALA), and eicosapentaenoic acid (EPA). Omega-3 fatty acids can be acquired by consuming the following oily, cold-water fish: salmon, sardines, tuna, mackerel, and herring.[58] One serving of salmon or mackerel could provide 1.5–3.5 g of omega-3 fatty acids. Omega-3 fatty acids are also available in vegetarian dietary choices. A number of different seeds and their oils and some nuts contain varying amounts of ALA. Flaxseeds (linseeds) and their oil typically contain ≈45–55% of fatty acids as ALA.[58] Omega-6 EFAs include linoleic acid (LA), gamma linoleic acid (GLA), dihomogamma-linoleic acid (DGLA), and arachidonic acid. Sources of omega-6 fatty acids include soybean oil, palm oil, grapeseed oil, sunflower oil, poultry, nuts, and cereals.[59] The omega-6 fatty acid linoleic acid (distinct from alpha linoleic acid) is the main polyunsaturated fatty acid in most Western diets and is typically consumed in 5- to 20-fold greater amounts than the omega-3 fatty acid, alpha linoleic acid.[60] Omega-3 derived from fish oil has a distinct fishy odor. Removal of the ester will remove the fish odor from the oil. Re-esterification of the omega-3 molecule may increase both the efficacy, as well as the serum concentration of omega-3.

Dosage

In a prospective randomized controlled trial, daily doses of 6 g of flaxseed oil (equivalent to 3.3 g/day of omega-3 fatty acids) resulted in a decrease in the RBC and plasma ratios of omega-6 to omega-3 fatty acids, compared to controls. Additionally, improvements in overall ocular surface disease index (OSDI) score, tear break-up time (TBUT), and meibum score were noted. This prospective clinical study found that dietary supplementation with omega-3 fatty acids induced a change in the fatty acid saturation content in meibum.[57,59]

In a small study, patients receiving lower doses of omega-3 fatty acids (450 mg of eicosapentaenoic acid, 300 mg of docosahexaenoic acid and 1000 mg of flaxseed oil) had an increase in aqueous tear secretion. No significant effect in meibum lipid composition or aqueous tear evaporation rate was reported, perhaps, due to the choice of active ingredients in the omega-3 dose, the trial length, and the dosing schedule in a population with chronic dry eye syndrome.[60] Review of dietary diaries of >32 000 patients enrolled in the Women's Health Study revealed that a higher dietary intake of omega-3 fatty acids is associated with a decreased incidence of dry eye syndrome in women. Also, low dietary intake of omega-3, a high omega-6 to omega-3 ratio, or both increase the risk of clinically diagnosed dry eye.[61] In clinical studies, supplementation with the combination of LA and GLA or with evening primrose oil (EPO), which contains both of these fatty acids, resulted in improvement of keratoconjunctivitis sicca syndrome.[62]

Side Effects

A tolerable upper intake level for omega-3 fatty acids has not been established. However, some studies have shown a possible increased risk of bleeding and hemorrhagic stroke following supplementation with high-dose omega-3. Individuals who have disorders involving bleeding, who have a tendency to bruise very easily, or who are taking blood thinners should consult their doctor before taking high doses of omega-3 fatty acids. Gastrointestinal distress, flatulence and eructation have all been reported as short-term side effects.

Medical Management of Ocular Surface Disease

Assessment of the patient with OSD requires a thorough history and examination. Many of these patients have seen numerous physicians and are desperate for relief. Despite the complexity of the evaluation and management, treatment of these patients is extremely gratifying. In each of these patients a multifaceted approach is recommended; both systemic and topical therapies are required.

The history must include a comprehensive review of the therapies tried, medical and surgical history, as well as a review of all systemic and topical medications. For example, a patient may not reveal a history of bariatric surgery without specific questioning, and have a resultant vitamin A deficiency. Once a complete history has been obtained, including the often overlooked contact lens history, a comprehensive examination of the ocular surface is required. Careful examination of the lids and lashes may reveal blepharitis, meibomian gland dysfunction, lid malposition, or punctal displacement. Tear evaluation includes tear break-up time and Schirmer testing, as well as an assessment of the height of the tear meniscus on the lower eyelid. Vital staining of the surface of the cornea and the conjunctiva, both bulbar and palpebral, including evaluation of corneal limbal staining, will aid in the diagnosis. Negative fluorescein staining reveals areas of epithelial elevation while late staining of the limbal cells may be seen in areas of corneal epithelial dysplasia.

In both the inflamed and dry ocular surface, systemic therapy is often required and should include the use of oral dietary supplementation with omega-3 fatty acids. Many patients cannot tolerate a maximal dosage of 3 g per day. Therefore, it is recommended that patients begin dietary supplementation with 1–2 g per day of omega-3 fatty acids and increase the dose as tolerated until they reach 3 g per day. Omega-3 fatty acids are concentrated in the walls of red blood cells and the serum. As a result of red blood cell turnover, 120 days of therapy are required for the maximum blood concentration. It is important to warn patients that a prolonged course of therapy is required prior to achieving positive results.

At the same time, it is imperative to assess the eyelid margins for blepharitis and meibomitis, both of which can result in exacerbation of ocular surface irritation, as well as the evaporative dry eye. Meibomitis can be difficult to diagnose without compressing the meibomian glands to evaluate their contents. Continual hygiene of the eyelash base and the meibomian gland orifice is the mainstay of treatment of these lid margin conditions. Eyelash shampoo in the shower, as opposed to warm compresses and lid scrubs, is recommended. In describing this technique to patients it is preferable to use the term eyelash shampoo, as it is not the lids that we want them to clean, but rather the eyelashes. Patients are instructed to shampoo the base of their lashes with a non-irritating dilute detergent (baby shampoo) on a washcloth at the end of their daily shower. The warm moist environment of the shower will provide the same effect as a warm compress, while the ease of the process increases patient compliance with this chronic therapy. In some patients a topical ointment (loteprednol) can be applied to the lashes at bedtime to soften the collarettes and decrease inflammation of the meibomian gland orifices. The oily effect of the ointment on the eyelid increases compliance with eyelash shampooing in the morning. In severe cases of blepharomeibomitis or recurrent chalazia, oral doxycycline 100 mg twice a day may be of use with a taper to 20 mg per day for long-term use. However, even in these low antiinflammatory doses the potential for systemic side effects remains, including photosensitivity. Topical azithromycin has been shown to have a role in the treatment of blepharitis, as well as the associated dry eye symptoms.[63–65]

In tear deficient OSD, it is necessary to use topical therapy to increase the tear volume. Artificial tear supplementation with a hydrogel that increases contact time with the ocular surface, as well as a low preservative toxicity profile is preferred (such as a preservative-free, Purite, or GenAqua-preserved artificial tear). In moderate or severe cases of OSD, punctal occlusion, either temporary or permanent, may be critical in stabilizing the ocular surface. A stepwise approach to punctal occlusion with initial occlusion of the inferior puncta will increase the tear volume and prolong tear contact time with the cornea and conjunctiva. It is important to simultaneously control the inflammatory status of the ocular surface to avoid prolonged contact of cytokine-filled tears with the already inflamed ocular surface. Additional closure of the upper puncta may be indicated after closure of the lower puncta in the severe dry eye patient. Placement of punctal plugs prior to permanent cauterization is warranted in the effort to avoid epiphora.

While an increase in tear volume may temporarily decrease irritation symptoms, it does not decrease the inflammation of the ocular surface. A topical steroid will have the quickest effect in reducing the ocular surface inflammation. However, due to the potential for side effects with long-term use of topical steroids, cyclosporine or other nonsteroidal antiinflammatory therapies should be considered. Coupling topical steroids with topical cyclosporine provides the beneficial effect of decreasing burning and stinging that may be seen in up to 18% of patients using cyclosporine alone.[66] Long-term use of topical cyclosporine will both reduce ocular inflammation and increase tear production. In blepharitis patients, chronic topical cyclosporine has been shown to improve patient symptoms.[20] In patients with keratinization of the eyelid margin, topical vitamin A ointment may be substituted for a topical steroid ointment and applied to the eyelid margin at bedtime.

In the patient with moderate to severe OSD and decreased tear production, topical corticosteroids along with doxycycline suppress metalloproteinases and cytokine activation.[67] The use of a topical steroid suspension (prednisolone acetate) may be contraindicated and a topical solution (prednisolone phosphate) preferred. The steroid suspension may result in further irritation of the ocular surface if the particulates in the suspension precipitate out and abrade the ocular surface. In addition, the particulates in the

suspension may combine with the mucus in the tear film of the aqueous deficient patient and result in filament formation. In these cases, the use of a topical steroid solution, such as prednisolone sodium phosphate is recommended. In recalcitrant OSD or patients who are steroid intolerant, topical tacrolimus ointment may be indicated for control of surface inflammation. In severe cases, autologous serum tears may also be useful, though long-term use is somewhat impractical.[68] However, in non-healing epithelial defects, autologous serum may be required to aid in healing of the epithelial defect and reduce the ocular surface inflammation. Future development of epithelial growth factors for clinical use may also play a role in refining the management of OSD.

Conclusion

Optimal medical management of the ocular surface requires fine-tuning the performance of its key players: the lids, lacrimal gland, cornea and conjunctiva. Understanding the pathophysiology driving various conditions affecting the health of the ocular surface serves as a guide for clinicians in developing a broad, multifaceted medical approach for the treatment of OSD. A careful understanding of the mechanism of action, delivery system, dosage and potential side effects of each treatment modality aids clinicians in their choice of medical treatments. Utilizing a stepwise approach and a thorough understanding of the medical options for both the clinician and the patient may help lead to increased compliance and improved outcomes while potentially avoiding the need for surgical intervention.

References

1. Tung CI, Kottaiyan R, Koh S, et al. Noninvasive, objective, multimodal tear dynamics evaluation of 5 over-the-counter tear drops in a randomized controlled trial. Cornea 2012;31:108–14.
2. Debbasch C, De La Salle SB, Brignole F, et al. Cytoprotective effects of hyaluronic acid and Carbomer 934P in ocular surface epithelial cells. Invest Ophthalmol Vis Sci 2002;43:3409–15.
3. Doughty MJ. Acute effects of chlorobutanol- or benzalkonium chloride- containing artificial tears on the surface of rabbit corneal epithelial cells. Optom Vis Sci 1994;71:562–72.
4. Ubels JL, Clousing DP, Van Haitsma TA, et al. Pre-clinical investigation of the efficacy of an artificial tear solution containing hydroxypropyl-guar as a gelling agent. Curr Eye Res 2004;28:437–44.
5. Hartstein I, Khwarg S, Przydryga J. An open-label evaluations of HP-Guar gellable lubricant eye drops for the improvement of dry eye signs and symptoms in a moderate dry eye adult population. Curr Med Res Opin 2005;21:255–60.
6. Foulks GN. Clinical evaluation of the efficacy of PEG/PG lubricant eye drops with gelling agent (HP-Guar) for the relief of the signs and symptoms of dry eye disease: a review. Drugs Today 2007;43:887–96.
7. Benitez-del-Castillo JM, Aranguez C, Garcia-Sanchez J. Corneal epithelial permeability and dry eye treatment. Adv Exp Med Biol 2002;506:703–6.
8. Dogru M, Tsubota K. Pharmacotherapy of dry eye. Expert Opin Pharmacother 2011;12:325–34.
9. Albietz JM, Lenton LM, McLennan SG, et al. A comparison of the effect of refresh plus and bion tears on dry eye symptoms and ocular surface health in myopic LASIK patients. CLAO J 2002;28:96–110.
10. Ridder WH 3rd, Lamotte JO, Ngo L, et al. Short-term effects of artificial tears on visual performance in normal subjects. Optom Vis Sci 2005;82:370–7.
11. McGhee CN. Pharmacokinetics of ophthalmic corticosteroids. Br J Ophthalmol 1992;76:681–4.

12. Roberts CW, Nelson PL. Comparative analysis of prednisolone acetate suspensions. J Ocul Pharmacol Ther 2007;23:182–7.

13. Rajpal RK, Digby D, D'Aversa G, et al. Intraocular pressure elevations with loteprednol etabonate; a retrospective chart review. J Ocul Pharmacol Ther 2011;27:305–8.

14. Awan MA, Agarwal PK, Watson DG, et al. Penetration of topical and subconjunctival corticosteroids into human aqueous humour and its therapeutic significance. Br J Ophthalmol 2009;93:708–13.

15. Dell SJ, Shulman DG, Lowry GM, et al. A controlled evaluation of the efficacy and safety of loteprednol etabonate in the prophylactic treatment of seasonal allergic conjunctivitis. Loteprednol Allergic Conjunctivitis Study Group. Am J Ophthalmol 1997;123:791–7.

16. Friedlaender MH, Howes J. A double-masked, placebo-controlled evaluation of the efficacy and safety of loteprednol etabonate in the treatment of giant papillary conjunctivitis. The Loteprednol Etabonate Giant Papillary Conjunctivitis Study Group I. Am J Ophthalmol 1997;123:455–64.

17. Controlled evaluation of loteprednol etabonate and prednisolone acetate in the treatment of acute anterior uveitis. Loteprednol Etabonate US Uveitis Study Group. Am J Ophthalmol 1999;127: 537–44.

18. Avunduk AM, Avunduk MC, Varnell ED, et al. The comparison of efficacies of topical corticosteroids and nonsteroidal anti-inflammatory drops on dry eye patients: a clinical and immunocytochemical study. Am J Ophthalmol 2003;136:593–602.

19. Pflugfelder SC, Maskin SL, Anderson B, et al. A randomized, double-masked, placebo-controlled, multicenter comparison of loteprednol etabonate ophthalmic suspension, 0.5%, and placebo for treatment of keratoconjunctivitis sicca in patients with delayed tear clearance. Am J Ophthalmol 2004;138:444–57.

20. Donnenfeld E, Pflugfelder SC. Topical ophthalmic cyclosporine: pharmacology and clinical uses. Surv Ophthalmol 2009;54: 321–38.

21. Kilic A, Gurler B. Topical 2% cyclosporine A in preservative-free artificial tears for the treatment of vernal keratoconjunctivitis. Can J Ophthalmol 2006;41:693–8.

22. Hingorani M, Moodaley L, Calder VL, et al. A randomized, placebo-controlled trial of topical cyclosporine A in steroid-dependent atopic keratoconjunctivitis. Ophthalmology 1998;105:1715–20.

23. Sall K, Stevenson OD, Mundorf TK, et al. Two multicenter, randomized studies of the efficacy and safety of cyclosporine ophthalmic emulsion in moderate to severe dry eye disease. CsA Phase 3 Study Group. Ophthalmology 2000;107:631–9.

24. Byun YJ, Kim TI, Kwon SM, et al. Efficacy of combined 0.05% cyclosporine and 1% methylprednisolone treatment for chronic dry eye. Cornea 2012;31:509–13.

25. Ianaro A, Ialenti A, Maffia P, et al. Anti-inflammatory activity of macrolide antibiotics. J Pharmacol Exper Ther 2000;292:156–63.

26. Amsden GW. Anti-inflammatory effects of macrolides – an underappreciated benefit in the treatment of community-acquired respiratory tract infections and chronic inflammatory pulmonary conditions? Rev J Antimicrob Chemother 2005;55:10–21.

27. Shinkai M, Rubin BK. Macrolides and airway inflammation in children. Paediatr Respir Re 2005;6:227–35.

28. Luchs J. Azithromycin in Durasite for the treatment of blepharitis. Clin Ophthalmol 2010;30:681–8.

29. Akpek EK, Vittitow J, Verhoeven RS, et al. Ocular surface distribution and pharmacokinetics of a novel ophthalmic 1% azithromycin formulation. J Ocul Pharmacol Ther 2009;25:433–9.

30. Friedlander MH, Protzko E. Clinical development of 1% azithromycin in DuraSite, a topical azalide anti-infective for ocular surface therapy. Clin Ophthalmol 2007;1:3–10.

31. Torkildsen G, O'Brien TP. Conjunctival tissue pharmacokinetic properties of topical azithromycin 1% and moxifloxacin 0.5% ophthalmic solutions: a single-dose, randomized, open-label, active-controlled trial in healthy adult volunteers. Clin Ther 2008; 30:2005–14.

32. Kim EC, Choi JS, Joo CK. A comparison of vitamin a and cyclosporine a 0.05% eye drops for treatment of dry eye syndrome. Am J Ophthalmol 2009;147:206–13.e3.

33. Herbort CP, Zografos L, Zwingli M, et al. Topical retinoic acid in dysplastic and metaplastic keratinization of corneoconjunctival epithelium. Graefes Arch Clin Exp Ophthalmol 1988;226:22–6.

34. Geerling G, Maclennan S, Hartwig D. Autologous serum eye drops for ocular surface disorders. Br J Ophthalmol 2004;88:1467–74.

35. Tsubota K, Goto E, Fujita H, et al. Treatment of dry eye by autologous serum application in Sjogren's syndrome. Br J Ophthalmol 1999; 83:390–5.

36. Goto E, Shimmura S, Shimazaki J, et al. Treatment of superior limbic keratoconjunctivitis by application of autologous serum. Cornea 2001;20:807–10.

37. Ogawa Y, Okamoto S, Mori T, et al. Autologous serum eye drops for the treatment of severe dry eye in patients with chronic graft-versus-host disease. Bone Marrow Transplant 2003;31:579–83.

38. Matsumoto Y, Dogru M, Goto E, et al. Autologous serum application in the treatment of neurotrophic keratopathy. Ophthalmology 2004;111:1115–20.

39. Rao K, Leveque C, Pflugfelder SC. Corneal nerve regeneration in neurotrophic keratopathy following autologous plasma therapy. Br J Ophthalmol 2010;94:584–91.

40. Noble BA, Loh RS, MacLennan S, et al. Comparison of autologous serum eye drops with conventional therapy in a randomised controlled crossover trial for ocular surface disease. Br J Ophthalmol 2004;88:647–52.

41. Jeng BH, Dupps Jr WJ. Autologous serum 50% eyedrops in the treatment of persistent corneal epithelial defects. Cornea 2009;28: 1104–8.

42. Koo JY, Fleisher AB, Abramovits W, et al. Tacrolimus ointment is safe and effective in the treatment of atopic dermatitis: results in 8000 patients. J Am Acad Dermatol 2005;53;S195–205.

43. Hooks M. Tacrolimus, a new immunosuppressant: a review of the literature. Ann Pharmacother 1994;28:501–11.

44. Attax-Fox L, Barkana Y, Iskhakov V, et al. Topical tacrolimus 0.03%ointment for intractable allergic conjunctivitis: an open label pilot study. Curr Eye Res 2008;33:545–9.

45. Joseph MS, Kaufman HE, Insler M. Topical tacrolimus ointment for treatment of refractory anterior segment inflammatory disorders. Cornea 2005;24:417–20.

46. Kymionis GD, Goldman D, Ide T, et al. Tacrolimus 0.03% ointment in the eye for the treatment of giant papillary conjunctivitis. Cornea 2008;27:228–9.

47. Garcia DP, Alperte JI, Cristobal JA, et al. Topical tacrolimus ointment for treatment of intractable atopic keratoconjunctivitis: A case report and review of the literature. Cornea 2011;30:462–4.

48. Miyazaki D, Tominaga T, Kakimaru-Hasegawa A, et al. Therapeutic effects of tacrolimus ointment for refractory ocular surface inflammatory diseases. Ophthalmology 2008;115:988–92.

49. Papas AS, Sherrer YS, Charney M, et al. Successful treatment of dry mouth and dry eye symptoms in Sjogren's syndrome patients with oral pilocarpine: a randomized, placebo-controlled, dose-adjustment study. J Clin Rheumatol 2004;10:169–77.

50. Akpek EK, Lindsley KB, Adyanthaya RS, et al. Treatment of Sjogren's syndrome-associated dry eye an evidence-based review. Ophthalmology 2011;118:1242–52.

51. Ramos-Casals M, Tzioufas AG, Stone JH, et al. Treatment of primary Sjogren syndrome: a systematic review. JAMA 2010 28;304: 452–60.

52. Maibach H. Second generation tetracyclines, a dermatologic overview: clinical uses and pharmacology. Cutis 1991;48:411–7.

53. Sloan B, Scheinfeld N. The use and safety of doxycycline hyclate and other second generation tetracyclines. Expert Opin Drug Saf 2008; 7:571–7.

54. Kircik LH. Doxycycline and minocycline for the management of acne: a review of efficacy and safety with emphasis on clinical implications. J Drugs Dermatol 2010;11:1407–11.

55. Sommer A. Vitamin a deficiency and clinical disease: an historical overview. J Nutr 2008;138:1835–9.

56. Lin P, Fintelmann RE, Khalifa YM, et al. Ocular surface disease secondary to vitamin A deficiency in the developed world: it still exists. Arch Ophthalmol 2011;129:798–9.

57. Macsai MS. The role of omega-3 dietary supplementation in blepharitis and meibomian gland dysfunction (an AOS thesis). Trans Am Ophthalmol Soc 2008;106:336–56.

58. Calder PC. Mechanisms of action of (n-3) fatty acids. J Nutr 2012; 142:592S–9S.

59. Rand AL, Asbell PA. Nutritional supplements for dry eye syndrome. Curr Opin Ophthalmol 2011;22:279–82.

60. Wojtowicz JC, Butovich I, Uchiyama E, et al. Pilot, prospective, randomized, double-masked, placebo-controlled clinical trial of an omega-3 supplement for dry eye. Cornea 2011;30:308–14.

61. Miljanovic B, Trivedi KA, Dana MR, et al. Relation between dietary n-3 and n-6 fatty acids and clinically diagnosed dry eye syndrome in women. Am J Clin Nutr 2005;82:887–93.

62. Barabino S, Rolando M, Camicione P, et al. Systemic linoleic and gamma-linolenic acid therapy in dry eye syndrome with an inflammatory component. Cornea 2003;22:97–101.

63. Veldman P, Colby K. Current evidence for topical azithromycin 1% ophthalmic solution in the treatment of blepharitis and blepharitis-associated ocular dyness. Int Ophthalmol Clin 2011;51:43–52.

64. Optiz DL, Tyler KF. Efficacy of azithromycin 1% ophthalmic solution for the treatments of ocular surface disease from posterior blepharitis. Clin Exp Optom 2011;94:200–6.

65. Haque RM, Torkildsen GL, Brubaker K, et al. Multicenter open-label study evaluating the efficacy of azithromycin ophthalmic solution 1% on the signs and symptoms of subjects with blepharitis. Cornea 2010;29:871–7.

66. Sheppard JD, Scoper SV, Samudre S. Topical lotoprednol pretreatment reduces cyclosporine stinging in chronic dry eye disease. J Ocul Pharmacol Ther 2011;27:23–7.

67. De Paiva CS, Corrales RM, Villarreal AL, et al. Corticosteroid and doxycycline suppress MMP-9 and inflammatory cytokine expression, MAPK activationin the corneal epithelium in experimental dry eye. Exp Eye Res 2006;83:526–35.

68. Alio JL, Abad M, Artola A, et al. Use of autologous platelet-rich plasma in the treatment of dormant corneal ulcers. Ophthalmology 2007;114:1286–93.

35 Contact Lenses for Ocular Surface Disease

DEBORAH S. JACOBS, LYNETTE K. JOHNS, and HONG-GAM LE

Introduction

Although contact lenses are typically thought of as a cosmetic option for the correction of refractive error, they can also play a therapeutic role after trauma, surgery, and in the treatment of ocular disease. The following is a brief review of the history of contact lens and the innovations that allowed for therapeutic use in ocular surface disease (OSD). The rationale behind and characteristics of various lenses that can be used for ocular surface disease will be reviewed, as will general approach to use, and a review of the prevention and treatment of complications. Finally, publications and experience with contact lens within various categories of ocular surface disease will be reviewed.

Because the market for therapeutic, as opposed to cosmetic, contact lenses is small, innovations, labeling, and marketing of contact lenses, for the most part, has been geared to cosmetic indications and correction of ammetropia rather than therapeutic applications. The few lenses developed specifically and only for therapeutic use (Plano T, Permalens, Protek) have generally been discontinued. Clinicians often will choose to use a lens 'off-label' based on familiarity, material, design, or immediate availability. The term 'bandage lens' is not typically part of United States Food & Drug Administration (FDA) labeling; labeling typically indicates if a lens is approved 'for therapeutic use' and 'as a bandage.'

History of Contact Lenses and Innovations Allowing for Therapeutic Use

The first description of contact lenses in the medical literature was a report on contact lenses by Adolf Eugene Fick in 1888.[1] Pearson,[2] in his review of the history of contact lenses, reports Karl Otto Himmler as the first manufacturer of contact lenses. Pearson describes reports of contact lenses ranging in diameter from 15 to 22 mm in 1888, 1888, and 1889 by Fick, Kalt, and Muller, respectively, all made of glass. Examining these early glass and then polymethyl methacrylate (PMMA) large-diameter lens designs retrospectively exposes various reasons for failure, most prominently, hypoxia related to the impervious nature of glass or PMMA. This problem was circumvented in the middle of the last century through the use of small diameter PMMA corneal lenses that allowed the majority of the cornea access to atmospheric oxygen, with some transmission to the area under the mobile contact lens via the tear film. Overwear syndrome could arise, due to hypoxia under

a tight or immobile lens. These lenses were used primarily for treatment of refractive error because there was invariably corneal touch and underlying hypoxia, both of which would be a challenge in the setting of ocular surface disease. Two innovations in material science allowed for contact lens to enter the therapeutic armamentarium: rigid gas-permeable polymers and soft hydrogels.

The introduction of rigid gas-permeable polymers into contact lens manufacturing allowed for better physiological tolerance of corneal lenses and the reintroduction of large-diameter scleral lens designs in the early 1980s.[3] Wide use of lenses made of these materials has been limited by challenges of corneal RGP lens fitting and the perception that a 'hard' lens cannot serve as a 'bandage.' Rigid gas-permeable scleral lenses that vault the cornea entirely can play a role in the treatment of ocular surface disease, as presented throughout the remainder of the chapter.

The introduction of hydrophilic gels for biologic use, and in particular for contact lens, by Czech chemist Otto Wichterle in the 1960s led to the availability of 'soft' lenses within a decade. Soft lenses are easily fitted, with greater range of tolerance for a given lens profile. The potential for therapeutic use was recognized contemporaneously with the introduction of soft contact lenses. In the decades that followed, modifications to materials, including increased water content or silicone for the sake of increased oxygen permeability, or modifications to improve wetting, were introduced in the field of soft contact lenses. Oxygen transmission has been held as the paragon for therapeutic lens, but mechanical interaction with the surface is also key to tolerance and clinical effectiveness. A North American survey of 'bandage' soft lens use by optometrists and ophthalmologist in 2002 found that 72% of respondents had prescribed soft contact lenses for therapeutic purposes, most typically for corneal wound healing and management of postoperative complications.[4]

In the conventional practice of contact lens fitting for correction of refractive error, the presence of ocular surface disease is a relative contraindication to contact lens wear. Nevertheless, contact lenses may be specifically indicated despite surface breakdown, history of infection, local or systemic immunosuppression, or the presence of underlying systemic disease, when the lens material, parameters of fit, and wear regimen are given thoughtful consideration.

In the 2007 Report of the International Dry Eye Workshop,[5] contact lens wear is among the treatment recommendations by severity level among level 3 interventions along with autologous serum tears and permanent punctal occlusion, with systemic treatment and surgery listed as level 4 interventions. Some are skeptical that a contact lens for ocular surface disease is therapeutic. One might ask how an object 'hard' or 'soft' can help an eye that is dry (and inflamed). Clinical observations are that an appropriately chosen, well-fitted therapeutic contact lens can:

- Promote corneal healing
- Provide mechanical protection and support
- Reduce desiccation
- Relieve pain.

Consideration of mechanisms underlying these observations, some of which remain part hypothetical, is beyond the scope of this chapter.

Characteristics of Soft Lenses Used for Treatment of Ocular Surface Disease

Important variables to consider in choosing a soft lens for OSD include material Dk and diameter. Labeled indications and wearing schedules are also variables to consider. Dk refers to the oxygen permeability of a given lens material. Dk is expressed in ISO/Fatt units $\times 10^{-11}(cm^3O_2)(cm)/[(sec(cm^2)(mmHg)]@35°C$. Convention is that it is reported as Dk/L or Dk/T for thickness of a −3.00 power lens of particular material and design. Among hydrogel soft lenses, water content, which is expressed as a percentage, has paradoxical implication for patients with aqueous tear deficiency. One might think that increased water content is better for a therapeutic lens in a dry eye patient, but this is not necessarily the case, as a higher water content soft lens may act as a sponge and be prone to problematic adherence.

The prototype therapeutic contact lens was the Bausch & Lomb Plano T, a hydrophilic hydrogel introduced in the 1970s specifically as a therapeutic lens. It had low water content (38%), low oxygen permeability (Dk 8.4), and was thick. Clinically, it reduced pain, promoted epithelialization, sealed leaks, and induced corneal edema (which was good for leaks but bad for other indications). The Permalens (CooperVision Inc, Fairport, NY) represented a significant advance with higher Dk value of 42. It was developed as an extended-wear lens for aphakia to be changed monthly, but its properties in low powers were advantageous over a Plano T lens for therapeutic indications. When programmed replacement and disposable lenses for correction of refractive error entered the marketplace, clinicians chose these for OSD because of immediate availability among trial inventories and relative low cost,[6,7] even though they were not labeled for therapeutic use. The Silsoft (Bausch & Lomb Inc, Rochester, NY) is the most gas-permeable soft lens (Dk 340); it is specifically approved for extended wear for the therapeutic indication of correction of pediatric aphakia. These lenses typically have required high lens plus power and larger diameter to support that power, all reducing availability of atmospheric oxygen to the cornea.[8]

In the last decade, very high Dk silicone hydrogel (SiHy) material and lenses have been developed and labeled specifically for therapeutic use in addition to cosmetic use. There have been reports of the utility of SiHy lenses as a therapeutic option across the spectrum of ocular surface

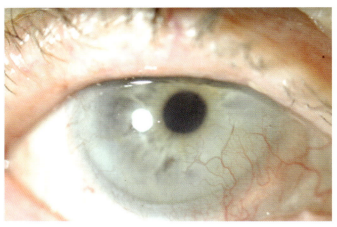

Figure 35.1 Extended wear of SiHy soft lens for comfort and vision in an 85-year-old physician with history of rosacea keratitis, nodular degeneration, and longstanding corneal neovascularization to AK incisions.

disease.[9,10] Epidemiologic studies have not found a lower rate of infection with these newer materials,[11,12] but there should be advantages conferred in OSD simply because of their higher oxygen transmission.

The authors recommend that clinicians choose a high Dk lens labeled for extended wear and/or therapeutic use as a first choice for therapeutic use in OSD (Fig. 35.1). Potential complications, including lens loss, lens deposits, discomfort, infectious keratitis and ulceration, and tight lens syndrome[7] should be reviewed. The risks and benefits of overnight wear should be reviewed with the patient and weighed against the alternatives for the treatment of their particular disease process. It is probably not advisable to use a daily disposable lens on an extended wear or therapeutic basis as they were not developed or manufactured for those uses.

Table 35.1 presents some lenses of historical and current interest, with their Dk, percentage water content, and labeling. Some soft lenses are labeled for therapeutic use on an extended wear basis. Others are labeled for extended wear, but not specifically for therapeutic use. Lenses labeled for daily wear could be used 'off-label' on an extended wear basis. Lenses labeled for extended wear on a cosmetic basis could be used 'off-label' on a therapeutic basis.

PRINCIPLES UNDERLYING FITTING OF A SOFT THERAPEUTIC LENS

Clinicians will typically choose from an inventory of trial lenses kept on hand for cosmetic correction of refractive error, or they may have an inventory of lenses ordered specifically for therapeutic use. If a range of base curves is available, one might choose based on whether the eye is a 'short' hyperopic eye or a 'longer' myopic eye, and if the cornea is known to be steep or flat. The fitter should be aware that corneal myopia requires a steep lens (smaller base curve), whereas a large myopic eye may require a flatter lens (larger base curve). If using keratometry readings, the flat K is used with respect to 45.00 diopters. A steeper base curve is used if flat K is >45.00 and flatter base curve if flat K is <45.00. Visible horizontal iris diameter can also change the starting point. The larger the cornea, the

Table 35.1   Soft Contact Lenses and RGP Materials

Trade Name	Material	Manufacturer	Availability	Diameter (mm)	Dk	H₂O %	Labeling
Plano T	Polymacon	Bausch & Lomb	Discontinued	14.5	8.4	38%	EWTh
Permalens	Perfilcon A	CooperVision	Discontinued	13.5–15.0	42	71%	EWTh
Proclear	Omafilcon A	CooperVision	Available	14.2	34	62%	DW
Kontur	Methafilcon A	Kontur Contact Lens	Available	15–24	18.8	55%	DW
Acuvue 2	Etafilcon A	VISTAKON	Available	14.0	28	58%	DW (2w)/EW (7d)
Air Optix Night & Day	Lotrafilcon A	Alcon Vision Care (CIBA)	Available	13.8	140	24%	DW/ EW (30d)/EWTh
PureVision	Balafilcon A	Bausch & Lomb	Available	14.0	91	36%	DW/EW (30d)
Acuvue Oasys	Senofilcon A	VISTAKON	Available	14.0	103	38%	DW/EW (7d)/EWTh
TrueEye	Narafilcon A	VISTAKON	Available	14.2	55	46%	DD
1 day Acuvue	Etafilcon A	VISTAKON	Available	14.2	28	58%	DD
Focus Dailies	Nelfilcon A	Alcon Vision Care (CIBA)	Available	13.8	26	69%	DD
Boston Equalens II (RGP material)	Oprifocon A	Bausch & Lomb	Available	Made to order	85	<1%	
Boston XO2 (RGP material)	Hexafocon B	Bausch & Lomb	Available	Made to order	141	<1%	DW
TYRO-97 (RGP material)	Hofocon A	Lagado	Available	Made to order	97	<1%	DW

DD, daily disposable; DW, daily wear; EW ,extended wear; EWTh, extended wear with therapeutic indications.

greater the sagittal depth, thus requiring a steeper base curve. Generally, a steeper lens is less likely to move or dislodge and more likely to be comfortable, compared to a flatter lens. If there is inadequate tear exchange and movement, the patient may develop 'tight lens syndrome' over the first day of wear, which will have deleterious effects as opposed to a therapeutic effect.

Typically, the lens is inserted by the clinician and fit assessed immediately and then after a period of wear, centration should be confirmed. To confirm tear exchange under the lens, the lens should move slightly with blink, but the edge should not traverse the limbus, with either blink or with eye movement to the extremes of gaze. The lens should be easily moved with pressure transmitted via the lower lid, commonly referred to as the 'push up' test. Excess movement indicates need for a steeper lens (smaller base curve). Inadequate movement will require a flatter lens (higher base curve). Finally, the lens should be comfortable; no 'adaptation' should be necessary. Edge design and modulus may contribute to tolerance or discomfort; so two lenses of identical radius, but different manufacture, material and design may differ in comfort to the patient. Relief of symptoms should exceed any lens awareness. If there is lens awareness or discomfort, then the lens is not likely to serve its therapeutic purpose, and an alternative lens should be trialed.

The authors recommend an in-office trial with observation for 20–30 minutes to ascertain that there is adequate movement after the lens settles, and to ensure that comfort and retention are satisfactory. If retention is a problem, due to extreme dryness, exposure, or abnormal lid function, then use of a tighter, steeper lens or larger-diameter lens may be warranted. It is advisable, when fitting for extended wear for therapeutic purposes, to evaluate the patient the next day to rule out tight lens, and to ascertain retention, particularly if the patient is not experienced with contact lens wear, insertion and removal. The patient should be

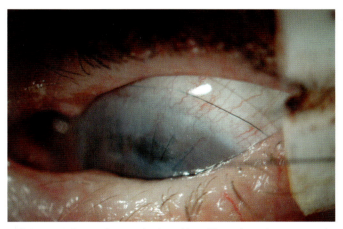

Figure 35.2 Large-diameter hydrogel lens (Kontur) used over sutured amniotic membrane graft used for poor healing after penetrating keratoplasty for sterile melt in ocular chronic graft-versus-host disease.

seen at appropriate intervals, decided on the basis of clinical judgment and product labeling, throughout the period that extended wear is required. Lens disinfection or exchange for a new lens should be undertaken at appropriate intervals by the patient, if he or she is experienced in contact lens wear, or at return visits to the clinician.

Very Large Diameter Soft Lenses

There are very-large-diameter hydrogel lenses (16–24 mm diameter) that have special utility in instances of OSD in which there is history or likelihood of poor soft lens retention. Profound aqueous deficiency, incomplete blink, lid abnormalities, eye rubbing, and exposure can all be contributory to poor retention (Fig. 35.2). Large-diameter soft lenses sold in range of base curves for a given diameter and the lenses with larger diameters will have central and peripheral zones of different diameters. Ideally, an assortment of diameters and curvatures are kept on hand, and best fit, tolerance, and retention are assessed with empiric trials. Large-diameter soft lenses in SiHy materials have recently become available on a custom-order basis.

Characteristics of Scleral Lenses Used for Treatment of Ocular Surface Disease

In 1983, Ezekiel[3] reported the use of gas-permeable material in a scleral or 'haptic' lens solving the problem of hypoxia in a large-diameter contact lens. This innovation was applied successfully in that decade in innovative large-diameter RGP lens designs at centers of excellence around the world.[13–15] The Dk of RGP materials has exceeded that of soft lens materials until the advent of SiHy materials for soft lenses in the past decade. Once hypoxia was conquered by these high-Dk RGP materials, lens suction was the next challenge. Suction was circumvented, literally, by fenestration, which allows for air ventilation, or by haptic design with channels or contours that allow for fluid ventilation with no intrusion of air bubbles. Air ventilation is often satisfactory for eyes with optical indications, such as keratoconus or post-keratoplasty astigmatism, but air bubble(s) are typically not well tolerated in ocular surface disease. Reports of utility of RGP scleral lenses for OSD in general have emerged over the past two decades.[13,14,16–19] Success with this modality is dependent on the motivation and skill set of the clinician, as well as access to specialty lens manufacturing lab. A true scleral lens, well-fitted, with features, including a fluid reservoir, little movement, and no corneal touch, can provide support and protection for the corneal epithelium beyond that offered by any soft lens, and can be tolerated and retained in setting in which a soft lens is not.

There is a category of specialty contact lenses that is called 'mini-scleral,' 'semi-scleral,' and 'corneoscleral' lenses. The definitions and distinctions are evolving, and classifications may be based on the diameter, characteristics of fit or both. Generally, these lenses are 13–16 mm, made of high-Dk materials, may contact the cornea at the apex or peripherally, and the principles of fit are similar to those for an RGP corneal lens rather than a true scleral lens.[20] These larger RGP lenses are sometimes included among reports of scleral lenses. Although they may be more easily fitted and initially well tolerated, a reduced bearing zone and deliberate or unrecognized corneal touch centrally and at the limbus make these lenses less appropriate for patients with ocular surface disease as they may induce erosion, scarring and neovascularization in areas of contact, compression, or impingement.

Typically, scleral lenses are inserted and removed on a daily-wear basis with overnight disinfection. Newer materials developed in the past decade for overnight orthokeratology and FDA approved for that use, might be used in a large-diameter lens on a daily or overnight regimen on an off-label basis. The challenges of fitting the eye and training the patient or caretaker in daily insertion and removal limit the use of scleral lenses as a short-term 'bandage lens.' In certain circumstances, continuous wear coupled with daily removal, disinfection, and reinsertion may be appropriate for support of the ocular surface.[21,22]

PROSE Treatment

PROSE (Prosthetic Replacement of the Ocular Surface Ecosystem) treatment is an interdisciplinary paradigm that uses custom-fabricated prosthetic devices to replace and/or enhance the function of the ocular surface ecosystem, improving vision, comfort, and supporting the ocular surface. The device used in PROSE treatment was approved by the FDA in 1994 for daily wear in the treatment of irregular astigmatism and ocular surface disorders. Over the past 20 years, the PROSE device has been referred to as the Boston Scleral Contact Lens, the Boston Scleral Lens, the Boston Scleral Lens Device, the Boston Scleral Lens Prosthetic Device, and the Boston Ocular Surface Prosthesis (BOS-P).

The critical design and fitting features in PROSE treatment are that the device is fitted with no corneal contact, with fluid ventilation, and with minimal movement. One of the design features that distinguishes a PROSE device from a conventional scleral lens is that the contour of a PROSE device is defined mathematically by software that uses spline functions rather than by a superposition of base curves, yielding front and back surface profiles that are malleable and junctionless. At insertion, the device is filled with sterile saline or artificial tears, which remains oxygenated, due to the gas permeability of the material (Fig. 35.3). This fluid exchanges minimally with the precorneal tear film because of the precision of the fit. PROSE devices are distinguished from conventional scleral lenses in the degree to which they are customized per eye in order to eliminate movement, conjunctival impingement, and tissue compression that might ultimately reduce patient comfort and physiological tolerance.

A PROSE device creates a transparent and smooth optical surface over the irregular, damaged or diseased cornea. It reestablishes a healthy ocular surface environment by creating an expanded artificial tear reservoir that provides constant lubrication while maintaining necessary oxygen supply. A PROSE device then supports the fragile ocular surface by shielding the cornea and conjunctiva against insult from the environment and lids. PROSE treatment promotes healing, improves vision by masking surface corneal irregularities, and mitigates pain and photophobia by supporting and stabilizing the ocular surface (Fig. 35.4).

A 2000 report[17] reviewed the experience with PROSE for treatment of OSD in 49 patients (76 eyes). Improvement in best-corrected visual acuity (defined as a gain of two or more Snellen lines) was observed in 40 (53%) of the eyes. Forty-five (92%) of 49 patients reported improvement in quality of life from reduction in photophobia and discomfort. In a report from 2010,[19] 101 consecutive patients seen in consultation for PROSE treatment in 2006 were reviewed. The full spectrum of corneal disease, including corneal ectasia and postoperative astigmatism is represented, but nearly half of patients (38 of 80) who completed fitting

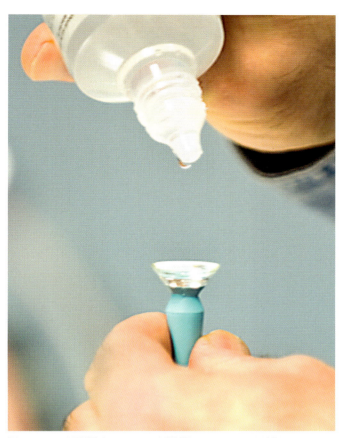

Figure 35.3 PROSE device being filled with sterile saline in preparation for insertion.

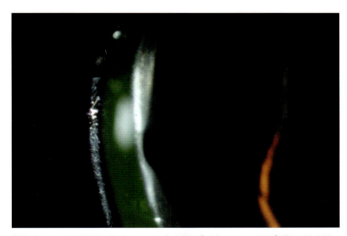

Figure 35.4 Fluorescein unmasks the fluid reservoir of this PROSE device in a patient with ocular surface disease and thinning from prior ulceration in Stevens–Johnson syndrome.

were referred for treatment of OSD. Mean visual acuity (VA) in the OSD cohort improved by −0.22 (logMAR). The authors report an increase in mean NEI VFQ-25[23,24] scores for the entire cohort from 57.0 to 77.8. Findings were similar for the OSD group, with only two patients recording a decrease in VFQ score in this group. Greater benefits in the VFQ subcategories of eye pain, photophobia, and role difficulties were seen in the OSD group than in the ectasia and

astigmatism subgroup. Cost effectiveness[25] of PROSE treatment in this cohort was also reported. As availability of PROSE treatment has increased, reports of clinical impact in cohorts with subgroups of OSD have arisen both in the United States[15] and abroad.[26]

Prevention and Treatment of Complications

Microbial keratitis, sterile melt, and corneal neovascularization are potential complications of contact lenses for ocular surface disease. In the absence of ocular surface disease, it is established that rates of infection is highest with extended wear, compared to daily wear regardless of soft lens type, and that RGP lens wear has the lowest infection rate.[11,12] Lens wear in the presence of punctate keratopathy or frank geographical defect of the corneal epithelium can be presumed to put the cornea at higher risk of infection, as would concurrent steroid use. There are no good data on prophylaxis or infection rate for contact lens use in the setting of OSD.

Approaches vary from one setting or clinical perspective to the next. Most clinicians would use antibiotic prophylaxis for any contact lens wear in the setting of a frank corneal epithelial defect, with agent/vehicle selected based on breadth of coverage, toxicity, cost, and availability. Later-generation fluoroquinolones and polymyxin/trimethoprim are good choices; aminoglycosides are sometimes chosen, but use in OSD should be limited, due to potential toxicity with continued use. Some clinicians favor institution of a reduced-frequency prophylactic regimen to avoid toxicity, but argument can be made for use at labeled frequency to avoid emergence of resistance. Some clinicians prescribe prophylactic antibiotics for any overnight wear in OSD, while other clinicians might prescribe antibiotics only if there is concurrent steroid use. It is practice at the authors' center, to use antibiotic prophylaxis only for overnight lens wear, in the setting of frank epithelial defect, regardless of lens type. The authors do not use antibiotic prophylaxis simply because of concurrent topical steroid use or for overnight wear in general, even in the presence of punctate keratopathy.

Infectious or sterile melt can accelerate under a lens, due to local hypoxia and/or stagnation of the precorneal tear film, which may contain lytic enzymes and toxic metabolites. Any patient fitted with a contact lens in the setting of an epithelial defect, or history of microbial or sterile ulceration, should be monitored closely, and warned to seek attention for any signs or symptoms of ulceration. Noncompliance may be a reason to seek an alternative other than therapeutic lens, such as tarsorrhaphy, in such cases.

Corneal neovascularization is a subacute complication of therapeutic contact lens wear, particularly in the setting of persistent epithelial defects, inflammatory processes, tight lens, or low Dk values. When neovascularization occurs, consideration must be given as to whether it is related to lens material, design and/or fit, or to the underlying disease, because treatment approaches vary, and lens discontinuation is not necessarily required. Vigilance and interdisciplinary collaboration between ophthalmology and optometry is required to avoid or treat this complication of contact lens wear when it arises in the setting of OSD. Maneuvers, such as switching to a higher-Dk lens, avoiding lens care products with epithelial toxicity, and introduction of topical steroid may allow for maintenance of the surface and regression of vessels without requiring the discontinuation of contact lens wear. At the authors' center, VEG-F inhibitors have been used as adjunct to PROSE treatment in the treatment of corneal neovascularization associated with OSD.[27]

An area of particular challenge is OSD in the setting of advanced glaucoma. Glaucoma patients may have surface breakdown resulting from either toxicity of topical agents, preservatives used in their formulation, and/or limbal stem cell deficiency (LSCD) from prior surgical interventions. Presence of a filtering bleb or tube shunt is a relative contraindication to contact lens wear in general and scleral lens fitting in particular because of risk of erosion and/or infection in an eye with direct communication between the anterior or posterior chambers and the subconjunctival space. The presence of the tube and plate(s) of a valve shunt may preclude a stable contact lens fit and may put the overlying conjunctiva at risk of erosion. Large-diameter hydrogel lenses are sometimes used for bleb leaks, and might be an appropriate choice for OSD in the presence of a filtering bleb or shunt. If a tube shunt is required for a patient with pre-existing cornea or OSD, it may be advisable to suggest to the surgeon pars plana entry for the tube and very posterior placement of the plates, using a long tube to facilitate subsequent-contact lens fitting and wear. PROSE devices can be fitted, with difficulty, in some patients with glaucoma tubes and trabeculectomies, which are usually relative contraindications to contact lens wear in general, particularly with scleral lens wear. Device modification after manufacture is the primary approach to dealing with limbal variants that are related to previous surgery.[28]

Contact Lens for Specific Ocular Surface diseases

RECURRENT EROSION SYNDROME

Soft contact lenses, on an extended wear basis, can result in satisfactory resolution of recurrent erosion syndrome (RES). A therapeutic lens is sometimes abandoned in favor of stromal micropuncture, superficial keratectomy with or without diamond burr polishing, or phototherapeutic keratectomy after a single trial of a suboptimal lens, or of well-fitted and tolerated lens worn for insufficient duration. Typically, months of wear, rather than weeks are required. Duration of wear in reports of effectiveness include 3 months,[29] and mean of 6 months.[30] If symptoms recur after discontinuation of lens wear it is this author's practice to double duration of wear prior to trial without lens. Lens selection, duration of therapy, frequency of exchange or disinfection, and use of antibiotic in the setting of treatment of RES vary from setting to setting.

PERSISTENT CORNEAL EPITHELIAL DEFECT (PED)

Contact lens wear is an important option in the treatment of a persistent corneal epithelial defect (PED).[31] Therapeutic

soft lens wear is used in normal eyes postoperatively in refractive surgery after surface ablation and in the case of traumatic and surgical wound leaks; in the latter cases, the local edema induced by a low-Dk lens might be desirable. In instances of a frank epithelial defect in the absence of a wound leak, a higher-Dk lens designed, manufactured, and labeled for extended wear or therapeutic use is advisable (Fig. 35.5). Appropriate fit may be a higher priority than material or labeling to achieve clinical tolerance. If prophylactic antibiotics are used, care should be taken to avoid drugs that are toxic. It is this author's opinion that topical steroids are not absolutely contraindicated in cases of PED treated with therapeutic contact lens, and that the risks of rebound inflammation must be weighed against the known risks of topical steroid use. Combination treatment with therapeutic lens and autologous serum eye drops may be more effective in PED than either treatment individually.[32,33]

Effectiveness of PROSE treatment for PED has been reported.[15,21] Recent experience with the use of non-preserved fluoroquinolones in the device reservoir for overnight wear in the setting of PED and daily monitoring have reduced the apparent rate of infection in PROSE treatment of PED. Extended wear of a PROSE device is effective in promoting the healing of a PED in some eyes that fail to heal

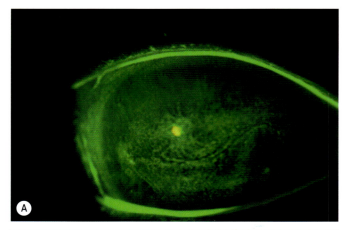

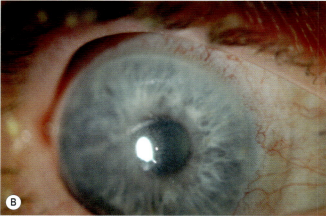

Figure 35.5 (**A**) Persistent epitheliopathy after pars plana vitrectomy. (**B**) High-Dk SiHy lens in place, to be worn overnight on a therapeutic basis.

after other therapeutic measures.[21,34] Infection was associated with extended wear, until the introduction of non-preserved fourth-generation fluoroquinolone antibiotics and the codification of device wear and hygiene regimens. Re-epithelialization appears to be supported by a combination of oxygenation, moisture, and protection of the fragile epithelium provided by the device.

LIMBAL STEM CELL DEFICIENCY (LSCD)

Therapeutic contact lenses have been reported as an adjunct to the treatment of LSCD of various etiologies. Soft contact lens therapy for aniridic ocular surface disease after penetrating keratoplasty has been reported.[35] Scleral lenses are reported as beneficial in LSCD of uncertain etiology[36] and in a case of ocular cicatricial pemphigoid.[37] PROSE treatment has been reported effective in the treatment of LSCD after treatment of conjunctival melanoma.[38] The specific type of lens for the specific entity is probably less important than the skill and experience of the clinician who is fitting lenses in these inflamed and sensitive eyes. All three reports involving epitheliopathy ascribed to LSCD, point to the capacity of a well-fitted scleral lens or PROSE device to improve clinical function by improving the environment at the ocular surface. Contact lens wear holds promise as a platform for expansion and transplantation of expanded stem cell populations. There is an early report on the use of an FDA-approved contact lens as the substrate and carrier of corneal stem cells in treatment of ocular surface melanoma and aniridia.[39]

STEVENS–JOHNSON SYNDROME (SJS)

A retrospective review from France, published in 2009 by Tougeron-Brousseau et al.,[40] details the authors' experience fitting scleral RGP lenses in a cohort of 39 consecutive patients. Sixty-seven eyes of the 39 patients diagnosed with Stevens–Johnson syndrome (SJS) or toxic epidermal necrolysis (TEN) were deemed candidates for scleral RGP wear at consultation. OSDI, NEI-VFQ-25, and VA were all outcome measures with the investigators finding significant improvement in all three categories. Mean follow-up was 33.3 months (range 16 to 54 months). The authors did not report on the patients they classified as non-candidates.

Patients with SJS/TEN have been described in the major reports[17,19,41] on PROSE treatment from the past two decades, although there has not been specific analysis of this disease subgroup. It is the authors' experience that PROSE treatment is life changing for patients suffering from the ocular sequelae of SJS. Typically, there is marked improvement in surface breakdown and debilitating photophobia (Fig. 35.6). PROSE treatment can heal a PED in SJS on full-time-wear basis, and then support the healed surface on a daily-wear basis.[21] The limiting factors for PROSE treatment in SJS are presence of symblephara to the cornea or limbus, and poor cooperation in children.

Rathi et al.[26] from India report their experience with PROSE treatment for 20 eyes in SJS patients who were treated primarily for relief of pain and photophobia and secondarily for improvement in vision. Although no method was taken to quantify the symptomatic relief, all patients reported a reduction in symptoms, and the authors

concluded that their findings regarding PROSE treatment of SJS patients was encouraging.

CHRONIC GRAFT-VERSUS-HOST DISEASE (CGVHD)

PROSE treatment has high impact in patients suffering from the ocular graft-versus-host disease (GVHD) as indicated in two reports from 2007. Jacobs and Rosenthal[42] report on the impact of PROSE treatment in cGVHD with benefit in comfort, vision, reading, and driving, and Takahide et al.[43] report on benefit on vision, clinical findings, and OSDI. Jupiter lenses (Medlens Innovations, Front Royal, VA, or Essilor Contact Lens, Inc., Dallas, TX)[44] and silicone hydrogel soft-contact lenses (Air Optix Night & Day, Alcon, Forth Worth, TX)[45] can also play a role in the management of GVHD. All four studies found improvement in symptoms, with Russo et al.[45] and Takahide et al.[43] both noting significant changes in OSDI scores. Ocular cGVHD is a disease for which scleral or soft lenses or PROSE treatment is an important option, since little else provides symptomatic relief for these patients. Until ocular cGVHD can be prevented or medically suppressed, therapeutic lens, and PROSE treatment in particular, is an important approach to improved quality of life in patients with cGVHD.

ALLERGY

Ocular surface disease associated with allergy can be treated with therapeutic contact lens wear. Large-diameter soft hydrogel lens wear contributed to the resolution of vernal ulcer in children.[46] Scleral RGP lenses had favorable response in management of the ocular surface and visual rehabilitation of 10 patients with medically controlled advanced atopic keratoconjunctivitis.[47] Atopic keratoconjunctivitis is a cause of disabling ocular surface disease and is not infrequently associated with keratoconus. PROSE treatment with its high degree of customization allows for the optical correction of keratoconus when there is coexistent atopy, which typically reduces contact lens tolerance.

EXPOSURE KERATOPATHY

Contact lens wear can reduce desiccation and resultant corneal surface breakdown in instances of anatomic or paralytic exposure keratitis. Underlying etiologies include cranial nerve VII dysfunction from Bell's palsy and tumor impingement or nerve damage following tumor resection, as with acoustic neuroma, schwannoma, or parotid gland tumors. Additional causes include trauma, history of cosmetic blepharoplasty or ptosis surgery, and thermal injury. Soft lenses are prone to the same desiccation as the ocular surface, so retention can be problematic. Hydrogel lenses of very large diameter offer increased retention. The benefits of PROSE treatment for exposure keratitis have been reported.[22,48,49]

A PROSE device is a valuable option for treatment of corneal exposure. Rosenthal and Croteau[50] reported success of PROSE treatment in 4 of 10 eyes with exposure (both paralytic and anatomic) when other measures, short of complete tarsorrhaphy, failed. In 2008, Lin et al.[49] described a case study in which PROSE treatment proved to be a useful adjunct in a patient with history of lymphoma

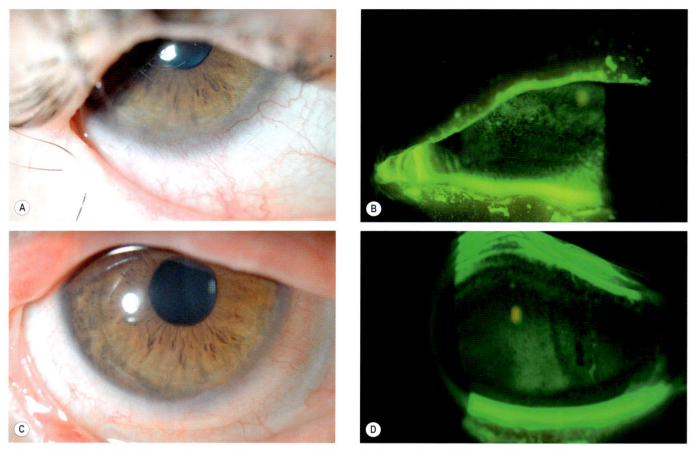

Figure 35.6 White light and fluorescein/blue light images of the right eye of a 9-year-old boy with history of Stevens–Johnson syndrome at age 5. (**A**) An image of the ocular surface in soft SiHy lens worn on a daily-wear basis for relief of symptoms of foreign body sensation and photophobia. (**B**) Staining pattern immediately upon removal. (**C**) The same eye with a PROSE device which offered greater relief. (**D**) Improved state of the ocular surface immediately after removal. (**C** and **D** also reveal greater capacity to cooperate for examination and photography.) BCVA has remained 20/25 OD and OS. Topical steroids have been used concurrently with soft lens and PROSE device wear. Mucous membrane grafting of keratinized lid margins has also been undertaken.

and cGVHD. The patient was treated for a secondary facial sarcoma with surgical and radiation therapy. PROSE treatment allowed for preservation of the ocular surface and the globe. PROSE treatment is an alternative to tarsorrhaphy in the management of both anatomic and paralytic exposure keratitis.

NEUROTROPHIC KERATOPATHY

Therapeutic soft contact lens wear is among the stepwise options for the treatment of neurotrophic keratopathy of various etiologies.[51] Patients with neurotrophic keratopathy are included in the reports of PROSE treatment for OSD and for PEDs.[15,21,34]

Conclusion

The successful treatment of ocular surface disease requires attention to four guiding principles. There must be treatment of underlying local processes, and there must be treatment of underlying systemic processes. The environment at the ocular surface must be optimized and this is

the role of the contact lens. Finally, adequate progenitor and amplifying stem cells must be present. Clinicians will serve their patients well to be familiar with the full range of therapeutic contact lens options for the treatment of OSD.

References

1. Fick AE. A contact lens. 1888. Arch Ophthalmol 1997;115: 120–1.
2. Pearson RM. Karl Otto Himmler, manufacturer of the first contact lens. Cont Lens Anterior Eye 2007;30:11–6.
3. Ezekiel D. Gas permeable haptic lenses. Br Contact Lens Assoc 1983;6:158–61.
4. Karlgard CC, Jones LW, Moresoli C. Survey of bandage lens use in North America, October-December 2002. Eye Contact Lens 2004; 30:25–30.
5. Management and therapy of dry eye disease: report of the Management and Therapy Subcommittee of the International Dry Eye WorkShop (2007). Ocul Surf 2007;5:163–78.
6. Lindahl KJ, DePaolis MD, Aquavella JV, et al. Applications of hydrophilic disposable contact lenses as therapeutic bandages. CLAO J 1991;17:241–3.
7. Bouchard CS, Trimble SN. Indications and complications of therapeutic disposable Acuvue contact lenses. CLAO J 1996;22:106–8.
8. Bendoriene J, Vogt U. Therapeutic use of silicone hydrogel contact lenses in children. Eye Contact Lens 2006;32:104–8.

9. Kanpolat A, Uçakhan OO. Therapeutic use of focus Night & Day contact lenses. Cornea 2003;22:726–34.

10. Lim L, Tan DT, Chan WK. Therapeutic use of Bausch & Lomb PureVision contact lenses. CLAO J 2001;27:179–85.

11. Stapleton F, Keay L, Edwards K, et al. The incidence of contact lens-related microbial keratitis in Australia. Ophthalmology 2008; 115:1655–62.

12. Dart JK, Radford CF, Minassian D, et al. Risk factors for microbial keratitis with contemporary contact lenses: a case-control study. Ophthalmology 2008;115:1647–54, 54 e1–e3.

13. Visser ES, Visser R, van Lier HJ, et al. Modern scleral lenses part I: clinical features. Eye Contact Lens 2007;33:13–20.

14. Visser ES, Visser R, van Lier HJ, et al. Modern scleral lenses part II: patient satisfaction. Eye Contact Lens 2007;33:21–5.

15. Gumus K, Gire A, Pflugfelder SC. The successful use of Boston ocular surface prosthesis in the treatment of persistent corneal epithelial defect after herpes zoster ophthalmicus. Cornea 2010;29: 1465–8.

16. Pullum K, Buckley R. Therapeutic and ocular surface indications for scleral contact lenses. Ocul Surf 2007;5:40–8.

17. Romero-Rangel T, Stavrou P, Cotter J, et al. Gas-permeable scleral contact lens therapy in ocular surface disease. Am J Ophthalmol 2000;130:25–32.

18. Severinsky B, Millodot M. Current applications and efficacy of scleral contact lenses – a retrospective study. J Optometry 2010;03: 158–63.

19. Stason WB, Razavi M, Jacobs DS, et al. Clinical benefits of the Boston Ocular Surface Prosthesis. Am J Ophthalmol 2010;149:54–61.

20. Ye P, Sun A, Weissman BA. Role of mini-scleral gas-permeable lenses in the treatment of corneal disorders. Eye Contact Lens 2007; 33:111–3.

21. Rosenthal P, Cotter JM, Baum J. Treatment of persistent corneal epithelial defect with extended wear of a fluid-ventilated gas-permeable scleral contact lens. Am J Ophthalmol 2000;130:33–41.

22. Kalwerisky K, Davies B, Mihora L, et al. Use of the Boston ocular surface prosthesis in the management of severe periorbital thermal injuries: a case series of 10 patients. Ophthalmology 2012;119: 516–21.

23. Mangione CM, Lee PP, Gutierrez PR, et al. Development of the 25-item National Eye Institute Visual Function Questionnaire. Arch Ophthalmol 2001;119:1050–8.

24. Raphael BA, Galetta KM, Jacobs DA, et al. Validation and test characteristics of a 10-item neuro-ophthalmic supplement to the NEI-VFQ-25. Am J Ophthalmol 2006;142:1026–35.

25. Shepard DS, Razavi M, Stason WB, et al. Economic appraisal of the Boston Ocular Surface Prosthesis. Am J Ophthalmol 2009;148: 860–8 e2.

26. Rathi VM, Mandathara PS, Dumpati S, et al. Boston ocular surface prosthesis: An Indian experience. Ind J Ophthalmol 2011;59: 279–81.

27. Jacobs DS, Lim M, Carrasquillo KG, et al. Bevacizumab for corneal neovascularization. Ophthalmology 2009;116:592–3; author reply 3–4.

28. Tanhehco T, Jacobs DS. Technological advances shaping scleral lenses: the Boston ocular surface prosthesis in patients with glaucoma tubes and trabeculectomies. Semin Ophthalmol 2010;25:233–8.

29. Fraunfelder FW, Cabezas M. Treatment of recurrent corneal erosion by extended-wear bandage contact lens. Cornea 2011;30:164–6.

30. Moutray TN, Frazer DG, Jackson AJ. Recurrent erosion syndrome – the patient's perspective. Cont Lens Anterior Eye 2011;34:139–43.

31. Blackmore SJ. The use of contact lenses in the treatment of persistent epithelial defects. Cont Lens Anterior Eye 2010;33:239–44.

32. Choi JA, Chung SH. Combined application of autologous serum eye drops and silicone hydrogel lenses for the treatment of persistent epithelial defects. Eye Contact Lens 2011;37:370–3.

33. Schrader S, Wedel T, Moll R, et al. Combination of serum eye drops with hydrogel bandage contact lenses in the treatment of persistent epithelial defects. Graefes Arch Clin Exp Ophthalmol 2006; 244:1345–9.

34. Rosenthal P, Cotter J. The Boston Scleral Lens in the management of severe ocular surface disease. Ophthalmol Clin N Am 2003; 16:89–93.

35. Ozbek Z, Raber IM. Successful management of aniridic ocular surface disease with long-term bandage contact lens wear. Cornea 2006; 25:245–7.

36. Schornack MM. Limbal stem cell disease: management with scleral lenses. Clin Exp Optom 2011.

37. Schornack MM, Baratz KH. Ocular cicatricial pemphigoid: the role of scleral lenses in disease management. Cornea 2009;28:1170–2.

38. Grover S, Jacobs DS, Colby KA. Boston Ocular Surface Prosthesis for persistent epitheliopathy after treatment of conjunctival melanoma. Cornea. 2010;29:459–61.

39. Di Girolamo N, Bosch M, Zamora K, et al. A contact lens-based technique for expansion and transplantation of autologous epithelial progenitors for ocular surface reconstruction. Transplantation 2009;87:1571–8.

40. Tougeron-Brousseau B, Delcampe A, Gueudry J, et al. Vision-related function after scleral lens fitting in ocular complications of Stevens–Johnson syndrome and toxic epidermal necrolysis. Am J Ophthalmol 2009;148:852–9 e2.

41. Schein OD, Rosenthal P, Ducharme C. A gas-permeable scleral contact lens for visual rehabilitation. Am J Ophthalmol 1990;109:318–22.

42. Jacobs DS, Rosenthal P. Boston scleral lens prosthetic device for treatment of severe dry eye in chronic graft-versus-host disease. Cornea 2007;26:1195–9.

43. Takahide K, Parker PM, Wu M, et al. Use of fluid-ventilated, gas-permeable scleral lens for management of severe keratoconjunctivitis sicca secondary to chronic graft-versus-host disease. Biol Blood Marrow Transplant 2007;13:1016–21.

44. Schornack MM, Baratz KH, Patel SV, et al. Jupiter scleral lenses in the management of chronic graft versus host disease. Eye Contact Lens 2008;34:302–5.

45. Russo PA, Bouchard CS, Galasso JM. Extended-wear silicone hydrogel soft contact lenses in the management of moderate to severe dry eye signs and symptoms secondary to graft-versus-host disease. Eye Contact Lens 2007;33:144–7.

46. Quah SA, Hemmerdinger C, Nicholson S, et al. Treatment of refractory vernal ulcers with large-diameter bandage contact lenses. Eye Contact Lens 2006;32:245–7.

47. Margolis R, Thakrar V, Perez VL. Role of rigid gas-permeable scleral contact lenses in the management of advanced atopic keratoconjunctivitis. Cornea 2007;26:1032–4.

48. Williams ZR, Aquavella JV. Management of exposure keratopathy associated with severe craniofacial trauma. J Cataract Refract Surg 2007;33:1647–50.

49. Lin SJ, Jacobs DS, Frankenthaler R, et al. An ocular surface prosthesis as an innovative adjunct in patients with head and neck malignancy. Otolaryngol Head Neck Surg 2008;139:589–91.

50. Rosenthal P, Croteau A. Fluid-ventilated, gas-permeable scleral contact lens is an effective option for managing severe ocular surface disease and many corneal disorders that would otherwise require penetrating keratoplasty. Eye Contact Lens 2005;31:130–4.

51. Pushker N, Dada T, Vajpayee RB, et al. Neurotrophic keratopathy. CLAO J 2001;27:100–7.

36 Ocular Surface Disease: Surgical Management

DAVID S. ROOTMAN, JUDY Y. F. KU and SONIA N. YEUNG

Introduction

Ocular surface dysfunction is the final common pathway that occurs as a result of an imbalance of ocular surface protective mechanisms. Each protective mechanism has its specific role, be it mechanical and/or physiological. Externally, the eyelids act as a physical barrier for protection of the ocular surface, and with each blink it distributes the tear film. Meanwhile, the corneal and conjunctival epithelia provide the biodefense system against microorganisms and proteolytic enzymes. The tear film is crucial, since it lubricates, protects and nourishes, as well as provides a smooth optical refractive surface. As in an orchestra, each component must function in concert to create a harmonious (and healthy) whole. For example, poor epithelial adherence to the basement membrane can lead to recurrent corneal erosion; lagophthalmos can lead to exposure keratopathy; these can all be exacerbated by the loss of corneal sensation and dry eyes.

When conventional medical therapy fails and/or secondary complications (such as persistent epithelial defect, scarring) occur, surgical intervention needs to be considered. The primary goals are to increase lubrication, to assist healing and epithelial adherence, to remove visually significant opacities and to restore sight with minimal side effects. This chapter reviews the current knowledge on various surgical procedures that assist in the protection and stabilization of the ocular surface in a variety of diseases.

ANTERIOR STROMAL PUNCTURE

History

In 1986, McLean and MacRae observed that recurrent corneal erosion (RCE) often followed superficial corneal trauma but was not seen after deep stromal laceration.[1] In light of this, they described the technique of anterior stromal puncture (ASP) for the treatment of RCE, which employed a 20G needle at the slit lamp to make multiple punctures through loose epithelium and Bowman's layer into the anterior stroma. This created a more secure bonding of the epithelium to the underlying basement membrane (BM), Bowman's layer, and stroma. This treatment has been shown to be effective, particularly in post-traumatic corneal erosions.

Indication

The therapeutic aim of ASP is to enhance epithelial adhesion to the BM by microscopic, superficial scar formation.

In RCE, the cause is thought to be failure of the wounded epithelial cells to adhere to the underlying stroma. This could be secondary to weak hemidesmosomal attachment, reduplication of the BM, the action of metalloproteinases,[2] and/or disruption of type VII collagen fibrils.[3]

ASP is a well-accepted treatment for RCE.[1,4,5] ASP induces reactive subepithelial fibrosis or production of extracellular matrix proteins, both of which may be responsible for increased adhesion of the epithelium.[6] Success rates of up to 80% have been reported in recalcitrant RCE.[1,4,5]

While phototherapeutic keratectomy (PTK) has also been shown to be effective, there are advantages of ASP over PTK. ASP can be easily performed in the office or outpatient setting with simple, inexpensive equipment and causes minimal discomfort. Moreover, there is a low risk of inducing visually significant scarring and changes in refraction.

Recently, ASP was reported to be used for RCE after laser in situ keratomileusis (LASIK), which helped in resolving secondary diffuse lamellar keratitis.[4] However, performing ASP immediately after LASIK may cause flap displacement and must be used judiciously.

Procedure

Anterior stromal puncture (ASP) is performed under topical anesthesia. Multiple superficial punctures are placed less than 0.5 mm apart in the affected area with a bent 25G needle attached to a 1- or 3-mL syringe. The needle can be bent at the tip with a needle holder to allow only superficial penetration into the cornea. Fluorescein can be instilled to define the affected area. Treatment is extended at least 1 mm into the normal epithelium bordering the lesion. Following the procedure, a bandage contact lens (BCL) is placed, and antibiotics drops are given until complete re-epithelialization. Usually, when ASP is begun, a much larger area of poorly adherent epithelium becomes visible.

ASP can also be performed with a short-pulsed Nd:YAG laser.[7] The Nd:YAG laser (1.8–2.2 mJ) is focused at the BM zone after epithelial debridement. Spots are placed in rows approximately 0.20–0.25 mm apart. The advantage of laser over needle puncture is that the laser puncture is more uniform, shallow and translucent. There may also be less corneal scarring, so the procedure can be repeated and can be used closer to the visual axis.[7]

Contraindications

Anterior stromal puncture may result in subepithelial scars, and its use is not advisable if the erosion encroaches on the visual axis since the resulting scar may result in glare and a reduction in vision. In addition, if performed over the pupil, ASP may induce multifocal scars and irregular topographic changes. In general, however, the scarring is minimal and has little effect on vision.

Key Surgical Points

- Avoid this procedure over the visual axis.
- The use of a bent 25G needle will lessen the chance of corneal perforation, while ensuring adequate puncture depth.
- This procedure may need to be repeated.

Complications

One of the major concerns with regard to the safety of ASP is corneal perforation. To address this concern, Rubinfeld and Laibson designed a specially bent needle for use on a disposable handle.[5] An insertion depth of 0.1 mm was found to be sufficient to cause a therapeutic, fibrocytic reaction.[6]

Another concern is scarring, due to deep stromal penetration, which may affect vision, especially if the visual axis is involved. Smaller-gauge needles have been used to minimize scarring but deeper incisions were reported with 27G or 30G needles.

ASP can be a safe and effective therapy if performed under a magnified view at the slit lamp.

PUNCTAL OCCLUSION

History

Occlusion of the nasolacrimal outflow tract was first described by Beetham in 1935.[8] He reported resolution of dry eye in eight eyes with filamentary keratitis with electrocautery or diathermy to occlude the puncta. In 1975, Freeman[9] proposed the use of punctal plugs to provide a reversible blockade of the nasolacrimal tract at the punctum. Semi-permanent and permanent punctal plugs are now widely used and are available in a range of sizes to ensure a good fit.

Indication

The principle behind punctal occlusion is the increase of the aqueous component of the tear film by blocking tear outflow and retention of both natural and artificial tears on the ocular surface. It has been shown to improve symptoms of lacrimal insufficiency. Tamponade is the most popular method, because surgery is not required and it is reversible.

Patients with severe keratoconjunctivitis sicca with or without underlying systemic collagen vascular disease often require permanent punctal occlusion. Punctal occlusion also plays a beneficial role in aqueous tear deficiencies secondary to ocular surface conditions, such as ocular cicatricial pemphigoid, Stevens–Johnson syndrome, and

Sjögren syndrome.[10,11] Dry eye secondary to reduced reflex tearing found in neurotrophic keratitis can also be effectively managed with this procedure. Finally, punctal occlusion may be beneficial in patients with dry eyes, due to increased evaporation from an exposed ocular surface. This may occur with lagophthalmos, exophthalmos seen with thyroid conditions, and following blepharoplasties. Other than dry eye syndromes, punctal occlusion has been shown to improve contact lens comfort and also may be helpful in the management of superior limbic keratoconjunctivitis.[12]

Punctal occlusion can dramatically improve the quality of life in many patients with moderate cases of dry eyes and can prevent visual loss in patients with severe cases of dry eyes.

Procedure

TEMPORARY PROCEDURES

Collagen Implants

Collagen implants provide temporary (usually less than 2 weeks) occlusion of the lacrimal drainage system. They are threaded into the canaliculus with jewelers' forceps. They can sometimes act as a test to see if more permanent methods would be beneficial or cause symptoms, such as epiphora.

Silicone Plugs

In this technique, the eye is anesthetized with a topical anesthetic. At the slit lamp, the size of the punctum is measured with a special gauge, which determines the size of plug to be used. The plug is inserted into the punctum until the domed head lies flush with the punctum. The inserter is then released and withdrawn. The plug can easily be removed with jeweler's forceps if its placement rubs against the conjunctiva or if epiphora results.

PERMANENT PROCEDURES

Thermal Methods

Thermal methods involve occlusion of the punctum by shrinking the canalicular walls with argon laser, cautery, or diathermy.[13,14] Even with thorough cauterization, the canaliculus may reopen in time. One of the most common techniques to accomplish permanent punctual closure is electrocautery. The eyelid adjacent to the punctum is infiltrated with local anesthetic (LA). A topical anesthetic is instilled in the cul-de-sac. The electrocautery instrument (Hyfrecator, Birtcher Corp., Los Angeles, CA) with a fine-needle tip is threaded into the punctum and along the canaliculus. The instrument is engaged while withdrawing the instrument slowly. The canaliculus is thermally de-epithelialized. Additional cautery may be performed at the punctal opening.

Thermal cauterization has been reported to be efficient in achieving punctal occlusion, with a reported recanalization rate of 26.1%.[10] Recently, a recanalization rate of 1.4% was reported with a high-heat-energy-releasing cautery device.[14] Thermal cauterization is performed similarly to electrocautery. Following LA, the loop tip of a disposable cautery is pinched together with sterile forceps to create a needle-tipped probe. This tip is resterilized at any time by turning the cautery on. If the probe does not insert into the canaliculus, the punctum is dilated with a dilator. The tip is threaded into the punctum and along the canaliculus. The instrument is then engaged while withdrawing the instrument slowly.

Contraindication/Cautions

Punctal occlusion is not indicated for all patients who have symptoms of dry eye. Many mild to moderate cases can be managed with the use of topical lubricating drops. Dry eye symptoms may manifest as a result of improperly fitted contact lenses; in these cases, a proper fitting will usually resolve the symptoms. Many commonly used oral medications with antihistaminic or anticholinergic properties can cause reversible ocular dryness. As such, punctal occlusion is not indicated when ocular dryness is a temporary condition.

Key Surgical Points

- Although permanent punctal occlusion can significantly reduce the symptoms of dry eye, epiphora can result with improper patient selection.
- Blepharitis and dry eyes frequently coexist and treatment of both is necessary.
- Patients with severe chronic dry eye or those who benefit from punctal plugs but experience repeated plug loss should be considered for permanent punctal occlusion.
- As occlusion of upper and lower puncta at the same time may increase the risk of epiphora, the procedures should be performed one at a time.
- Even with cautery, permanent punctal occlusion may not be achieved and the procedure may need to be repeated.
- If granulation around a silicone plug is noted, it should resolve with removal of the punctual plug.

Complications

Punctal plugs can cause ocular discomfort and complications,[15,16] such as punctum enlargement, loss or migration or extrusion of the implant, epiphora, pyogenic granuloma, local inflammatory reaction to silicone, dacryocystitis, and canaliculitis.[16,17]

Granuloma formation is thought to be caused by local stimulation by the plug. Intracanalicular plugs are associated with higher rate of granulation tissue formation in the lacrimal tract when, compared with other forms of punctal plugs. Cases have been reported in which plug migration inside the lacrimal passage resulted in peripheral inflammations and infections, requiring surgical removal.[18]

Epithelial irritation caused by the exposed portion of the plug coming into contact with the cornea and conjunctiva may occur. Removing the plug or placing the plug with one of a different configuration may help.

PHOTOTHERAPEUTIC KERATECTOMY

History

The laser–tissue phenomenon of photoablation was first demonstrated in 1983 by Trokel and Srinivasan,[19] who were working on the ultraviolet 193-nm excimer laser. Its potential role in refractive and therapeutic corneal surgery was quickly recognized. The excimer laser underwent extensive preclinical trials before it was applied to human eyes, and it is now being used for photorefractive keratectomy (PRK), LASIK and PTK.

Excimer laser PTK utilizes 193-nm wavelength ultraviolet light to break the molecular bonds in corneal tissue, in turn ablating the anterior stroma in a highly predictable fashion. It was approved by the FDA in 1995 for the treatment of visually significant anterior corneal pathologies, namely superficial corneal dystrophies, epithelial basement membrane dystrophy (EBMD) with irregular corneal surfaces, corneal scars and opacities.[20]

Advantages

The main advantages of PTK over mechanical superficial keratectomy (SK) include precise tissue ablation with minimal damage to the surrounding tissues, a smooth residual bed for corneal re-epithelialization, and repeatability of the treatment. Compared to lamellar or penetrating keratoplasty (PKP), it is also less invasive, with more rapid visual recovery. PTK can be performed before or after PKP and does not impair the prognosis of PKP.[21]

Disadvantages

Phototherapeutic keratectomy may ablate normal tissue at a different rate from scar tissue, which may result in an irregular surface. Hence, masking agents are often used to fill in any irregular troughs to achieve a smoother surface. In contrast, a surgical plane between normal and abnormal tissue is more readily identified during mechanical SK, which provides a better surgical dissection.

Indications

Phototherapeutic keratectomy is best utilized for corneal pathologies affecting the epithelium or anterior 10–20% of the corneal stroma. For safety reasons, the residual corneal bed thickness must be greater than 300 μm at the end of the procedure. The indications for PTK can be separated into four broad categories,[20] although they often overlap:

- superficial opacities, e.g. granular dystrophy (Fig. 36.1), scars from trauma or keratitis, post-PRK haze (Fig. 36.2)
- elevated lesions or irregularities of the corneal surface, e.g. Salzmann's nodular degeneration (SND), keratoconus nodules
- EBMD, e.g. RCE

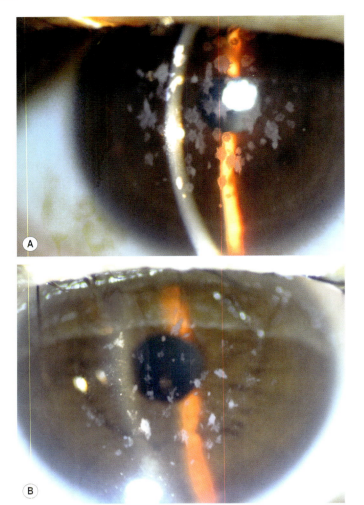

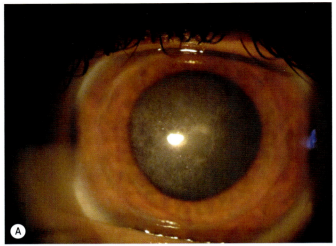

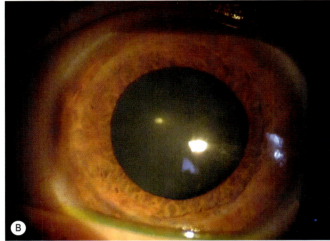

Figure 36.1 Granular dystrophy treated with PTK and PRK. (**A**) A 46-year-old woman with decreased best-corrected visual acuity (BCVA) of 20/40 (+0.50/−2.75 × 13) from granular dystrophy in the left eye. (**B**) After transepithelial PTK combined with PRK treatment, at 1 month postoperatively, there was a significant reduction in density of opacities. The BCVA improved to 20/30 with significant reduction in refractive error (−0.50/−0.25 × 141).

Figure 36.2 A 41-year-old man with previous IntraLase™ enabled keratoplasty and post PRK haze in the left eye. (**A**) Subepithelial and superficial stromal haze centrally, in a honeycomb reticular pattern. This was visually significant (BCVA 20/40−1). (**B**) Post PTK with MMC. At day 4 the central graft was clear and the epithelium has healed. His BCVA improved to 20/25−2.

- Others
  - painful bullous keratopathy
  - band keratopathy
  - post-LASIK complications, e.g. flap striae.

Contraindications

It is important to identify patients who have conditions that predispose them to delayed epithelial healing and who would not be suitable candidates for PTK. They include immunocompromised individuals and patients with anesthetic corneas, severe dry eyes or uncontrolled uveitis.[20] Others may require additional procedures prior to PTK, e.g. a patient with lagophthalmos secondary to paralytic ectropion may require ectropion repair first. Any deep corneal pathology requiring removal of more than 20–30% of corneal thickness may be more suitable for anterior lamellar keratoplasty rather than PTK. If

there is significant thinning in the treatment zone, PTK may predispose them to ectasia and hence should be avoided.

Preoperative Assessment

All patients should be assessed carefully to determine suitability for PTK. There are four main areas that the surgeon should consider: (1) whether the corneal pathology is amenable to PTK treatment anatomically, (2) the patient's healing ability after surgery, (3) whether the goal of the PTK treatment is achievable, and (4) tailoring a surgical approach to the pathology. As with all surgeries, it is important to establish realistic expectations with the patient. For example, for a patient with granular dystrophy, the goal of PTK is often not a crystal-clear cornea, but rather improvement in vision so that one could delay or even avoid keratoplasty.

PATIENT HISTORY

Once the diagnosis is established, one should clarify the chief complaints. For example, in a patient with RCE, how frequent and how long are the painful episodes? Were they amenable to medical therapy? This will give some guidance as to whether the symptoms will likely be alleviated with PTK. Past ocular and medical history are important to determine whether the patient has potential corneal healing abnormalities, such as neurotrophic corneas (e.g. herpes simplex or herpes zoster keratitis), previous corneal grafts, exposure keratopathy, collagen vascular conditions (e.g. rheumatoid arthritis) and diabetes mellitus. Certain systemic immunosuppressive agents may also prevent healing after PTK. In addition, those with a history of herpes simplex keratitis (HSK) are at risk of recurrence after PTK.

EXAMINATION

A thorough examination should be performed to: (1) confirm the diagnosis, (2) ensure that the symptoms and signs correlate (e.g. that the level of visual loss corresponds to the severity of the corneal opacity), (3) detect other co-morbidities that may be responsible for poor vision (e.g. glaucoma, maculopathy), and (4) evaluate the corneal abnormality in detail.

Using slit lamp biomicroscopy, one should determine the size, depth, location, and density of the corneal abnormality, as well as any corneal thinning. In general, PTK is most suited to patients with superficial stromal opacities without significant irregularity and thinning, and those with small, central, elevated corneal lesions not amenable to SK.[22] If the lesion is deep enough that the residual corneal thickness approaches 300 μm, one should exercise caution. In this scenario, either lamellar or penetrating keratoplasty may be the preferred treatment.

IMAGING

Recent advancements in anterior segment imaging technology can be useful in the surgical planning of these cases. Subtle surface irregularities can be difficult to detect clinically. Corneal topography can highlight any irregularities of the cornea and document any irregular astigmatism. Pentacam® tomography (OCULUS Optikgerate GmbH, Watzlar, Germany) also provides Scheimflug imaging, which can illustrate the depth of the corneal lesions, although the resolution is limited. High-frequency ultrasound biomicroscopy may be of more use for large lesions. High-resolution anterior segment optical coherence tomography is a quick, non-contact imaging modality that can provide pachymetric mapping of corneal opacities.[23] It could potentially result in more accurate resection of tissues during PTK. Sometimes, accurate depth is difficult to determine with these modalities as they all are subject to posterior shadowing which may overestimate the depth of lesions.

Procedure

For PTK, the surgical technique varies depending on the characteristics of the pathology. This includes the size, shape, location, density and depth of the lesions.

The general principles are:

- Maintain a smooth surface if possible, e.g. a patient with granular dystrophy with a smooth epithelium could be treated with transepithelial PTK, in which case the epithelium is used as the masking agent.
- In those with loose epithelium (e.g. RCE) or elevated lesions (e.g. SND), mechanical debridement (or with adjunctive 20–50% alcohol for 5–10 seconds) with a blade should be utilized prior to PTK.
- Remove the least amount of tissue to achieve the desired results by frequently stopping and checking the results under the microscope or the slit lamp before proceeding with further laser treatments.
- Maintain centration of the treatment zone to avoid inducing irregular astigmatism.
- Use a controlled amount of modulating or masking agent to achieve a uniform corneal surface (e.g. artificial tears or balanced saline solution).
- For superficial opacities, the goal is to clear as much of the opacity centrally as possible while resisting the temptation to ablate deeper tissues (which can result in excessive induced hyperopia).
- For RCE, only aim to remove 5–6 μm of the Bowman's membrane.
- For focal corneal scars, one may partially treat any induced refractive error, or use an opaque mask (e.g. use a specifically shaped weckcell sponge) if the treatment will remove tissue in an area where it is not desirable.

In general, the treatment zone should be tailored to the abnormality. For example, granular dystrophy could be treated with a larger treatment zone of around 6–7 mm diameter, while a 2-mm Salzmann's nodule centrally should be treated with a 2–3-mm spot size. After laser ablation has been completed, topical antibiotics and steroids are applied along with a soft bandage contact lens (BCL). However, some advocate the use of a pressure patch rather than a BCL if there is a history of HSK or in a neurotrophic cornea. The patient should be reviewed frequently until re-epithelialization is complete. For RCE patients, after removal of the BCL, the use of hyperosmotic 5% sodium chloride ointment at bedtime may reduce the recurrence of erosions.

Adjunct Therapy

In recent years, mitomycin C (MMC) has been shown to be effective in reducing the occurrence of corneal haze following excimer laser ablation.[24] Corneas requiring PTK are inherently at higher risk of haze, due to the presence of stimulated fibroblasts, surface irregularities (e.g. SND) and potential suboptimal healing ability (e.g. RCE). The ideal concentration and duration of MMC exposure remains controversial. Depending on the surgeon's preference and the pathology, the dosage may range from 0.001% to 0.04%, with a duration of application between 12 seconds to 2 minutes.[24] For high-risk patients, such as PTK post-corneal transplant or repeat treatments, the authors recommend 0.02% with a minimum application of 30 seconds.

Hyperopic shifts are common after PTK, due to central flattening, particularly in those with deeper ablations.[25] This could be managed post-PTK with contact lenses or sequential hyperopic PRK treatment. If the patient has pre-existing hyperopia, one could combine PTK and hyperopic PRK treatment at the same time. With deeper ablations, one could perform a simple anti-hyperopic ablation concurrent with the PTK treatment. The authors recommend setting the laser with a standard +1.00 D treatment (ablation zone 9 mm, correction diameter 5 mm) to smooth out the mid periphery and increase the peripheral zone treated and the curvature. Others recommend using the joystick to maneuver a 2 mm diameter circular spot around the periphery of the central ablation (between 5 and 6 mm) to smooth out the edge of the ablation zone, thus counteracting the induced hyperopia.[26]

Outcomes

The outcome of PTK in RCE is related to the etiology, with traumatic etiology (success rate 74.4–80.0%) being better than EBMD (success rate 53.8%).[27] In general, several studies have reported good results in anterior corneal dystrophies of the Bowman's and stroma.[28,29] However, recurrences are not uncommon, especially in Reis–Buckler and granular dystrophy.[28] Fortunately, recurrences are often superficial and amenable to repeat PTK with good results. One must distinguish the difference between early haze from laser ablation (homogenous opacity over ablation zone) and recurrences (more heterogeneous with patterns resembling the underlying dystrophy).[28] There are also reports of differential prognosis depending on the genotypes of the corneal dystrophy, with Gly623Arg mutation responding better to PTK.[30] Others have shown success in treating lattice dystrophy,[28] SND,[31] keratoconus nodules,[32] LASIK flap striae[33] and symptomatic bullous keratopathy.

Key Surgical Points

- Careful selection of patients who are good candidates for PTK avoids any disappointments or unwanted complications.
- PTK is best for corneal pathologies affecting the epithelium or anterior 10–20% of the stroma.
- For patient safety, the residual corneal bed thickness must be greater than 300 μm.
- Try to maintain a smooth surface during PTK; either perform a transepithelial PTK if able, or use masking agents.
- Remove the least amount of tissue required to achieve the intended goal.
- Be aware of hyperopic shift and try and correct it within the same setting if possible.

Complications

In the immediate postoperative period, delayed epithelial healing can present a challenge. The time to re-epithelialization ranges between 2 and 6 days.[34] Poor healing can be associated with more severe consequences, such as scarring, irregular astigmatism and infection. Induced hyperopia is the most common refractive change.[35] However, induced myopia and irregular astigmatism have also been reported. Combined symptomatic and morphologic recurrence for RCE related to EBMD occurs in 14% of patients.[36] Other side effects post-PTK include haze, graft rejection and reactivation of HSK.

SUPERFICIAL KERATECTOMY

History

Treatment of RCE with superficial debridement of loose epithelium was reported as early as 1900.[37] This, combined with chemical cautery, was advocated by Chandler in 1944, as he recognized that the pathology is one of epithelial adherence.[37] However, this resulted in clouding of the cornea. Few decades later, Buxton and Fox reported their series of SK in patients with EBMD in 1983.[38] They performed a total superficial epithelial keratectomy from limbus to limbus with a blade and then applied diamond drill to areas of persistent abnormalities. Eleven out of 13 patients were relieved of their symptoms. However, given the potential limbal stem cell damage from the large debridement, others advocate sparing of the peripheral corneal epithelium.[39]

Indications

Superficial keratectomy involves mechanical excision of the epithelium, Bowman's membrane and superficial stroma with a sharp blade or a rotating diamond burr. This procedure is inexpensive, requires commonly used instruments and does not tend to induce significant refractive changes. It works well in a selected group of patients with ocular surface diseases not amenable to medical treatment. The advantage of mechanical debridement is that the surgical planes are clearer, potentially creating a smoother surface, especially for superficial elevated lesions. The primary indications include superficial corneal scars, SND and RCE.

Procedure

This is performed under topical or local anesthesia. It can be performed at the slit lamp or under an operating microscope in a minor operating room. For RCE, use a sharp instrument (e.g. a 64 Beaver blade) to debride the loose epithelium in a sheet, combined with gentle wiping with a cellulose sponge. Care should be taken to leave a 12-mm rim of peripheral corneal epithelium to avoid stem cell damage. This can be combined with the use of a fine diamond burr to polish in a gentle circular motion in the affected areas, which is shown to reduce recurrence rates with similar efficacy to PTK.[40–42] For elevated lesions, such as a Salzmann's nodule, grasp the nodule with a toothed forceps, e.g. Colibri, and dissect with a crescent or a 64 beaver blade. Scraping with the blade at 90 degrees to the surface of the cornea will often reveal a clear plane of

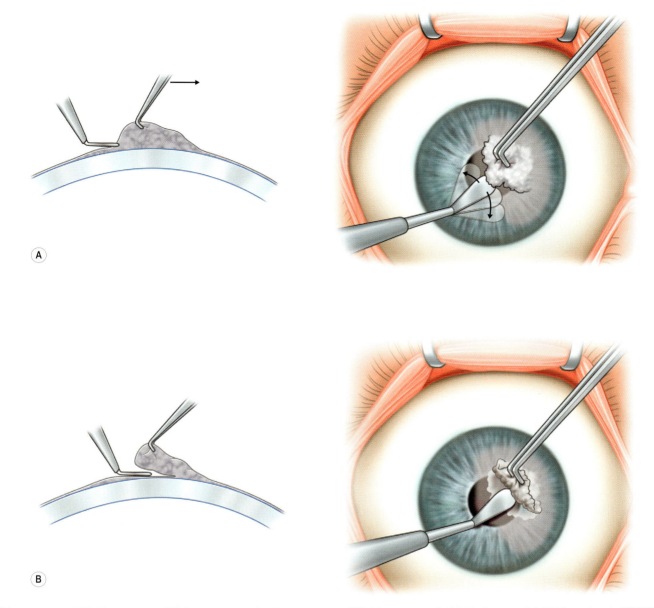

Figure 36.3 Superficial keratectomy for a Salzmann's nodule. (**A**) Scrape with a blade to reveal a clear plane of dissection (**B**) before advancing forward. Place a bandage contact lens at the end and leave it until epithelialization occurs.

dissection at the level of the Bowman's membrane, leaving a smooth bed (Fig. 36.3. Some also promote the use of MMC intraoperatively to prevent recurrence and haze.[42] A soft BCL is then applied and the patient is commenced on topical antibiotics for 1 week and topical steroids on a tapering regimen over 2–3 weeks. Frequent review is required until the epithelium is healed.

Key Surgical Points

- Care must be taken to leave a peripheral 1–2-mm rim of corneal epithelium to avoid stem cell damage.
- When using the diamond burr, apply in gentle small circular motions to avoid inducing irregular astigmatism.

- For those with SND, one might consider using MMC to prevent recurrent and haze.

Outcomes

In general, SK with or without diamond burr polishing is thought to be a safe and cost-effective treatment option. In RCE associated with EBMD, diamond burr polishing has been shown to be as efficacious as PTK, and it has a lower recurrence rate of 11.1% compare to 26.7% in the PTK group.[42] Diamond burr SK is also thought to be more effective, compared to epithelial debridement alone, with less recurrences and the need for repeated surgical interventions.[41] In a retrospective study of patients with SND treated with SK combined with MMC, there were no recurrences and most had improvement in their symptoms.[43]

Complications

Similar to PTK, early postoperative complications include delayed epithelialization and infection. Care needs to be taken to avoid induced astigmatism after diamond burr SK by using only gentle small circular motions.[44] Postoperative subepithelial haze was reported in around 23–26% of patients, which can occur at any time after surgery for RCE.[45,46]

TARSORRHAPHY

Tarsorrhaphy is closure of the eyelids via an adhesion between the two upper and lower lid margins, which reduces corneal exposure and evaporation of the tear film while minimizing friction between the eyelid and ocular surface during blinking. It is, therefore, an effective procedure for patients requiring prolonged surface protection for persistent corneal epithelial defects, secondary to neurotrophic keratopathy following herpes simplex or herpes zoster disease, exposure keratopathy (e.g. paralytic ectropion in seventh nerve palsy), keratoconjunctivitis sicca and corneal melt. It should be used in conjunction with the appropriate medical therapy.

Tarsorrhaphy can be either temporary or permanent, depending on the expectant recovery phase of the underlying condition. For example, a patient with Bell's palsy, who is expected to have some recovery of the facial nerve function over the ensuring few weeks, requires a temporary tarsorrhaphy. Meanwhile, a patient with an anesthetic cornea and a large neurotrophic ulcer may require a permanent tarsorrhaphy.

Temporary Suture Tarsorrhaphy

Temporary suture tarsorrhaphy was first described by Koenig and Harris[47] in 1991, with various modifications published since then, including without the bolsters[48] and a drawstring technique.[49] The most common type is a partial lateral tarsorrhaphy, which permits examination of the ocular surface and preserves the patient's visual axis. If additional protection is required, one could also add a medial tarsorrhaphy. Often, complete temporary closure may be needed to achieve epithelial healing and should not be withheld.

PROCEDURE

1. Assess the amount of tarsorrhaphy that is required (usually one-third to one-quarter length of the eyelid).
2. Infiltrate the eyelids with 2–3 mL of LA with 1:100000 epinephrine (for hemostasis). Flip over the lid and inject above the superior tarsus and below the inferior tarsus to achieve complete anesthesia.
3. Prepare two 1–1.5-cm silicone or rubber bolsters. These prevent erosion of the sutures through the eyelids and aid eversion of the lids to prevent trichiasis.

4. Use a double-armed 5-0 nylon or 6-0 silk suture (the authors prefer nylon as it is easier to remove later on), pass them through one of the bolsters completely at one end, then through the skin 3–4 mm from the upper eyelid margin, into the tarsus, and exits at the gray line of the upper lid. The needle is then passed through the lower lid gray line and exits 2–3 mm inferior to the lid margin. Repeat the same maneuver with the other end of the needle, but displace it laterally. Tie the sutures externally over the bolsters. Ensure that there are no sutures internally that could cause further irritation of the ocular surface.
5. One modification is the drawstring method[49] which allows complete closure but also easy access to the ocular surface. This technique uses three bolsters, two 2 cm and one 1 cm sections. The first step is as described above, but using the two 2-cm bolsters. Then the two suture arms below the lower lid margin are passed through the 1-cm bolster. This is tied, but 2–3 cm of slack is left in the suture to allow the surgeon to loosen the bolsters (move the smaller bolster away from the larger bolster) and examine the ocular surface as required. In the interim, the loop can be taped to the skin with steri-strips.

Permanent Tarsorrhaphy

Permanent tarsorrhaphy involves the removal of the mucocutaneous margins of the upper and lower lids to create an inter-marginal lid adhesion. Although it is more permanent, it is reversible.

PROCEDURE

1. As with temporary tarsorrhaphy, infiltrate the eyelids with local anesthetic with epinephrine.
2. Use a sharp blade (e.g. No.11 stab blade) and split the eyelids down the gray line, approximately 2–3 mm deep. Then make two relieving incisions perpendicular to the gray line incision, directed posteriorly.
3. Use Westcott scissors to excise a strip of the posterior eyelid margin in both the upper and the lower lids.
4. Appose the denuded posterior lid margin using multiple interrupted 5-0 or 6-0 Vicryl mattress sutures through the tarsus and tie the knots anteriorly away from the cornea.
5. Close the anterior lamellar with multiple interrupted 6-0 vicryl or 6-0 double-armed nylon through a bolster (as for temporary tarsorrhaphy) as it everts the lid during healing. The nylon and bolster can be removed after 2 weeks.

Postoperatively, topical antibiotic ointment is applied to the eyelids for 2 weeks. The lid margin will be fused laterally, but this can be reversed at any stage by dividing across the intermarginal adhesion.

Botox Tarsorrhaphy

Botulinum toxin was first used for ocular disorders for the treatment of strabismus. In 1987, Adams and Kirkness[50] identified that temporary induced ptosis from injection of botulinum toxin into the levator palpebrae superioris (LPS) could act as a protector of a compromised ocular surface. For patients unwilling or medically unable to undergo a surgical procedure, such as suture tarsorrhaphy, this may be an alternative. It provides a complete ptosis and the ocular surface is easily accessible to the examiner and for instilling drops. However, it has the expense of the neurotoxin, it is mildly invasive, with more obvious appearance asymmetry. It also commits the patient to monovision for 6–9 weeks until the ptosis recovers.

There are several types of botulinum toxin, but the majority of studies were based on Dysport (Ipsen, Slough, United Kingdom) and Type A Botox (Allergan, Irvine, California). These are not bioequivalent; hence, one must be careful when reconstituting the drug and should also be aware of the difference in concentrations. The suggested relative bioequivalence or per-unit strength ratio of Dysport compared to Botox is $3:1$.[51] The earlier reports described administration of the botulinum toxin with a 25-mm needle, through the eyelid, aiming at the levator palpebrae superioris muscle belly.[50,52,53] The toxin doses were 0.0625 ng for Dysport[50,52] and 2.5–5 units for Botox.[53] The mean duration of ptosis ranged between 6.5 and 8.5 weeks. However, this was associated with 24–80% superior rectus underaction,[50,52,53] which could exacerbate exposure keratopathy. A recent report suggested a more anterior chemodenervation of the LPS, which was associated with no superior rectus dysfunction.[54] In this approach, the clinician used a tuberculin syringe and a half-inch 26G or 30G needle and placed the needle tip near the anterior orbital roof just behind the superior orbital rim in the mid-pupillary axis before injection. The mean effective dose was 12.5 units and the mean ptosis duration was 9.2 weeks. In general, the time from injection to complete ptosis is 3.6–4 days.[53] The patient should be continued on appropriate topical medications as prescribed by the surgeon.

Other Modalities

Other types of tarsorrhaphies that have been described which may be useful in selected patients. Cyanoacrylate adhesion of the eyelids is an easy and effective method of closing the palpebral aperture.[55] However, it does not permit easy examination of the eye and its duration is unpredictable (range 1–15 days). This may be useful as a short-term solution in those who have contraindications or are unwilling to have other surgical procedures (e.g. on anticoagulants). Mulhern and Rootman described the use of the Stamler temporary lid splints,[56] which are inexpensive, non-invasive and easy to apply. However, these only last for a short period of time (average 3–7 days) and require frequent re-application. Their role is limited to application in those patients requiring a total therapeutic ptosis for a short period of time (less than 2 weeks) and to those who are able to return, or to be taught how to reapply the splint.

Key Surgical Points

- The decision on the type of tarsorrhaphy depends on the diagnosis and the expected recovery time.

- For temporary and permanent suture tarsorrhaphy, avoid leaving any internal sutures that may inadvertently rub against the ocular surface.
- Using the drawstring technique can make it easier to access and examine the ocular surface.
- For botulinum toxin ptosis, one must be mindful of which serotype and product, as they are not all bioequivalent.

Outcomes

In general, temporary and permanent suture tarsorrhaphies are successful in achieving re-epithelialization. A series evaluating the outcome of suture tarsorrhaphies in a cohort of cornea and external eye disease patients showed that 90.9% of the epithelial defects completely resolved. The mean time to healing after tarsorrhaphy was 18 days.[57] When comparing lateral tarsorrhaphy to patching in persistent post-keratoplasty epithelial defects, the epithelial healing was significantly faster (7.61 veersus 12.6 days) and the patients were more comfortable in the lateral tarsorrhaphy group.

Botox ptosis is effective in inducing complete ptosis in 75% of cases,[52] although in some cases the patient may require a second injection to achieve the desired result.

Complications

Complications of suture temporary tarsorrhaphy include premature separation of tarsorrhaphy, trichiasis and cellulitis. When reversing permanent tarsorrhaphy, the lid margins can scar and deform with possible secondary cicatricial entropion. Beware of doing a lateral tarsorrhaphy in patients with a sixth nerve palsy as it may exacerbate the exposure. In patients with central melting, it may be better to completely close the lid fissure, as a lateral tarsorrhaphy may exacerbate the exposure and melting. Superior rectus underaction is the most commonly reported side effect (68–80%) following Botox ptosis, leading to hypotropia and reduced Bell's phenomenon.[50,52] This could exacerbate exposure keratopathy. The mean recovery time of superior rectus underaction was reported to be 6 weeks, although 16% persisted beyond resolution of ptosis.[52] Diplopia occurs in 16–24%, with some persisting beyond the resolution of the ptosis.

CONJUNCTIVAL FLAPS
History

Conjunctival flaps have been used in the treatment of corneal diseases since the 1800s. Described in the German literature in the 1877, Gundersen[58,59] reported the largest series and described his technique for thin conjunctival flaps in 1958. He advocated their use for corneal ulcerations and thinning disorders, such as neuroparalytic keratitis, marginal ulcerations, relapsing erosions, and herpetic ulcers. In the early 1900s this procedure was used to reinforce cataract wounds.[58]

Indication

The treatment of recalcitrant corneal surface disease can be a challenge. Although local and systemic treatment is often successful, there are situations in which medical or surgical therapy may fail, with resultant recurrent epithelial breakdown and stromal ulceration. In specific situations, the conjunctival flap is effective and definitive treatment for persistent ocular surface disease.[59–62] Patients are relieved of pain, frequent regimen of topical medication, as well as more invasive surgery or enucleation.

The purpose of a conjunctival flap is to restore the integrity of a chronically compromised corneal surface,[63,64] and provide metabolic and mechanical support for corneal healing.[63,65] They do not add tectonic support and should not be used in very thin or perforated corneas. Conjunctival flaps act as biologic patches, conferring a trophic effect because of the nutritional and immunologic supply by its vascular connective tissue. A conjunctival flap will often provide comfort, reduce the ocular inflammation, and promote healing in these patients. This is particularly helpful in the setting of a blind painful eye where the flap can provide a new ocular surface for the placement of a cosmetic scleral shell (Fig. 36.4).

The most common indication for the use of a conjunctival flap is in the management of a persistent sterile corneal ulcer. Quite often, this chronic breach of corneal surface integrity has not responded to extensive lubrication, patching, a bandage contact lens, or a tarsorrhaphy. This may be a result of sensory denervation of the cornea (i.e. neurotrophic keratitis, paralysis of the seventh cranial nerve leading to exposure keratitis, corneal anesthesia following herpes zoster ophthalmicus, or metaherpetic ulceration following chronic HSK) or limbal stem cell deficiency. Ectatic thinning of the cornea near the limbus may also be managed with a conjunctival flap as long as the cornea is not excessively thinned.

A conjunctival flap is rarely used in the management of microbial keratitis. Marginal fungal ulcers unresponsive to antimycotic therapy have been successfully treated with conjunctival flaps.[66,67] This treatment is not appropriate in the setting of an active suppurative infection that is in danger of perforation.[67] A repeat graft is generally preferable once the inflammation associated with graft infections

has resolved. In cases where medical treatment has been exhausted, a conjunctival flap may offer a more effective means to resolve the infection.[68] A repeat graft can then be safely performed at a later date.

In the technique described by Gunderson,[58,59] coverage of the entire cornea with the conjunctiva obstructed any view of the anterior chamber[58,69] and precluded monitoring of corneal disease progression. In addition, this procedure was challenging in patients with short fornices and had the potential to cause ptosis.[58] It also required a more careful and extensive surgical procedure in the operating room. Any buttonholes or traction could ultimately lead to flap failure. In cases where only partial coverage of the cornea is required, a selective partial conjunctival flap tailored to cover the desired part of the diseased cornea provides an alternative to a total conjunctival flap.[58] This is particularly helpful if the patient has short fonices. Visualization of the anterior segment is not limited with this technique, and therefore, progression of corneal disease can be monitored. Intraocular pressure can also be accurately measured. Following stabilization of the ocular surface with either a total or partial conjunctival flap, PKP may be considered.

Procedure

TYPES OF CONJUNCTIVAL FLAPS

Total Conjunctival Flap

The most commonly employed technique for a total conjunctival flap is described by Gundersen[58] or modifications thereof.[60,70] Anesthesia may be local or general, but retrobulbar anesthesia is adequate in mos casest. Before the procedure, it is important to evaluate the availability and mobility of the conjunctiva. Conjunctival scarring in the area to be mobilized may preclude the success of this procedure.

After placement of the lid speculum, a 7-0 silk traction suture is placed through the peripheral cornea at the superior limbus (Fig. 36.5A). This allows the surgeon to control the globe and rotate it downward to expose the entire upper bulbar conjunctiva. Removal of the corneal epithelium can be performed after mobilization of the conjunctival flap. However, if done first, it is completed in a bloodless field and ensures it is not forgotten.

Next, the conjunctival flap is mobilized. A caliper is used to measure at least 14 mm from and concentric to the superior limbus into the fornix, the area necessary to cover the cornea. The incision is carried from medial to lateral canthal area superiorly in an arc (Fig. 36.5B). The conjunctiva is then ballooned up with a subconjunctival injection of 1% lidocaine with epinephrine (Fig. 36.5C). Some surgeons prefer not to inject subconjunctivally as it swells the Tenon's capsule and makes dissection more difficult. The injection site should not reside within the area to be used to cover the cornea. With the globe rotated downward, an incision in the previously marked superior fornix is made, avoiding the underlying Tenon's capsule (Fig. 36.5D). A very thin flap of conjunctiva is dissected downward towards the limbus without creating buttonholes (Fig. 36.5E). When the limbus is reached, the resultant flap is freed with a 360-degree

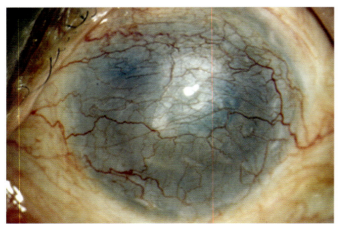

Figure 36.4 A total conjunctival flap covering the ocular surface.

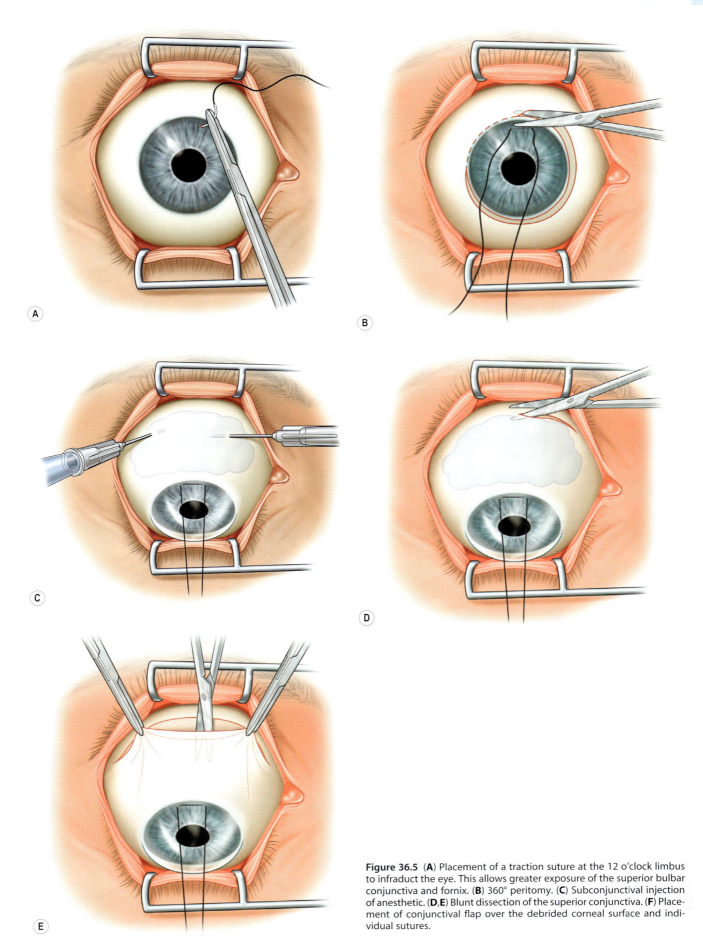

Figure 36.5 (**A**) Placement of a traction suture at the 12 o'clock limbus to infraduct the eye. This allows greater exposure of the superior bulbar conjunctiva and fornix. (**B**) 360° peritomy. (**C**) Subconjunctival injection of anesthetic. (**D,E**) Blunt dissection of the superior conjunctiva. (**F**) Placement of conjunctival flap over the debrided corneal surface and individual sutures.

Continued on following page

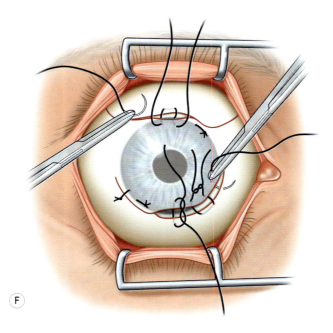

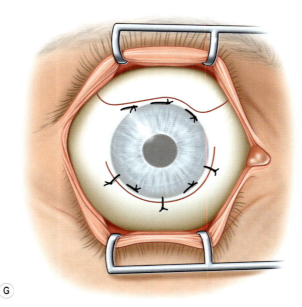

Figure 36.5 (Continued) **(G)** Multiple sutures in place. (Reproduced with permission from Krachmer JH, Mannis MJ, Holland EJ. Cornea. 3rd ed. Elsevier Inc; 2011. Figure 145.2.)

peritomy. Bleeding in the dissection bed is controlled with cautery.

The traction suture is released and the conjunctival flap is pulled down over the cornea (Fig. 36.5F). Relaxing incisions may help to release tension. Finally, the flap is sutured into place with Vicryl or nylon sutures placed in the superficial sclera just outside the limbus (Fig. 36.5G).

Although most authors agree that the procedure of choice is performing thin conjunctival flaps, without Tenon's capsule,[60] there are special situations in which a keratectomy is necessary and where Tenon's capsule may

be useful to occupy the space.[71] Sanitato et al.[66] reported on a thick conjunctival flap with Tenon's capsule for the treatment of peripheral corneal mycotic abscesses. The thicker flaps do thin out over time, thereby improving the overall appearance.

Bridge Flap

A bridge flap is used to cover focal central or paracentral corneal defects (Fig. 36.6A). This technique is similar to a Gundersen flap except that the width of the flap to be dissected is measured to be large enough to cover the corneal lesion (typically 20–30% larger). The corneal epithelium is removed in the area to be covered. Following appropriate measurements and marking in the superior bulbar conjunctiva, a thin flap is dissected from periphery to limbus, and released with a limited peritomy (Fig. 36.6B). The flap is then mobilized to cover the corneal lesion and fixed into place with Vicryl or nylon sutures (Fig. 36.6C).

Pedicle Flap

This flap is used to cover lesions near the limbus. After an LA, the corneal epithelium is removed from the area to be covered. As with a bridge flap, the size of the pedicle should be 20–30% larger than the lesion to be covered (Fig. 36.7A). Following appropriate measurements and marking in the conjunctiva to be used, a thin flap is dissected, mobilized to cover the corneal lesion, and fixed with nylon or Vicryl sutures (Fig. 36.7B,C).

Simple Advancement Flaps

This flap may also be used to cover lesions near the limbus and can be used with a lamellar patch graft. After an LA, a limited peritomy is performed in the area of interest (Fig. 36.8A,B). The conjunctiva is dissected to create a flap without tension, which is then pulled forward into place to cover the corneal lesion. Nylon or Vicryl sutures may be used to fix the flap into place (Fig. 36.8C,D).

Contraindication

Total conjunctival flaps should not be used in frank perforations. Once the flap is in place, the integrity of the anterior chamber cannot be monitored and, in general, a flap will not seal a perforation.

Key Surgical Points

- The key to creating a proper conjunctival flap involves selection of the appropriate site, mobilization of the flap without traction, and preservation of the flap's blood supply. The surgeon should determine preoperatively how much conjunctiva is available. If necessary, an inferior flap may be combined to provide adequate coverage.
- If possible, bridge flaps should be created vertically rather than horizontally to prevent the flap displacement by the action of the lid. The flap must be maintained in position by mattress sutures into the stroma.
- A small hole in a conjunctival flap will enlarge if the flap is under tension. If necessary, the hole may be closed

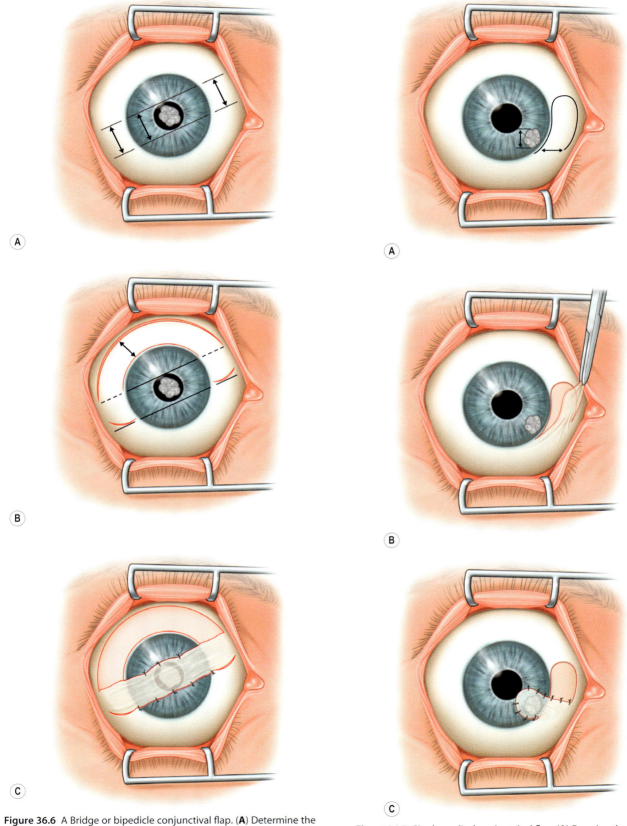

Figure 36.6 A Bridge or bipedicle conjunctival flap. (**A**) Determine the width of pedicle by measuring the lesion. (**B**) Width of flap should be 20–30% greater than diameter of corneal lesion. (**C**) Flap sutured into place. (Reproduced with permission from Krachmer JH, Mannis MJ, Holland EJ. Cornea. 3rd ed. Elsevier Inc; 2011. Figure 145.3.)

Figure 36.7 Single-pedical conjunctival flap. (**A**) Examine the lesion to determine size of flap. (**B**) Thin flap is dissected. (**C**) Suture flap to debrided corneal surface. (Reproduced with permission from Krachmer JH, Mannis MJ, Holland EJ. Cornea. 3rd ed. Elsevier Inc; 2011. Figure 145.4.)

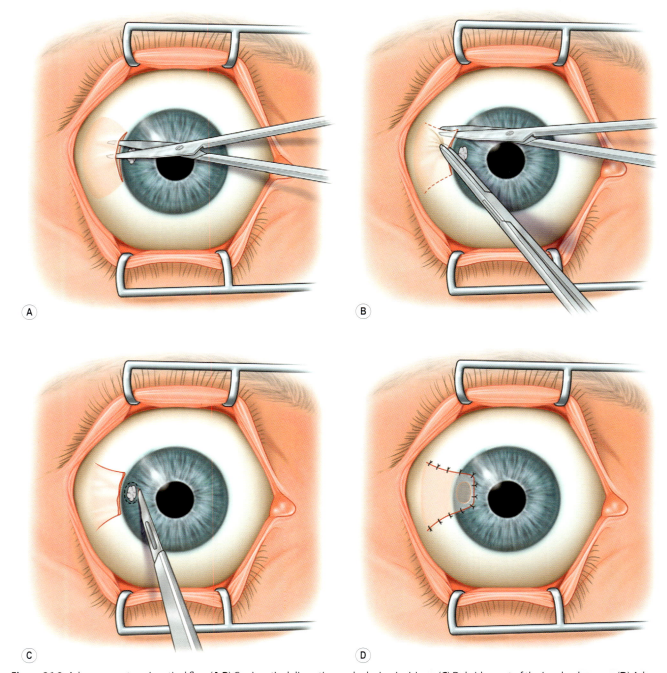

Figure 36.8 Advancement conjunctival flap. (**A,B**) Conjunctival dissection and relaxing incisions. (**C**) Debridement of the involved cornea. (**D**) Advancement conjunctival flap with sutures in place. (Reproduced with permission from Krachmer JH, Mannis MJ, Holland EJ. Cornea, 3rd ed. Elsevier Inc; 2011. Figure 145.5.)

using 11-0 nylon on a vascular needle suturing the conjunctiva to the underlying cornea. If necessary, a buttonhole may be moved off the cornea by shifting the whole flap medially or laterally.

- Epithelial cysts may form underneath the flap secondary to inadequate removal of corneal epithelium during the procedure. These may be excised as necessary.
- Over time, there may be corneal vascularization and scarring underneath a conjunctival flap. This can influence the success of subsequent transplantation.

Complications

Postoperative complications of conjunctival flaps include buttonholing of the conjunctiva, retraction of the flap, and formation of granulomas and inclusion cysts. Ptosis has been reported as a complication of conjunctival flap surgery.[58,60] Gundersen thought the ptosis was caused by the incorporation of Tenon's capsule within the flap or insufficient dissection of the flap from its lateral and

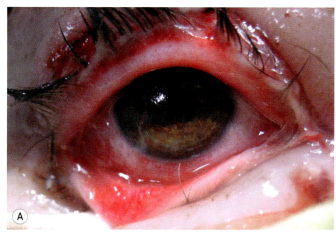

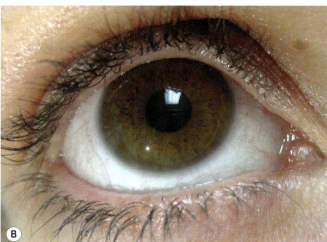

Figure 37.3 (**A**) Severe inflammation of the conjunctiva and eyelid margins in acute Stevens–Johnson syndrome. Amniotic membrane was applied to the eyes and eyelids 5 days into the illness as described in Figure 37.4 and the video supplement to this text. The 6-month postoperative outcome is shown in (**B**). Vision was 20/20 in both eyes with minimal dry eye symptoms. (Reproduced from Gregory DG. Treatment of acute Stevens–Johnson syndrome and toxic epidermal necrolysis using amniotic membrane: a review of 10 consecutive cases. Ophthalmology 2011;118:908–14, with permission of *Ophthalmology*.)

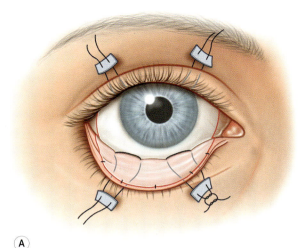

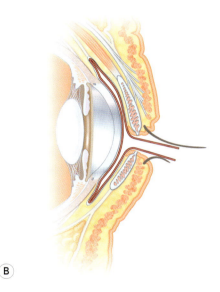

Figure 37.4 Schematic depiction of AM covering the lid margins, tarsal conjunctiva and entire ocular surface. The technique may be used for acute chemical burns or acute Stevens–Johnson syndrome. Each lid is treated with an individual AM sheet and then a separate sheet is applied to the ocular surface (**A**: front view; **B**: side view). (Reproduced from Meller D, Pires RT, Tseng SC. Ex vivo preservation and expansion of human limbal epithelial stem cells on amniotic membrane cultures. Br J Ophthalmol 2002;86:463–71, with permission of *Ophthalmology*.)

In SJS and TEN, AM has proven very effective if applied within the first 10 days of the illness, with the concept of 'the earlier the better' (Fig. 37.3). First described in 2002,[9] two subsequent case series have shown good outcomes with the use of AM applied to the lids, palpebral conjunctiva and entire ocular surface.[10,11] The method of application is similar in both chemical burns and SJS (Fig. 37.4). The surgical technique is described in detail in a video supplement to this text. Acute SJS cases that need AM treatment are characterized by extensive areas of epithelial sloughing on the lid margins, palpebral conjunctiva or cornea. It is important to inspect the fornices carefully with fluorescein stain. Extensive epithelial sloughing on the lid margins and palpebral conjunctiva puts the patient at high risk for scarring and loss of the normal mucosal epithelium. This can lead to severe dry eye problems and malpositioning of the lid margins and eyelashes. Scarred surfaces on the tarsal conjunctiva have been associated with long-term visual problems due to chronic blink-related microtrauma to the

cornea.[12] A Prokera™ can be used for corneal sloughing, but if there is extensive sloughing of the bulbar conjunctiva as well, it is important to cover the entire ocular surface with a sheet of AM, rather than just a Prokera™. Although, it is easy to place and can be helpful in cases with limited bulbar conjunctival involvement, a Prokera™ alone is not adequate treatment in SJS – the palpebral conjunctiva and lid margins must also receive AM grafting. A separate symblepharon ring should be placed over the eye once all the AM has been sutured into place if a Prokera™ has not been used on the ocular surface.

In the setting of a high-risk cornea transplant, a Prokera™ may speed healing of the epithelial defect on the graft and limit inflammation in the immediate postoperative

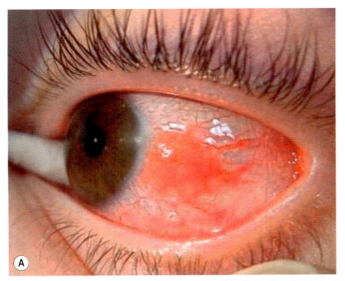
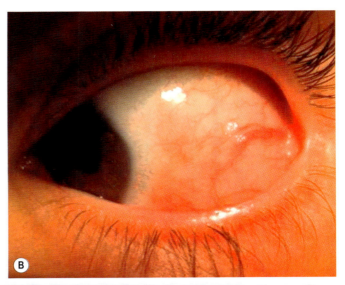

Figure 37.5 Amelanotic nevus in a 9-year-old child, preoperatively (**A**) and 3 months post excision with fibrin glue fixated amniotic membrane grafting over the resultant conjunctival defect (**B**). Amniotic membrane is particularly helpful in such cases to minimize pain.

period, likely enhancing graft survival. A Prokera™ is like a therapeutic contact lens for eyes with a disordered tear film and ocular surface and can be a helpful part of the treatment approach for many non-healing corneal epithelial defects. Any significant anatomical problems, such as symblepharon or entropion, should be addressed prior to any corneal transplantation. Optimizing the lubrication and decreasing the exposure of the ocular surface via tear supplements, punctal occlusion and partial tarsorrhaphy will further increase the chances for successful healing.

Permanent Graft

Amniotic membrane can also be used as a permanent graft to facilitate healing of areas where epithelium and subepithelial tissues have been damaged or removed. It is generally preferable to use a patient's own tissue for grafting, but this is not always feasible if the area to be treated is large, or if prior surgeries or disease have caused a relative lack of normal tissue that may be harvested for grafting purposes.

Following the excision of conjunctival tumors, AM may be placed over the ensuing epithelial defect. Fibrin glue fixation of AM and the subsequent decreased inflammation result in faster healing and less discomfort, which is particularly helpful in pediatric cases (Fig. 37.5). The edges of the AM should be tucked under any surrounding conjunctiva to help prevent dislodgement and to facilitate epithelial migration over of the graft.

For non-healing corneal epithelial defects with ulceration, multiple layers of AM 'pancakes' may be stacked in the defect to fill the hole.[13] The pancakes may be secured using sutures or fibrin glue. The area must then be covered with a larger sheet of AM or a Prokera™ to prevent dislodgement of the stacked AM grafts (Fig. 37.6).

Amniotic membrane transplantation has also proven useful in symblepharon repair and fornix reconstruction.

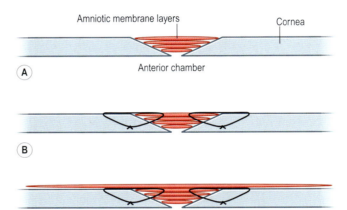

Figure 37.6 Schematic drawing showing the orientation of the amniotic membrane (AM) grafts in the ulcer bed. (**A**) Application of a few layers of AM. (**B**) Sutures anchoring the AM to the cornea (may also be done with fibrin glue in place of sutures). (**C**) AM patch covering the entire cornea. (Reproduced from Solomon A, Meller D, Prabhasawat P, et al. Amniotic membrane grafts for nontraumatic corneal perforations, descemetoceles, and deep ulcers. Ophthalmology 2002;109:694–703, with permission of *Ophthalmology*.)

The scarred tissue should first be completely freed from its adhesions to the globe and extraocular muscles. The fibrotic subconjunctival tissue should then be carefully dissected away and removed from the overlying conjunctiva. No conjunctiva is removed. Rather, it is allowed to retract into the fornix and is used to form the palpebral conjunctiva. It can be fixated to the back surface of the lid using double-armed, full-thickness sutures passed through the lid from the conjunctival side and tied on the external surface over a bolster (Fig. 37.7).[14] Any exposed extraocular muscles can be wrapped with AM to minimize adhesions and restrictive strabismus. Sponges soaked in a dilute concentration of

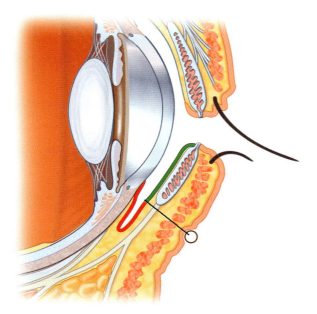

Figure 37.7 Schematic drawing showing a surgical strategy for symblepharon repair and fornix reconstruction. The scarred conjunctiva is freed up from the sclera and cornea and allowed to retract to become the palpebral conjunctiva (*green*). Subconjunctival scar tissue is removed from the underside of the retracted conjunctiva and the conjunctiva is fixated to the back surface of the lid using a double-armed suture (*gray line*) passed full-thickness through the lid and tied externally on the skin over a bolster (*gray circle*). The remaining epithelial defect in the fornix and on the sclera is filled in with either a conjunctival autograft or an amniotic membrane graft if sufficient conjunctiva is unavailable (*pink*). (Reproduced from Kheirkhah A, Blanco G, Casas V, et al. Surgical strategies for fornix reconstruction based on symblepharon severity. Am J Ophthalmol 2008;146:266–75, with permission of the *American Journal of Ophthalmology*.)

mitomycin C (0.2 mg/mL) can be applied to the underside of the conjunctiva surrounding the area of bare sclera that was previously covered by scar tissue. Using a dilute concentration for a short duration (30–60 seconds) and avoiding the application of mitomycin C directly to the sclera helps decrease the risk of late complications, such as scleral thinning and scleral necrosis. The bare sclera can then be covered with a conjunctival autograft from the fellow eye, or AM can be used if an autograft is not feasible. If an autograft is used, covering the harvest site with AM can minimize scarring and pain.

The use of AM in place of a conjunctival autograft in pterygium surgery has been somewhat controversial. When used to cover the conjunctival epithelial defect following pterygium excision, autografts have been shown to yield a very low recurrence rate.[15] Amniotic membrane grafts have been used as a substitute for the autograft, with the main advantage being decreased operative time. The recurrence rates are significantly higher, however, even if adjunctive mitomycin C is applied to the sclera or conjunctiva intraoperatively.[16] Pterygium recurrences can cause significant ocular morbidity and can be challenging to repair. Preventing recurrence should be the top priority when considering the different surgical techniques. Autografts are highly safe and effective, though the surgery is more tedious and time-consuming. The patients are often relatively young adults and the eye is otherwise healthy. With its significant history

of late complications, applying mitomycin C in a primary pterygium case seems an unwarranted risk. Fixating the autograft with fibrin glue rather than sutures helps decrease the operative time and improves patient comfort.

Conclusion

Whether used as a temporary patch or as a permanent graft, AM has proven to be an extremely helpful tool in ocular surface surgery. The ability to fixate AM with fibrin glue has increased surgical efficiency and patient comfort. Prokera™ offers a simple, but often effective, means of decreasing corneal inflammation and promoting epithelial healing without scarring. Amniotic membrane's ability to suppress inflammation has been shown to prevent the potentially disastrous damage that can occur in acute Stevens–Johnson syndrome. Amniotic membrane has limitations, however. Other disordered aspects of the ocular surface, such as dryness and exposure, must also be addressed if outcomes are to be successful. When possible, using a patient's own tissue for permanent grafting is ideal. In some instances, however, adequate tissue for an autologous graft may be unavailable. Additionally, in cases of conjunctival tumor excision it is not advisable to cover resultant bare sclera with an autograft. In these cases, AM promotes healing and minimizes the scarring and pain that would likely occur if the excision site was simply left bare. After an initial explosion of described uses, the role of AM in ocular surface surgery is becoming more well defined, and it has improved outcomes in a wide variety of settings. Knowledge of its uses and limitations is crucial for surgeons who treat disease of the ocular surface.

References

1. de Rotth A. Plastic repair of conjunctival defects with fetal membranes. Arch Ophthalmol 1940;23:522–5.
2. Dua HS, Gomes JAP, King AJ, et al. The amniotic membrane in ophthalmology. Surv Ophthalmol 2004;49:51–77.
3. Tseng SCG, Espana EM, Kawakita T, et al. How does amniotic membrane work? Ocul Surf 2004;2:177–87.
4. Liu J, Sheha H, Fu Y, et al. Update on amniotic membrane transplantation. Expert Rev Ophthalmol 2010;5:645–61.
5. Meller D, Dabul V, Tseng SCG. Expansion of conjunctival epithelial progenitor cells on amniotic membrane. Exp Eye Res 2002;74:537–45.
6. Koizumi N, Fullwood NJ, Bairaktaris G, et al. Cultivation of corneal epithelial cells on intact and denuded human amniotic membrane. Invest Ophthalmol Vis Sci 2000;41:2506–13.
7. Meller D, Pires RT, Tseng SCG. Ex vivo preservation and expansion of human limbal epithelial stem cells on amniotic membrane cultures. Br J Ophthalmol 2002;86:463–71.
8. Meller D, Pires RT, Mack RJ, et al. Amniotic membrane transplantation for acute chemical or thermal burns. Ophthalmology 2000;107:980–90.
9. John T, Foulks GN, John ME, et al. Amniotic membrane in the surgical management of acute toxic epidermal necrolysis. Ophthalmology 2002;109:351–60.
10. Shammas MC, Lai EC, Sarkar JS, et al. Management of acute Stevens–Johnson syndrome and toxic epidermal necrolysis utilizing amniotic membrane and topical corticosteroids. Am J Ophthalmol 2010;149:203–13.
11. Gregory DG. Treatment of acute Stevens–Johnson syndrome and toxic epidermal necrolysis using amniotic membrane: a review of 10 consecutive cases. Ophthalmology 2011;118:908–14.
12. Di Pascuale MA, Espana EM, Liu DT, et al. Correlation of corneal complications with eyelid cicatricial pathologies in patients with

Stevens–Johnson syndrome and toxic epidermal necrolysis syndrome. Ophthalmology 2005;112:904–12.

13. Solomon A, Meller D, Prabhasawat P, et al. Amniotic membrane grafts for nontraumatic corneal perforations, descemetoceles, and deep ulcers. Ophthalmology 2002;109:694–703.

14. Kheirkhah A, Blanco G, Casas V, et al. Surgical strategies for fornix reconstruction based on symblepharon severity. Am J Ophthalmol 2008;146:266–75.

15. Hirst LW. Prospective study of primary pterygium surgery using pterygium extended removal followed by extended conjunctival transplantation. Ophthalmology 2008;115:1663–72.

16. Luanratanakorn P, Ratanapakorn T, Suwan-apichon O, et al. Randomised controlled study of conjunctival autograft versus amniotic membrane graft in pterygium excision. Br J Ophthalmol 2006;90: 1476–80.

OCULAR SURFACE TRANSPLANTATION

38 *Preoperative Staging of Ocular Surface Disease*

ANDREA Y. ANG, GARY S. SCHWARTZ, and EDWARD J. HOLLAND

Introduction

Diseases that affect the ocular surface have many etiologies and present at different stages of evolution and severity. There are several ocular and non-ocular factors that must be taken into consideration when deciding upon the optimal type and timing of surgical treatment. The most important ocular factors are laterality of disease, the extent of limbal stem cell deficiency (LSCD), and the extent of conjunctival disease. Additional factors include the extent of stromal scarring, mechanical eyelid problems, and other vision-limiting disease, including glaucoma and retinal disease. Non-ocular factors that should be considered include age, systemic health, and personality factors.

Ocular Factors

LATERALITY

Bilateral causes of LSCD include congenital diseases, such as aniridia, and autoimmune or inflammatory diseases, such as Stevens–Johnson syndrome (SJS), ocular cicatricial pemphigoid (OCP), and atopic keratoconjunctivitis. Most acquired causes of LSCD may be unilateral or bilateral, including chemical or thermal injuries, contact lens-induced keratitis (CLIK), and iatrogenic causes, such as ocular surgery and toxic medications.

Performing either ocular stem cell transplantation (OSST) or keratoprosthesis (KPro) surgery commits the patient to long-term regular follow-up visits, and potential complications. Patients with unilateral disease who are functioning well with good vision in the fellow eye may choose not to undergo surgery. Other patients with unilateral disease may undergo surgery to restore binocular vision or to treat a chronically painful or cosmetically unacceptable diseased eye. In true unilateral disease the treatment of choice is a conjunctival limbal autograft (CLAU) from the fellow healthy eye. The fellow eye should be examined carefully for any signs of ocular surface disease, and in cases of asymmetric bilateral disease, such as CLIK or chemical injury, the fellow eye should not be used as donor tissue for CLAU.

If the diseased eye is the patient's only eye, the surgeon should consider a stem cell transplant rather than a KPro. In OSST, complications result in loss of the surface only, and there is less potential for sight-threatening complications, compared with KPro surgery.

EXTENT OF LIMBAL STEM CELL DEFICIENCY

Limbal stem cell deficiency (LSCD) may be partial or total. In congenital aniridia or in diseases with ongoing chronic inflammation, partial LSCD can progress over time to total LSCD. As seen in Figure 38.1, a patient with a severe alkaline chemical injury progresses over time from active conjunctival inflammation to partial LSCD and then total LSCD. If the visual axis remains unaffected in partial LSCD, the patient may not require transplantation and may be treated medically and monitored for progression. In quiet eyes, with small areas of conjunctival invasion, patients may benefit from sequential conjunctival epitheliectomy in the hope that the residual normal stem cells may repopulate the ocular surface. If several clock hours or more of LSCD exists, then a sectoral OSST may be used to treat that area of LSCD. In total LSCD, the only treatment options are complete OSST for restoration of the ocular surface with or without optical keratoplasty, or a KPro for visual rehabilitation.

EXTENT OF CONJUNCTIVAL INVOLVEMENT

The ocular surface diseases most difficult to treat are those that have both limbal stem cell and conjunctival involvement, such as in SJS and OCP. The conjunctiva itself is necessary for a healthy ocular surface, since it provides the mucin for a stable tear film and contains the lymphoid tissue to fight infection. Moreover, its structure of redundant folds allows for free movement of the eye within the orbit. Conjunctival disease may cause mucin–tear deficiency, subepithelial fibrosis, foreshortening of conjunctival fornices, symblepharon, ankyloblepharon, and in the most severe cases, keratinization of the ocular surface.

Activity of Inflammation

In patients with conjunctival involvement, a distinction must be made between previously inflamed conjunctiva and current active inflammation. The conjunctival inflammation from chemical/thermal injuries tends to subside slowly over a period of several months from the initial insult. In comparison, in autoimmune diseases, such as SJS or OCP, there tends to be a chronic background level of inflammation and associated exacerbations of conjunctival inflammation when the disease in active. When the conjunctiva is actively inflamed, there is an increase in immune mediators at the ocular surface. If surgery is performed during active inflammation, there is an increased risk of delayed epithelial healing, corneal melt, and immune rejection postoperatively.

It is important to manage the inflammation preoperatively and wait until the eye is quiet before performing the OSST or KPro. For chemical/thermal injuries, the authors recommend waiting at least 1 year after the initial insult. For autoimmune diseases, the underlying systemic disease should be optimally controlled and the ocular

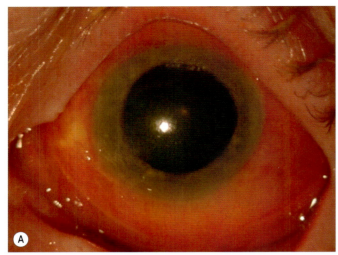

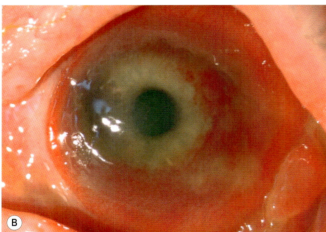

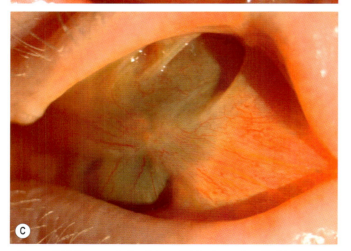

Figure 38.1 Severe alkaline injury. (**A**) Acute conjunctival inflammation 1 week after the injury. (**B**) Same eye showing progression to partial limbal stem cell deficiency at 1 month. (**C**) Same eye showing progression to total conjunctivalization and symblepharon formation.

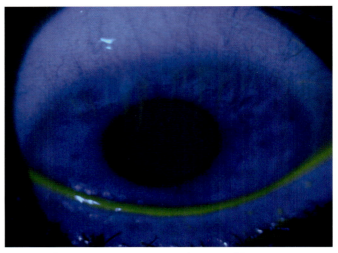

Figure 38.2 Stage Ia ocular surface failure in a patient with contact-lens induced keratitis. Note the late fluorescein staining superiorly demonstrating the partial LSCD.

Table 38.1   Classification of Ocular Surface Disease

	Normal Conjunctiva (Stage a)	Previously Inflamed Conjunctiva (Stage b)	Inflamed Conjunctiva (Stage c)
Partial stem cell deficiency (stage I)	Iatrogenic, CIN, contact lens (stage Ia)	History of chemical or thermal injury (stage Ib)	Mild SJS, OCP, recent chemical injury (stage Ic)
Total/ subtotal stem cell deficiency (stage II)	Aniridia, severe contact lens and iatrogenic (stage IIa)	History of severe chemical or thermal injury (stage IIb)	Severe SJS, OCP, recent chemical or thermal injury (stage IIc)

Classification system of ocular surface disease based on the extent of stem cell deficiency and the presence or absence of conjunctival inflammation. (Adapted from Schwartz GS et al. Ocular surface disease: medical and surgical management. New York: Springer-Verlag; 2002.)

inflammation minimized with topical and often systemic anti-inflammatory agents before proceeding with surgery.

Schwartz et al.[1] proposed a classification system of ocular surface disease based on the extent of stem cell deficiency (stage I or II) and the presence or absence of conjunctival inflammation (stage a, b, or c) (Table 38.1). CLIK and aniridia are examples of stage Ia or IIa disease with partial/ total stem cell deficiency but normal conjunctiva, as shown in Figures 38.2 and 38.3. A quiet eye with previous chemical or thermal injury would be an example of either stage Ib or IIb, depending on the extent of limbal stem cell loss, as shown in Figure 38.4. A chronically inflamed eye from OCP or SJS would be an example of either stage Ic or IIc disease, as shown in Figures 38.5 and 38.6.

Keratolimbal allograft (KLAL) replaces limbal stem cells only, whereas a living-related conjunctival limbal allograft (lr-CLAL) replaces both limbal stem cells and conjunctival goblet cells. Therefore, patients with conjunctival, as well as limbal involvement may benefit more from an lr-CLAL or combined KLAL/lr-CLAL (the Cincinnati procedure)[2] as opposed to a KLAL alone to help increase mucin production for a healthier ocular surface.

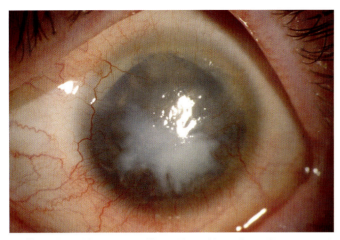

Figure 38.3 Stage IIa ocular surface failure in a patient with congenital aniridia. Note the total LSCD and anterior stromal scarring, with normal conjunctiva.

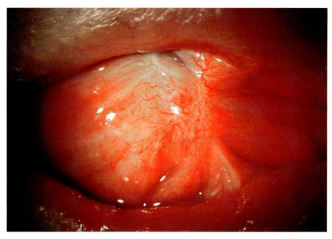

Figure 38.6 Stage IIc ocular surface failure in a patient with a history of severe alkali injury, showing total LSCD and chronic conjunctival inflammation.

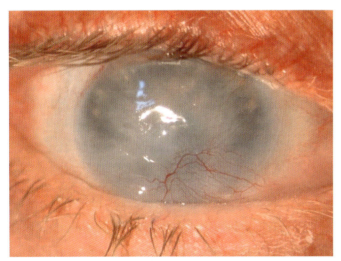

Figure 38.4 Stage IIb ocular surface failure in a patient with past chemical injury. Note the total LSCD, corneal stromal scarring, and resolved conjunctival inflammation.

Tear Film Abnormalities

A healthy tear film is essential for epithelial healing after OSST and for prevention of corneal melts after KPro surgery. Tears contain growth factors, immunoglobulins, and electrolytes, and prevent desiccation of the ocular surface.[3] The mucin component of tears is produced by the goblet cells of the conjunctiva, which may be deficient in conjunctival disease. The aqueous component is produced by the glands of Wolfring and Krause, which may be damaged by conjunctival disease causing subepithelial fibrosis and forniceal foreshortening. Similarly, conjunctival fibrosis may scar the lacrimal ductules that secrete aqueous from the lacrimal gland, further compounding aqueous deficiency. The lipid component may be deficient from damage caused from scarring of the tarsus.

The health of the tear film must be assessed preoperatively to help determine which OSST procedure or which KPro procedure is most likely to succeed. For example, patients with keratinization and dryness of the ocular surface would likely fail KLAL alone, or the cornea may melt with a Boston Type 1 KPro. Either a combined KLAL/lr-CLAL (which replaces conjunctival goblet cells) or a Boston Type 2 or osteo-odonto-keratoprosthesis (OOKP) would be a more appropriate choice.

EXTENT OF STROMAL SCARRING

More than half the patients undergoing stem cell transplantation will require a future keratoplasty for visual rehabilitation.[4] A keratoplasty may not be necessary if the corneal scarring is superficial and removed with the superficial keratectomy when performing stem cell transplantation. In diseases characterized by progressive LSCD, such as aniridia, the authors recommend that OSST be performed prior to the onset of stromal scarring in patients with significant epithelial disease.[5] If corneal transplantation is necessary and the endothelium is normal, then a deep anterior lamellar keratoplasty (DALK) is preferred over a penetrating keratoplasty (PK). The epithelium should be allowed to heal completely, and ocular surface inflammation allowed to subside before keratoplasty is performed. Patients should

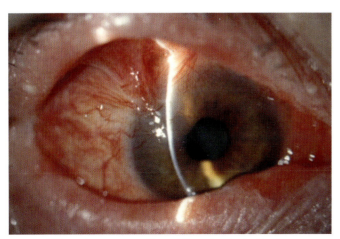

Figure 38.5 Stage Ic ocular surface failure in an SJS patient, showing chronic conjunctival inflammation and partial LSCD.

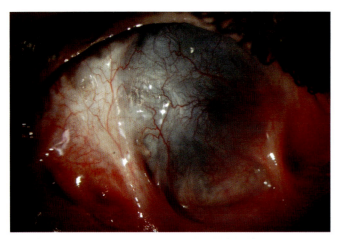

Figure 38.7 Total surface failure and symblepharon formation after chemical injury.

be informed of the longer time-frame required to achieve visual improvement with OSST and keratoplasty, compared to the more immediate visual improvement with KPro.

MECHANICAL EYELID PROBLEMS

Conjunctival inflammation and scarring may cause foreshortening of the fornices, symblepharon, ankyloblepharon, distichiasis, trichiasis, entropion or ectropion. Disorders of the lid–lash complex may cause microtrauma and perpetuate chronic inflammation through the mechanical rubbing of lashes against the ocular surface.[6] Ectropion or lagophthalmos can cause exposure keratopathy and delay healing post-OSST, or predispose to corneal melting post-KPro surgery. Symblepharon and loss of fornices make it difficult to retain a bandage contact lens that is necessary to prevent corneal melting after KPro implantation. Figure 38.7 shows symblepharon formation after chemical injury.

Eyelid abnormalities should be assessed and surgically corrected prior to or at the time of ocular surface reconstruction surgery. In patients with chronic inflammation who are at high risk of corneal melt, a lateral tarsorrhaphy should be performed at the time of OSST or KPro surgery.

OTHER OCULAR DISEASE: GLAUCOMA AND RETINAL DISEASE

Glaucoma

Ocular stem cell transplantation (OSST) and KPro surgery may cause glaucoma or contribute to the progression of pre-existing glaucoma. The UC Davis study[7] showed that glaucoma is the major cause of long-term vision loss after KPro implantation. Many patients have pre-existing glaucoma from diseases, such as congenital aniridia or chemical/thermal injuries and may already have had surgical treatment, usually in the form of a glaucoma drainage device. Patients should be assessed by a glaucoma specialist preoperatively, and their IOP should be well controlled prior to OSST or KPro surgery. Given the difficult in measuring IOP after KPro surgery and the high risk of developing glaucoma, some surgeons have a lower threshold for placement of a glaucoma drainage device prior to KPro implantation.

End-stage glaucoma is a contraindication for OSST and KPro surgery, since it is possible that postoperative spikes in IOP may snuff out a borderline optic nerve.

Retina

In congenital aniridia, most patients suffer from some degree of foveal or optic nerve hypoplasia. It is important to assess the patient's visual potential by clarifying what the patient's vision was prior to developing aniridic keratopathy. If the patient has a definite history of worsening of vision after the keratopathy developed, it would then be sensible to proceed with ocular reconstructive surgery. If the patient's limiting factor is the retina or optic nerve, it is unlikely they will benefit from surgery unless the purpose is to alleviate chronic pain.

Non-Ocular Factors

AGE

The age of the patient is important in deciding between OSST or KPro in a patient who may be suitable for either procedure. For example, a younger aniridic may prefer a KPro so that they do not have to take immunosuppression; however, this exposes a younger patient to many years of the risk of sight-threatening complications, such as progression of glaucoma, corneal melt and extrusion, and endophthalmitis. An OSST may require immunosuppression, but complications of OSST generally result in loss of the surface only, and not loss of the eye.

Although elderly patients are likely to have more co-morbidities, many do not require immunosuppression for OSST, since they have a dampened immune response. In the authors' experience, younger age is the strongest risk factor for OSST rejection.[4]

SYSTEMIC HEALTH

Immunosuppression is necessary to prevent immune rejection in OSST. Immunosuppression can be co-managed with a renal transplant team or rheumatologist using a steroid-sparing regimen of tacrolimus and mycophenolate mofetil.[8] Absolute contraindications for systemic immunosuppression are patients with a history of malignancy within 5 years, as well as significant co-morbidities, such as diabetes, uncontrolled hypertension, renal insufficiency, congestive heart failure, and other organ failure.

PERSONALITY FACTORS

Patients who are candidates for OSST or KPro surgery must be willing and able to comply with long-term regular follow-up. Patients undergoing OSST must be compliant with their immunosuppression medication and laboratory follow-up. Noncompliance with immunosuppression has been shown to increase the risk of immune rejection and surface failure.[4] Patients undergoing KPro implantation must be compliant with bandage contact lens wear and the use of long-term prophylactic antibiotics. Patients who have been noncompliant with previous treatment or who do not comprehend the importance of complying with follow-up and medications should not undergo OSST or KPro surgery.

Conclusion

Both ocular and non-ocular factors must be assessed in order to decide on the optimal treatment for a particular patient. The laterality, extent of LSCD and conjunctival involvement, tear film abnormalities, extent of stromal scarring, mechanical eyelid problems, and other vision-limiting ocular disease must be assessed. These factors are considered on the background of the age, systemic health, and personality of the patient.

References

1. Schwartz GS, Gomes JAP, Holland EJ. Preoperative staging of disease severity. In: Holland EJ, Mannis MJ, editors. Ocular surface disease: medical and surgical management. New York: Springer-Verlag, 2002: 158–167.

2. Biber JM, Skeens HM, Neff KD, et al. The Cincinnati procedure: technique and outcomes of combined living-related conjunctival limbal allografts and keratolimbal allografts in severe ocular surface failure. Cornea 2011;30:765–71.

3. Management and Therapy Subcommittee members of the International Dry Eye Workshop. Management and therapy of dry eye disease: Report of the Management and Therapy Subcommittee of the International Dry Eye Workshop (2007). Ocul Surf 2007;5:163–78

4. Ang AY, Chan CC, Biber JM, et al. Ocular surface stem cell transplantation rejection: incidence, characteristics, and outcomes. Cornea 2013; 32:229–36.

5. Holland EJ, Djalilian AR, Schwartz GS. Management of aniridic keratopathy with keratolimbal allograft: a limbal stem cell transplantation technique. Ophthalmology 2003;110:125–30.

6. Di Pascuale MA, Espana EM, Liu DT, et al. Correlation of corneal complications with eyelid cicatricial pathologies in patients with Stevens–Johnson syndrome and toxic epidermal necrolysis syndrome. Ophthalmology 2005;112:904–12.

7. Greiner MA, Li JY, Mannis MJ. Longer-term vision outcomes and complications with the Boston Type 1 keratoprosthesis and the University of California, Davis. Ophthalmology 2011;118:1543–50.

8. Holland EJ, Mogilishetty GM, Skeens HM, et al. Systemic immunosuppression in ocular surface stem cell transplantation: Results of a 10-year experience. Cornea 2012;31:655–61.

39 The Classification of Ocular Surface Transplantation

SHERAZ M. DAYA and EDWARD J. HOLLAND

Introduction

The ocular surface of the eye is a complex functional unit consisting of several elements that all interrelate. These include the eyelids, lubrication, conjunctiva and cornea. Homeostasis of the ocular surface is vital for the maintenance of good corneal epithelium, which in turn ensures good corneal clarity and vision. Lids provide protection to the ocular surface, as well as distribution of tears through a wiper-type action picking up tears from the lower lid meniscus and distributing this across the corneal surface. Lubrication is important in terms of content, osmolality and quantity.[1] Normal conjunctiva provides mucins from goblet cells along with cytokines and the corneal limbus has been recognized and accepted as the source of limbal stem cells for the replacement of normal corneal phenotype.[2-3]

Numerous techniques to rehabilitate the ocular surface have developed over the last two decades. Rehabilitation of the ocular surface includes improving the ocular surface environment and, in particular, ensuring control of inflammation, good lubrication, lid closure and elimination of keratinization and symblephara. Restoration of the normal corneal phenotype and appropriate corneal clarity is highly dependent on a good environment.[4] A number of transplantation techniques have been employed over the years, and many have been described with various terminology, including autologous and allograft conjunctival transplantation,[5-7] keratoepithelioplasty,[8] homotransplantation of limbal cells,[9] limbal transplantation,[10] and autologous[11] and allograft limbal transplantation.[12-15] These terms are not always clear in terms of tissue source (auto- or allogeneic) and precise anatomic location. Limbal transplantation, for instance, can be conjunctival alone or corneoscleral.[16] Additionally, in the last 15 years tissue engineered techniques have become more popular and include culture and expansion of presumed stem cells and transplantation back to the host or to another recipient.[17-27]

Clarity of communication is necessary as is the ability to accurately compare outcomes of these innovative procedures. Holland and Schwartz, recognizing the need for common terminology, provided a rationale for common nomenclature illustrating a variety of techniques described in the literature, often using similar terminology.[16] The authors proposed a classification based on: (1) anatomic source of the tissue and (2) genetic source (autologous, allogeneic and living related). Since the publication in1996, further developments have resulted in the description of more techniques, as well as new sources of tissue[28-35] along with the introduction of cell culture techniques.[36-44] In order to include all current techniques and procedures, the Cornea Society felt there was a need for an internationally agreed nomenclature. This nomenclature was established by an international group of cornea surgeons involved in ocular surface transplantation through an initial steering committee (Table 39.1) and once ratified by the Board of the Cornea Society was published in *Cornea*.[45] A literature search was performed to ascertain types of ocular surface rehabilitative procedures reported for which inclusion in the new nomenclature. The committee agreed to expand on the principles initially proposed by Holland and Schwartz in 1996.[16] The nomenclature was based on the following criteria: (1) *anatomic source* of the tissue being transplanted, (2) *genetic source* – autologous or allogeneic and to reflect histocompatability in the latter group, whether living-related or not, and (3) *cell culture* techniques. Types of procedures were broadly categorized by the anatomic type, source, and whether it was tissue engineered (Box 39.1). Further categorization according to anatomic type of tissue,

Table 39.1 Steering and International Committee

Co-Chairs	Sheraz M. Daya (United Kingdom)
	Edward J. Holland (United States of America)
Initial Steering Group	Shigeru Kinoshita (Japan)
	Jose Gomes (Brazil)
	Donald Tan (Singapore)
	Ali Djalilian (United States of America)
Wider International Panel	Clara Chan (Canada)
	Eric Donnenfeld (United States of America)
	Harminder Dua (United Kingdom)
	Friedrich Kruse (Germany)
	Mark Mannis (United States of America)
	Ray Tsai (Taiwan)
	Paolo Rama (Italy)
	Kazuo Tsubota (Japan)

Box 39.1 Tissue Type, Anatomic and Tissue Engineered

Type of tissue transplanted
 Conjunctival
 Limbal
 Other mucosal
Ex-vivo tissue engineered
 Ex vivo cultivated *conjunctival* transplantation
 Ex vivo cultivated *limbal* transplantation
 Other ex vivo cultivated *mucosal* transplantation

Table 39.2   Classification of Surgical Procedures for Ocular Surface Rehabilitation

Procedure	Abbrev.	Donor	Transplanted Tissue
Conjunctival Transplantation			
Conjunctival autograft	CAU	Fellow eye	Conjunctiva
Cadaveric conjunctival allograft	c-CAL	Cadaveric	Conjunctiva
Living-related conjunctival allograft	lr-CAL	Living relative	Conjunctiva
Living non-related conjunctival allograft	lnr-CAL	Living non-relative	Conjunctiva
Limbal Transplantation			
Conjunctival limbal autograft	CLAU	Fellow eye	Limbus/conjunctiva
Cadaveric conjunctival limbal allograft	c-CLAL	Cadaveric	Limbus/conjunctiva
Living-related conjunctival limbal allograft	lr-CLAL	Living relative	Limbus/conjunctiva
Living non-related conjunctival limbal allograft	lnr-CLAL	Living non-relative	Limbus/conjunctiva
Keratolimbal autograft	KLAU	Fellow eye	Limbus/cornea
Keratolimbal allograft	KLAL	Cadaveric	Limbus/cornea
Other Mucosal Transplantation			
Oral mucosa autograft	OMAU	Recipient	Oral mucosa
Nasal mucosa autograft	NMAU	Recipient	Nasal mucosa
Intestine mucosa autograft	IMAU	Recipient	Intestinal mucosa
Peritoneal mucosa autograft	PMAU	Recipient	Peritoneum

Table 39.3   Classification of Tissue Engineered Surgical Procedures for Ocular Surface Rehabilitation

Procedure	Abbrev.	Donor	Transplanted Tissue
Ex Vivo Cultivated Conjunctival Transplantation			
Ex vivo cultivated conjunctival autograft	EVCAU	Recipient eye(s)	Conjunctiva
Ex vivo cultivated cadaveric conjunctival allograft	EVc-CAL	Cadaveric	Conjunctiva
Ex vivo cultivated living-related conjunctival allograft	EVlr-CAL	Living relative	Conjunctiva
Ex vivo cultivated living non-related conjunctival allograft	EVlnr-CAL	Living non-relative	Conjunctiva
Ex Vivo Limbal Transplantation			
Ex vivo cultivated limbal autograft	EVLAU	Recipient eye(s)	Limbus/cornea
Ex vivo cultivated cadaveric limbal allograft	EVc-LAL	Cadaveric	Limbus/cornea
Ex vivo cultivated living-related limbal allograft	EVlr-LAL	Living relative	Limbus/cornea
Ex vivo cultivated living non-related limbal allograft	EVlnr-LAL	Living non-relative	Limbus/cornea
Other Ex Vivo Cultivated Mucosal Transplantation			
Ex vivo cultivated oral mucosa autograft	EVOMAU	Recipient	Oral mucosa

namely conjunctival, limbal and other mucosal grafts is listed in Table 39.2. Tissue engineered procedures are listed in Table 39.3 and classified according to anatomic source of tissue.

Anatomic Type

The principle anatomic sources of tissue for ocular surface rehabilitative procedures are either conjunctiva or limbus. The use of peritonea[46–48] and rectal mucosa[28] as sources of cells have been described, requiring the inclusion of a third category of 'other mucosal' tissue. Conjunctival tissue is increasingly recognized as an important contributor to the welfare of the ocular surface and felt to be necessary in cases where there is concomitant conjunctival deficiency.[49] The provision of mucins from goblet cells, as well as cytokines, contributes to the milieu and equilibrium of the ocular surface. Conjunctival tissue is not to be confused with limbal conjunctival tissue and is confined to bulbar and forniceal conjunctiva only. There have been reports suggesting the fornix as a source of conjunctival stem cells and there may be some theoretical advantage of using fornix over bulbar conjunctiva; however, as this has not been demonstrated scientifically, the committee chose not to further classify the source of conjunctiva.[50]

Limbal tissue has been demonstrated to have stem cell characteristics and can be divided into two main anatomic types, including limbal conjunctiva and keratolimbal tissue. The latter includes a combination of anterior corneal tissue and scleral tissue. Conjunctival limbal tissue is procured from either the fellow eye or a living relative. The rationale for procuring only conjunctiva and not cornea, although the former is felt to have a lower quantity of stem cells, is to preserve the donor limbus. There is an added advantage in that the graft contains bulbar conjunctival tissue as well, which is useful in cases where conjunctival deficiency may also be present.

Other mucosal tissue, including buccal,[29,30] nasal,[33,34] rectal[28] and peritoneal[46-48] have been used to populate the palpebral conjunctiva and recreate the fornix. Autologous buccal mucosa has also been used with good success in tissue engineering techniques.[31,32,35]

Source

Histocompatibility is an important parameter that influences graft success.[7] Autologous tissue, if such a source is available, is the best source; however, it is not possible in bilateral disease. The next best source of tissue is a best-matched living relative or, at a minimum, a parent or offspring, in which case half the haplotype will be in common.[51,52] Non-related tissue can be either living or cadaveric and viability of the latter often depends on the preservation technique used.[53] Attempts to ensure better histocompatibility by tissue marching can be performed and a non-related living donor can be used. The source of tissue that is used (autologous, living-related or cadaveric) is included in the nomenclature for both the tissue transplantation and tissue engineered sections (see Tables 39.2 and 39.3).

Tissue Engineered Grafts

Tissue engineered grafts are a more recent and exciting addition to the armamentarium of ocular surface procedures. A number of reports have demonstrated the value of 'ex vivo' cell cultivation techniques.[17-27,36-44] Theoretical advantages include a large volume of cells without the inclusion of highly antigenic tissue as a carrier. Additionally, the loss of antigen-presenting cells further decreases the chance of acute and chronic immune rejection.[26] Similar anatomic origins of tissue, as well as genetic sources (autologous, living related, non-related and cadaveric) are used in the nomenclature.

Human amniotic membrane has been used as a substrate for epithelial growth[36,54] or tissue filler,[55,56] as well as a biologic dressing.[57-62] Although discussed by the steering committee, amniotic membrane was not included in the nomenclature. The importance of the use of amniotic membrane as an adjuvant in ocular surface rehabilitation is acknowledged; however, it is not included in the nomenclature, as no donor cells are contributed. In tissue engineering techniques, there have been reports of use of amniotic membrane as a substrate for growth,[21-23,25-27,38] and others have used other substrates[24,39-43] or none at all.[35,44] The influence of the carrier or growth substrate on outcomes has yet to be determined and in time this may require inclusion in the nomenclature.

As is the case with classification systems and nomenclature, periodic review will be required to embrace new and emerging techniques, and this will be conducted by the Cornea Society as the need arises. Meanwhile, to ensure clear communication and understanding, the cornea community is encouraged to use the Cornea Society nomenclature for ocular surface rehabilitative procedures.

References

1. Tsubota K, Tseng SCG, Nordlund ML. Anatomy and physiology of the ocular surface. In: Holland EJ, Mannis MJ, editors. Ocular surface disease medical and surgical management. New York: Springer-Verlag; 2002. p. 3–15.
2. Davanger M, Evensen A. Role of the pericorneal papillary structure in renewal of corneal epithelium. Nature 1971;229:560–1.
3. Schermer A, Galvin S, Sun TT. Differentiation-related expression of a major 64K corneal keratin in vivo and in culture suggests limbal location of corneal epithelial stem cells. J Cell Biol 1986;103:49–62.
4. Dilly PN. Structure and function of the tear film. Adv Exp Med Biol 1994;350:239–47.
5. Thoft RA. Conjunctival transplantation. Arch Ophthalmol 1977;95:1425–7.
6. Vastine DW, Stewart WB, Schwab IR. Reconstruction of the periocular mucous membrane by autologous conjunctival transplantation. Ophthalmology 1982;89:1072–81.
7. Kwitko S, Raminho D, Barcaro S, et al. Allograft conjunctival transplantation for 8 bilateral ocular surface disorders. Ophthalmology 1995;102:1020–5.
8. Thoft RA. Keratoepithelioplasty. Am J Ophthalmol 1984;97:1–6.
9. Pfister RR. Corneal stem cell disease: concepts, categorization, and treatment by auto- and homotransplantation of limbal stem cells. CLAO J 1994;20:64–72.
10. Jenkins C, Tuft S, Liu C, et al. Limbal transplantation in the management of chronic contact-lens-associated epitheliopathy. Eye 1993;7:629–33.
11. Kenyon KR, Tseng SCG. Limbal autograft transplantation for ocular surface disorders. Ophthalmology 1989;96:709–22; discussion 722–3.
12. Tsai RJ, Tseng SCG. Human allograft limbal transplantation for corneal surface reconstruction. Cornea 1994;13:389–400.
13. Tsubota K, Toda I, Saito H, et al. Reconstruction of the corneal epithelium by limbal allograft transplantation for severe ocular surface disorders. Ophthalmology 1995;102:1486–96.
14. Holland EJ. Epithelial transplantation for the management of severe ocular surface disease. Trans Am Ophthalmol Soc 1996;19:677–743.
15. Croasdale CR, Schwartz GS, Malling JV, et al. Keratolimbal allograft: recommendations for tissue procurement and preparation by eye banks, and standard surgical technique. Cornea 1999;18:52–8.
16. Holland EJ, Schwartz GS. The evolution of epithelial transplantation for severe ocular surface disease and a proposed classification system. Cornea 1996;15:549–56.
17. Schrader S, Notara M, Beaconsfield M, et al. Tissue engineering for conjunctival reconstruction: established methods and future outlooks. Curr Eye Res 2009;34:913–24.
18. Vemuganti GK, Kashyap S, Sangwan VS, et al. Ex-vivo potential of cadaveric and fresh limbal tissues to regenerate cultured epithelium. Ind J Ophthalmol 2004;52:113–20.
19. Shortt AJ, Secker GA, Notara MD, et al. Transplantation of ex vivo cultured limbal epithelial stem cells: a review of techniques and clinical results. Surv Ophthalmol 2007;52:483–502.
20. Daya SM, Watson A, Sharpe JR, et al. Outcomes and DNA analysis of ex vivo expanded stem cell allograft for ocular surface reconstruction. Ophthalmology 2005;112:470–7.
21. Grueterich M, Espana EM, Touhami A, et al. Phenotypic study of a case with successful transplantation of ex vivo expanded human limbal epithelium for unilateral total limbal stem cell deficiency. Ophthalmology 2002;109:1547–52.
22. Koizumi N, Rigby H, Fullwood NJ, et al. Comparison of intact and denuded amniotic membrane as a substrate for cell-suspension culture of human limbal epithelial cells. Graefes Arch Clin Exp Ophthalmol 2007;245:123–34.
23. Pellegrini G, Traverso CE, Franzi AT, et al. Long-term restoration of damaged corneal surfaces with autologous cultivated corneal epithelium. Lancet 1997;349:990–3.
24. Rama P, Bonini S, Lambiase A, et al. Autologous fibrin-cultured limbal stem cells permanently restore the corneal surface of patients with total limbal stem cell deficiency. Transplantation 2001;72:1478–85.
25. Sangwan VS, Vemuganti GK, Singh S, et al. Successful reconstruction of damaged ocular outer surface in humans using limbal and conjunctival stem cell culture methods. Biosci Rep 2003;23:169–74.

26. Schwab IR, Reyes M, Isseroff RR. Successful transplantation of bioengineered tissue replacements in patients with ocular surface disease. Cornea 2000;19:421–6.

27. Shimazaki J, Aiba M, Goto E, et al. Transplantation of human limbal epithelium cultivated on amniotic membrane for the treatment of severe ocular surface disorders. Ophthalmology 2002;109:1285–90.

28. Mahatme VH. Rectal mucous membrane graft for dry eye syndrome. Ind J Ophthalmol 1999;47:129–31.

29. Hosni FA. Repair of trachomatous cicatricial entropion using mucous membrane graft. Arch Ophthalmol 1974;91:49–51.

30. Shore JW, Foster CS, Westfall CT, et al. Results of buccal mucosal grafting for patients with medically controlled ocular cicatricial pemphigoid. Ophthalmology 1992;99:383–95.

31. Nakamura T, Inatomi T, Sotozono C, et al. Transplantation of cultivated autologous oral mucosal epithelial cells in patients with severe ocular surface disorders. Br J Ophthalmol 2004;88:1280–4.

32. Inatomi T, Nakamura T, Koizumi N, et al. Midterm results on ocular surface reconstruction using cultivated autologous oral mucosal epithelial transplantation. Am J Ophthalmol 2006;141:267–75.

33. Kuckelkorn R, Schrage N, Redbrake C, et al. Autologous transplantation of nasal mucosa after severe chemical and thermal eye burns. Acta Ophthalmol Scand 1996;74:442–8.

34. Wenkel H, Rummelt V, Naumann GO. Long-term results after autologous nasal mucosal transplantation in severe mucus deficiency syndromes. Br J Ophthalmol 2000;84:279–84.

35. Nishida K, Yamato M, Hayashida Y, et al. Corneal reconstruction with tissue-engineered cell sheets composed of autologous oral mucosal epithelium. N Engl J Med 2004;351:1187–96.

36. Meller D, Dabul V, Tseng SCG. Expansion of conjunctival epithelial progenitor cells on amniotic membrane. Exp Eye Res 2002;74:537–45.

37. Ang LP, Sotozono C, Koizumi N, et al. A comparison between cultivated and conventional limbal stem cell transplantation for Stevens–Johnson Syndrome. Am J Ophthalmol 2007;143:178–80.

38. Tsai RJ, Li LM, Chen JK. Reconstruction of damaged corneas by transplantation of autologous limbal epithelial cells. N Engl J Med 2000;343:86–93.

39. Rama P, Matuska S, Paganoni G. Limbal stem-cell therapy and long-term corneal regeneration. N Engl J Med 2010;363:174–55.

40. Nishida K, Yamato M, Hayashida Y, et al. Functional bioengineered corneal epithelial sheet grafts from corneal stem cells expanded ex vivo on a temperature-responsive cell culture surface. Transplantation 2004;77:379–85.

41. Benhabbour SR, Sheardown H, Adronov A. Cell adhesion and proliferation on hydrophilic dendritically modified surfaces. Biomaterials 2008;29:4177–86.

42. Deshpande P, Notara M, Bullett N, et al. Development of a surface modified contact lens for transfer of cultured limbal epithelial cells for ocular surface diseases. Tissue Eng Part A 2009;15:2889–902.

43. Notara M, Bullet NA, Deshpande P, et al. Plasma polymer coated surfaces for serum-free culture of limbal epithelium for ocular surface disease. J Mater Sci Mater Med 2007;18:329–38.

44. Ang LP, Tan DT, Cajucom-Uy H, et al. Autologous cultivated conjunctival transplantation for pterygium surgery. Am J Ophthalmol 2005;139:611–9.

45. Daya SM, Chan CC, Holland EJ. Cornea Society Nomenclature for Ocular Surface Rehabilitative Procedures. Cornea 2011;30:1115–9.

46. Nath K, Shukla BR, Nema HV, et al. Auto-peritoneum as a conjunctival substitute. Ind J Ophthalmol 1964;12:75–81.

47. Allen JH. The use of peritoneum as a substitute for conjunctiva in plastic surgery: a preliminary report. Am J Ophthalmol 1953;36:1249–52.

48. Malhotra M. Plastic repair of conjunctiva with peritoneum transplantation. Br J Ophthalmol 1957;41:616–21.

49. Kruse FE. Classification of ocular surface disease. In: Holland EJ, Mannis MJ, editors. Ocular surface disease medical and surgical management. New York: Springer-Verlag; 2002. p. 16–36.

50. Wei ZG, Cotsarelis G, Sun TT, et al. Label-retaining cells are preferentially located in fornical epithelium: implications on conjunctival epithelial homeostasis. Invest Ophthalmol Vis Sci 1995;36:236–46.

51. Scocco S, Kwitko S, Rymer S, et al. HLA-matched living-related conjunctival limbal allograft for bilateral ocular surface disorders: long-term results. Arq Bras Oftalmol 2008;71:781–7.

52. Daya SM, Ilari FA. Living related conjunctiva limbal allograft for the treatment of stem cell deficiency. Ophthalmology 2001;108:126–33; discussion 133–4.

53. Croasdale CR, Schwartz GS, Malling JV, et al. Keratolimbal allograft: recommendations for tissue procurement and preparation by eye banks, and standard surgical technique. Cornea 1999;18:52–8.

54. Tseng SCG, Prabhasawat P, Barton K, et al. Amniotic membrane transplantation with or without limbal allografts for cornea surface reconstruction in patients with limbal stem cell deficiency. Arch Ophthalmol 1998;116:431–41.

55. Lee SH, Tseng SCG. Amniotic membrane transplantation for persistent epithelial defects with ulceration. Am J Ophthalmol 1997;123:303–12.

56. Paridaens D, Beekhuis H, van Den Bosch W, et al. Amniotic membrane transplantation in the management of conjunctival malignant melanoma and primary acquired melanosis with atypia. Br J Ophthalmol 2001;85:658–61.

57. Shimazaki J, Yang HY, Tsubota K. Amniotic membrane transplantation for ocular surface reconstruction in patients with chemical and thermal burns. Ophthalmology 1997;104:2068–76.

58. Azuara-Blanco A, Pillai CT, Dua HS. Amniotic membrane transplantation for ocular surface reconstruction. Br J Ophthalmol 1999;83:399–402.

59. Honovar SG, Bansal AK, Sangwan VS, et al. Amniotic membrane transplantation for ocular surface reconstruction in Stevens-Johnson syndrome. Ophthalmology 2000;107:975–9.

60. Gomes JA, dos Santos MS, Cunha MC, et al. Amniotic membrane transplantation for partial and total limbal stem cell deficiency secondary to chemical burn. Ophthalmology 2003;110:466–73.

61. Solomon A, Espana EM, Tseng SCG. Amniotic membrane transplantation for reconstruction of the conjunctival fornices. Ophthalmology 2003;110:93–100.

62. Barabino S, Rolando M, Bentivoglio G, et al. Role of amniotic membrane transplantation for conjunctival reconstruction in ocular cicatricial pemphigoid. Ophthalmology 2003;110:474–80.

njunctival Limbal Autograft

N J. WIFFEN

ongress in 1964, José
ograft of limbus from
al burns as a prepara-
He noted that this
helium but the mech-
ampelli et al. reported
rized opaque corneas
ng of limbus from the
ique in more detail at
Plastic Conference in
me time later that the
stem cells responsible
ated, and Kenyon and
fts of conjunctiva and
unilateral limbal defi-
bal autografts (CLAU)
n system for epithelial
nd and Schwartz in
any reports describing
role of CLAU in man-
ace disease has been

U) is indicated for man-
total unilateral limbal

y include varying com-
the cornea, with associ-
ular pannus, persistent
d scarring or stromal
on, chronic or recurrent

ry, as in aniridia, or sec-
uma, multiple surgeries,
-induced keratopathy, or
a.

of limbal autografts has
he form of an ipsilateral
is little evidence that the
ny benefit over a standard
other forms of unilateral
harvested from the other
chemical injury is prob-
enario. Figure 40.1 dem-
cular surface with CLAU

Preoperative Assessment and Considerations

It has been recognized that the state of the rest of the ocular surface is critical to the outcome of limbal transplantation. Preoperative assessment must include thorough examination of the ocular adnexa and ocular surface. The nature of chemical injuries and many of the other causes of limbal deficiency is such that other ocular surface or adnexal problems are commonly associated. Two important considerations in determining management are whether the condition is unilateral or bilateral and whether there is conjunctival involvement.[5]

Lid malposition, symblepharon, and trichiasis all need to be dealt with prior to limbal transplantation. The most common pre-existing problem is that of dry eye and this is a major prognostic factor.[11] If aqueous tear function is inadequate, then punctal occlusion should be performed. Blepharitis or ocular surface inflammation should be controlled optimally before surgery if possible.

In chemical injury cases, timing of CLAU is an important factor. CLAU may be performed either in the acute phase to aid healing or later once the cornea has conjunctivalized and inflammation has settled. In the acute phase, a limbal graft will not survive if the limbus is ischemic, and Tenon's advancement may be required. In addition, the inflammation that occurs in the acute and subacute stages of a chemical injury will often cause the CLAU to fail. Therefore it is advisable to wait until the inflammation has resolved before performing a CLAU. The delay in CLAU surgery is especially critical as the fellow eye can only be used once as a donor.

Intraocular pressure should be estimated, taking into account that tonometry may not be accurate with an abnormal ocular surface and cornea. Secondary glaucoma is common in the context of chemical injuries and steroid-related intraocular pressure rises may occur postoperatively. It is easy to overlook glaucoma when there are severe ocular surface problems, and loss of vision may occur even when epithelial transplantation is successful.

An assessment of the visual potential of the affected eye is required. If the eye has no visual potential, then it is not sensible to risk the donor eye, when another procedure, such as a conjunctival flap, may stabilize the ocular surface and provide comfort. Thorough discussion with the patient of the risks and benefits of surgery are required. In particular, the risk to the donor eye needs to be discussed. If the fellow eye has a history of trauma, then a careful examination of the conjunctiva, limbus and cornea is critical before recommending a CLAU. In addition, a history of long-term contact lens wear can result in subclinical damage to the limbal stem cells and may be a contraindication for CLAU.

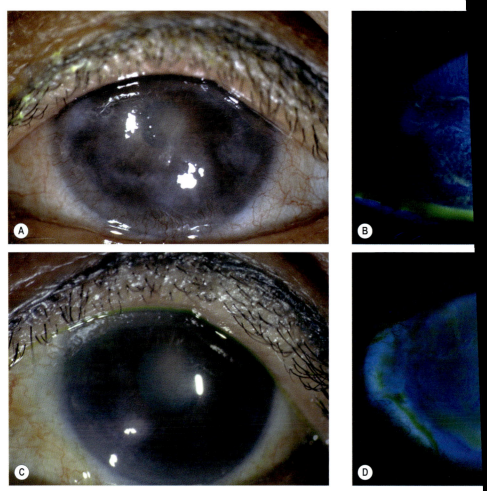

Figure 40.1 Conjunctival limbal autograft (CLAU) in chronic phase of unilateral chemical injury. (**A, B**) Pre□ valization of entire cornea. (**C, D**) Photographs at 6 weeks post CLAU. Note the smooth surface but some p□

Surgical Technique

Surgery may be performed under local or general anesthetic but the patient will need to be able to manage having both eyes operated on both during and after the procedure under local anesthetic.

Both eyes are prepped and draped. A well-fitting specu□ lum is required. At the start of surgery vasoconstriction may be achieved with topical epinephrine 1/10000 or, with apraclonidine 0.5% (Iopidine) or brimonidine 0.1% (Alphagan P) to avoid pupil dilation.

RECIPIENT PREPARATION

It is best to prepare the recipient eye first so that bleeding can be controlled. For complete limbal deficiency, a 360° limbal peritomy is performed with Westcott scissors (Fig. 40.2A). The conjunctiva is undermined to allow it to be recessed several millimeters in the superior and inferior locations. The pannus on the cornea will be easily removed except where the stroma has been damaged. In those areas

it will be more adherent □ section or scraping with □ With full conjunctivaliz□ adherence of the limbal □ removed around the lim□ required, to minimize fur□ ally stop with the wait d□ bed can be prepared for t□ ocular surface is moisten□ the eye closed or covered □

DONOR PREPARATION

Several techniques have b□ tion and fixation.[6] The ge□ 3 clock-hours (60–90°) □ inferior locations of the d□

The corneal extent of th□ an inked 10 or 11-mm tr□ concentric to the end of th□ diamond knife or the trep□

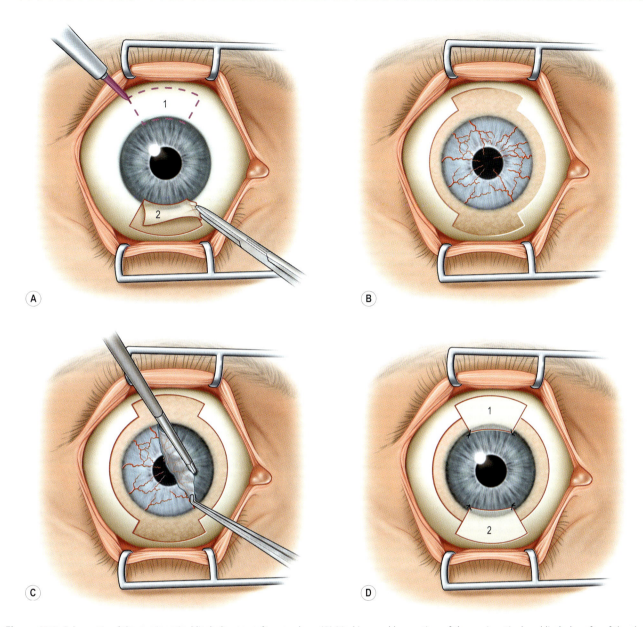

Figure 40.2 Schematic of the conjunctival limbal autograft procedure. (**A**) Marking and harvesting of the conjunctival and limbal grafts of the donor tissue at 12 and 6 o'clock. (**B**) Preparation of the recipient site with a 360° peritomy and resection of the conjunctiva at 12 and 6'clock for placement of the donor tissue. (**C**) Superficial keratectomy of the recipient cornea. (**D**) Placement of the CLAU grafts.

the cornea to a shallow depth to provide a discrete central edge. The diamond knife can be used to create discrete vertical nasal and temporal edges to the dissection as well. The conjunctival extent of the donor is marked with a pen in a fashion to allow easy orientation once it is transferred. The size of the conjunctiva section of the CLAU depends on the status of the injured eye. If there is primarily limbal deficiency and the conjunctiva is healthy appearing, a small conjunctival carrier section (2–3 mm) is all that is needed to carry the limbal cells. If the fellow eye has significant conjunctival disease with scarring and symblepharon formation, the conjunctival section should be larger to provide conjunctival epithelial and goblet cells. This section can be 4–6 mm superiorly, where there is redundant conjunctiva.

The conjunctiva is dissected, leaving as much Tenon's as possible, down to the adherence at the limbus. Some prefer to elevate conjunctiva with subconjunctival injection of balanced salt solution or anesthetic solution but it is not necessary. Conjunctiva is best handled with non-toothed or Moorfields forceps to avoid tissue damage. Westcott scissors are used to undermine the conjunctiva and it is easiest to do this with the conjunctiva under tension. That can be achieved by making the vertical incisions to the limbus first, then undermining between and then cutting the posterior conjunctival edge last.

Once the conjunctiva is undermined up to the limbus it can be reflected over the cornea and a crescent, or similar, blade is used to undermine the stroma to a shallow depth at the limbus up to the prepared corneal edges. It helps to have an assistant gently elevate the conjunctiva so that the blade tip can be seen just beneath the surface. If the corneal edges have not been scored at the start, the donor can be freed with straight Vannas scissors or the edge of the crescent blade, though the edge tends to me more irregular with this technique.

The donor tissue is transferred epithelial side up to a sterile dish and kept wet with balanced salt solution. If superior and inferior autografts are to be used, then the process is repeated for the inferior graft.

The donor site may be left as is, or the bulbar conjunctiva advanced toward the limbus and sutured or glued to reduce the size of the epithelial defect. The speculum is removed and the eye is closed while the tissue is secured in the recipient eye.

PLACEMENT OF THE DONOR TISSUE

The recipient limbus can be prepared in the same fashion as the donor to provide a discrete corneal edge for the donor tissue to butt against. Care is needed not to make the recipient bed too deep or there will be a step up at the corneal edge that will inhibit epithelial healing. Otherwise, the donor tissue may be just placed on the recipient limbus (Fig. 40.2D). Fibrin glue is applied to the recipient and the donor tissue placed in anatomical position and smoothed out. Alternatively, the graft is sutured in place at each end to the sclera either with 10-0 polyglactin (Vicryl) or 10-0 nylon. Braided polyglactin, though easier to handle, causes more tissue reaction and inflammation and loosens very quickly. The corners of the conjunctival part of the graft are then tacked to episclera and the recipient conjunctival edge with enough tension to keep it evenly spread out. Even with glue, it is prudent to place sutures at each end of the graft to prevent any chance of it dislodging. The donor conjunctival edge can be approximated carefully to the recessed recipient conjunctiva with sutures of just two single throws of 10-0 polyglactin as it should not be under tension. It is important for the assistant to keep the surface wet with balanced salt solution during this part of the procedure. A viscoelastic can be used to protect the surface but it tends to make suturing somewhat more difficult as the fine suture material sticks to it.

Subconjunctival and/or topical antibiotic and steroid are applied to both eyes. Bandage contact lenses are applied and the recipient eye has a patch and shield applied until the first postoperative day. The donor eye can be left open and topical therapy with antibiotic, steroid and lubricants started the same day.

Postoperative Management

Preservative-free topical steroid and antibiotics are given every 2–4 hours for the first week and then reduced as the surface heals. The bandage lenses are removed once the epithelium has closed and is stable.

There is generally some immediate swelling of the transplanted conjunctiva. The graft typically revascularizes within 5 days; there is then gradual thinning of the conjunctiva over weeks. Corneal epithelium extends from the central edges of the graft in a convex pattern and progresses

centrally over days (Fig. 40.3). The rate of healing depends on the state of the ocular surface at the time of transplantation and presumably other general factors, such as the age of the patient. The advancing edges of the corneal epithelium meet in the central cornea and may produce a typical healing line. The last part to heal is usually in the 3 and 9 o'clock zones of the peripheral cornea when superior and inferior grafts are used. If the conjunctival epithelium reaches the limbus before the corneal epithelium has healed, it may need to be removed by sequential sector conjunctival epitheliectomy (SSCE) as suggested for management of partial limbal deficiency[9] to prevent recurrent conjunctivalization of the cornea.

The donor site heals with slight thinning and some superficial vascularization of the cornea (Fig. 40.4).

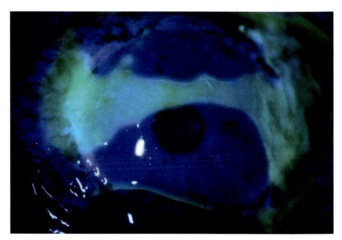

Figure 40.3 Conjunctival limbal autograft for limbal deficiency after multiple surgeries for conjunctival melanosis. Photograph at 5 days post surgery showing healing epithelium from superior and inferior grafts heading toward corneal centre. Note the conjunctival epithelial defects in the horizontal meridian.

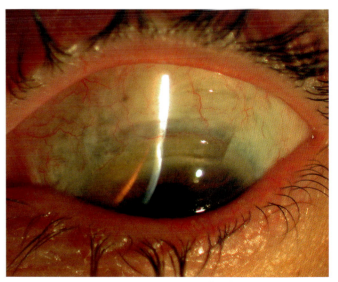

Figure 40.4 Conjunctival limbal autograft donor site at 1 year after surgery. Note mild thinning and some vascularization but smooth and clear adjacent cornea.

Problems

Complications may occur with CLAU surgery and have been reviewed recently.[12] These may relate to case selection and preoperative management, as well as to surgical technique. Damage to the donor eye is a major concern. There is one report of limbal deficiency developing in a donor eye in a case of contact lens-induced epitheliopathy that was not strictly unilateral.[13]

There has been one report of medium-term attenuation in viability of CLAU with progressive conjunctival ingrowth within a year of transplantation in three consecutive cases.[14] This has not been reported elsewhere.

Variations and Combination with other Procedures

It is not clear what minimum amount of limbus is required to provide a stable and clear surface in cases of total limbal deficiency. Given that in many clinical situations only a few clock hours of normal limbus are required to keep a cornea clear, it should not always be necessary to transplant 180° of limbus from the donor. However, the situation in the affected eye is not normal. Liang et al. have reported a satisfactory outcome from transplanting 60° of limbus combined with amniotic membrane transplantation.[8]

It has been suggested that amniotic membrane may facilitate expansion of remaining limbal stem cells in chemical injuries and it may do so in the autograft situation. Amniotic membrane transplantation has been used extensively in combination with CLAU and may reduce inflammation on the ocular surface, as well as providing a better environment for the corneal epithelium to recover.[8]

CLAU has been combined with penetrating or lamellar keratoplasty, either at the same time or subsequent to healing of the corneal surface, but there is little information about the longer-term success of keratoplasty in combined cases versus delayed keratoplasty.[7]

In cases of severe unilateral conjunctival and limbal disease with significant symblepharon formation, CLAU has been combined with keratolimbal allograft tissue (KLAL) at the 3 and 9 o'clock meridian (modified Cincinnati procedure) to prevent failure from conjunctival invading from the 3 and 9 o'clock meridians.[15] These patient require systemic immunosuppression to prevent rejection of the KLAL tissue. However, the duration of immunosuppression is shorter than in those patients with complete allografts.

The Future

Although the risk to the donor eye with CLAU is small, the procedure may be superseded by use of ex vivo expansion of limbal stem cells once systems for that are better defined and standardized. However, there may still be circumstances where transplantation of the limbal stem cell niche itself may be required or where CLAU is preferable as conjunctiva is also required.

References

1. Barraquer J. Panel Three Discussion. In: King JH, McTigue JW, editors. The Cornea World Congress. Washington: Butterworths; 1965. p. 354.
2. Strampelli B, Restivo Manfridi ML. Total keratectomy in leukomatous eye associated with autograft of a keratoconjunctival ring removed from the controlateral normal eye. Ann Ottalmol Clin Ocul 1966; 92:778–86.
3. Strampelli B. Ring autokeratoplasty. In: Rycroft PV, editor. Corneo-plastic surgery. Oxford: Pergamon Press; 1969. p. 253–75.
4. Kenyon KR, Tseng SCG. Limbal autograft transplantation for ocular surface disorders. Ophthalmology 1989;96:709–23.
5. Holland EJ, Schwartz GS. The evolution of epithelial transplantation for severe ocular surface disease and a proposed classification system. Cornea 1996;15:549–56.
6. Basti S, Rao SK. Current status of limbal conjunctival autograft. Curr Opin Ophthalmol 2000;11:224–32.
7. Cauchi PA, Ang GS, Azuara-Blanco A, et al. A systematic literature review of surgical interventions for limbal stem cell deficiency in humans. Am J Ophthalmol 2008;146:251–9.
8. Liang L, Sheha H, Li J, et al. Limbal stem cell transplantation: new progresses and challenges. Eye 2009;23:1946–53.
9. Dua HS, Miri A, Said DG. Contemporary limbal stem cell transplantation – a review. Clin Exp Ophthalmol 2010;38:104–17.
10. Kheirkhah A, Hashemi H, Adelpour M, et al. Randomized trial of pterygium surgery with mitomycin C application using conjunctival autograft versus conjunctival-limbal autograft. Ophthalmology 2012;119:227–32.
11. Santos MS, Gomes JA, Hofling-Lima AL, et al. Survival analysis of conjunctival limbal grafts and amniotic membrane transplantation in eyes with total limbal stem cell deficiency. Am J Ophthalmol 2005; 140:223–30.
12. Baradaran-Rafii AA, Eslani MM, Jamali JH, et al. Postoperative complications of conjunctival limbal autograft surgery. Cornea 2012;31: 893–9.
13. Jenkins C, Tuft S, Liu C, et al. Limbal transplantation in the management of chronic contact-lens-associated epitheliopathy. Eye 1993;7: 629–33.
14. Basti S, Mathur U. Unusual intermediate-term outcome in three cases of limbal autograft transplantation. Ophthalmology 1999;106: 958–63.
15. Chan CC, Biber JM, Holland EJ. The modified Cincinnati procedure: combined conjunctival-limbal autografts and keratolimbal allografts for unilateral severe ocular surface failure. Cornea 2012;31: 1264–72.

41 Living-Related Conjunctival–Limbal Allograft (lr-CLAL) Transplantation

ELHAM GHAHARI, ALIREZA BARADARAN-RAFII, and ALI R. DJALILIAN

Indications

In bilateral limbal stem cell deficiency (LSCD), a limbal allograft transplant utilizing donor tissue from a living relative (living-related conjunctival–limbal allograft; lr-CLAL) is an option that may be considered as an alternative or in combination with a keratolimbal allograft (KLAL). The lr-CLAL procedure utilizes normal limbal tissue on a conjunctival carrier that is harvested from one eye of a patient's living relative and transplanted to the diseased eye of the recipient. This procedure offers two distinct advantages over KLAL. First, in contrast to a KLAL graft which only includes viable limbal tissue, the lr-CLAL graft also includes a significant amount of healthy conjunctiva. The transplanted conjunctiva makes lr-CLAL particularly useful in patients with combined limbal and conjunctival deficiency, such as cicatrizing conjunctival diseases, including mucous membrane pemphigoid (MMP) and Stevens–Johnson syndrome (SJS). In many of the cicatrizing conjunctival cases, it may actually be beneficial to combine the lr-CLAL procedure with KLAL (i.e. the 'Cincinnati procedure') in order to provide enough limbal stem cells and the necessary conjunctiva for ocular surface rehabilitation. The other main advantage of lr-CLAL over KLAL is that it provides an opportunity for immunologic matching of the donor and the recipient. Although systemic immunosuppression is still necessary after lr-CLAL, matching the donor and recipient can potentially reduce the risk of immune rejection and the need for continued long-term systemic immunosuppression. The disadvantage of lr-CLAL, compared to KLAL is that the amount of tissue is limited, with fewer limbal stem cells transplanted. In addition there are gap areas between transplanted tissue with the lr-CLAl that can allow invasion of conjunctiva over the cornea in some cases. Lr-CLAL alone may be a particularly attractive option for patients with some residual limbal function, such that 360 degrees of limbal transplantation is not necessary or in cases without severe conjunctival disease.

Surgical Procedure

DONOR EYE

A thorough eye examination should be performed in all potential donors. If there is any ocular surface disease, history or suspicion of glaucoma (probability of future trabeculectomy) or history of long-term contact lens use (probability of limbal stem cell compromise), the donor should be excluded. The designated donor is then screened for hepatitis B and C, syphilis, and human immunodeficiency virus. They are also ABO and human leukocyte antigen (HLA I and II) typed and the best-matched consenting relative is selected for donation.

Harvesting the donor tissue is essentially the same as in CLAU. This procedure is typically done under local anesthesia using subconjunctival injection of xylocaine plus epinephrine. In some cases, retrobulbar/peribulbar anesthesia may be necessary. Two 60-degrees arcs of limbal lenticule, each spanning 2–3 clock hours, are harvested from one or both eyes of donor at 12 or 6 o'clock positions. A gentian violet surgical marking pen may be used to mark the conjunctival portions of the grafts (Fig. 41.1). The dissection can be started with lamellar dissection from the corneal side approximately 1 mm anterior and extending 2 mm posterior to the limbus, leaving behind the Tenon's capsule as much as possible. Alternatively, as the authors prefer, the dissection can be started on the conjunctiva and carried forward towards the limbus about 1–1.5 mm onto the cornea in a superficial manner. Care should be taken to avoid buttonholing of the donor tissue. Dissection onto the peripheral cornea past the palisades of Vogt is critical in order to obtain limbal stem cells. Amputation of the tissue peripheral to this landmark with result in the harvesting of conjunctiva only.

Typically, a 5-mm conjunctival skirt is harvested; however, the amount of the conjunctiva can be increased if the recipient eye also requires symblepharon repair and fornix reconstruction. After excising the donor tissue, the surrounding conjunctiva is undermined and advanced anteriorly and sutured with 10-0 nylon (or dissolvable suture) to close or partially close the conjunctival defect. Although the donor sites heal quickly, closing the defect enhances patient comfort and reduces likelihood of localized pannus formation.[1]

RECIPIENT EYE

The surgical procedure of lr-CLAL is identical to CLAU.[1] Surgery is done under general or retrobulbar/peribulbar anesthesia. After a 360-degree conjunctival peritomy, subconjuntival scar tissues are removed as much as possible, which typically results in the recession of the conjunctival edge to 3–5 mm from the limbus. Hemostasis is achieved

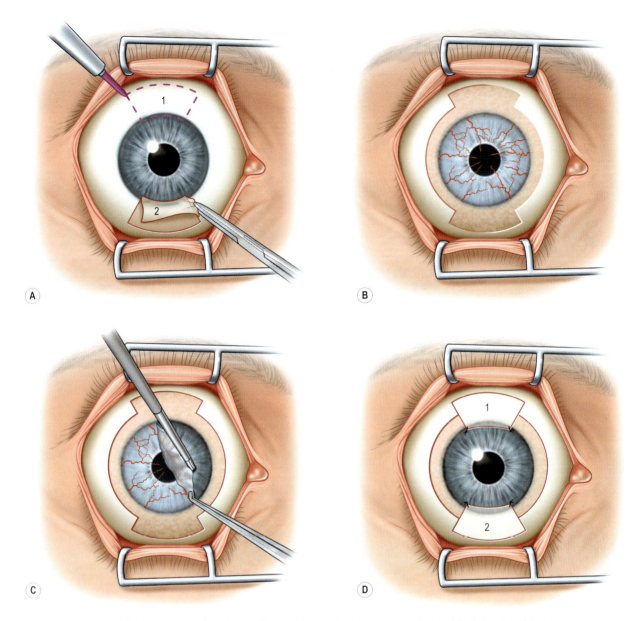

Figure 41.1 Schematic of the lr-CLAL procedure. (**A**) Marking and harvesting of the conjunctival and limbal grafts of the donor tissue at 12 and 6 o'clock. (**B**) Preparation of the recipient site with a 360° peritomy and resection of the conjunctiva at 12 and 6'clock for placement of the donor tissue. (**C**) Superficial keratectomy of the recipient cornea. (**D**) Placement of the CLAL grafts.

with mild wet-field cautery or dilute epinephrine (1 : 10 000). Corneal pannus is removed with special caution not to perforate the cornea. Donor grafts are sutured to the recipient eye at the corresponding anatomic sites by interrupted 10-0 nylon sutures. As an alternative to using sutures, the lr-CLAL grafts can also be directly fibrin glued onto the prepared bed.[2,3] This approach has the potential to decrease operative time, increase ease of technique, and improve patient comfort postoperatively. The surgical site may be covered with an overlain amniotic membrane or a high-DK bandage contact lens. At the end of surgery, upper and lower punctal occlusion and lateral tarsorrhaphy may be performed to protect grafts from the mechanical trauma of blinking, as well as from evaporative moisture loss in the early postoperative period in the more severe cases (Fig. 41.2).

CINCINNATI PROCEDURE

The Cincinnati procedure combines lr-CLAL and KLAL.[4] This procedure is considered for patients with both limbal and conjunctival deficiency. The Cincinnati procedure is useful in the management of eyes with cicatrizing conjunctival diseases and total limbal deficiency, such as SJS, OCP, and some chemical injuries. It improves the outcome by adding goblet cells and mucin production to the surface, providing barriers to symblepharon formation, and creating better fornices to allow for a better contact lens fitting, if required. The Cincinnati procedure uses only one corneoscleral rim, which is divided into two 180-degree KLAL segments. The harvested living-related tissue is typically sutured in the 12- and 6-o'clock meridians followed by the cadaveric donor segments which are placed at the 3- and

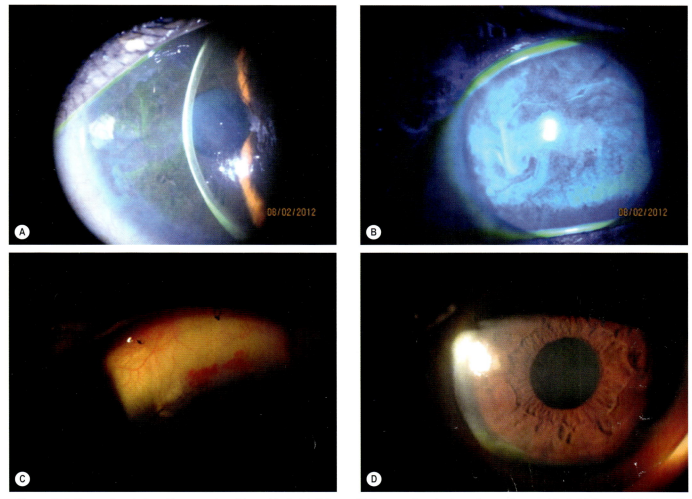

Figure 41.2 Contact lens-induced keratopathy with total limbal deficiency. (**A**) Preoperative photograph revealing total limbal failure with thickened abnormal corneal epithelium. (**B**) Preoperative photograph with fluorescein stain demonstrating diffuse late staining. (**C**) One month postoperative photograph of superior LR-CLAL segment. (**D**) Three month postoperative photograph showing normal corneal epithelium.

9-o'clock meridians (Fig. 41.3). The potential disadvantages, compared with KLAL alone are the risks to the donor, the time required to identify and test the donor, and the increased antigen load to the recipient. The advantages of the Cincinnati procedure are the increased amount of stem cells transplanted, the covering of the limbus with donor tissue for 360 degrees and the conjunctival and goblet cells that are provided. This procedure results in improved outcomes on those most challenging patients with severe ocular surface disease – those patients with severe conjunctival deficiency and limbal deficiency (Fig. 41.4).[4]

Postoperative Management

The basic principles of postoperative management after lr-CLAL are quite similar to KLAL and include controlling inflammation and preventing immune rejection, prophylaxis against infection, and assurance of adequate ocular surface lubrication.

After surgery, topical antibiotic and steroid drops (preferably preservative-free) are used 4–6 times a day. The former is discontinued when corneal epithelialization is complete, while the latter are continued indefinitely with the dosage adjusted according to ocular surface inflammation. Typically, a wave of progressive epithelium appears in front of each transplanted lenticule 1–2 days after surgery. They usually meet together after 7–10 days. Topical preservative-free artificial tears are used liberally to provide adequate lubrication of the ocular surface. Autologous serum drops are sometimes used during the first 2–3 months. High-DK bandage soft contact lenses may be used if the tear film is compromised or there is mild exposure.

The systemic immunosuppressive regimen is similar to KLAL and includes mycophenolate mofetil (1–2 g/day) and tacrolimus (4–8 mg/day) in twice a day dosing. The doses are adjusted according to ocular surface inflammation, trough levels and systemic adverse effects in collaboration with a transplant specialist. Oral prednisolone 0.5–1 mg/kg/day is started and tapered down during 6–8 weeks while inflammation decreases. Tapering of tacrolimus is started at 6–12 months based on the level of inflammation. In some patients, with an HLA-matched donor tissue, the taper may be started sooner while in

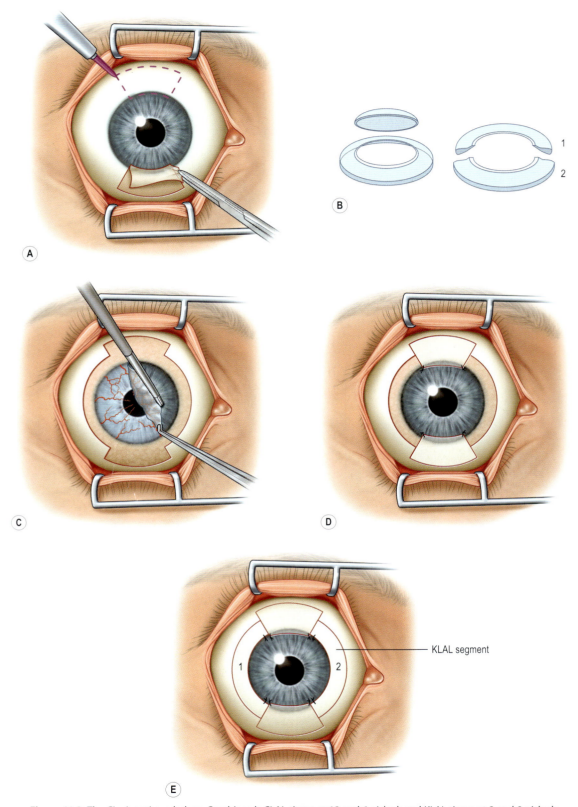

Figure 41.3 The Cincinnati prodedure. Combines lr-CLAL tissue at 12 and 6 o'clock and KLAL tissue at 3 and 9 o'clock.

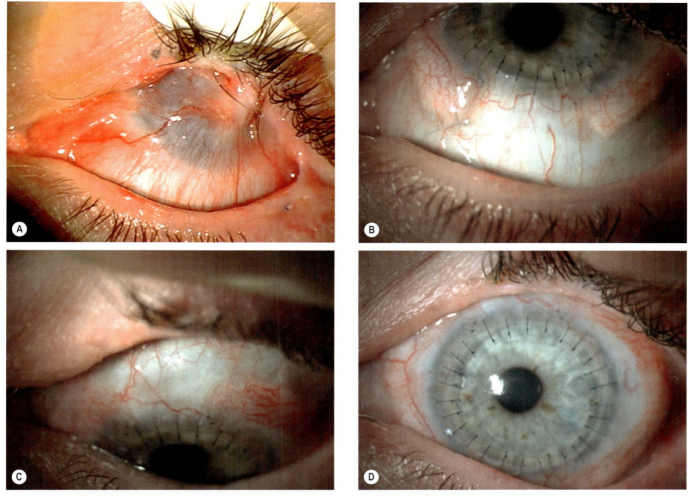

Figure 41.4 The Cincinnati procedure. (**A**) Preoperative photograph of severe chemical injury with conjunctival scarring, symblepharon, total limbal deficiency and corneal scarring. (**B**) Postoperative photograph showing the inferior lr-CLAL section and the 3 and 9 o'clock KLAL sections. (**C**) Postoperative photograph showing the superior lr-CLAL section. (**D**) Penetrating keratoplasty after a successful Cincinnati procedure.

patients with underlying inflammatory diseases it may be necessary to continue indefinitely on a maintenance dose.[4,5]

REJECTION

Acute rejection is the most common postoperative complication of lr-CLAL, occurring in 25% to 33% of cases.[6] Acute rejection typically presents with conjunctival injection, graft swelling and engorgement, with a progressively moving epithelial rejection line (Fig. 41.5).[7–9] Chronic rejection typically presents more insidiously as graft thinning with progressive corneal conjunctivalization/vascularization.

Acute rejections can be treated with an increase in dosage and frequency of topical and systemic steroids. Subconjunctival injection of triamcinolone may also be used. They are tapered according to reduction of ocular surface inflammation, vessel engorgement, local chemosis and disappearance of the epithelial rejection line.[5,7] Chronic rejection is treated with an increase in dosage of systemic immunosuppressives medication

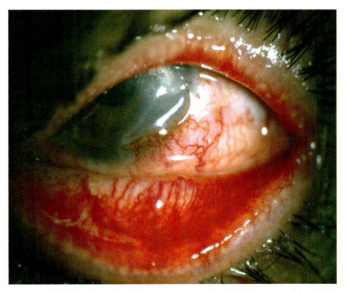

Figure 41.5 Acute epithelial rejection after lr-CLAL in an eye with stem cell deficiency, due to mustard gas keratopathy. Note graft edema, hyperemia, and progressive epithelial rejection line.

There are a few studies that suggest HLA matching may be useful in reducing the risk of rejection in lr-CLAL. In a prospective study of allogeneic conjunctival transplantation in 12 cases of bilateral ocular surface disorders, fewer rejection episodes and a better outcome was seen in patients who underwent identical or haploidentical HLA-matched grafts, compared with non-matched grafts.[10] Similar findings were observed in eight patients with severe chemical burns and SJS who underwent lr-CLAL from HLA-matched and unmatched donors. These studies suggest that HLA matching may play a role in graft survival.

Outcomes

Healing of the corneal epithelial defect and appearance of a smooth transparent epithelial surface are considered clinical success (Fig. 41.6).[8] Failure is defined as the presence of abnormally high fluorescein permeability with diffuse late-staining epithelium, recurrence of conjunctivalization, neovascularization, or persistent epithelial defects.[11,12]

The survival rate of lr-CLAL has been reported between 14% to 91.6%.[5,8,10,13,14,15] This wide range in outcomes is due, in part, to differences in inclusion criteria, follow-up periods, immunosuppression regimens, and success criteria. In a study with a mean follow-up of 48.7 months, 1 year after surgery visual acuity improved in 46.2%, and a stable corneal surface was achieved in 84.6% of the eyes. At the final follow-up, 66.6% of the eyes that had gained visual acuity 1 year after surgery maintained an improved visual acuity, and 93.9% still had a stable corneal surface.[11] In another study with a mean follow-up of 32 months, the success rate was reportedly as high as 89%.[16]

Complications

Donor eyes complications in lr-CLAL are rare and donor sites typically recover very well, without complication with re-epithelialization of the peripheral denuded limbus, within several days[17]. Donor sites may be partially re-epithelialized by conjunctival epithelium with some associated vessels in the periphery; however, this rarely leads to conjunctival growth beyond the excised area. Other possible complications are localized haze, pseudopterygium, filamentary keratitis, microperforation, abnormal epithelium, progressive conjunctivalization, corneal depression and subclinical limbal stem cell deficiency. Closing the conjunctival gap either by advancing the conjunctiva or with amniotic membrane and reducing the postoperative inflammation may reduce the risk of such complications in the donor eye. Excision and transplantation of more than six clock hours is best avoided for fear of precipitating limbal stem cell deficiency in the donor.

Intraoperative complications of the recipient eye include damage to the muscle during symblepharon release, bleeding during superficial keratectomy and corneal perforation. In most situations, putting the limbal tissue at 6 and 12-o'clock positions is important to have a constant coverage by upper and lower lids with a good spreading of tear film. Chronic exposure will lead to thinning, progressive vascularization and final failure of donor lenticules. Donor

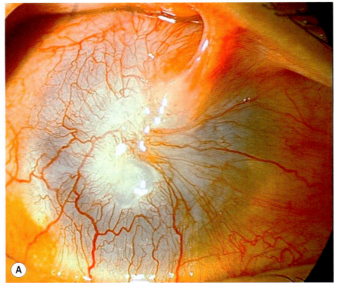

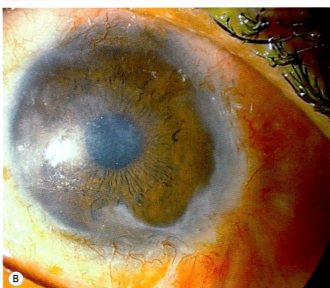

Figure 41.6 (A) Preoperative photograph showing 360 degrees of limbal stem cell deficiency and symblepharon formation in an eye with severe bilateral chemical burn. **(B)** One and one-half year after symblepharon repair and lr-CLAL from both eyes of his brother. Note remarkable clarity of the cornea and regression of corneal vascularization.

limbal tissue should be adequately trimmed and thinned. Thee placing of thick limbal grafts presents a barrier for epithelial cells by creating a large the step. It may also result in improper distribution of the tear film with subsequent dellen formation. Applying amniotic membrane may help reduce the step between thick or poorly trimmed limbal tissue and the ocular surface. Limbal alignment is important to prevent exposure and cutting limbal grafts during trephination in probable future keratoplasty. Very small limbal grafts can lead to PED, sectoral conjunctivalization, thinning and perforation. Proper suturing and timely suture removal are necessary to prevent dislodging of the donor tissue by the shearing action of the lids and to avoid injury to the growing epithelial edge.[18]

Progressive horizontal conjunctivalization and vascularization from gap areas may occur in some eyes. Sequential sector conjunctival epitheliectomy can be carried out when host conjunctival epithelium encroaches onto the cornea. The Cincinnati procedure, which combines lr-CLAL and KLAL, can prevent this complication.

References

1. Dua HS, Miri A, Dalia G, et al. Contemporary limbal stem cell transplantation – a review. Clin Exp Ophthalmology 2010;38:104–17.
2. Nassiri N, Pandya HK, Djalilian AR. Limbal allograft transplantation using fibrin glue. Arch Ophthalmol 2011;129:218–22.
3. Santos MS, Gomes JA, Hofling-Lima AL, et al. Survival analysis of conjunctival limbal grafts and amniotic membrane transplantation in eyes with total limbal stem cell deficiency. Am J Ophthalmol 2005;140:223–30.
4. Biber JM, Skeens HM, Neff KD, et al. The Cincinnati procedure: technique and outcomes of combined living-related conjunctival limbal allografts and keratolimbal allografts in severe ocular surface failure. Cornea 2011;30:765–71.
5. Javadi MA, Baradaran-Rafii AR. Living-related conjunctival–limbal allograft for chronic or delayed-onset mustard gas keratopathy. Cornea 2009;28:51–7.
6. Kwitko S, Marinho D, Barcaro S, et al. Allograft conjunctival transplantation for bilateral ocular surface disorders. Ophthalmology 1995;102:1020–5.
7. Daya SM, Ilari L. Living related conjunctival limbal allograft for the treatment of stem cell deficiency. Ophthalmology 2001;108:126–34.
8. Gomes JAP, Santos MS, Ventura AS, et al. Amniotic membrane with living related corneal limbal/conjunctival allograft for ocular surface reconstruction in Stevens–Johnson syndrome. Arch Ophthalmol 2003;121:1369–74.
9. Sangwan VS, Fernandes M, Bansal AK, et al. Early results of penetrating keratoplasty following limbal stem cell transplantation. Ind J Ophthalmol 2005;53:31–5.
10. Rao SK, Rajagopal R, Sitalakshmi G, et al. Limbal allografting from related live donors for corneal surface reconstruction. Ophthalmology 1999;106:822–8.
11. Reinhard T, Spelsberg H, Henke L, et al. Long-term results of allogeneic penetrating limbo-keratoplasty in total limbal stem cell deficiency. Ophthalmology 2004;111:775–82.
12. Scocco C, Kwitko S, Rymer S, et al. HLA-matched living-related conjunctival limbal allograft for bilateral ocular surface disorders: long-term results. Arq Bras Oftalmol 2008;71:781–7.
13. Liang L, Sheha H, Li J, et al. Limba Stem cell transplantation: new progresses and challenges. Eye 2009;23:1946–53.
14. Wylegala E, Dobrowolski D, Tarnawska D, et al. Limbal stem cells transplantation in the reconstruction of the ocular surface: 6 years experience. Eur J Ophthalmol 2008;18:886–90.
15. Miri A, Al-Deiri B, Dua HS. Long-term outcomes of autolimbal and allolimbal transplants. Ophthalmology 2010;117:1207–13.
16. Fernandes M, Sangwan VS, Rao SK, et al. Limbal stem cell transplantation. Ind J Ophthalmol 2004;52:5–22.
17. Miri A, Said DG, Dua HS. Donor Site Complications in Autolimbal and Living-Related Allolimbal Transplantation. Ophthalmology 2011;118:1265–71.
18. Baradaran-Rafii A, Eslani M, Jamali H, et al. postoperative complications of conjunctival limbal autograft surgery. Cornea 2012;31:893–9.

42 *Keratolimbal Allograft*

CLARA C. CHAN and EDWARD J. HOLLAND

Background

Keratolimbal allograft (KLAL) is a technique in which allogeneic cadaveric limbal stem cells are transplanted to a recipient eye with severe ocular surface disease using peripheral donor cornea as a carrier.[1] A number of techniques for KLAL have been reported, many of which describe strategies to facilitate harvesting the donor limbal grafts and donor tissue dissection. One of the earliest techniques, termed 'keratoepithelioplasty,' was to dissect the limbal tissue from a whole globe.[2] Tsubota and co-workers reported the use of stored corneoscleral rims for limbal stem cell transplantation, which allowed for better coordination of surgery after suitable donor tissue was retrieved.[3] Holland and Schwartz further modified the technique to use two stored corneoscleral rims instead of one, in order to fashion a contiguous ring of KLAL lenticules around the recipient limbus, which doubled the quantity of limbal stem cell supply and created a barrier to conjunctivalization.[4] Djajilian reported a conjunctival-based thin KLAL technique which employed fibrin glue alone to secure the limbal allografts using minimal or no peripheral scleral skirt.[5]

Optical keratoplasty, either deep anterior lamellar keratoplasty (DALK) or penetrating keratoplasty (PK), may be required after KLAL, if deeper corneal stromal scarring is present. Sundmacher et al. have described a procedure termed homologous penetrating central limbokeratoplasty, in which a stored corneoscleral rim is intentionally trephined off-center to create a penetrating keratoplasty button.[6] Using this technique, approximately 30–40% of the graft circumference contains limbal stem cells, and the patient benefits from receiving a clear penetrating graft along with limbal stem cells in a single operation. However, in severe cases of LSCD, it may be more beneficial to have limbal stem cells through 360 degrees. Performing optical keratoplasty as a staged procedure at least 3–6 months after KLAL allows for decreased ocular surface inflammation and stabilization of the corneal epithelium.

Indications

Keratolimbal allograft surgery is performed in patients who have no suitable living-related donor and have either bilateral LSCD or unilateral LSCD and fear damage to the healthy fellow eye (Fig. 42.1). Patients need to be suitable candidates for systemic immunosuppression, which is crucial to the success of KLAL in stabilizing the ocular surface and restoring a normal corneal epithelium phenotype.[7–9]

KLAL is ideal for diseases, such as aniridia, contact lens wear-related LSCD, and iatrogenic LSCD that affect mainly the limbus with minimal to no involvement of the conjunctiva.[1,7,10] Patients with total LSCD require 360-degree KLAL, while those with sectoral LSCD may require only sectoral KLAL.

In patients with mild chemical injuries, Stevens–Johnson syndrome (SJS) or ocular cicatricial pemphigoid (OCP) and who have LSCD with mild to moderate conjunctival inflammation, it is best if the eye is allowed to quiet for at least a year or more prior to KLAL surgery in order to increase the chances of graft survival. The success rate of KLAL decreases with increasing conjunctival inflammation, such as in severe cases of chemical injuries, SJS, or OCP.[1] In these cases, there is chronic conjunctival inflammation and scarring, decreased mucin and aqueous tear deficiency, and great potential for keratinization of the ocular surface. Since KLAL alone does not provide any healthy conjunctiva, for these severe cases of ocular surface disease, one can use in conjunction with two KLAL segments from one donor corneoscleral rim, living-related conjunctival limbal allograft (lr-CLAL) for bilateral disease and conjunctival limbal autograft (CLAU) for unilateral disease (Fig. 42.2).[11,12]

Preoperative Considerations

Prior to any limbal stem cell transplantation procedure, including KLAL, it is crucial that any lid functional abnormalities, exposure, and severe aqueous tear deficiency, be addressed. Eyelid abnormalities, such as lagophthalmos, misdirected lashes, malpositioned or keratinized lid margins, should be operated on prior to KLAL. The prognosis for KLAL is poor in patients with an abnormal or absent blink reflex, as persistent epithelial defects may develop with risk of scarring and infection. Patients with severe aqueous tear deficiency lack essential tear components and may benefit from autologous serum drops used regularly after KLAL.

Patients, such as those after chemical injury, who have glaucoma or uncontrolled intraocular pressure, should undergo glaucoma drainage device implantation prior to KLAL, since multiple glaucoma medications may contribute to additional ocular surface toxicity (Fig. 42.3). Long-term use of topical corticosteroids to prevent graft rejection will also further aggravate any pre-existing glaucoma.

KLAL is contraindicated in patients with significant keratinization of the ocular surface.[1] Uncontrolled severe inflammation is another poor prognostic factor for KLAL. Amniotic membrane grafts may be used in conjunction with KLAL to suppress inflammation and facilitate epithelialization.[9] Finally, systemic immunosuppression medications plays an important role and patient compliance must be assured prior to KLAL, since noncompliance has been shown to be the main reason for graft rejection and failure.[13]

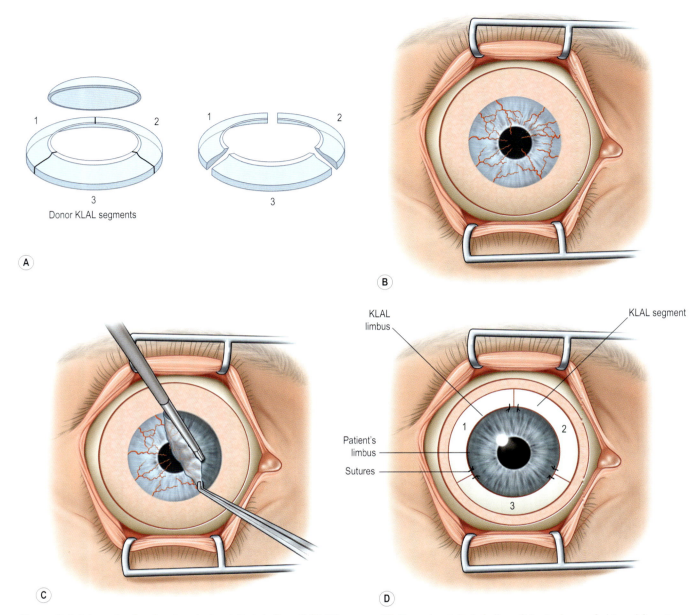

Figure 42.1 Schematic of major steps to keratolimbal allograft (KLAL) surgery. (**A**) Donor keratolimbal allograft lenticules are fashioned from two cadaver corneoscleral rims with the central 7.5 mm of cornea removed by trephination. (**B**) Conjunctival peritomy for 360 degrees and tenectomy is performed and the conjunctiva retracts. (**C**) Abnormal corneal epithelium and fibrovascular pannus are removed by superficial dissection using blunt and sharp techniques such as with a 64 Beaver blade. (**D**) KLAL lenticules are secured to the recipient limbus using 10-0 nylon sutures and tissue glue.

Donor Tissue Considerations

TISSUE SELECTION

Donor tissue supplied by an eye bank and stored in Optisol™ has greatly facilitated the ease of planning for KLAL procedures. However, the surgeon must communicate with the eye bank regarding availability of tissue and educate the staff regarding the special tissue requirements for KLAL. In contrast to the standard emphasis on preserving corneal endothelium and stroma for penetrating keratoplasty (PK) and endothelial keratoplasty (EK), for tissue to be used in KLAL, the donor limbal epithelium needs to be protected

from any trauma. 'Excellent epithelium' is an important specification and if the corneal epithelial layer appears entirely normal, the surgeon may be reassured that the limbal stem cells have undergone minimal harm during procurement.

Based on the authors' experience with supply of KLAL tissue from the Minnesota Lions Eye Bank, in addition to the Eye Bank Association of America guidelines, the following donor tissue selection guidelines have provided high-quality donor KLAL tissue:

- No active infection and no prior ventilator exposure in the donor

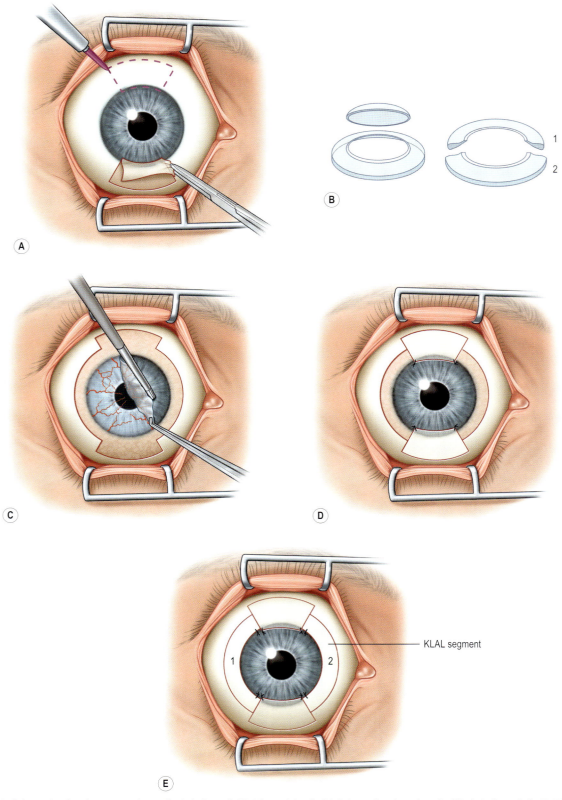

Figure 42.2 Schematic of major steps to keratolimbal allograft (KLAL) combined with living-related conjunctival limbal allograft (lr-CLAL) or conjunctival limbal autograft (CLAU) surgery. (*Top left*) Donor conjunctival limbal tissue is harvested. (*Top right*) Donor KLAL lenticules are fashioned from one cadaver corneoscleral rim with the central 7.5 mm of cornea removed by trephination. (*Middle left*) Conjunctival peritomy for 360 degrees and tenectomy is performed and the conjunctiva retracts. Abnormal corneal epithelium and fibrovascular pannus are removed by superficial dissection using blunt and sharp techniques such as with a 64 Beaver blade. (*Middle right*) lr-CLAL or CLAU donor tissue is secured to the recipient using 10-0 nylon sutures at the limbus and tissue glue. (*Bottom*) KLAL lenticules are secured to the recipient limbus using 10-0 nylon sutures and tissue glue.

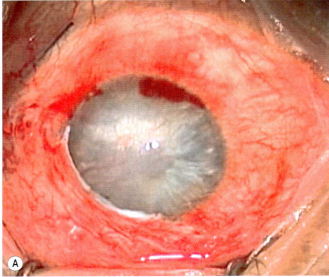

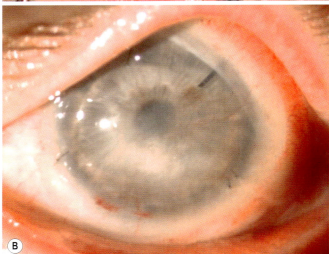

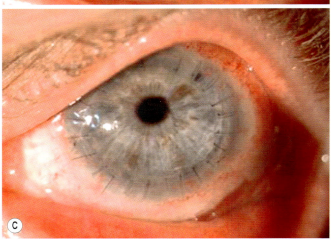

Figure 42.3 (**A**) Severe ocular surface failure with both limbal stem cell and conjunctival deficiency due to chemical and thermal injury. Visual acuity was hand motions. Glaucoma drainage device implantation was performed 3 months before ocular surface stem cell transplantation. (**B**) Three months after keratolimbal allograft. Note the stable ocular surface with reduced conjunctival inflammation and residual corneal stromal scarring. The glaucoma drainage device is positioned at 2 o'clock with a suture in situ. (**C**) Penetrating keratoplasty (PK) is performed 3 months after keratolimbal allograft has stabilized the ocular surface. Three months after PK, best corrected visual acuity measured 20/40.

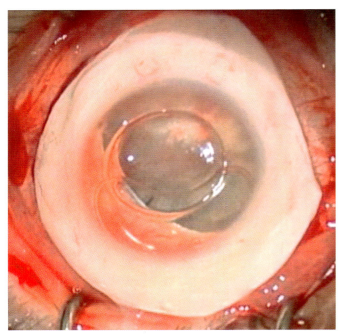

Figure 42.4 Donor corneoscleral rim after trephination of central 7.5 mm of central cornea. Note the excellent epithelium quality and the 3–4-mm skirt of peripheral conjunctiva along with a 4–5-mm scleral rim to ensure minimal damage to the limbal area during donor tissue preparation.

- Donor age 5 to 70 years (preferably younger than 50 years)
- Minimal time from donor death to tissue preservation
- Implantation of KLAL tissue 5–7 days from death of donor.

EYE BANK TISSUE PREPARATION

Another difference from tissue preparation for PK or EK is that a 3–4-mm skirt of peripheral conjunctiva along with a 4–5-mm scleral rim is left on the corneoscleral rim for KLAL transplantation (Fig. 42.4). Leaving both this conjunctival and scleral rim minimizes damage to the limbal area and provides some goblet cells which are often deficient in recipient eyes. There has been no evidence to indicate any increased risk of infection by leaving the conjunctival rim intact.

For 360-degree limbal coverage using KLAL tissue, the corneoscleral rims from both eyes of the same donor are used for one recipient eye. In cases in which KLAL is performed in conjunction with living-related conjunctival limbal allograft ('Cincinnati procedure') or conjunctival limbal autograft ('Modified Cincinnati procedure') surgery, only one corneoscleral rim is needed.[11,12]

Surgical Technique

GENERAL CONSIDERATIONS

Keratolimbal allograft surgery provides healthy limbal stem cells to the host limbus. Since most tissue supply is prepared and delivered by an eye bank, the use of peripheral corneo-scleral tissue with overlying conjunctiva allows for the safe transfer and securing of stem cells to the recipient limbus.

In general, retrobulbar anesthesia with a seven cranial nerve block or general anesthesia is administered. Figure 42.1 and the associated video footage demonstrate key steps of the KLAL procedure (Video 1), which has been further adapted from the original corneoscleral crescent technique of Holland and Schwartz.[4,7]

PREPARATION OF THE DONOR TISSUE

The central cornea of each corneoscleral rim is excised with a 7.5-mm trephine as in routine keratoplasty. Under a surgical microscope, the rim is then sectioned into two halves and trimmed to leave approximately 2–3 mm of sclera peripheral to the limbus. The posterior sclera and corneal stroma, including Descemet's membrane and endothelium of each segment are removed by lamellar dissection using a sharp rounded crescent blade and curved Vannas scissors. The prepared KLAL lenticules are then placed in storage media solution.

If the surgeon does not have an assistant to provide countertraction during tissue preparation, he or she may utilize cyanoacrylate glue to stabilize the KLAL scleral bed onto a sterile plastic platform followed by a thin strip of viscoelastic near the anterior edge of the lenticule during donor dissection of the anterior corneal stroma and donor conjunctival limbal tissue.[5]

PREPARATION OF THE RECIPIENT EYE

A 360° conjunctival peritomy is performed, including release of any symblephara that are present at the limbus. The conjunctiva is allowed to recess 2–3 mm from the limbus. This often occurs naturally due to previous tension from scarring. Tenon's capsule is often extremely thick in these eyes due to chronic inflammation and may be liberally excised with care taken to preserve the overlying conjunctiva. In the rare event that excess conjunctiva is present, a conservative amount may be trimmed. Topical epinephrine (1:10000 dilution) and wet-field cautery are used to control for hemostasis and to allow for better visualization of the surgical field. Abnormal corneal epithelium and fibrovascular pannus are then removed by superficial keratectomy using a No. 64 Beaver or equivalent crescent blade, taking care to avoid cutting deep into stroma.

PLACEMENT OF THE DONOR TISSUE

Each KLAL segment may be secured at the limbal edge using two 10-0 nylon sutures cut very short. The segments may then be trimmed as needed so that they do not overlap. Fibrin tissue glue is applied to secure the base of the KLAL lenticules to the recipient sclera and to ensure that the conjunctiva sits abutting the posterior edge of the KLAL lenticule. During suturing, the KLAL tissue should be protected from trauma with a viscoelastic coating. If the donor tissue is very thin, fibrin glue alone may be used to secure the lenticules (Fig. 42.5).

It is crucial to place the three donor segments immediately adjacent to one another to avoid any gaps between

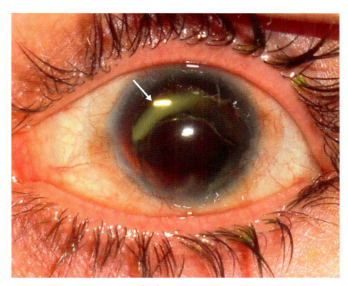

Figure 42.5 Photograph of left eye in patient with aniridia 1.5 years after conjunctival-based thin keratolimbal allograft and subsequent cataract extraction and intraocular lens implant. Note the residual Sommering's ring and the faint outline of the KLAL (*arrows*).

tissues, which could allow conjunctival invasion onto the surface. The authors recommend that the host and donor conjunctiva be well approximated to each other or to have the host conjunctiva slightly pulled over the donor conjunctiva. This avoids the possibility of host conjunctival growth under the grafts while also preventing the formation of inclusion cysts.

Postoperative Care

LOCAL MANAGEMENT AND SYSTEMIC IMMUNOSUPPRESSION

At the conclusion of the KLAL procedure, subconjunctival corticosteroids and cefazolin are injected into the recipient eye. A 16.0 or 18.0-mm (9.8-mm base curve) soft bandage contact lens (BCL) (Kontur Contact Lens, Co, Richmond, CA) is placed, and a protective patch and shield is taped on for 4 hours. At home, the patient removes the patch and shield and begins the standard topical medications used after routine PK: topical cyclosporine 0.05% twice daily (for the duration of the patient's follow-up), difluprednate (or prednisolone acetate 1%) four times daily (for the first 3 months then tapered by 1 drop per month according to the degree of ocular surface inflammation), a fourth-generation fluoroquinolone four times daily (until the corneal epithelium is healed and at which time the BCL is also removed), and frequent non-preserved artificial tears.

Systemic immunosuppression must be used in patients after KLAL to prevent immune rejection of the allograft tissue and to manage the chronic inflammation present in eyes with severe ocular surface disease. Inflammation may lead to destruction of transplanted stem cells in the short and long term. A regimen consisting ideally of systemic steroids, tacrolimus, and mycophenolate mofetil has been used with good success to increase graft survival.[5,8,9] Triple treatment consisting of systemic steroids, cyclosporine, and azathioprine has previously been used. Co-management with an organ transplant specialist with experience in the use of these immunosuppression medications is highly recommended.

OPTICAL KERATOPLASTY

After achieving a stable ocular surface with KLAL (see Fig. 42.3Bb), subsequent optical keratoplasty may be performed to clear any deep stromal scarring (see Fig. 42.3C). It is advisable to wait at least 3–6 months to achieve a stable ocular surface before proceeding with PK or DALK. There are technical challenges in corneal transplantation after ocular surface stem cell transplantation. Usually, larger-diameter trephinations (approximately 9.5 to 11 mm) are sized to abut the border of the KLAL tissue. Donor buttons should be oversized by 0.5 mm, since eyes with chronic inflammation or cicatricial disease from chemical injury often contract after trephination of the host cornea. Deep bites should be employed with 24 interrupted 10-0 nylon sutures to ensure that the donor and host cornea are fully approximated, avoiding suturing just to the superficial KLAL segment.[14]

Outcomes

Graft survival rates for KLAL range from 33% to 84%.[15] The use of systemic immunosuppression after KLAL is required to decrease the risk of graft failure secondary to rejection. This subject is discussed more extensively in Chapter 46.

The best results after limbal stem cell transplantation are achieved with adequate triple systemic immunosuppression. In a study of 31 eyes of 23 patients with aniridia after KLAL with follow-up of 12 to 117 months, 23 eyes (74.2%) achieved a stable ocular surface, and overall mean visual acuity improved from 20/1000 to 20/165.[7] A study of 19 eyes from 16 patients demonstrated a KLAL survival rate of 76.9% after a follow-up of 31 months.[5] Fifteen eyes (78.9%) showed an improvement in vision of two or more Snellen lines. Another study of 12 eyes from 10 patients with follow up of 36 to 91 months after KLAL reports a stable ocular surface achieved in 83%.[9]

In evaluating the success of KLAL, it is also important to consider the length of follow-up. Three to four months after PK, a healthy-appearing ocular surface may be populated by the transplanted adult epithelial cells of the donor cornea only. It can be a year or more before the limbal stem cells are called upon to repopulate the ocular surface. Hence, more than 1 year of follow-up after KLAL is needed to pass judgment on the procedure's success.

References

1. Holland EJ. Epithelial transplantation for the management of severe ocular surface disease. Trans Am Ophthalmol Soc 1996;94: 677–743.
2. Thoft RA. Keratoepithelioplasty. Am J Ophthalmol 1984;97:1–6.
3. Tsubota K, Toda I, Saito H, et al. Reconstruction of the corneal epithelium by limbal allograft transplantation for severe ocular surface disorders. Ophthalmology 1995;102:1486–96.
4. Croasdale CR, Schwartz GS, Malling JV, et al. Keratolimbal allograft: recommendations for tissue procurement and preparation by eye banks, and standard surgical technique. Cornea 1999;18:52–8.
5. Nassiri N, Pandya HK, Djalilian AR. Limbal allograft transplantation using fibrin glue. Arch Ophthalmol 2011;129:218–22.
6. Reinhard T, Sundmacher R, Spelsberg H, et al. Homologous penetrating central limbo-keratoplasty (HPCLK) in bilateral limbal stem cell insufficiency. Acta Ophthalmol Scand 1999;7:663–7.
7. Holland EJ, Djalilian AR, Schwartz G. Management of aniridic keratopathy with keratolimbal allograft: a limbal stem cell transplantation technique. Ophthalmology 2003;110:125–30.
8. Holland EJ, Mogilishetty G, Skeens HM, et al. Systemic immunosuppression in ocular surface stem cell transplantation: results of a 10-year experience. Cornea 2012;31:655–61.
9. Liang L, Sheha H, Tseng SC. Long-term outcomes of keratolimbal allograft for total limbal stem cell deficiency using combined immunosuppressive agents and correction of ocular surface deficits. Arch Ophthalmol 2009;127:1428–34.
10. Schwartz GS, Holland EJ. Iatrogenic limbal stem cell deficiency. Cornea 1998;17:31–7.
11. Biber JM, Skeens HM, Neff KD, et al. The Cincinnati procedure: technique and outcomes of combined living-related conjunctival limbal allografts and keratolimbal allografts in severe ocular surface failure. Cornea 2011;30:765–71.
12. Chan CC, Biber JM, Holland EJ. The modified Cincinnati procedure: combined conjunctival limbal autografts and keratolimbal allografts for severe unilateral ocular surface failure. Cornea 2012;31: 655–61.
13. Andrea AY, Chan CC. Biber JM, et al. Ocular surface stem cell transplantation rejection: incidence, characteristics, and outcomes. Cornea 2012, June 4.
14. Biber JM, Neff KD, Holland EJ, et al. Corneal transplantation in ocular surface disease. In: Krachmer JH, Mannis MJ, Holland EJ, editors. Cornea, vol. 2. 3rd ed. London: Elsevier; 2010. p. 1755–8.
15. Cauchi PA, Ang GS, Azuara-Bianco A, et al. A systematic literature review of surgical interventions for limbal stem cell deficiency in humans. Am J Ophthalmol 2008;146:251–9.

43 Tissue Engineering for Reconstruction of the Corneal Epithelium

URSULA SCHLÖTZER-SCHREHARDT, NARESH POLISETTI,
JOHANNES MENZEL-SEVERING, and FRIEDRICH E. KRUSE

Introduction

Over the past several years tissue engineering has become a rapidly growing field of research with strong translational potential into clinical practice through application of adult stem cells (SC) and biomaterial sciences. It is believed that SC, with their inherent plasticity, could be utilized to regenerate the natural complexity present in native tissue, while providing factors required for lineage maintenance and differentiation. Thus, the basic strategy of tissue engineering is the construction of a biocompatible scaffold that in combination with SC and bioactive molecules replaces and regenerates damaged cells or tissues.[1]

The cornea is composed of three layers, an outer stratified, rapidly regenerating epithelium, the underlying stroma, and an inner single-layered endothelium. Homeostasis of corneal epithelial cells is an important prerequisite not only for the integrity of the ocular surface, but also for corneal transparency and visual function (Fig. 43.1A,C). The continuous renewal of the corneal epithelium is provided by a population of adult SC located in the basal epithelium of the transitional zone between cornea and conjunctiva, the limbus (Fig. 43.1B).[2] Stem cell maintenance and function are controlled by various intrinsic and extrinsic factors provided by a unique local microenvironment or niche.[3] Limbal stem cells (LSC) and their progeny reside within small clusters in the basal epithelium in close relationship with specific extracellular matrix components, stromal fibroblasts, blood vessels, and nerves providing increased levels of growth and survival factors. Limbal SC can divide both symmetrically to self-renew and asymmetrically to produce daughter transiently amplifying cells that migrate centripetally to populate the basal layer of the corneal epithelium and eventually become post-mitotic terminally differentiated epithelial cells (Fig. 43.1B). Limbal SC can be identified by positive expression of putative stem/progenitor cell markers, including ABCG2, ΔNp63α, Bmi1, CEBPδ, OCT4, Lgr5, cytokeratin K15, and N-Cadherin, and the absence of corneal epithelial differentiation markers, such as cytokeratins K3 and K12.[4]

Dysfunction or loss of the LSC population in combination with an impairment of their niche, due to different inherited or acquired conditions may result in partial or total limbal stem cell deficiency (LSCD), which has severe consequences for ocular surface integrity and visual function (Fig. 43.1D). A range of inflammatory eye conditions (e.g. Stevens – Johnson syndrome, mucous membrane pemphigoid), degenerative processes (e.g. recurrent pterygia), hereditary causes (e.g. congenital aniridia), and chemical or thermal trauma, can lead to chronic epithelial healing defects associated with conjunctival epithelial ingrowth, neovascularization, inflammation, ulceration and scarring, and ultimately to functional blindness.[5,6] These conditions are contraindications for conventional corneal transplantation, i.e., a full-thickness corneal graft, because the ocular surface will not re-epithelialize properly without replenishment of the depleted stem cell pool. Therefore, corneal repair may be possible only by addressing the epithelial disorder through layer-specific stem cell-based approaches to corneal surface reconstruction. Reconstruction of the stratified ocular surface epithelium, particularly in patients with bilateral LSCD, is critical to restore vision and represents one of the most challenging problems in clinical ophthalmology.

Current tissue engineering approaches for reconstruction of the corneal epithelium utilize adult SC, usually LSC derived from a small tissue biopsy from either the patient (autologous) or a donor (allogeneic), followed by their ex vivo expansion in culture on a natural scaffold, usually human amniotic membrane, and generation of three-dimensional epithelial constructs for transplantation.[7] Differences in culture techniques include the use of explant or single-cell suspension systems, the presence or absence of a mouse 3T3 fibroblast feeder layer, the type of substrate, and the optional application of airlifting to promote epithelial differentiation and stratification. In their attempt to improve and standardize this therapeutic approach, researchers have focused on the optimization of culture conditions in order to replicate the in vivo stem cell niche and to preserve stemness, on the introduction of safer culture procedures to avoid the use of xenobiotics, on the exploration of alternative autologous stem cell sources for treatment of bilateral surface disorders, and on the evaluation of novel scaffolds to aid SC expansion and enhance transplantation efficacy. The challenges to create a tissue-engineered corneal epithelial equivalent include generating a biocompatible, mechanically stable, and optically transparent construct, which supports SC growth and maintenance in culture and after transplantation.

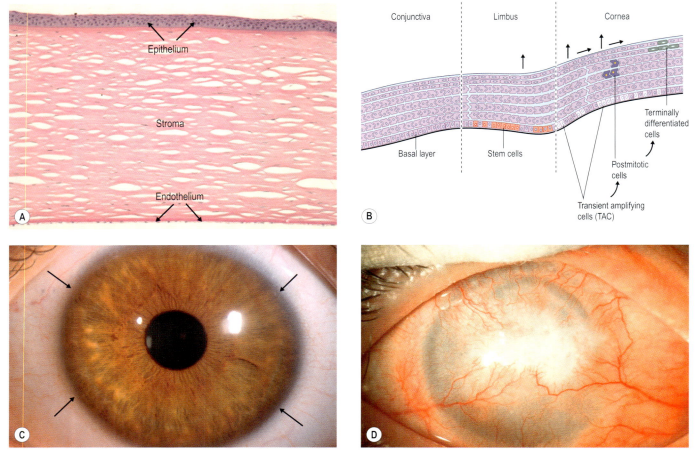

Figure 43.1 The ocular surface. (**A**) Light microscopic image of a section through a human cornea showing its composition of a stratified surface epithelium, stroma, and single-layered endothelium (periodic acid–Schiff staining). (**B**) Schematic concept of limbal location of corneal stem cells and transient amplifying cells. (**C**) Clinical appearance of a healthy human cornea (*arrows indicate corneal limbus*). (**D**) Clinical appearance of a patient with severe limbal stem cell insufficiency showing conjunctivalization and vascularization of the corneal surface. (Fig. 1B: Reproduced from: Schlötzer-Schrehardt U, Kruse FE. Identification and characterization of limbal stem cells. Exp Eye Res 2005;81:247–64. With permission from Elsevier.)

Stem Cell Sources for Corneal Epithelial Reconstruction

Limbal SC have been extensively investigated for their ex vivo culture and subsequent transplantation efficacy in clinical application. In addition, cultured oral mucosal epithelial SC have been used for the treatment of LSCD in patients with bilateral ocular surface disease.[8] Cell types other than LSC or oral mucosal epithelial SC, including conjunctival epithelial SC,[9–11] hair follicle SC,[12,13] mesenchymal SC,[14–16] immature dental pulp SC,[17] umbilical cord SC,[18] and embryonic SC[19] have been additionally proposed as alternative autologous SC sources for tissue engineering and already provided promising results in vitro and in vivo preclinical animal studies. It is clearly desirable to use autologous cells for tissue engineering, as this avoids the risk of allogeneic immune rejection and the need for immunosuppression.

Conditions mimicking the in vivo LSC niche, such as limbal fibroblast conditioned media, have been used to induce a corneal epithelial-like phenotype in constructs derived from non-corneal SC sources.[12,16,20] The suitability of epithelial constructs as a corneal epithelium

replacement is usually evaluated by expression of typical corneal epithelial differentiation markers (cytokeratins K3 and K12) and the ability to reconstruct the damaged ocular surface by providing sufficient mechanical stability and optical transparency.

LIMBAL EPITHELIAL STEM/PROGENITOR CELLS

A major tissue engineering strategy for reconstruction of the corneal epithelium is based on ex vivo expansion of autologous SC taken from the limbus of the patient's contralateral healthy eye in unilaterally affected patients.[21,22] This cultured limbal epithelial transplantation (CLET) appears to be a promising treatment modality for LSCD with an overall success rate of 75% up to 119 months follow-up.[23–26] The most widely used expansion method is the explant culture system, in which a small limbal biopsy (1–2 mm²) is placed on a carrier, usually amniotic membrane, and the limbal epithelial cells then migrate out of the biopsy and proliferate to form an epithelial sheet (Fig. 43.2). However, outgrowths from human limbal explants show a rapid decline in proliferative potential,[27] and use of limbal epithelial cell suspensions appears to increase the proportion of SC in the culture system.[28]

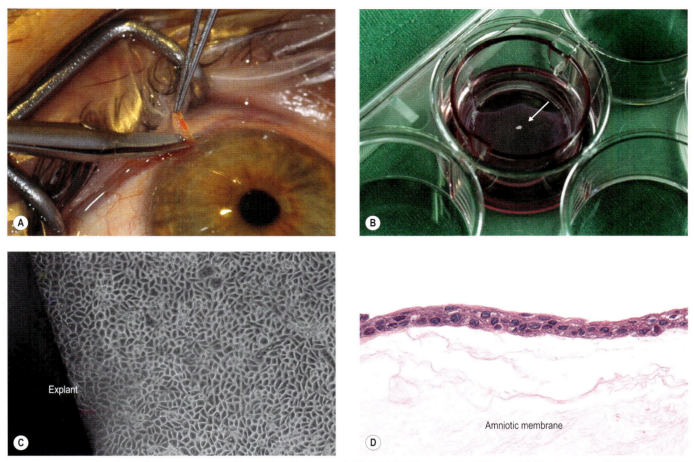

Figure 43.2 Ex vivo expansion of human limbal stem cells on human amniotic membrane. (**A**) Harvest of a 1×2-mm biopsy from the superior limbus of the healthy eye from a patient with unilateral limbal stem cell deficiency. (**B**) Explant culture of a limbal biopsy (*arrow*) on human amniotic membrane. (**C**) Outgrowth of an epithelial monolayer from the explant. (**D**) Multilayered epithelial sheet growing on amniotic membrane after 2 weeks in culture.

An essential prerequisite of epithelial grafts for long-term restoration of the ocular surface is the presence of an adequate number of stem cells.[4,29,30] Since the pioneering work by Rheinwald and Green,[31] studies have confirmed that long-term survival of epithelial SC is possible if co-cultured with embryonic fibroblast feeder cells, which appear to reproduce aspects of the SC niche in vitro. This strategy led to the development of a culture system that involves enrichment of LSC by clonal growth on an inactivated mouse 3T3 fibroblast feeder layer before being seeded onto transplantable carriers to produce epithelial sheets.[22,32] Preoperative demonstration of ΔNp63-positive cells within epithelial grafts has been considered as a means of quality control for transplantation.[25,33–35]

Over the past years there have been various modifications of culture techniques. Important parameters that influence cell proliferation and differentiation include growth factors, serum and calcium concentrations, type of matrix coating, and substrate stiffness as indicated by the elastic modulus.[32,36] Culture of epithelial cells at the air–liquid interface (airlifting) has addressed the in situ environment of the cornea thereby promoting epithelial cell differentiation and stratification.[37] Hypoxic conditions coupled with air exposure have been shown to further enhance LSC proliferation.[38]

Moreover, co-culture of LSC and adherent mesenchymal niche cells expressing embryonic SC markers has been reported to promote the preservation of a LSC phenotype.[39] Recent approaches aim at establishing genetically modified cells, such as telomerase immortalized corneal epithelial cells,[40] and at replacing potentially hazardous xenobiotics, such as fetal calf serum and murine feeder cells, by materials of human origin[41–43] or using serum- and feeder-free culture systems.[44]

Nevertheless, at present, the most common method for clinical application uses LSC, human amniotic membrane or fibrin as substrates, and mouse 3T3 fibroblast feeder layers. Alternative sources of non-corneal adult SC and novel scaffolds are currently under extensive investigation.

NON-CORNEAL EPITHELIAL STEM/PROGENITOR CELLS

For treatment of patients with bilateral ocular surface disease, strategies may utilize autologous SC from stratified epithelia of other areas of the body. Recent progress in this field suggests that conjunctival epithelium,[9–11] oral mucosal epithelium,[8,45,46] epidermis,[47] and hair follicle[12,32] may serve as alternative sources of autologous adult SC of related lineage, which can be used to construct an artificial corneal epithelium and to reconstruct the ocular surface in animal models and patients with LSCD.

Oral mucosal epithelium has attracted much attention as an autologous epithelial stem cell source and cultured oral mucosal epithelial transplantation (COMET) has already been used for restoration of the corneal surface in patients with bilateral LSCD.[8,45,46,47,48] A recent study by Nakamura and coworkers showed promising long-term clinical results of COMET with an improved visual acuity in 10 eyes (53%) at 36 months postoperatively.[49] However, peripheral neovascularization is commonly seen in COMET, and the long-term clinical success of this technique still requires detailed investigation. It has also been reported that oral mucosal epithelial cell grafts rarely transdifferentiate to a corneal epithelial phenotype, as indicated by lacking expression of cytokeratin K12.[8]

The discovery of various, not yet completely defined SC populations in the epithelial and mesenchymal compartment of the hair follicle, has encouraged research into utilizing the hair follicle as a source of adult multipotent SC for regenerative medicine.[50] The hair follicle bulge region represents a major repository of multipotent keratinocyte SC, which have the potential to differentiate into hair follicle, sebaceous gland, and epidermis (Fig. 43.3A,B). The potential of murine hair follicle-derived adult SC to transdifferentiate into corneal epithelial-like cells has been recently shown by Blazejewska et al.[12] When exposed to a limbus-specific environment using conditioned medium from limbal stromal fibroblasts and laminin V-coated culture dishes, hair follicle-derived SC could be reprogrammed in vitro into a corneal epithelial phenotype expressing corneal epithelial differentiation markers K12 and Pax6 (Fig. 43.3C–F). Using a transgenic reporter mouse model, which allowed for the detection of K12 expression in vivo, the transplanted corneal epithelial constructs provided evidence of corneal epithelial transdifferentiation and were able to reconstruct the ocular surface of LSCD mice (Fig. 43.4).[13] These data highlight the promising therapeutic potential of these plastic and readily accessible SC to treat bilateral LSCD.

MESENCHYMAL STEM CELLS

Other proposed sources of SC for reconstruction of the corneal epithelium include bone marrow-derived mesenchymal SC,[14,15,51,52] adipose tissue-derived mesenchymal SC[53] and dental pulp SC.[17]

Studies by Ye et al.[15] have implied that locally recruited mesenchymal SC may play a role in corneal epithelial healing following alkali injury in a rabbit model and justified the idea that transplantation of mesenchymal SC could be used to treat corneal epithelial defects. Whereas injection of human mesenchymal SC under transplanted amniotic membrane did not provide an improved corneal surface, compared to controls,[52] the ocular surface of chemically burned rat eyes was repaired when mesenchymal SC were transplanted as an intact sheet.[14] However, their differentiation into corneal epithelial cells was not confirmed, leading these and other authors to suggest that the therapeutic effect of mesenchymal SC transplantation was rather associated with the inhibition of inflammation and

angiogenesis than with mesenchymal to epithelial transdifferentiation.[54] Though co-culture with corneal fibroblasts stimulated mesenchymal SC to express K3 and K12 and to transdifferentiate into a corneal epithelial phenotype in vitro and in vivo.[16,51] Adipose tissue-derived mesenchymal SC, isolated from human orbital fat tissue, were also shown to differentiate into a corneal epithelial lineage when exposed to proper environmental stimuli, such as co-culture with corneal epithelial cells.[53] Finally, human dental pulp stem cells, which represent a type of mesenchymal SC from dental pulp of deciduous teeth, have been shown to share key features with LSC and to have the capacity to differentiate into and reconstruct the corneal epithelium in rabbits after chemical burn.[17]

Further studies are definitely needed to confirm the value of mesenchymal SC as a cell source for corneal epithelial repair.

EMBRYONIC STEM CELLS

Embryonic SC remain largely unexplored for corneal regenerative applications. In one study, mouse embryonic SC cultured on collagen type IV were found to transdifferentiate into corneal epithelial cells and to re-epithelialize the chemically injured corneas of mice within 24 hours of application.[19] In a follow-up study, Ueno et al.[55] transplanted Pax6-transfected embryonic SC to damaged corneas with even better efficacy. Corneal restoration was achieved and no teratomas were observed. The group also used embryonic SC obtained from cynomolgous monkeys, which are more similar to human cells.[56] Similarly, human embryonic SC cultured on type IV collagen using limbal fibroblast conditioned medium were found to express corneal epithelial markers, such as K3 and K12, in vitro.19 These studies provide initial data to support further investigation of embryonic SC in corneal epithelial tissue engineering.

Scaffolds for Corneal Epithelial Reconstruction

Function and survival of the expanded SC and the successful establishment of a tissue-engineered corneal epithelium are highly dependent on the structural and biochemical support from the underlying substrate. Although human amniotic membrane has been widely used for LSC expansion and transplantation, a range of alternative biological, biosynthetic or synthetic carriers suitable for SC culture and transplantation has been tested for corneal epithelial tissue engineering in preclinical or clinical applications. A suitable scaffold for corneal epithelial reconstruction should have non-immunogenic and non-inflammatory properties, provide optical transparency and mechanical stability, and promote cell attachment and proliferation.

BIOLOGICAL SCAFFOLDS

Human Amniotic Membrane

The most widely used substrate for corneal epithelial reconstruction is the human amniotic membrane (HAM), i.e., the innermost membrane of the fetal sac, which can be obtained from healthy volunteers during routine caesarean sections

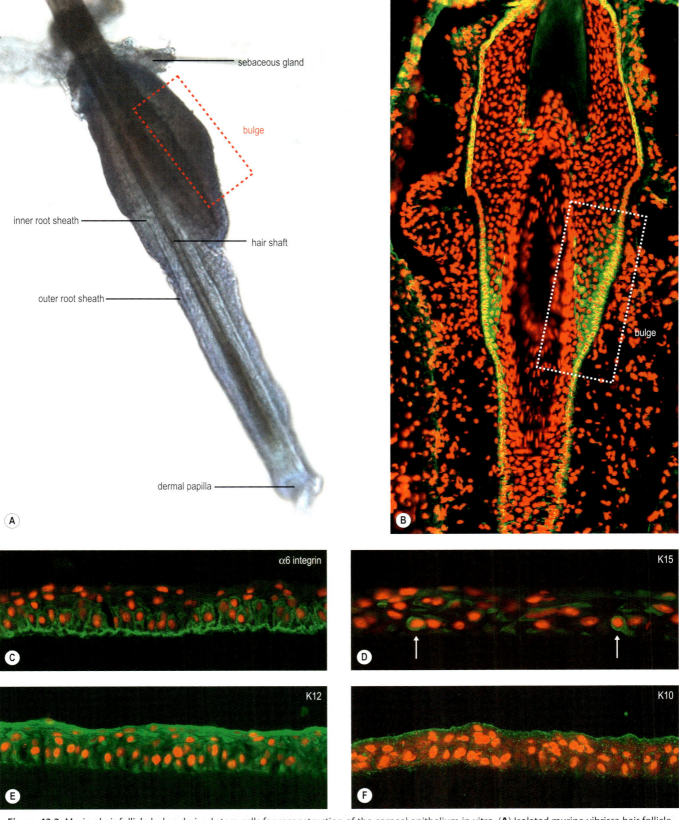

Figure 43.3 Murine hair follicle bulge-derived stem cells for reconstruction of the corneal epithelium in vitro. (**A**) Isolated murine vibrissa hair follicle with bulge region harboring the epithelial stem cells. (**B**) Expression of cytokeratin K15, a putative epithelial stem and progenitor cell marker, in the hair follicle bulge region. (**C–F**) Phenotypic appearance of hair follicle-derived, fibrin-based epithelial constructs showing positive expression of α6 integrin, a putative stem and progenitor cell marker, in the basal layer (**C**), expression of the stem cell marker K15 (*arrows*) in few single basal cells (**D**), expression of the corneal epithelial differentiation marker K12 throughout all epithelial layers (**E**), and expression of the epidermal differentiation marker K10 in the most superficial cell layer (**F**). (Fig 3A–F: Reproduced from: Blazejewska EA, Schlötzer-Schrehardt U, Zenkel M, et al. Corneal limbal microenvironment can induce transdifferentiation of hair follicle stem cells into corneal epithelial-like cells. Stem Cells 2009;27:642–52. With permission from AlphaMed Press.)

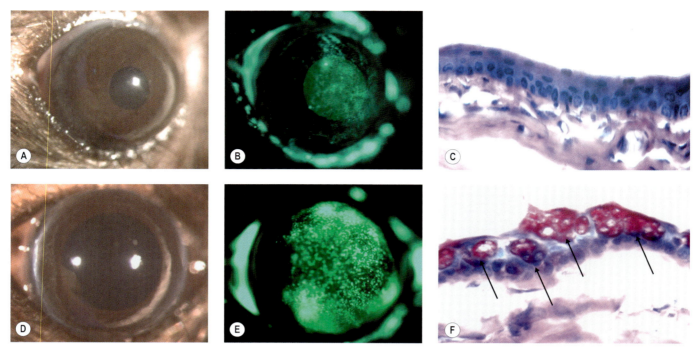

Figure 43.4 Murine hair follicle bulge-derived stem cells for ocular surface reconstruction in a rabbit model of limbal stem cell deficiency in vitro (**A–C**, transplanted eye; **D–F**, untransplanted control eye). (**A,B**) Transplantation of the epithelial construct to the limbal stem cell deficient eye resulted in re-establishment of a transparent ocular surface (**A**) and epithelial barrier function as revealed by a decrease in fluorescein uptake in the ocular surface (**B**) when compared with untransplanted controls (**D,E**). (**C,F**) Periodic acid Schiff staining of excised corneas demonstrated reconstruction of a regular corneal epithelial surface 4 weeks after transplantation with little to no conjunctival goblet cells present (**C**); however, without transplantation, the ocular surface is entirely covered by goblet cells (arrows) indicating conjunctival epithelial ingrowth (**F**). (Fig. 4A–F: Reproduced from Meyer-Blazejewska EA, Call MK, Yamanaka O, et al. From hair to cornea: toward the therapeutic use of hair follicle-derived stem cells in the treatment of limbal stem cell deficiency. Stem Cells 2011;29:57–66. With permission from AlphaMed Press.)

(Fig. 43.5A).[57] It is composed of a single-layered epithelium, which rests on a thick basement membrane and an avascular stroma (Fig. 43.5B). In addition to its structural stability and elasticity, it has anti-immunogenic, antiangiogenic and anti-inflammatory properties, and contains a variety of growth factors and cytokines promoting epithelialization.[58] HAM basement membrane composition shows extensive similarities with that of the human cornea and limbus (Fig. 43.5C,D),[59] supporting the notion of HAM serving as a surrogate niche for ex vivo expansion of LSC.[35,60] However, the preparation of HAM is not standardized, and it has been used fresh or frozen, and as an intact or epithelially denuded membrane. Epithelially denuded HAM exposing its BM appears to provide a superior niche for LSC proliferation and phenotypic maintenance.[61] On the other hand, a progressive decline in the number of epithelial progenitor cells was observed during ex vivo expansion on HAM, suggesting limitations in its suitability as a surrogate limbal niche.[3]

Despite its extensive and successful clinical use in ocular surface reconstruction, HAM has several disadvantages, such as great intra- and interdonor tissue variability and poor standardization. Regional variations in growth factor concentrations and differences in protein expression profiles, dependent on donor age, race, length of pregnancy, and HAM processing and storage, affect not only composition and physical structure of the membrane but also clinical outcome.[62] Additional shortcomings, such as low transparency, donor-associated risk of infections, inconsistent supply, high costs, and wrinkling during culture and

transplantation, have encouraged efforts to develop alternative substrates for LSC expansion and ocular surface reconstruction.[63] Still, HAM serves as a gold standard in all studies exploring the potential of novel scaffolds with respect to their mechanical and cell growth-supporting properties. In addition, attempts have been made to modify the HAM itself, e.g. by freeze-drying, coating with fibrin, or cross-linking with a polyvinyl alcohol (PVA) hydrogel, to enhance mechanical stability.[63]

Lens Capsule

Human anterior lens capsules obtained from patients undergoing cataract surgery were used as substrate for cultivation of LSC after removal of the lens epithelium in one study.[64]

Acellular and Cellular Corneal Tissue

Although the main field of application of decellularized corneas may be the development of artificial corneas, they have also been used as biological scaffolds to support the growth and differentiation of cultured limbal epithelial cells and to reconstruct the corneal epithelium and anterior stroma ('hemicornea').[65] Such tissue-derived scaffolds provide an appropriate extracellular matrix for the functional reconstruction of tissues, such as the stratified corneal epithelium. For decellularization of animal, i.e. bovine or porcine, or human cadaver corneas, research groups have used various processing methods, including detergent- and non-detergent based approaches.[65,66] Such tissue-processing

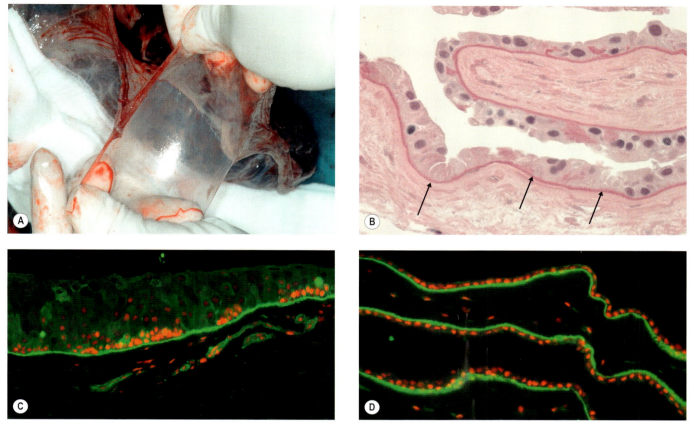

Figure 43.5 Human amniotic membrane as carrier in corneal epithelial reconstruction. (**A**) Human amniotic membrane. (**B**) Light microscopic appearance of human amniotic membrane showing its composition of a single-layered epithelium, a prominent basement membrane (*arrows*), and an avascular stroma (periodic acid – Schiff staining). (**C,D**) Similarities in immunohistochemical staining for agrin between epithelial basement membranes of the human limbus (**C**) and fresh amniotic membrane (**D**). (Fig. 5D: Reproduced from: Dietrich-Ntoukas T, Hofmann-Rummelt C, Kruse FE, et al. Comparative analysis of the basement membrane composition of the human limbus epithelium and amniotic membrane epithelium. Cornea 2012;31:564–9. With permission from Lippincott Williams & Wilkins.)

methods can, in fact, be applied to xenografts because the essential components of the remaining extracellular matrix are often conserved between species. Consistently, transplantation experiments in rabbit eyes showed these biological constructs to be immunologically inert with mechanical and optical properties of native corneal tissue.

Reconstruction of a tissue-engineered human hemicornea using human keratoplasty lenticules as a biological scaffold resulted in natural corneal grafts for clinical applications.[67] The lenticule stroma revealed an intact collagen architecture and viable keratocytes which maintained the phenotypic appearance of quiescent fibroblasts. Limbal SC expanded onto keratoplasty lenticules gave rise to a stratified keratinized epithelium morphologically similar to that of normal cornea without any alterations of their clonogenic potential.

Therefore, acellular or cellular hemi-corneas, may provide a scaffold that can support the combined growth of corneal epithelial cells and stromal fibroblasts for ocular surface reconstruction, avoiding the necessity of a feeder layer for SC expansion. The development of a tissue-engineered human hemicornea might offer new therapeutic perspectives to patients affected by LSCD with stromal scarring.

BIOSYNTHETIC SCAFFOLDS

Fibrin Gels

Fibrin sealant or fibrin 'glue' is a natural serum-derived component of wound repair that is being utilized with increasing frequency in surgical applications. It is commercially available as a two-component system, which is prepared by diluting defined volumes of stock solutions of fibrinogen and thrombin of human origin in order to form a gel of standardized thickness.[12] Aprotinin, a protease inhibitor, is added to the culture medium in order to prevent fibrinolysis by cultured cells.

Fibrin-based scaffolds have been used as suitable substrate for cultivating LSC and have been shown to promote epithelial adhesion, proliferation and migration, and to support the maintenance of a SC phenotype (Fig. 43.6).[25,32,68,69] The fibrin-based epithelial constructs offer mechanical stability, resiliency, and good transparency, and appear to be completely degraded within few days after transplantation. Hence, fibrin-based epithelial constructs have been successfully used in the treatment of LSC deficiency.[25,70] In their large series, Rama and colleagues[25] reported that 82/107 eyes (76.6%) were considered as a success based on their ability to maintain a stable, avascular

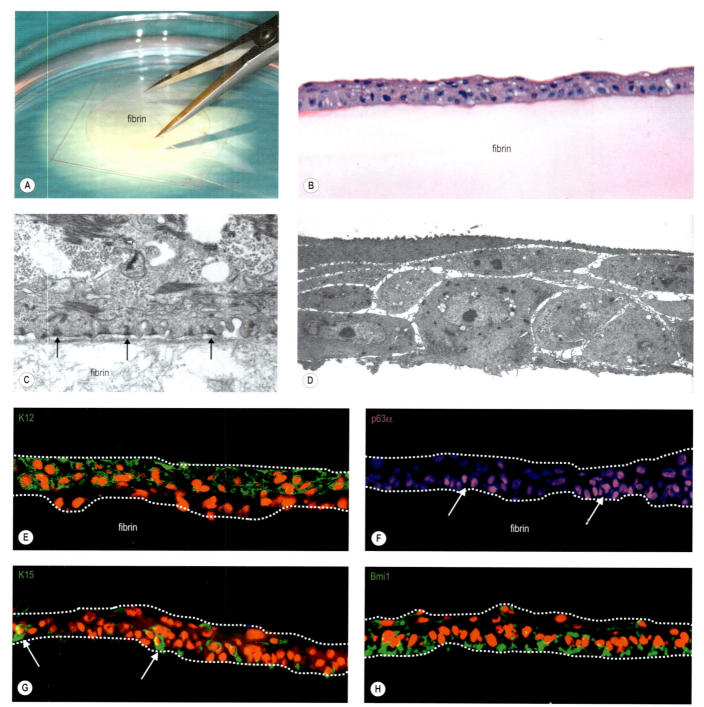

Figure 43.6 Fibrin gels as carrier in corneal epithelial reconstruction. (**A**) Fibrin gel (about 50 μm thick and 200 mm in diameter) prepared by diluting defined volumes of fibrinogen and thrombin. (**B**) Light micrograph showing a fibrin-based multilayered epithelial cell sheet formed by ex vivo expanded limbal stem cells (periodic acid – Schiff staining). (**C,D**) Transmission electron micrographs showing multilayered epithelial sheets consisting of a cuboid basal cell layer and two to three suprabasal layers of elongated cells (**D**); basal cells adhere to the fibrin carrier by hemidesmosomes (*arrows*) and newly produced basement membrane (**C**). (**E–H**) Immunofluorescence analysis showed that K12 expression was restricted to superficial cell layers (**E**), whereas positive staining for the stem and progenitor cell markers p63α (**F**), K15 (**G**), and Bmi-1 (**H**) was observed in clusters of mainly basally located cells (*arrows*). (Fig. 6B,D,F,H: Reproduced from Meyer-Blazejewska EA, Kruse FE, Bitterer K, et al. Preservation of the limbal stem cell phenotype by appropriate culture techniques. Invest Ophthalmol Vis Sci 2010;51:765–74. With permission from Association for Research in Vision and Ophthalmology.)

and transparent corneal surface for a mean follow-up period of 2.91 years (range 1–10 years).

In essence, distinct advantages of this biomatrix include its commercial availability, clinical approval, standardization, easy manipulation, complete and rapid bioadsorbance, and good mechanical and optical qualities. In view of these favorable properties, it is surprising that fibrin gels have not been used more widely for reconstruction of the corneal epithelium.[26]

Collagen Scaffolds

In view of the major structural roles played by collagen in different tissues, such as the corneal stroma, research has focused on developing novel biomaterials to mimic the fibrillar architecture as a scaffold for replacing the native collagenous extracellular matrix or for supporting adhesion and growth of overlying cells. Animal-derived and recombinant collagens, especially type I, are acknowledged as one of the most useful biomaterials available and are widely used for tissue engineering. They are used either in their native fibrillar form or after denaturation in variously fabricated forms, such as sheets of variable thickness.[71] Thus, this natural biopolymer has been a commonly used constituent of bioengineered corneal tissue replacements.[63] Collagen gels used as a cellular substrate are suitable carriers for corneal epithelial reconstruction to replace HAM (Fig. 43.7). For example, a novel source of collagen from fish scales was used to fabricate collagen scaffolds of good mechanical strength and optical transparency for ex vivo expansion of LSC.[72]

However, hydrated collagen gels contain a large proportion of water and are inherently weak. Collagen can be cross-linked using different methods to produce a rather stable hydrogel with improved mechanical properties. Carbodiimide-crosslinked recombinant human collagen type III was used as a substrate for LSC in culture.[73] The hydrogels revealed a tensile strength, refractive index,

transmission and backscatter properties that were similar to that of the native cornea, and supported growth, stratification, and stemness of LSC in culture. Similarly, type I collagen gels cross-linked with riboflavin and UV light were found to support LSC adhesion, proliferation, and formation of multilayered epithelial sheets, while preserving a stem cell phenotype in the basal epithelial layers. Preliminary transplantation experiments in a rabbit model confirmed their biocompatibility and optical transparency (Petsch et al., manuscript in preparation). However, chemical cross-linking may reduce biocompatibility and cell-based remodeling of the collagen scaffold, and may lower the rate of degradation.

Vitrification is a potential alternative method to chemical cross-linking, and consists of evaporation of fluid from the collagen gel at low temperatures to yield a thin (about 20 μm thick), rigid, glass-like platelet, which can be rehydrated to obtain a transparent collagen membrane, with improved mechanical properties.[74] These vitrigel membranes are composed of high-density collagen fibrils, equivalent to connective tissues in vivo, e.g. Bowman's layer of the corneal stroma. They have superior optical properties to other collagen substrates and have been used successfully as a matrix for keratinocyte and limbal epithelial cell culture and transplantation of stratified epithelial sheets.[75,76] Recently, this group has used collagen vitrigel membranes for developing a corneal epithelial model for an ocular irritancy evaluation as an alternative to the Draize eye irritation test.[77]

Another elegant strategy to improve the mechanical quality of collagen scaffolds is plastic compression of collagen hydrogels, which results in thin, semitransparent membranes with enhanced mechanical strength. Collagen fibers within compressed gels were found to be densely packed and more evenly arranged than those of conventional collagen gels, resembling collagen fibers within the normal corneal stroma. Incorporated corneal fibroblasts

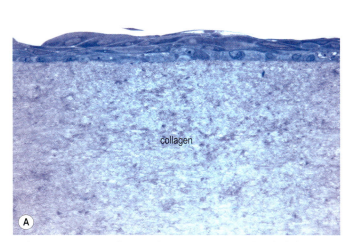

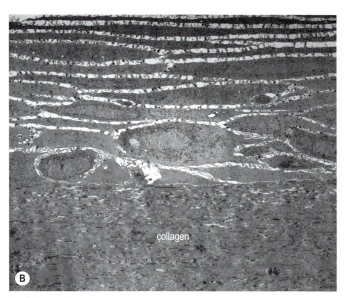

Figure 43.7 Type I collagen gels as carrier in corneal epithelial reconstruction. (**A**) Light micrograph showing a collagen-based multilayered epithelial sheet formed by ex vivo expanded limbal stem cells (semithin section; toluidine blue staining). (**B**) Transmission electron micrograph showing a multilayered epithelial sheet consisting of a cuboid basal cell layer and several suprabasal layers of elongated cells.

obviously remain viable after compression and exert a beneficial microenvironmental effect on cultivated surface epithelial cells. Consistently, these cellular constructs have been shown to offer suitable substrates for reconstituting a stratified corneal epithelial cell sheet with phenotypic features closely resembling that of a normal corneal epithelium[78,79] In addition, an increased mechanical stiffness of the collagen substrates, induced by compression, has been shown to promote cell growth and to influence the phenotype of cultured LSC by increasing expression of the differentiation marker K3 compared with uncompressed gels.[80] The elastic modulus, which is a measure of tissue stiffness, was found to be 2900 Pa of compressed collagen gels, compared to 3 Pa of conventional collagen gels. Compressed collagen gels were thus suggested to represent a significant improvement over conventional collagen gels and to serve as an excellent biomimetic scaffold for the construction of an artificial corneal epithelium.

Collagen hydrogels are composed of a randomly arranged network of collagen fibrils. However, aligned sheets of collagen fibers allow for the construction of scaffolds that better mimic the dense and regularly structured connective tissue, such as the corneal stroma. The process of electrospinning, which is commonly used to produce synthetic polymer nanofibers, can also be used to achieve an alignment of type I collagen fibers. This method uses an electric field to control the deposition of collagen fibers from solutions that are combined with synthetic polymers, which may, however, not be applicable for cell culture purposes.[81] Recently, electrospun aligned collagen I fibers have been produced using a less toxic solvent and have been used for cultivation of corneal fibroblasts.[82,83] Such a construct appears to provide an appropriate viable scaffold material with improved optical properties for corneal stroma replacement, but its suitability for LSC expansion remains to be investigated.

Keratin Films

Keratins are a group of cysteine-rich structural proteins formed in epithelial cells of vertebrates. Keratin obtained from hair or wool has been proposed as an appropriate material for producing films or scaffolds for cell cultivation and tissue engineering.[84] Transparent keratin films were engineered by a multistep procedure, including keratin extraction, neutral and alkaline dialysis, drying and a curing process, and were composed of a nanoparticulate keratin structure. The film characteristics could be varied by changing the protein composition, adding softening agents or varying the curing temperature and duration. Films based on human hair keratin showed improved biomechanical strength and light transmission as compared with HAM, but provided comparable conditions for corneal epithelial cell adhesion and proliferation. It has been suggested that keratin films may represent a new, promising alternative for ocular surface reconstruction, but further investigations need to be undertaken.

Silk Fibroin

Silk fibroin is a structural protein obtained from the cocoon of the domesticated silkworm (*Bombyx mori*). It is a particularly useful material in corneal bioengineering as it can be prepared as membranes of defined thickness and material

characteristics, which are mechanically robust, highly transparent, porous, degradable, and easy to handle.[85,86] Their biocompatibility was confirmed in rabbit corneas for up to 6 months.[87] Silk fibroin films have also been shown to support the adhesion and growth of LSC in vitro, and epithelial multilayers constructed on silk fibroin retained comparable numbers of progenitor cells to those grown on HAM.[88,89] Surface modifications, such as collagen coating or RGD-coupling appear to improve cell attachment and proliferation. It may also be used as a depot for biologically active molecules. Due to its fibrous structure, this biomaterial offers important benefits not only for corneal epithelial reconstruction but also for regeneration of the corneal stroma.[90]

Chitosan

Chitosan is a linear polysaccharide composed of randomly distributed β-(1-4)-linked D-glucosamine and N-acetyl-D-glucosamine. Chitosan is produced commercially by deacetylation of chitin, which is the structural element in the exoskeleton of crustaceans and cell walls of fungi. Novel polymeric hydrogel scaffolds based on blends of chitosan and other biopolymers, such as hydroxypropylcellulose, polycaprolactone, collagen, and elastin, have been fabricated for corneal epithelial tissue engineering.[91] Blending two polymers provides the chance to develop novel biomaterials with superior properties to that of the individual components. Comparing various combinations, hydrogels prepared from chitosan – collagen blend, cross-linked with genipin, provided adequate mechanical properties and the most promising scaffolds for corneal epithelial cell culture by supporting the formation of a regular stratified epithelial layer.

Three-dimensional porous collagen-GAG-chitosan matrices have been used as a scaffold for the combined cultivation of epithelial cells and fibroblasts enabling the reconstruction of a 'hemicornea' composed of a surface epithelium in combination with a connective tissue equivalent.[92]

SYNTHETIC SCAFFOLDS

Nanofibers

Since allogenic biological materials may be associated with a risk of rejection, current research activities focus on the development of novel biosynthetic carriers for ocular surface epithelial cell replacement. Synthetic polymers, including polyesters, polyglycolide (PGA), polyurethanes, polyester amide, etc., are alternatives to conventional biomaterials because their manufacturing process involves a high potential for modifications, which makes custom design possible.

Electrospinning is a widely used technique for the production of nanofibers from various natural or synthetic polymers. By adjusting the processing conditions and the composition of the polymer solution, the properties of the resultant nanofibrous networks, including fiber diameter, porosity, mechanical properties and surface topography, can be tightly controlled. Electrospun nanofibers have been proposed as a biocompatible cell culture substrate. The structure of the nanofibrous network mimics the fibrillar architecture of the extracellular matrix, and the high surface area to volume ratio has been shown to support adhesion, proliferation and differentiation of various cell types.[93]

Currently, electrospun nanofibers fabricated from poly-ε-caprolactone (PCL) dissolved in trifluoroethanol have been studied as a potential scaffold for LSC expansion.[94] The polymer, consisting of fibers about 130 nm in diameter with a pore size of 0.2–4.0 μm and a tensile strength of 1.75 MPa, proved to be biocompatible and to support LSC attachment, proliferation, and differentiation into a normal corneal epithelial phenotype. Epithelial cells infiltrated the nanofibers and formed a three-dimensional corneal epithelium, which was viable for two weeks. Similarly, 3D-nanofiber scaffolds prepared from polyamide 6/12 (PA6/12) by electrospun technology, have been shown to represent a suitable scaffold for expansion of LSC, and were able to reconstruct the ocular surface of mouse eyes. Co-transfer with mesenchymal SC, which have immunosuppressive properties, significantly inhibited local inflammatory reactions and supported the healing process.[95] A comparison of randomly oriented and aligned nanofiber scaffolds showed better corneal epithelial cell growth on randomly arranged networks.[96]

Therapeutic Contact Lens

In 2007, Di Girolamo and coworkers provided proof-of-concept that human limbal epithelial cells could be directly expanded on a standard siloxane-hydrogel contact lens used as a bandage for patients after pterygium surgery.[97] This material (Lotrafilcon A) sustained proliferation, migration and differentiation of limbal cells in the presence of autologous serum and without 3T3 feeder cells. In a follow-up pilot study, autologous limbal or conjunctival SC were expanded and cell-laden contact lenses were transferred to the damaged corneal surface of three patients with LSCD. After removal of the contact lenses 2–3 weeks later, a stable corneal epithelial surface was restored in all patients.[98] One year after transplantation, clinical results showed establishment of a healthy corneal surface and significant improvement in visual acuity. The authors suggested that autologous SC transfer using a FDA-approved contact lens may provide a safe and convenient therapeutic strategy for patients with LSCD.

Other researchers have used acrylic acid-coated contact lenses to improve cell attachment and facilitate the delivery of cultured limbal epithelial cells in animal models.[99]

Carrier-Free Epithelial Cell Sheets

While the majority of LSC transplantation strategies involve the use of a scaffold to supports the transplanted cell sheet, some have employed carrier-free methods in which intact cell sheets are transplanted without an underlying supportive membrane.

ENZYMATIC SUBSTRATE DEGRADATION

Higa and colleagues[24,100] have developed a technique for generating carrier-free corneal epithelial sheets using a commercial biodegradable fibrin sealant as culture substrate. They seeded corneal epithelial cells onto a fibrin matrix that was later enzymatically digested by intrinsic proteases to create a stratified epithelial sheet, which could be transplanted onto the corneal surface of rabbit eyes without sutures. These epithelial sheets seemed to contain more differentiated epithelial cells than those cultivated on HAM, while retaining similar levels of colony-forming progenitor cells. This technique was subsequently adopted for the cultivation and transplantation of carrier-free oral mucosal epithelial cell sheets.[101] The results showed that the success rates of COMET at 12 months after surgery were 62.5% in the substrate-free sheet group and only 43.8% in the HAM control group.

Carrier-free epithelial cell sheets can be also produced by cultivating corneal epithelial cells in culture dishes coated with biodegradable type I collagen and subsequent release of the multilayered cell sheet by using collagenase digestion.[102]

TEMPERATURE-RESPONSIVE SUBSTRATES

Temperature-responsive synthetic polymers, e.g. poly-N-isopropylacrylamide, chemically immobilized in thin films on cell culture surfaces, exhibit reversible hydration and dehydration of their polymer chains in response to temperature changes. They facilitate cell adhesion and growth at normal cell culture conditions at 37°C, whereas, by lowering the temperature below 30°C, they can reversibly alter their hydration properties, prompting complete detachment of adherent cells, without the use of proteolytic enzymes.[103] Taking advantage of this elegant technique, Nishida et al.[104] have developed carrier-free corneal epithelial cell sheets that have been transplanted directly to the ocular surface of rabbit eyes without sutures. Subsequent preclinical studies demonstrated the great potential of this method for carrier-free transplantation, which ensures optimal preservation of cell-cell junctions and basement membrane components produced during cultivation.[105,106]

Similar temperature-responsive culture wells, the UpCell®-Inserts (CellSeed Inc, Tokyo, Japan), have been used to manufacture Cultured Autologous Oral Mucosal Epithelial Cell-Sheets (CAOMECS), transparent, resistant and rapidly bioadhesive cell sheets.[107,108] Suture-free transplantation of CAOMECS has been proposed for the treatment of total bilateral LSCD, in patients with moderate or severe symptoms, for whom any other treatment options are not applicable. The safety and efficacy of CAOMECS transplantation has been recently confirmed in a clinical study, showing a successful clinical outcome, defined by a stable avascular ocular surface, in 16/25 patients (64%) one year after grafting.[108]

Mebiol gel, a synthetic copolymer comprised of thermoresponsive polymer poly-N-isopropylacrylamide-co-n-butyl methacrylate and hydrophilic polymer polyethylene glycol (PEG), is hydrophilic below 20°C and forms a hydrophobic hydrogel at 37°C.[109] The sol-gel transition temperature can be controlled by altering the chemical composition of the thermoreversible gelation polymer. Human LSC cultured on Mebiol gel in the absence of a 3T3 feeder layer, showed a high proliferative capacity and a limbal SC phenotype, as indicated by expression of ABCG2 and p63.[110] Transplantation of hydrogel-based epithelial cell sheets showed high transparency of the construct and restoration of a nearly normal ocular epithelial surface in rabbit eyes.[111]

CENTRIFUGATION-CONSTRUCTED CORNEAL EPITHELIAL SHEET (CCCES)

Zhang and coworkers developed a centrifugal cell seeding method for the rapid and efficient construction of corneal epithelial sheets for reconstruction of the ocular surface in a rabbit model of LSCD.[112] Corneal epithelial sheets were constructed by applying centrifugal driving force, and orthogonal design experiments were used to optimize centrifugation parameters for cell seeding. In vitro experiments showed the rapid construction of three-layered epithelial sheets, which displayed the characteristics of a normal corneal epithelium. In vivo, CCCES successfully reconstructed the cornea epithelium in a rabbit model of LSCD.

Conclusion

Within recent years, there have been significant developments in treating ocular surface disorders, especially LSCD, by using SC-based approaches in combination with various biomaterials or synthetic substrates for corneal epithelial tissue engineering. In particular, the LSC, together with oral mucosal epithelial SC, have been widely investigated for their ex vivo culture and subsequent transplantation in clinical applications. Currently, cultivated limbal epithelial transplantation (CLET) and cultivated oral mucosal epithelial transplantation (COMET) are still the only widely applied tissue engineered SC-based therapies in ophthalmology which have been clinically validated. The most advanced approaches for engineering epithelial constructs in clinical applications are the transplantation on biodegradable fibrin gels or human amniotic membranes, as well as the use of temperature-responsive polymer surfaces to generate carrier-free cell sheets. These therapies have been proven to be beneficial at avoiding sight-threatening complications in patients with LSCD. However, in view of limited tissue supply, the focus of current research in this field has turned to the search for alternative easily accessible autologous SC sources appropriate for corneal epithelial regeneration, such as hair follicle-derived SC. Autologous tissue is evidently a preferable transplant material for long-term graft persistence avoiding the risk of immune-mediated rejection and the need for immunosuppression.

Although these progresses are expected to steadily improve clinical outcomes in patients with ocular surface disorders, further improvements, such as standardization of culture conditions and development of xenobiotic-free culture systems, are required to further advance this therapeutic strategy. In particular, investigations into xenobiotic-free culture systems are ongoing, and will likely be crucial for the widespread application of LSC transplantation. Moreover, tissue engineering strategies must include a kind of quality control verifying the preservation of SC during the culture process in order to ensure functionality and long-term regeneration of the transplants. These techniques must be evaluated for long term success to determine if they will be as efficacious as the standard limbal SC transplantation techniques of Conjunctival Limbal Allograft, Living Related Conjunctival Limbal Allograft and Keratolimbal Allograft. In addition the significant additional cost of tissue engineering must be part of the evaluation.

Further challenges that remain, include elucidation of signaling pathways that determine stem cell function and fate in vivo and in vitro. Future trends are the development of biomimetic scaffolds that not only provide structural support for living cells, but also can serve as a delivery system for drugs, growth factors or signaling molecules that may further promote cell function and tissue regeneration.

References

1. Polak JM, Bishop AE. Stem cells and tissue engineering: past, present, and future. Ann N Y Acad Sci 2006;1068:352–66.
2. Cotsarelis G, Cheng SZ, Dong G, et al. Existence of slow-cycling limbal epithelial basal cells that can be preferentially stimulated to proliferate: implications on epithelial stem cells. Cell 1989;57:201–9.
3. Li W, Hayashida Y, Chen YT, et al. Niche regulation of corneal epithelial stem cells at the limbus. Cell Res 2007;17:26–36.
4. Pellegrini G, Rama P, Mavilio F, et al. Epithelial stem cells in corneal regeneration and epidermal gene therapy. J Pathol 2009;217:217–28.
5. Dua HS, Saini JS, Azuara-Blanco A, et al. Limbal stem cell deficiency: concept, aetiology, clinical presentation, diagnosis and management. Indian J Ophthalmol 2000;48:83–92.
6. Burman S, Sangwan V. Cultivated limbal stem cell transplantation for ocular surface reconstruction. Clin Ophthalmol 2008;2:489–502.
7. Selvam S, Thomas PB, Yiu SC. Tissue engineering: current and future approaches to ocular surface reconstruction. Ocul Surf 2006;4:120–36.
8. Nishida K, Yamato M, Hayashida Y, et al. Corneal reconstruction with tissue-engineered cell sheets composed of autologous oral mucosal epithelium. N Engl J Med 2004;351:1187–96.
9. Tanioka H, Kawasaki S, Yamasaki K, et al. Establishment of a cultivated human conjunctival epithelium as an alternative tissue source for autologous corneal epithelial transplantation. Invest Ophthalmol Vis Sci 2006;47:3820–7.
10. Ono K, Yokoo S, Mimura T, et al. Autologous transplantation of conjunctival epithelial cells cultured on amniotic membrane in a rabbit model. Mol Vis 2007;13:1138–43.
11. Ang LP, Tanioka H, Kawasaki S, et al. Cultivated human conjunctival epithelial transplantation for total limbal stem cell deficiency. Invest Ophthalmol Vis Sci 2010;51:758–64.
12. Blazejewska EA, Schlötzer-Schrehardt U, Zenkel M, et al. Corneal limbal microenvironment can induce transdifferentiation of hair follicle stem cells into corneal epithelial-like cells. Stem Cells 2009;27:642–52.
13. Meyer-Blazejewska EA, Call MK, Yamanaka O, et al. From hair to cornea: toward the therapeutic use of hair follicle-derived stem cells in the treatment of limbal stem cell deficiency. Stem Cells 2011;29:57–66.
14. Ma Y, Xu Y, Xiao Z, et al. Reconstruction of chemically burned rat corneal surface by bone marrow-derived human mesenchymal stem cells. Stem Cells 2006;24:315–21.
15. Ye J, Yao K, Kim JC. Mesenchymal stem cell transplantation in a rabbit corneal alkali burn model: engraftment and involvement in wound healing. Eye 2006;20:482–90.
16. Jiang TS, Cai L, Ji WY, et al. Reconstruction of the corneal epithelium with induced marrow mesenchymal stem cells in rats. Mol Vis 2010;16:1304–16.
17. Gomes JA, Geraldes Monteiro B, Melo GB, et al. Corneal reconstruction with tissue-engineered cell sheets composed of human immature dental pulp stem cells. Invest Ophthalmol Vis Sci 2010;51:1408–14.
18. Reza HM, Ng BY, Gimeno FL, et al. Umbilical cord lining stem cells as a novel and promising source for ocular surface regeneration. Stem Cell Rev 2011;7:935–47.
19. Homma R, Yoshikawa H, Takeno M, et al. Induction of epithelial progenitors in vitro from mouse embryonic stem cells and application for reconstruction of damaged cornea in mice. Invest Ophthalmol Vis Sci 2004;45:4320–6.

20. Ahmad S, Stewart R, Yung S, et al. Differentiation of human embryonic stem cells into corneal epithelial-like cells by in vitro replication of the corneal epithelial stem cell niche. Stem Cells 2007;25:1145–55.

21. Lindberg K, Brown ME, Chaves HV, et al. In vitro propagation of human ocular surface epithelial cells for transplantation. Invest Ophthalmol Vis Sci 1993;34:2672–9.

22. Pellegrini G, Traverso CE, Franzi AT, et al. Long-term restoration of damaged corneal surfaces with autologous cultivated corneal epithelium. Lancet 1997;349:990–3.

23. Shortt AJ, Secker GA, Notara MD, et al. Transplantation of ex vivo cultured limbal epithelial stem cells: a review of techniques and clinical results. Surv Ophthalmol 2007;52:483–502.

24. Higa K, Shimazaki J. Recent advances in cultivated epithelial transplantation. Cornea 2008;27(Suppl. 1):S41–7.

25. Rama P, Matuska S, Paganoni G, et al. Limbal stem-cell therapy and long-term corneal regeneration. N Engl J Med 2010;363:147–55.

26. Baylis O, Figueiredo F, Henein C, et al. 13 years of cultured limbal epithelial cell therapy: a review of the outcomes. J Cell Biochem 2011;112:993–1002.

27. Li W, Hayashida Y, He H, et al. The fate of limbal epithelial progenitor cells during explant culture on intact amniotic membrane. Invest Ophthalmol Vis Sci 2007;48:605–13.

28. Koizumi N, Cooper LJ, Fullwood NJ, et al. An evaluation of cultivated corneal limbal epithelial cells, using cell-suspension culture. Invest Ophthalmol Vis Sci 2002;43:2114–21.

29. De Luca M, Pellegrini G, Green H. Regeneration of squamous epithelia from stem cells of cultured grafts. Regen Med 2006;1:45–57.

30. Pellegrini G, Rama P, De Luca M. Vision from the right stem. Trends Mol Med 2010;17:1–7.

31. Rheinwald JG, Green H. Serial cultivation of strains of human epidermal keratinocytes: the formation of keratinizing colonies from single cells. Cell 1975;6:331–43.

32. Meyer-Blazejewska EA, Kruse FE, Bitterer K, et al. Preservation of the limbal stem cell phenotype by appropriate culture techniques. Invest Ophthalmol Vis Sci 2010;51:765–74.

33. Pellegrini G, Dellambra E, Golisano O, et al. p63 identifies keratinocyte stem cells. Proc Natl Acad Sci USA 2001;98:3156–61.

34. Di Iorio E, Barbaro V, Ruzza A, et al. Isoforms of DeltaNp63 and the migration of ocular limbal cells in human corneal regeneration. Proc Natl Acad Sci USA 2005;102:9523–8.

35. Tsai RJ, Tsai RY. Ex vivo expansion of corneal stem cells on amniotic membrane and their outcome. Eye Contact Lens 2010;36:305–9.

36. Eberwein P, Steinberg T, Schulz S et al. Expression of keratinocyte biomarkers is governed by environmental biomechanics. Eur J Cell Biol 2011;90:1029–40.

37. Ban Y, Cooper LJ, Fullwood NJ, et al. Comparison of ultrastructure, tight junction-related protein expression and barrier function of human corneal epithelial cells cultivated on amniotic membrane with and without air-lifting. Exp Eye Res 2003;76:735–43.

38. Li C, Yin T, Dong N, et al. Oxygen tension affects terminal differentiation of corneal limbal epithelial cells. J Cell Physiol 2011;226:2429–37.

39. Chen SY, Hayashida Y, Chen MY, et al. A new isolation method of human limbal progenitor cells by maintaining close association with their niche cells. Tissue Eng Part C Methods 2011;17:537–48.

40. Robertson DM, Kalangara JP, Baucom RB, et al. A reconstituted telomerase-immortalized human corneal epithelium in vivo: a pilot study. Curr Eye Res 2011;36:706–12.

41. Chen YT, Li W, Hayashida Y, et al. Human amniotic epithelial cells as novel feeder layers for promoting ex vivo expansion of limbal epithelial progenitor cells. Stem Cells 2007;25:1995–2005.

42. Notara M, Haddow DB, MacNeil S, et al. A xenobiotic-free culture system for human limbal epithelial stem cells. Regen Med 2007;2:919–27.

43. Omoto M, Miyashita H, Shimmura S, et al. The use of human mesenchymal stem cell-derived feeder cells for the cultivation of transplantable epithelial sheets. Invest Ophthalmol Vis Sci 2009;50:2109–15.

44. Shortt AJ, Secker GA, Rajan MS, et al. Ex vivo expansion and transplantation of limbal epithelial stem cells. Ophthalmology 2008;115:1989–97.

45. Nakamura T, Kinoshita S. Ocular surface reconstruction using cultivated mucosal epithelial stem cells. Cornea 2003;22:S75–80.

46. Inatomi T, Nakamura T, Koizumi N, et al. Midterm results on ocular surface reconstruction using cultivated autologous oral mucosal epithelial transplantation. Am J Ophthalmol 2006;141:267–75.

47. Yang X, Moldovan NI, Zhao Q, et al. Reconstruction of damaged cornea by autologous transplantation of epidermal adult stem cells. Mol Vis 2008;14:1064–70.

48. Ang LP, Nakamura T, Inatomi T, et al. Autologous serum-derived cultivated oral epithelial transplants for severe ocular surface disease. Arch Ophthalmol 2006;124:1543–51.

49. Nakamura T, Takeda K, Inatomi T, et al. Long-term results of autologous cultivated oral mucosal epithelial transplantation in the scar phase of severe ocular surface disorders. Br J Ophthalmol 2011;95:942–6.

50. Tiede S, Kloepper JE, Bodò E, et al. Hair follicle stem cells: walking the maze. Eur J Cell Biol 2007;86:355–76.

51. Gu S, Xing C, Han J, et al. Differentiation of rabbit bone marrow mesenchymal stem cells into corneal epithelial cells in vivo and ex vivo. Mol Vis 2009;15:99–107.

52. Reinshagen H, Auw-Haedrich C, Sorg RV, et al. Corneal surface reconstruction using adult mesenchymal stem cells in experimental limbal stem cell deficiency in rabbits. Acta Ophthalmol 2011;89:741–8.

53. Ho JH, Ma WH, Tseng TC, et al. Isolation and characterization of multi-potent stem cells from human orbital fat tissues. Tissue Eng Part A 2011;17:255–66.

54. Oh JY, Kim MK, Shin MS, et al. The anti-inflammatory and anti-angiogenic role of mesenchymal stem cells in corneal wound healing following chemical injury. Stem Cells 2008;26:1047–55.

55. Ueno H, Kurokawa MS, Kayama M, et al. Experimental transplantation of corneal epithelium-like cells induced by Pax6 gene transfection of mouse embryonic stem cells. Cornea 2007;26:1220–7.

56. Kumagai Y, Kurokawa MS, Ueno H, et al. Induction of corneal epithelium-like cells from cynomolgus monkey embryonic stem cells and their experimental transplantation to damaged cornea. Cornea 2010;29:432–8.

57. Gomes JA, Romano A, Santos MS, et al. Amniotic membrane use in ophthalmology. Curr Opin Ophthalmol 2005;16:233–40.

58. Tseng SCG, Espana EM, Kawakita T, et al. How does amniotic membrane work? Ocul Surf 2004;2:177–87.

59. Dietrich-Ntoukas T, Hofmann-Rummelt C, Kruse FE, et al. Comparative analysis of the basement membrane composition of the human limbus epithelium and amniotic membrane epithelium. Cornea 2012;31:564–9.

60. Grueterich M, Espana EM, Tseng SCG. Ex vivo expansion of limbal epithelial stem cells: amniotic membrane serving as a stem cell niche. Surv Ophthalmol 2003;48:631–46.

61. Koizumi N, Rigby H, Fullwood NJ, et al. Comparison of intact and denuded amniotic membrane as a substrate for cell-suspension culture of human limbal epithelial cells. Graefes Arch Clin Exp Ophthalmol 2007;245:123–34.

62. Dua HS, Rahman I, Miri A, et al. Variations in amniotic membrane: relevance for clinical applications. Br J Ophthalmol 2010;94:963–4.

63. Levis H, Daniels JT. New technologies in limbal epithelial stem cell transplantation. Curr Opin Biotechnol 2009;20:593–7.

64. Galal A, Perez-Santonja JJ, Rodriguez-Prats JL, et al. Human anterior lens capsule as a biologic substrate for the ex vivo expansion of limbal stem cells in ocular surface reconstruction. Cornea 2007;26:473–8.

65. Shafiq MA, Gemeinhart RA, Yue BY, et al. Decellularized human cornea for reconstructing the corneal epithelium and anterior stroma. Tissue Eng Part C Methods 2012;18:340–8.

66. Ponce Márquez S, Martínez VS, McIntosh Ambrose W, et al. Decellularization of bovine corneas for tissue engineering applications. Acta Biomater 2009;5:1839–47.

67. Barbaro V, Ferrari S, Fasolo A, et al. Reconstruction of a human hemicornea through natural scaffolds compatible with the growth of corneal epithelial stem cells and stromal keratocytes. Mol Vis 2009;15:2084–93.

68. Han B, Schwab IR, Madsen TK, et al. A fibrin-based bioengineered ocular surface with human corneal epithelial stem cells. Cornea 2002;21:505–10.

69. Talbot M, Carrier P, Giasson CJ, et al. Autologous transplantation of rabbit limbal epithelia cultured on fibrin gels for ocular surface reconstruction. Mol Vis 2006;12:65–75.

70. Rama P, Bonini S, Lambiase A, et al. Autologous fibrin-cultured limbal stem cells permanently restore the corneal surface of patients with total limbal stem cell deficiency. Transplantation 2001;72: 1478–85.

71. Cen L, Liu W, Cui L, et al. Collagen tissue engineering: development of novel biomaterials and applications. Pediatr Res 2008;63: 492–6.

72. Krishnan S, Sekar S, Katheem MF, et al. Fish scale collagen–a novel material for corneal tissue engineering. Artif Organs 2012;36: 829–35.

73. Dravida S, Gaddipati S, Griffith M, et al. A biomimetic scaffold for culturing limbal stem cells: a promising alternative for clinical transplantation. J Tissue Eng Regen Med 2008;2:263–71.

74. Takezawa T, Ozaki K, Nitani A, et al. Collagen vitrigel: a novel scaffold that can facilitate a three-dimensional culture for reconstructing organoids. Cell Transplant 2004;13:463–73.

75. McIntosh Ambrose W, Salahuddin A, So S, et al. Collagen Vitrigel membranes for the in vitro reconstruction of separate corneal epithelial, stromal, and endothelial cell layers. J Biomed Mater Res B Appl Biomater 2009;90:818–31.

76. McIntosh Ambrose W, Schein O, Elisseeff J. A tale of two tissues: stem cells in cartilage and corneal tissue engineering. Curr Stem Cell Res Ther 2010;5:37–48.

77. Takezawa T, Nishikawa K, Wang PC. Development of a human corneal epithelium model utilizing a collagen vitrigel membrane and the changes of its barrier function induced by exposing eye irritant chemicals. Toxicol In Vitro 2011;25:1237–41.

78. Levis HJ, Brown RA, Daniels JT. Plastic compressed collagen as a biomimetic substrate for human limbal epithelial cell culture. Biomaterials 2010;31:7726–37.

79. Mi S, Chen B, Wright B, et al. Plastic compression of a collagen gel forms a much improved scaffold for ocular surface tissue engineering over conventional collagen gels. J Biomed Mater Res A 2010; 95:447–53.

80. Jones RR, Hamley IW, Connon CJ. Ex vivo expansion of limbal stem cells is affected by substrate properties. Stem Cell Res 2012; 8:403–9.

81. Buttafoco L, Kolkman NG, Engbers-Buijtenhuijs P, et al. Electrospinning of collagen and elastin for tissue engineering applications. Biomaterials 2006;27:724–34.

82. Wray LS, Orwin EJ. Recreating the microenvironment of the native cornea for tissue engineering applications. Tissue Eng Part A 2009;15:1463–72.

83. Phu D, Wray LS, Warren RV, et al. Effect of substrate composition and alignment on corneal cell phenotype. Tissue Eng Part A 2011;17:799–807.

84. Reichl S, Borrelli M, Geerling G. Keratin films for ocular surface reconstruction. Biomaterials 2011;32:3375–86.

85. Lawrence BD, Marchant JK, Pindrus MA et al. Silk film biomaterials for cornea tissue engineering. Biomaterials 2009;30:1299–308.

86. Lawrence BD, Pan Z, Weber MD, et al. Silk film culture system for in vitro analysis and biomaterial design. J Vis Exp 2012;24:62.

87. Higa K, Takeshima N, Moro F, et al. Porous silk fibroin film as a transparent carrier for cultivated corneal epithelial sheets. J Biomater Sci Polym Ed 2011;22:2261–76.

88. Chirila T, Barnard Z, Zainuddin A, et al. Bombyx mori silk fibroin membranes as potential substrata for epithelial constructs used in the management of ocular surface disorders. Tissue Eng Part A 2008;14:1203–11.

89. Bray LJ, George KA, Ainscough SL, et al. Human corneal epithelial equivalents constructed on Bombyx mori silk fibroin membranes. Biomaterials 2011;32:5086–91.

90. Bray LJ, George KA, Hutmacher DW, et al. A dual-layer silk fibroin scaffold for reconstructing the human corneal limbus. Biomaterials 2012;33:3529–38.

91. Grolik M, Szczubiałka K, Wowra B, et al. Hydrogel membranes based on genipin-cross-linked chitosan blends for corneal epithelium tissue engineering. J Mater Sci Mater Med 2012;23:1991–2000.

92. Auxenfans C, Builles N, Andre V, et al. Porous matrix and primary-cell culture: a shared concept for skin and cornea tissue engineering. Pathol Biol 2009;57:290–8.

93. Kubinová S, Syková E. Nanotechnologies in regenerative medicine. Minim Invasive Ther Allied Technol 2010;19:144–56.

94. Sharma S, Mohanty S, Gupta D, et al. Cellular response of limbal epithelial cells on electrospun poly-ε-caprolactone nanofibrous scaffolds for ocular surface bioengineering: a preliminary in vitro study. Mol Vis 2011;17:2898–910.

95. Zajicova A, Pokorna K, Lencova A, et al. Treatment of ocular surface injuries by limbal and mesenchymal stem cells growing on nanofiber scaffolds. Cell Transplant 2010;19:1281–90.

96. Yan J, Qiang L, Gao Y, et al. Effect of fiber alignment in electrospun scaffolds on keratocytes and corneal epithelial cells behavior. J Biomed Mater Res A 2011 [Epub ahead of print].

97. Di Girolamo N, Chui J, Wakefield D, et al. Cultured human ocular surface epithelium on therapeutic contact lenses. Br J Ophthalmol 2007;91:459–64.

98. Di Girolamo N, Bosch M, Zamora K, et al. A contact lens-based technique for expansion and transplantation of autologous epithelial progenitors for ocular surface reconstruction. Transplantation 2009;87:1571–8.

99. Deshpande P, Notara M, Bullett N, et al. Development of a surface-modified contact lens for the transfer of cultured limbal epithelial cells to the cornea for ocular surface diseases. Tissue Eng Part A 2009;15:2889–902.

100. Higa K, Shimmura S, Kato N, et al. Proliferation and differentiation of transplantable rabbit epithelial sheets engineered with or without an amniotic membrane carrier. Invest Ophthalmol Vis Sci 2007; 48:597–604.

101. Hirayama M, Satake Y, Higa K, et al. Transplantation of cultivated oral mucosal epithelium prepared in fibrin-coated culture dishes. Invest Ophthalmol Vis Sci 2012;53:1602–9.

102. Ke Q, Wang X, Gao Q, et al. Carrier-free epithelial cell sheets prepared by enzymatic degradation of collagen gel. J Tissue Eng Regen Med 2011;5:138–45.

103. Schmaljohann D, Oswald J, Jørgensen B, et al. Thermo-responsive PNiPAAm-g-PEG films for controlled cell detachment. Biomacromolecules 2003;4:1733–9.

104. Nishida K, Yamato M, Hayashida Y, et al. Functional bioengineered corneal epithelial sheet grafts from corneal stem cells expanded ex vivo on a temperature-responsive cell culture surface. Transplantation 2004;77:379–85.

105. Hayashida Y, Nishida K, Yamato M, et al. Transplantation of tissue-engineered epithelial cell sheets after excimer laser photoablation reduces postoperative corneal haze. Invest Ophthalmol Vis Sci 2006;47:552–7.

106. Yang J, Yamato M, Nishida K, et al T. Cell delivery in regenerative medicine: the cell sheet engineering approach. J Control Release 2006;116:193–203.

107. Yamato M, Utsumi M, Kushida A, et al. Thermo-responsive culture dishes allow the intact harvest of multilayered keratinocyte sheets without dispase by reducing temperature. Tissue Eng 2001;7: 473–80.

108. Burillon C, Huot L, Justin V, et al. Cultured autologous oral mucosal epithelial cell sheet (CAOMECS) transplantation for the treatment of corneal limbal epithelial stem cell deficiency. Invest Ophthalmol Vis Sci 2012;53:1325–31.

109. Vemuganti GK, Fatima A, Madhira SL, et al. Limbal stem cells: application in ocular biomedicine. Int Rev Cell Mol Biol 2009;275:133–81.

110. Sudha B, Madhavan HN, Sitalakshmi G et al. Cultivation of human corneal limbal stem cells in Mebiol gel–A thermo-reversible gelation polymer. Indian J Med Res 2006;124:655–64.

111. Sitalakshmi G, Sudha B, Madhavan HN, et al. Ex vivo cultivation of corneal limbal epithelial cells in a thermoreversible polymer (Mebiol Gel) and their transplantation in rabbits: an animal model. Tissue Eng Part 2009;15:407–15.

112. Zhang W, Xiao J, Li C, et al. Rapidly constructed scaffold-free cornea epithelial sheets for ocular surface reconstruction. Tissue Eng Part C Methods 2011;17:569–77.

44 Cultured Limbal Epithelial Stem Cells for Reconstruction of the Corneal Epithelium

JOHANNES MENZEL-SEVERING, BJOERN BACHMANN, and FRIEDRICH E. KRUSE

Introduction

The possibility to serially propagate limbal epithelial stem cells (LESCs) in the cell culture laboratory has made these cells amenable to further study in vitro, but has also been used as a therapeutic approach. Cultivated sheets of LESCs can be transplanted with the aim of reconstructing a stem cell-deficient corneal surface. A recent study followed 112 patients with ocular surface disease due to corneal burns which received transplantation of autologous LESCs expanded on a fibrin gel. Clinical success (defined as a transparent, avascular and stable corneal surface) was seen in more than 75% of the study eyes.[1] Cultured limbal epithelium has also been used to treat other causes of limbal stem cell deficiency with varying success rates.[2] Although there is currently a lack of evidence to show that transplantation of cultivated LESCs is superior to conventional techniques involving whole limbal tissue transplants, there are theoretical advantages. In this chapter, the authors outline the concept and practice of cultured LESCs for reconstruction of the corneal surface and provide an overview of its current clinical significance and potential.

History and Rationale

Transplantation of healthy limbal tissue for treatment of total limbal stem cell deficiency can be obtained from the contralateral eye,[3,4] a relative of the patient, or from the eye of a cadaveric donor. There is a very low risk for the healthy eye of a living donor unless repeated limbal biopsies are required. Therefore, the concept of ex vivo expansion of LESCs is regarded as a potential beneficial to increase cell yields prior to transplantation, allowing the size of the limbal biopsy to be reduced (Figs 44.1, 44.2). In exceptional cases, using this technique, autologous LESCs can also be obtained from a small, healthy region of a partially stem cell-deficient eye.[5] In addition, cultured sheets of allogeneic epithelium have been purported to be less prone to immune rejection, since antigen-presenting cells are deemed to be absent following cell culture.

Human corneal epithelium was first grown successfully in culture in 1977. This was made possible by the use of the 3T3 co-culture method, which had been described 2 years earlier by Rheinwald and Green.[3,4] They reported that in the presence of mouse embryonic 3T3 fibroblasts, which had been growth-arrested by irradiation, single epithelial cells

showed clonal expansion and could be serially propagated in vitro. However, it was not until 20 years later that transplantation of autologous, cultured limbal epithelial cells was shown to be beneficial in clinical cases of limbal stem cell deficiency. In 1997, Pellegrini and coworkers successfully transplanted cultured cell sheets obtained from autologous limbal tissue in two patients with alkali burns. Since then, numerous studies have focused on transplantation of cultured limbal epithelium.[6,7] These interventions were performed in a number of different conditions, using different culture systems and yielding varying, yet promising results (see below).

Currently it remains unclear what the precise mechanisms are by which grafting cultivated LESCs contributes to ocular surface healing. One would expect transplanted LESCs to improve the corneal surface by replenishing the depleted stem cell pool. However, Daya et al.[8] determined the genotype of corneal epithelial cells following their transplantation to the corneal surface in humans, and were unable to detect donor DNA from as early as 1 month postoperatively. This may mean that rather than integrating into the recipient corneal surface (re-integration theory), transplanted corneal epithelium may allow or actively stimulate the recovery of an endogenous stem cell population (biological bandage theory).

Isolation Methods

The two main techniques available for isolation and ex vivo expansion of corneal epithelium are the explant culture system and the somewhat more common suspension culture system. The former consists of placing a piece of limbal tissue (e.g. 2×2 mm) in culture as a whole (Fig. 44.3). The latter uses enzymatic digestion to remove the epithelial cells from the limbal tissue (Fig. 44.4). In this system, dispase is most frequently used to digest the epithelial basement membrane, while trypsin is employed subsequently to disrupt intercellular adhesions, producing a suspension of epithelial cells. Epithelial outgrowth from the explant or clonal growth around single isolated LESCs can be observed when appropriate culture conditions are being used (see below). Favorable clinical results have been obtained in a number of studies using either isolation strategy, and although limbal epithelial cell suspensions may contain a higher proportion of stem cells, clinical superiority of either of the two methods has not been formally established.[2]

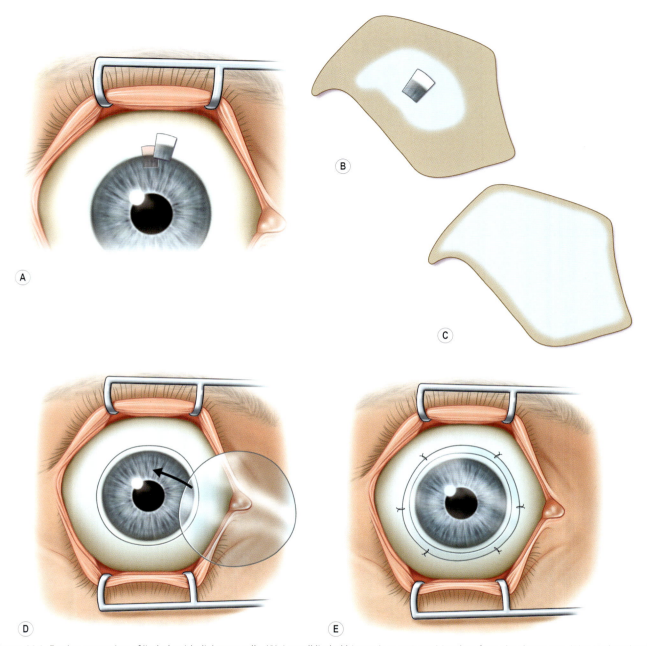

Figure 44.1 Ex vivo expansion of limbal epithelial stem cells. (**A**) A small limbal biopsy (e.g. 1×2 mm) is taken from the donor eye. (**B**) It is placed onto a suitable substrate (e.g. amniotic membrane or fibrin gel) for cultivation. (**C**) The expanded epithelial cell sheet may then be transferred to the recipient ocular surface. (**D**) Scar tissue is removed from the diseased corneal surface prior to applying the transplant. (**E**) The graft is held in place on the ocular surface by sutures. (From Shortt AJ, Tuft SJ, Daniels JT. Ex vivo cultured limbal epithelial transplantation. A clinical perspective. Ocul Surf 2010;8:80–90; courtesy of Ethis Communications.)

Baylis et al. have proposed that impression cytology should be performed on the donor eye to rule out subclinical LESC deficiency, which could be made manifest by performing a limbal biopsy or which may predict culture failure.[6] Also, several studies have suggested an uneven distribution of LESCs along the limbus.[9] Knowledge regarding the localization of LESCs is important for targeting limbal biopsies to stem cell-rich regions. Most frequently, LESCs have been proposed to be more abundant in the superior and inferior limbal regions. However, the lack of definitive markers for unequivocal identification of LESCs continues to hamper the development of efficient methods not only for isolation, but also for propagation and delivery of LESCs. When cells are harvested from a living donor, the limbal palisades should be identified, and a specimen of 1–6 mm^2 is obtained under local anesthesia (see Fig. 44.2). Although this technique maximizes the yield of clonogenic LESCs and therefore, the chances of successfully initiating an LESC culture, it remains unknown whether it also has a positive effect on the clinical performance of the graft.

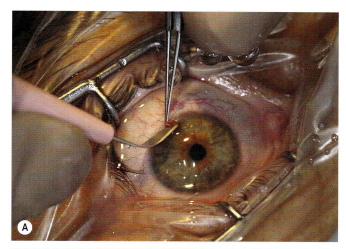

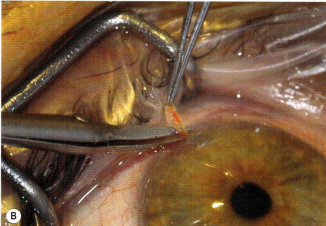

Figure 44.2 Harvesting a limbal biopsy for ex vivo expansion from the eye of a living donor. Under local anesthesia, a limbal biopsy of approximately 1×2 mm is obtained from the 12 o'clock position. (See supplementary video 1 for the full procedure.) The excised tissue is placed in culture medium during transport to the cell culture laboratory.

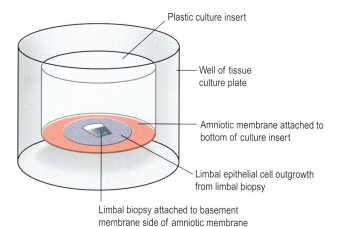

Figure 44.3 The explant culture system. The limbal specimen is placed on amniotic membrane and air dried for a few minutes, thereby allowing adhesion of the explant to its substrate. Subsequently, the tissues are covered with cell culture medium. Limbal epithelium can then migrate from the limbal biopsy to the surface of the amniotic membrane. Not shown: growth-arrested 3T3 fibroblasts can also be added to the bottom of the culture well in a coculture system. (From: Shortt AJ, Secker GA, Notara MD, et al. Transplantation of ex vivo cultured limbal epithelial stem cells: a review of techniques and clinical results. Surv Ophthalmol 2007;52:483–502.)

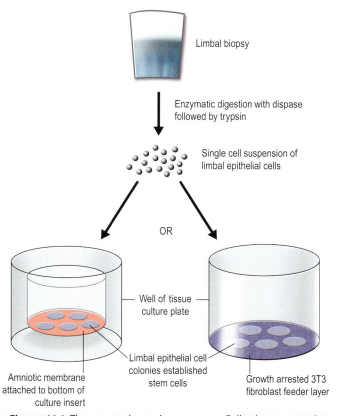

Figure 44.4 The suspension culture system. Following enzymatic release of single epithelial cells from the limbal tissue specimen, these cells are cultured either on amniotic membrane (*left*) or on growth-arrested 3T3 feeder cells. (From: Shortt AJ, Secker GA, Notara MD, et al. Transplantation of ex vivo cultured limbal epithelial stem cells: a review of techniques and clinical results. Surv Ophthalmol 2007;52:483–502.)

In a similar vein, where cadaveric corneal tissue needs to be relied upon, the duration of storage of ocular tissue in the eye bank has been suggested to negatively influence the rate of successfully initiating LESC cell culture; however, this has not been shown to affect the suitability of successfully established cell sheets for transplantation.[2] Likewise, characteristics of tissue donors may influence attachment, survival and proliferation of LESCs. It has been reported that donor age has an influence on putative limbal stem cell markers, as well as morphological niche parameters, and that colony forming efficiency of LESCs declines with age.[10,11] Additionally, it has been shown that corneal wound healing is impaired in diabetes mellitus, and limbal basal cells from diabetic human donors have been suggested to express fewer putative stem cell markers than those from normal subjects.[12] This exemplifies that LESCs may be affected by systemic disease present in the donor. Again, whether this is likely to affect culture and transplantation of human limbal epithelial cells remains to be determined.

The Limbal Stem Cell Niche in Culture

Transplantation of limbal epithelium is deemed a stem cell therapy. This notion is supported, for instance, by the observation that a minimum of 3000 transplanted putative limbal stem cells was associated with a higher success rate in patients with ocular surface disease due to chemical and thermal burns.[1] However, expanded limbal epithelial cell sheets contain a considerable fraction of differentiated daughter cells (Fig. 44.5). Also, LESCs have only a finite life span when propagated in culture, although one of the most important features describing stem cell populations is that of indefinite self-renewal. The current conception is that the maintenance of limbal stem cells is governed by a number of intrinsic, but also extrinsic factors, the latter of which are provided in vivo by the local microenvironment present at the corneoscleral limbus. Rather than being a mere transition zone between cornea and sclera, the limbus provides some unique anatomical specializations that are believed to be important for maintaining the stem cell population (see Chapter 5). In addition to a protective limbal anatomy, signals received from extracellular matrix and surrounding cells are believed to contribute to regulating LESC function and fate. For instance, extracellular matrix components were found to be expressed differentially in different areas of the ocular and corneal surface and may play a role in regulating LESC proliferation and differentiation.[13] Likewise, soluble factors secreted by limbal fibroblasts have been proposed to have regulatory effects on limbal basal epithelium. The notion of adjacent structures and cells influencing stem cell behavior corresponds well to what has

been termed the 'stem cell niche.' A system which removes LESCs from their niche to expand the cells for transplantation will need to replicate the stem cell niche in order to retain 'stemness' of the cells.

The limbal stem cell niche may also play a role during engraftment of cultivated LESCs onto the recipient corneal surface. In the case of keratolimbal allograft or conjunctival limbal graft, both LESCs and the underlying tissue containing putative niche components are transplanted. This, however, is not the case where only sheets of cultured epithelium are transferred. As is discussed in the next section, amniotic membrane has received considerable attention for its potential as an LESC carrier that may replace certain niche factors both during cell culture and on the recipient ocular surface.

Amniotic Membrane as a Culture Substrate

In the first two cases of cultured LESC transplantation reported by Pellegrini and coworkers, transfer of the cultured epithelial sheet to the recipient ocular surface was performed using petroleum gauze in one patient, while a soft contact lens served as a carrier in the other. Subsequent works have frequently used fibrin gels. These gels have been shown to support LESC growth and attachment in culture, while they are degraded within 24 hours following transplantation (Fig. 44.6). However, these matrices do not actively contribute to the preservation of stem cell properties during expansion and engraftment. To provide a surrogate niche for LESCs throughout ex vivo culture and after transfer to the ocular surface, amniotic membrane (AM) has become a popular substrate. AM is the innermost membrane of the fetal sac, which can be obtained from healthy volunteers during routine caesarean sections. Properties which make AM well suited for ocular surface reconstruction are its avascularity, relative transparency, low immunogenicity, expression of anti-inflammatory and antiangiogenic proteins, as well as growth factors (see Chapter 37). AM can therefore, act both as a culture substrate in vitro and as a carrier for LESC transfer and attachment to the corneal surface. AM has been used successfully as a substrate for LESC expansion and transplantation for more than a decade. Growth factors that convey favorable properties for LESC maintenance and expansion are produced by the AM stroma and particularly the amniotic epithelium. Among these growth factors are keratocyte, hepatocyte, epidermal, nerve and basic fibroblast growth factor, as well as members of the transforming growth factor family (Fig. 44.7).

Frequently, prior to applying limbal epithelial cells, the amniotic epithelium is removed by physical scraping or enzymatically to expose the underlying thick basement membrane. Basement membrane components that are present in AM and which may support LESC growth and adhesion include collagen IV and laminin isoforms, as well as fibronectin.[14] These properties aid in the formation of confluent, well-attached, stratified sheets of epithelium of a corneal phenotype.[15] However, it has been suggested that AM with an intact epithelial layer may be more suitable for maintaining LESCs in their undifferentiated

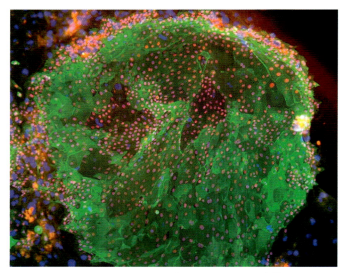

Figure 44.5 Immunohistochemical image of a limbal stem cell-derived clonal growth on a feeder layer of murine 3T3 fibroblasts. Cells in the center of the clones stain positive for desmoglein (*green*), which plays a role in the assembly of mature intercellular junctions and therefore, serves as an indicator for differentiated epithelial cells. Cells at the external boundaries of the clones stain positive for the nuclear transcription factor p63 (*red*), which has been suggested to be a marker of heavily proliferative limbal progenitor cells. (Photograph courtesy of Ursula Schlötzer-Schrehardt.)

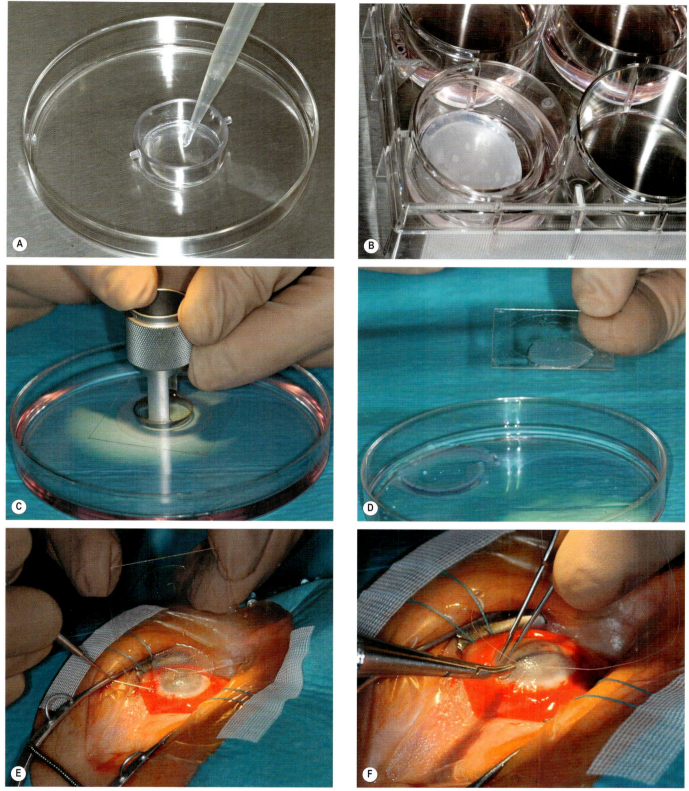

Figure 44.6 Transplantation of cultured limbal epithelium on fibrin gel. (**A**) Fibrin gel is prepared in a plastic mold by adding fibrinogen and thrombin. (**B**) Following polymerization, the fibrin gel is placed in a cell culture insert on top of a feeder layer of growth-arrested 3T3 fibroblasts. The explant (alternatively, a cell suspension obtained following enzymatic dissociation) is placed on the surface of the fibrin gel, covered in medium and cultured for approximately 2–3 weeks until a confluent monolayer has formed. (**C, D**) A 16-mm trephine is used to excise the central area of the gel. (**E**) Following 360° conjunctival peritomy and removal of precorneal fibrovascular tissue, the fibrin gel carrying the cultured epithelium is transferred to the ocular surface. (**F**) Peripherally, the graft is placed into a conjunctival pocket and fixed using single sutures. Postoperatively, a therapeutic contact lens and/ or tarsorrhaphy may be used to protect the transplanted epithelium. (See supplementary video 2 for the full procedure.)

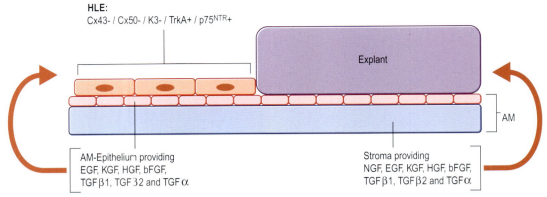

HLE:
Cx43- / Cx50- / K3- / TrkA+ / p75^{NTR}+

Explant

AM

AM-Epithelium providing
EGF, KGF, HGF, bFGF,
TGFβ1, TGFβ2 and TGFα

Stroma providing
NGF, EGF, KGF, HGF, bFGF,
TGFβ1, TGFβ2 and TGFα

Figure 44.7 Limbal epithelial cells cultured on human amniotic membrane using the explant culture system. Following outgrowth from the limbal explant, limbal epithelial cells form a monolayer on top of the devitalized amniotic membrane epithelium. An additional feeder layer is not required when using non-denuded amniotic membrane, likely due to the higher level of growth factors derived from the amniotic epithelium. The limbal epithelial cells are negative for the expression of differentiation markers connexin 42 and keratin 3. (Modified from Grueterich M, Espana EM, Tseng SCG. Ex vivo expansion of limbal epithelial stem cells: amniotic membrane serving as a stem cell niche. Surv Ophthalmol 2003;48:631–46.)

state, as it appears to result in propagation of smaller cells (putative progenitor cells)[16] and preservation of a limbal phenotype.[14]

Hence, the optimal method of preparing AM for LESC culture remains unclear. This extends also to methods used for AM preservation. It has been argued that fresh AM (stored at 4°C) may be able to contribute more of its bioactive factors; however, also cryopreserved and lyophilized membrane have been used successfully.[17] While glycerol is used widely as a cryoprotective agent, Shortt et al. have suggested that it results in poor retention of putative stem cell markers and epithelial cell morphology. Instead, it has been proposed that the use of balanced saline solution may be superior with respect to the mentioned parameters.[18] Protocols for the preparation of AM also differ in terms of the method used for reducing infectious risk. Here, antibiotic treatment, peracetic acid, and gamma irradiation have all been used in the context of LESC expansion.[19]

Although certainly useful for ocular surface reconstruction, AM does carry infectious risks which, despite costly screening of donors plus disinfection/sterilization, cannot be fully eliminated. Additional shortcomings, such as biological variability, inconsistent supply and only relative transparency have encouraged efforts to develop alternative, biomimetic substrates for expansion of LESCs. These substrates may be engineered to incorporate additional, more specific limbal niche components (see Chapter 43).

Culture Media

The growth potential of human epidermal cells has been characterized by the type of colony that forms in culture: holoclones contain cells showing high clonogenic capacity, meroclones include a larger fraction of cells that have a more limited capacity for proliferation, and paraclones consist of cells that are still closer to terminal differentiation. This typical growth pattern is also seen in epithelial cells obtained from the corneoscleral limbus (Fig. 44.8). In addition to the culture substrates discussed above, the media used for ex vivo expansion have been shown to play

an important role in preserving stem cell properties of cultured LESCs.[10] Optimal culture conditions for LESCs would be expected to yield a high proportion of stem cell-containing holoclones. A typical composition of limbal epithelial stem cell culture medium is listed in Table 44.1. Different variations of this formulation have been used in a number of clinical trials to evaluate LESC grafts. However, it has been proposed that the high calcium content of DMEM/F12 promotes rapid growth but leads to early differentiation.[10] Since LESCs have been described as slow-cycling cells, it seems logical that culture conditions which achieve high rates of proliferation may not be expanding stem cells, but rather supporting the growth of transient amplifying progenitors. Instead, a growth medium containing low calcium concentration of 0.03 mM was shown to support an undifferentiated phenotype. This culture medium, however, contains bovine pituitary gland extract and may therefore, not be suitable for clinical use due to the potential risk of transmitting infectious agents of animal origin. Other investigators have proposed that the medium supplement B-27 is suitable for cultivating LESCs in a serum-free culture system without unknown xenobiotic factors to reduce this risk.[20].

Currently, there is no universally accepted standard protocol for ex vivo preparation of cultivated LESCs. Despite the use of several medium supplements, successful expansion of LESCs still relies on the presence of murine 3T3 feeder cells, amniotic membrane, or both. It appears likely that increased understanding of limbal stem cell biology will lead to further modification of the culture conditions, with the aim of better preserving stem cells.

Airlifting has been used by some investigators to produce coherent sheets of multilayered epithelium for transfer to the ocular surface. This technique consists of raising the monolayer of epithelial cells that forms during submersion in culture medium to the air – liquid interface to induce stratification. However, this procedure may result in the loss of stem cells within the cultured sheet due to increased differentiation cues. Other investigators have, therefore, proposed the transfer of a single-cell suspension to the recipient ocular surface.[21] The idea of stem cell-containing eye drops illustrates that the development of cell-based therapies for

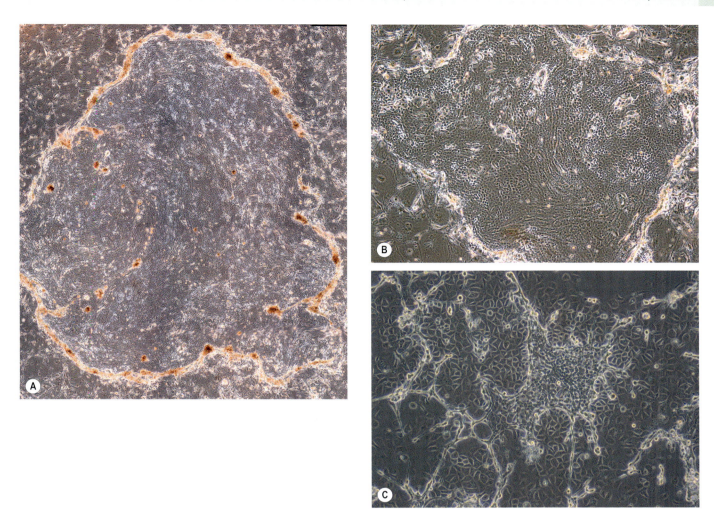

Figure 44.8 Limbal epithelial cells cultured on a feeder layer of 3T3 fibroblasts. Clonal growth occurs in three different patterns. (**A**) Holoclones have large, almost circular colonies with smooth boundaries. These clones are likely to contain large numbers of LESCs. (**B**) Meroclones are somewhat smaller in size with more irregular boundaries. Cells from these clones are more restricted in their proliferative potential and are deemed to be transient amplifying cells. (**C**) Paraclones are small and possess highly irregular boundaries; they contain cells that are close to terminal differentiation. (Photographs courtesy of Ewa Meyer-Blazejewska.)

Table 44.1   Example of Limbal Epithelial Stem Cell Growth and Expansion Medium[2,4]

Medium Constituent	Final Concentration	Description
Dulbecco's modification of Eagle's medium (DMEM)		Basal medium
Ham's nutrient mixture F-12	25%	DMEM and F-12 have also been used at a ratio of 1:1
Fetal bovine serum	10%	The use of human autologous serum has also been reported[30]
Insulin	5 µg/mL	Reduces serum requirements
Hydrocortisone	0.4 µg/mL	Improves epithelial cell growth and morphology
Cholera toxin	0.1 nM	Stimulates DNA synthesis
Adenine	0.18 mM	Enhances colony formation
Transferrin	5 µg/mL	Stimulates stem cell replication
Tri-iodothryronine	2 nM	Reduces serum requirements
Epidermal growth factor	10 ng/mL	Promotes migration and cell spreading; inhibits differentiation
Antibiotics/antimycotics	e.g. penicillin (100 IU/mL), streptomycin (100 µg/mL), amphotericin B (25 µg/mL)	Optional

(From Shortt AJ, Tuft SJ, Daniels JT. Ex vivo cultured limbal epithelial transplantation. A clinical perspective. Ocul Surf 2010;8:80–90. and Osei-Bempong C, Henein C, Ahmad S. Culture conditions for primary human limbal epithelial cells. Regen Med 2009;4:461–70.)

the treatment of ocular surface disease falls within the scope of activities of regulatory authorities that supervise the development and distribution of medicinal products. Regulatory issues surrounding the transition of cultured LESCs from bench to bedside are discussed in the following section.

Regulatory Requirements

To ensure product safety and consistency, routine use of cultured cells for therapeutic purposes in humans underlies strict regulation from the relevant authorities in many countries. In the European Union, the legal framework for procurement and processing of tissues and cells for the production of biological therapeutics is provided by the EU Tissue and Cells Directive, with a national regulatory authority in each member state being responsible for implementing the exigencies of this directive. In the United States, the Food and Drug Administration is responsible for enforcing Good Manufacturing Practice (GMP) in the production of cell-based therapies. To comply with regulatory requirements, informed consent must be obtained from the donor (or next of kin), and serological screening must be performed for transmissible diseases.[22] The need for serological testing is extended also to patients planned for autologous treatment to avoid pathogen transmission to laboratory staff or other specimens during processing. To minimize any risk of transmitting zoonotic diseases, of tumorigenesis or of precipitating immunologic rejection, it has repeatedly been postulated that products intended for cell therapy at the ocular surface should be free from xenobiotics.[23] However, the actual risk is difficult to quantitate, and other authors argue that fetal calf serum and murine 3T3 feeder cells may be suitable to provide highly reproducible culture conditions for delivery of cultured LESC of consistent quality.[24]

GMP regulations also require that preparation of LESC sheets be carried out in a dedicated cleanroom environment. The establishment, accreditation and maintenance of a dedicated facility for GMP-compliant preparation of cultured LESC grafts require a significant amount of resources. From the angle of health economics, and to make cultured LESC treatment available to patients at smaller centers, the development of suitable systems for distribution of grafts would be advantageous.

Clinical and Surgical Management and Outcomes

Transplantation of cultured LESCs is indicated primarily in cases of unilateral or bilateral total limbal stem cell deficiency, where an area of healthy limbus available at a donor eye may benefit from the risk reduction offered by the smaller biopsy.

It has been suggested that the local tissue environment may be an important factor determining graft success.[24] This notion is supported by the somewhat poorer results seen when ocular surface disease is associated with inflammation and severe dry eye.[2] Hence, the recipient ocular surface may require pretreatment to optimize the

conditions for the cultured LESC graft. Most importantly, this involves assessment of the ocular adnexa and subsequent correction of any lid dysfunction, treatment of dry eye disease, as well as thorough control of ocular surface inflammation.[25] To avoid complications during surgery, preoperative pachymetry is recommended in cases where corneal thickness cannot be assessed reliably at the slit lamp.[2]

The host ocular surface is surgically prepared by performing a 360° conjunctival peritomy and removing any remaining epithelium and fibrovascular tissue which may cover the diseased cornea (see Fig. 44.6 and supplementary video 2). At this stage in some studies, mitomycin C is applied topically for a brief period.[6] If significant corneal stromal thinning or scarring is present, a full-thickness or anterior lamellar corneal graft may need to be performed simultaneously or subsequent to the surface reconstruction procedure (Fig. 44.9). The cultured LESC graft is transferred to the corneal surface and sutured in place. For mechanical protection of the graft during the postoperative period, available options are therapeutic contact lenses, a secondary layer of amniotic membrane and/or temporary lid closure.

Postoperative care routinely involves administration of topical unpreserved steroid and broad-spectrum antibiotics. In addition, corticosteroids may also be administered systemically with the objective of controlling inflammation and preventing allograft rejection. Intravenous methylprednisolone can be given postoperatively for 3 days; however, most studies used a 1-month course of betamethasone or prednisolone (1 mg/kg/day).[7] Although it has not been shown specifically that systemic immunosuppression is able to reduce the risk of immune rejection following cultured LESC transplantation, it is known that allogeneic limbal epithelial cells can become the target of an immunological reaction.[26] Therefore, long-term immunosuppression may be of value and should be considered following cultured LESC transplantation (see Chapter 46). However, in view of the report that donor DNA could not be detected on host ocular surfaces 9 months after transplantation, it can be argued that immunosuppression should not be continued beyond this point.[8] Immunosuppression is commonly achieved using oral cyclosporine A; however, there is no consensus as to what dose should be administered and when or if treatment should be reduced or discontinued. Additional topical cyclosporine A or systemic cyclophosphamide have been used in some studies, but again it remains unclear whether this yields any further reduction of the risk of immune rejection.[7]

Assessment of the ocular surface integrity is widely regarded the most relevant measure to judge the success of a cultured LESC graft. There is no general consensus as to how successful restoration of corneal epithelium should be determined clinically. Most studies rely on epithelial transparency and superficial vascularization, but often the parameters used to assess LESC deficiency pre- and postoperatively remain unspecified. Rama et al. developed a scoring system to assess the severity of LESC deficiency.[27] This assessment relies on clinical findings, as well as the cytokeratin expression of corneal epithelial cells obtained via impression cytology and may therefore, offer an objective measure of ocular surface improvement. Other authors

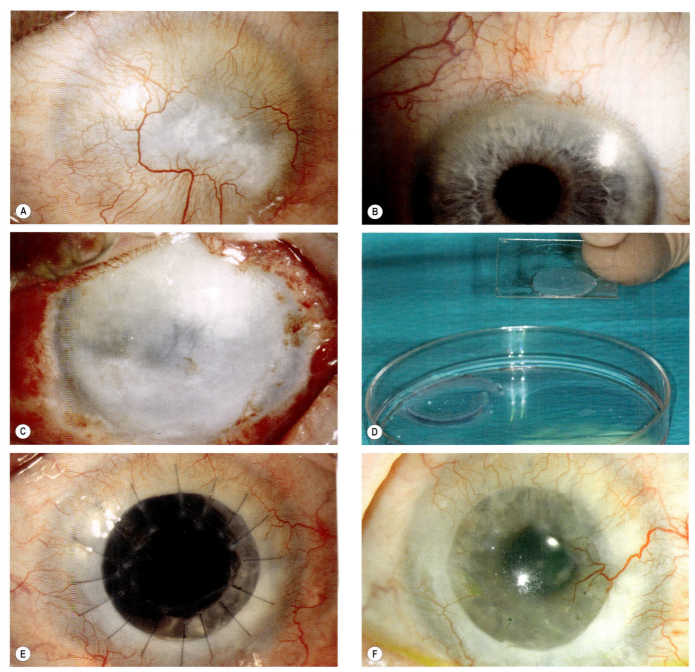

Figure 44.9 Clinical course of a patient with a 25-year history of unilateral caustic burn, who underwent autologous transplantation of ex vivo expanded limbal epithelium. (**A**) Preoperative findings: the ocular surface trauma caused severe limbal stem cell deficiency with subsequent precorneal scarring and vascularization. (**B**) A small limbal biopsy was obtained from the uninjured fellow eye, leaving only minor irritation 1 day after the procedure. Full recovery of this donor eye was seen during follow-up visits (not shown). The limbal biopsy was expanded on fibrin gel and transplanted to the surface of the diseased eye 2 weeks after the limbal biopsy (see supplementary videos for the surgical procedures). (**C**) Immediate postoperative findings, showing the transplanted epithelial cell sheet attached to the recipient ocular surface. (**D**) The same eye photographed 6 months after the surgery, showing a stable corneal epithelium with some recurrent vascularization and residual stromal scarring. (**E**) After the ocular surface had remained stable for a period of 2 years, penetrating keratoplasty was performed to improve visual acuity. (**F**) Six years after the initial operation, superficial corneal vascularization is seen to be progressing slowly; however, the central cornea remains clear and the corneal epithelium is intact.

have advocated the use of confocal microscopy to detect the presence of conjunctival epithelium on the corneal surface.[18] This method correlated well with impression cytology findings, and does not carry the risk of damaging the reconstructed epithelium.

In contrast to many other medical or surgical procedures in ophthalmology, visual acuity is considered only a secondary end point in many studies of LESC transplantation. This stems from the fact that, frequently, considerable stromal scarring impedes immediate visual recovery following ocular surface treatment. Instead, while reconstruction of the ocular surface by cultured LESC transplantation paves the way for subsequent surgery which may restore visual function, reduction of ocular symptoms has been reported from various studies.[6] It has recently been suggested that quality of life should be included as an outcome measure for LESC transplantation, as this may allow a combined and structured measure of useful vision, ocular discomfort and also cosmesis.[28]

The most common underlying condition in patients who received cultured LESC grafts is chemical or thermal trauma, which accounts for 75% of the patients reported.[6] Upon reviewing clinical studies on cultured LESC transplantation, independent groups found a generally favorable outcome with around 75% of all published cases being classified as clinically successful.[6,7] This is despite the fact that the published evidence on clinical results of cultured LESC transplantation is limited by inconsistent inclusion criteria, culture protocols, and outcome measures. Systematic meta-analysis of success rates of cultured LESC grafts is therefore, not feasible at this stage.

Adverse events have been reported from a number of studies that transplanted cultured LESCs. Among the most frequently reported adverse events were bleeding (2.8%) and perforation (1.3%).[6] Out of a total of 150 cases reviewed by Shortt et al.,[7] infectious keratitis occurred in five patients, all of whom had received cultured limbal allografts and were therefore, immunosuppressed. In another five eyes, epithelial rejection of allografts was observed despite systemic immunosuppression. As a result, graft failure occurred in three of the five eyes. Kaplan – Meier analyses indicate that, generally, failure occurs predominantly within the first 1–2 years of grafting.

Outlook

Since the early successes in LESC culture, a multitude of clinical trials has examined their clinical usefulness for the reconstruction of the corneal epithelium. Results are favorable across many studies, and follow-up data have been recorded for periods up to 10 years in some cases.[1] Molecular characterization of LESCs and the limbal stem cell niche are likely to translate into improved culture techniques in the future. However, only in conjunction with thorough understanding of the mechanisms of action of LESC transplantation in vivo and through coordinated efforts for clinical evaluation and implementation will defined culture conditions lead to clinical success in reconstruction of the corneal epithelium. Studies to compare cultured LESC grafts to other methods of limbal stem cell transplantation (which consume fewer resources for their preparation) are

missing.[29] Currently, there is no standard protocol for clinical grading of LESC deficiency, and no consensus on how outcomes of cultured LESC transplantation should be reported, impeding direct comparison between studies on cultured LESC transplantation. At the time of writing, efforts are under way within the LESC research community to compile such a set of standards for clinical and research applications. Furthermore, randomized, multicenter trials are required in order to standardize and optimize the available protocols for LESC expansion and transplantation.

While it is likely that cultured LESCs reduce the risk that a limbal biopsy poses to the donor eye, there are no reliable data to quantitate the remaining risk. In addition, allogeneic transplants carry inherent risks, such as disease transmission, immune rejection or the sequels of systemic immunosuppression. For these reasons, substantial research efforts have been directed towards establishing autologous cultured transplants of adult progenitor cells harvested from other body sites (e.g. hair follicle, dental pulp, bone marrow or buccal mucosa).

References

We apologize to those authors whose works have not been cited due to space limitation. Recent findings are referenced; the older evidence is discussed in the reviews cited.

1. Rama P, Matuska S, Paganoni G, et al. Limbal stem-cell therapy and long-term corneal regeneration. N Engl J Med 2010;363: 147–55.
2. Shortt AJ, Tuft SJ, Daniels JT. Ex vivo cultured limbal epithelial transplantation. A clinical perspective. Ocul Surf 2010;8:80–90.
3. Ahmad S, Osei-Bempong C, Dana R, et al. The culture and transplantation of human limbal stem cells. J Cell Physiol 2010;225: 15–9.
4. Osei-Bempong C, Henein C, Ahmad S. Culture conditions for primary human limbal epithelial cells. Regen Med 2009;4:461–70.
5. Sangwan VS, Vemuganti GK, Iftekhar G, et al. Use of autologous cultured limbal and conjunctival epithelium in a patient with severe bilateral ocular surface disease induced by acid injury: a case report of unique application. Cornea 2003;22:478–81.
6. Baylis O, Figueiredo F, Henein C, et al. 13 years of cultured limbal epithelial cell therapy: a review of the outcomes. J Cell Biochem 2011;112:993–1002.
7. Shortt AJ, Secker GA, Notara MD, et al. Transplantation of ex vivo cultured limbal epithelial stem cells: a review of techniques and clinical results. Surv Ophthalmol 2007;52:483–502.
8. Daya SM, Watson A, Sharpe JR, et al. Outcomes and DNA analysis of ex vivo expanded stem cell allograft for ocular surface reconstruction. Ophthalmology 2005;112:470–7.
9. O'Callaghan AR, Daniels JT. Concise review: limbal epithelial stem cell therapy: controversies and challenges. Stem Cells 2011;29: 1923–32.
10. Meyer-Blazejewska EA, Kruse FE, Bitterer K, et al. Preservation of the limbal stem cell phenotype by appropriate culture techniques. Invest Ophthalmol Vis Sci 2010;51:765–74.
11. Notara M, Shortt AJ, O'Callaghan AR, et al. The impact of age on the physical and cellular properties of the human limbal stem cell niche. Age (Dordr) 2012. [Epub ahead of print].
12. Saghizadeh M, Soleymani S, Harounian A, et al. Alterations of epithelial stem cell marker patterns in human diabetic corneas and effects of c-met gene therapy. Mol Vis 2011;17:2177–90.
13. Schlötzer-Schrehardt U, Dietrich T, Saito K, et al. Characterization of extracellular matrix components in the limbal epithelial stem cell compartment. Exp Eye Res 2007;85:845–60.
14. Grueterich M, Espana EM, Tseng SCG. Ex vivo expansion of limbal epithelial stem cells: amniotic membrane serving as a stem cell niche. Surv Ophthalmol 2003;48:631–46.
15. Koizumi N, Rigby H, Fullwood NJ, et al. Comparison of intact and denuded amniotic membrane as a substrate for cell-suspension culture of human limbal epithelial cells. Graefes Arch Clin Exp Ophthalmol 2007;245:123–34.

16. Shortt AJ, Secker GA, Lomas RJ, et al. The effect of amniotic membrane preparation method on its ability to serve as a substrate for the ex-vivo expansion of limbal epithelial cells. Biomaterials 2009; 30:1056–65.

17. Dua HS, Rahman I, Miri A, et al. Variations in amniotic membrane: relevance for clinical applications. Br J Ophthalmol 2010;94:963–4.

18. Shortt AJ, Secker GA, Rajan MS, et al. Ex vivo expansion and transplantation of limbal epithelial stem cells. Ophthalmology 2008; 115:1989–97.

19. Nakamura T, Yoshitani M, Rigby H, et al. Sterilized, freeze-dried amniotic membrane: a useful substrate for ocular surface reconstruction. Invest Ophthalmol Vis Sci 2004;45:93–9.

20. Yokoo S, Yamagami S, Usui T, et al. Human corneal epithelial equivalents for ocular surface reconstruction in a complete serum-free culture system without unknown factors. Invest Ophthalmol Vis Sci 2008;49:2438–43.

21. Li CJ, Ashraf FM, Rana TS, et al. Long-term survival of allogeneic donor cell-derived corneal epithelium in limbal deficient rabbits. Curr Eye Res 2001;23:336–45.

22. Daniels JT, Secker GA, Shortt AJ, et al. Stem cell therapy delivery: treading the regulatory tightrope. Regen Med 2006;1:715–9.

23. Schwab IR, Johnson NT, Harkin DG. Inherent risks associated with manufacture of bioengineered ocular surface tissue. Arch Ophthalmol 2006;124:1734–40.

24. Pellegrini G, Rama P, De Luca M. Vision from the right stem. Trends Mol Med 2010;17:2177–90.

25. DeSousa JL, Daya S, Malhotra R. Adnexal surgery in patients undergoing ocular surface stem cell transplantation. Ophthalmology 2009; 116:235–42.

26. Cooper LJ, Fullwood NJ, Koizumi N, et al. An investigation of removed cultivated epithelial transplants in patients after allocultivated corneal epithelial transplantation. Cornea 2004;23:235–42.

27. Rama P, Bonini S, Lambiase A, et al. Autologous fibrin-cultured limbal stem cells permanently restore the corneal surface of patients with total limbal stem cell deficiency. Transplantation 2001;72:1478–85.

28. Miri A, Mathew M, Dua HS. Quality of life after limbal transplants. Ophthalmology 2010;117:638, e1–3.

29. Cauchi PA, Ang GS, Azuara-Blanco A, et al. A systematic literature review of surgical interventions for limbal stem cell deficiency in humans. Am J Ophthalmol 2008;146:251–9.

30. Nakamura T, Ang LP, Rigby H, et al. The use of autologous serum in the development of corneal and oral epithelial equivalents in patients with Stevens – Johnson syndrome. Invest Ophthalmol Vis Sci 2006; 47:909–16.

45 Non-Ocular Sources for Cell-Based Ocular Surface Reconstruction

TAKAHIRO NAKAMURA

Introduction

The concept of 'ocular surface reconstruction' (OSR) is widely accepted in the field of ophthalmology, and our understanding of the role of the ocular surface has greatly improved, due to the basic science and clinical research carried out in this field. Over the past 30 years, there have been several scientific discoveries, such as the identification of corneal epithelial stem cells, the establishment of novel methods for epithelial culturing, and a deep understanding of the extracellular matrices, all of which have enabled us to adopt novel surgical procedures to treat severe ocular surface disease. However, despite the success of these surgical procedures, several clinical problems still remain. Firstly, transplantation of corneal epithelial cells from donors requires sufficient donor material, and secondly, that procedure carries the risk of rejection. Consequently, postoperative systemic immunosuppression is required for allografts in order to prevent inflammation and rejection. This chapter describes a history and an attempt to overcome the problems of allogeneic OSR by using oral epithelial cells as a substitute for corneal epithelial cells. In addition, recent advancements, current developments, and future challenges related to OSR using the transplantation of epithelial cells of non-ocular surface origin will also be discussed.

Development of Cultivated Oral Mucosal Epithelial Transplantation (COMET, Preclinical Trail)

THE SUCCESSFUL CULTURE OF RABBIT ORAL MUCOSAL EPITHELIAL CELLS

The problem of allograft rejection is the main reason that we decided to develop a new method of autologous oral mucosal epithelium transplantation for OSR.[1] In our laboratory experiment, epithelial cells from the oral mucosa began to form colonies on the denuded AM within 3 days. At 3 weeks, the cultivated oral epithelial cells showed 4–5 layers of stratification, were well differentiated (Fig. 45.1A), and appeared very similar to in vivo normal corneal epithelium (Fig. 45.1B).[1]

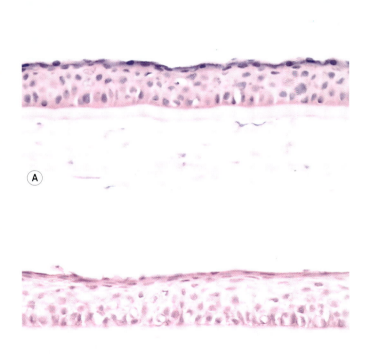

(A)

(B)

Figure 45.1 Light micrographs showing cross-sections of normal corneal epithelial cells (**A**) and rabbit cultivated oral mucosal epithelial cells on amniotic membrane (**B**) stained with hematoxylin and eosin. The cultivated oral mucosal epithelial sheet had 4–5 layers of stratified, well-differentiated cells and appeared very similar to in vivo normal corneal epithelium. (Modified from Nakamura T, Endo K, Cooper LJ, et al. The successful culture and autologous transplantation of rabbit oral mucosal epithelial cells on amniotic membrane. Invest Ophthalmol Vis Sci 2003;44:106–16.)

CELL BIOLOGICAL CHARACTERISTICS OF THE RABBIT CULTIVATED ORAL MUCOSAL EPITHELIAL SHEET

Cytokeratins play an important structural and protective role in maintaining the integrity of the epithelium of the anterior segment of the eye. Defined subsets of individual

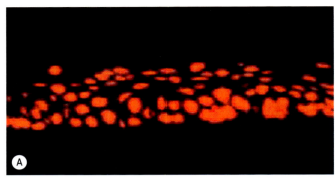

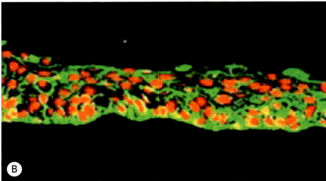

Figure 45.2 Keratin 3 was expressed in all epithelial layers of the cultivated oral mucosal sheet, whereas cornea-specific keratin 12 immunostaining was not found in these cultivated oral mucosal epithelial cells. (Modified from Nakamura T, Endo K, Cooper LJ, et al. The successful culture and autologous transplantation of rabbit oral mucosal epithelial cells on amniotic membrane. Invest Ophthalmol Vis Sci 2003;44:106–16.)

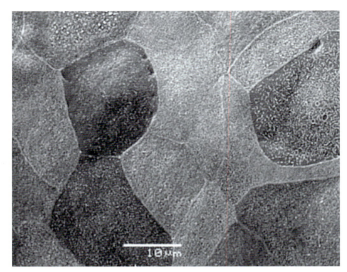

Figure 45.3 Scanning electron micrograph of rabbit cultivated oral mucosal epithelial sheet. The cells appear healthy and well formed with distinct cell boundaries. (Modified from Nakamura T, Endo K, Cooper LJ, et al. The successful culture and autologous transplantation of rabbit oral mucosal epithelial cells on amniotic membrane. Invest Ophthalmol Vis Sci 2003;44:106–16.)

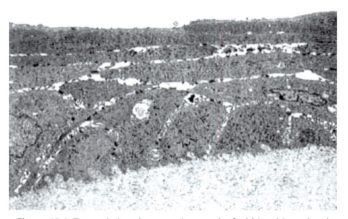

Figure 45.4 Transmission electron micrograph of rabbit cultivated oral mucosal epithelial sheet. The culture formed 5–6 layers of a healthy well-stratified epithelial cell layer. (Modified from Nakamura T, Endo K, Cooper LJ, et al. The successful culture and autologous transplantation of rabbit oral mucosal epithelial cells on amniotic membrane. Invest Ophthalmol Vis Sci 2003;44:106–16.)

cytokeratin pairs are characteristically expressed, depending on the type of epithelial cell tissue and level of differentiation. In this study, we used immunohistochemistry to demonstrate that the keratin 1/10 pair, which is involved in the physiological keratinization process in the epidermis, is not expressed in any layers of the cultivated oral epithelial sheet. We also found that the keratin 4/13 pair, which is observed in nonkeratinized, stratified epithelia, is expressed in the superficial and intermediate layers of the cultivated oral epithelial cells. These results led us to believe that the oral epithelial cells cultivated on AM have the characteristics of nonkeratinized mucosa, not keratinized mucosa. Immunohistochemical examination revealed no cornea-specific keratin 12 expression in any layers of the cultivated oral epithelial sheets (Fig. 45.2A), whereas cornea-specific keratin 3 was expressed in all epithelial layers of the cultivated oral epithelial sheet (Fig. 45.2B). Even though the cells of the cultivated oral epithelial sheet are not able to become corneal epithelial cells, we suggest that they might have the potential ability to become cornea-like epithelial cells under proper in vitro culture conditions.

MORPHOLOGICAL CHARACTERISTICS OF THE RABBIT CULTIVATED ORAL MUCOSAL EPITHELIAL SHEET

Electron microscopic results of the cultivated oral mucosal epithelial sheet are of particular interest. Examination by use of a scanning electron microscope (SEM) revealed that rabbit oral epithelial cells appeared healthy and well formed with tightly opposed cell junctions (Fig. 45.3). The cultivated oral cells were similar in size and appearance to rabbit corneal epithelial cells. Transmission electron microscopy (TEM) confirmed that the cultivated oral epithelial sheet was very similar in appearance to that of corneal epithelium, and very different from conjunctiva and oral mucosa. Like corneal epithelium, it had 4–5 layers of stratified cells which were differentiated into columnar, wing, and squamous cells (Fig. 45.4). Both our SEM and TEM results show clearly that our oral mucosal cells, cultivated on AM, resemble normal corneal epithelial cells more closely than any other cell type.

In regard to the growth of cultivated oral mucosal epithelial cells, the method of how the basal cells attach to the underlying AM, as well as whether or not the superficial cells develop a normal barrier function, are both important questions. Our TEM results showed that the cultivated oral mucosal epithelial sheet attached to the basement membrane via hemidesmosomal junctions. Adjacent cells in the cultivated oral sheet are also joined with numerous desmosomal junctions, and what appear to be tight junctions are evident between the most superficial cell layers. From these findings, we believe that the cells of the cultivated oral mucosal epithelial sheet have similar junctional specializations to those of in vivo corneal epithelial cells.

The anterior surface of normal corneal epithelium has numerous folds in the anterior epithelial cell membranes in the form of microvilli, together with a glycocalyx layer. Another key point for carrying out successful cultivated oral epithelial sheet transplantation is elucidation of how the most superficial cells contact the tear – ocular surface interface. SEM revealed that the apical surface of the cultivated oral epithelial cells is covered with numerous microvilli, almost identical to those found on corneal epithelial cells. Interestingly, we also found evidence of a cell-surface glycocalyx, similar in appearance to the glycocalyx present on the surface of corneal epithelial cells. These findings encouraged us to carry out the transplantation of cultivated oral mucosal epithelial cells.

SUCCESSFUL TRANSPLANTATION OF THE RABBIT CULTIVATED ORAL MUCOSAL EPITHELIAL SHEET

After the successful culture of rabbit oral mucosal epithelial cells on AM, we tried to reconstruct the damaged corneal surfaces by transplantation of autologous cultivated oral mucosal epithelial cells in order to test the viability of using these cells as a substitute for cultivated corneal epithelial cells. At 48 hours after surgery, most of the area of the transplanted cultivated oral mucosal epithelial sheet possessed intact epithelium. At 10 days after transplantation, the ocular surface covered by the transplanted epithelium was intact and without defects, thus suggesting that the autologous transplantation of cultivated oral mucosal epithelia is a viable procedure for ocular surface reconstruction (Fig. 45.5). Histological examination of the transplanted sheets at 10 days after surgery revealed that the sheets were well adhered to the host corneal stroma, with no evidence of subepithelial cell infiltration or stromal edema. Superficial cells of the transplanted sheets had nuclei, indicating that they were indeed nonkeratinized mucosal epithelial cells.

Therefore, we successfully generated a well-stratified and differentiated rabbit cultivated oral mucosal epithelial sheet. Moreover, we successfully performed autologous transplantation of these cells onto keratectomized rabbit corneas. Hence, we believe that autologous transplantation of rabbit cultivated oral mucosal epithelial sheet is a feasible method for OSR.

THE SUCCESSFUL CULTURE OF HUMAN ORAL MUCOSAL EPITHELIAL CELLS

We next focused our attention on cultivating human oral mucosal epithelial cells using our previously reported

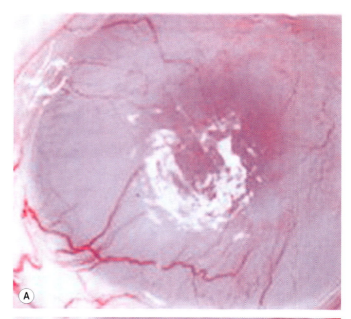

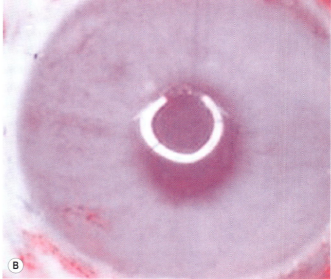

Figure 45.5 Slit lamp photographs of rabbit taken before transplantation (**A**) and 10 days after transplantation (**B**). Before transplantation, ocular surface had total limbal stem cell destruction. Forty-eight hours after surgery, most of the corneal surface was covered with transplanted cultivated oral mucosal epithelial cells. (Modified from Nakamura T, Endo K, Cooper LJ, et al. The successful culture and autologous transplantation of rabbit oral mucosal epithelial cells on amniotic membrane. Invest Ophthalmol Vis Sci 2003;44:106–16.)

culture methods for rabbit oral mucosal epithelial cells, yet with several modifications. It should be noted that it was quite difficult to cultivate human oral mucosal epithelial cells using the previously reported culture technique for rabbit oral epithelial cells, and therefore, the culture process did require some modification. In the end, and as a result of the modification, we were able to successfully generate a well-stratified and differentiated human cultivated oral mucosal epithelial sheet (Fig. 45.6). Light microscopy revealed that the human cultivated oral mucosal epithelial cells were very similar in appearance to normal corneal epithelial cells. Moreover,

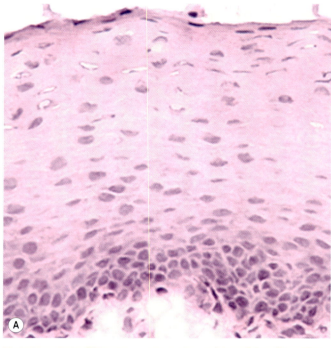

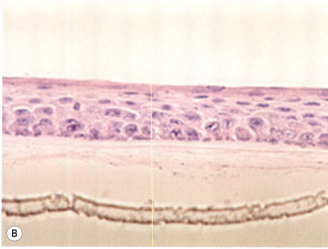

Figure 45.6 Light micrographs showing cross-sections of human normal oral mucosal epithelial cells (**A**) and human cultivated oral mucosal epithelial cells on amniotic membrane (**B**) stained with hematoxylin and eosin. The cultivated oral mucosal epithelial sheet had 5–6 layers of stratified, well-differentiated cells and appeared very similar to in vivo normal corneal epithelium. (Modified from Nakamura T, Inatomi T, Sotozono C, Amemiya T, Kanamura N, Kinoshita S. Transplantation of cultivated autologous oral mucosal epithelial cells in patients with severe ocular surface disorders. Br J Ophthalmol 2004;88:1280–4.)

immunohistochemistry confirmed the presence of keratins 4/13 and 3 in the human cultivated oral mucosal epithelial cells, similar to those found in the rabbit model.

SUCCESSFUL XENOTRANSPLANTATION OF THE HUMAN CULTIVATED ORAL MUCOSAL EPITHELIAL SHEET

After the successful culture of human oral mucosal epithelial cells, we attempted to reconstruct rabbit keratectomized corneas through the xenotransplantation of a human cultivated oral mucosal epithelial sheet to evaluate the physiological functions of these sheets in the early postoperative stage. Observation of the transplanted sheets was performed only for the first 2 postoperative days, as it is generally thought that after epithelial transplantation, especially xenotransplantation, acute epithelial rejection often occurs, even though intensive postoperative immunosuppression is performed. Rabbit corneas grafted with the human cultivated oral mucosal epithelial cells were clear, and were all epithelialized at 48 hours after surgery. From these results, and although the long-term outcome of such transplantation has yet to be elucidated, we believe that human cultivated oral mucosal epithelial sheets can function as an ocular surface epithelium, and that human COMET is a feasible method of OSR.

We investigated whether it was possible to reconstruct the corneal surface using autologous mucosal epithelium of non-ocular surface origin. To that end, we were successful in generating both rabbit and human cultivated oral mucosal epithelial sheets from biopsy-derived oral mucosal tissues, as well as transplanting these cultivated oral mucosal epithelial cells onto rabbit corneas. In the final analysis, we believe that the transplantation of cultivated oral mucosal epithelial cells represents an effective technique for OSR in patients with severe OSD.

Transplantation of Cultivated Oral Mucosal Epithelial Cells in Patients with Severe OSD (Clinical Trial)

INITIAL CLINICAL RESULTS

In the past, several researcher groups investigated the possibility of using oral mucosa for OSR. Ballen reported that oral mucosal grafts which included both epithelium and subepithelial tissues, heavily vascularized with early fibrosis.[2] In addition, Gipson et al. reported that in vivo oral epithelium, freed of underlying connective tissue, was not maintained in the central avascular corneal regions.[3]

We investigated the possibility of reconstructing the human ocular surface using autologous mucosal epithelium of non-ocular-surface origin. Using rabbits, we have already established a surgical method for transplanting cultivated autologous oral mucosal epithelial cells.[1] We next applied this method in six eyes of four patients with severe OSD.[4]

Preoperatively, all patients were followed up in regard to their adherence to the requirements for tooth decay treatment, no alcohol or tobacco use, and regular brushing and iodine gargle. The culture process was performed according to the previous method. After removing abnormal conjunctivalized tissues on the corneal surface using surgical scissors, subconjunctival fibroblasts were treated with mitomycin C followed by vigorous repeated washing with saline. The cultivated oral mucosal epithelial sheet was transplanted onto the corneal surface of the damaged eye and secured with 10-0 nylon sutures at the limbus. Postoperatively, ofloxacin and dexamethasone eye drops were instilled four times a day; the doses were tapered to a maintenance dose at 2 to 3 months, depending on the severity of postoperative inflammation. Betamethasone and cyclophosphamide, administered to prevent postoperative inflammation and conjunctival fibrosis, were stopped 1 to 2 months after surgery.

At 48 hours post transplant, the entire corneal surface of all six eyes was free of epithelial defects, indicating complete survival of the transplanted cultivated oral mucosal epithelium. Visual acuity was improved in all eyes. During follow-up (13.8 ± 2.9 months), the ocular surface remained stable, although all eyes showed mild peripheral neovascularization. Therefore, autologous cultivated oral mucosal epithelial sheets can be transplanted to treat severe CSD (Fig. 45.7). This initial clinical study represents a first step toward assessing the feasibility of transplanting autologous cultivated epithelial transplants of non-ocular-surface origin.

MID-TERM CLINICAL RESULTS

We next present the mid-term clinical data on 15 eyes of 12 patients transplanted with cultivated autologous oral mucosal epithelial sheets.[5] We also assessed their clinical outcomes, with special reference to postoperative neovascularization.

Cultivated autologous oral mucosal epithelial sheets were successfully generated from all 12 patients. Two days after transplantation, 14 of the 15 eyes demonstrated total re-epithelialization on the cornea; the one exception was an eye in which the quality of the cultivated sheet was judged as fair prior to transplantation. During the mid-term follow-up (20 months), the ocular surface was stable with no major complications in the cultivated sheet in 10 of 15 eyes, and the ectopically transplanted cultivated oral mucosal epithelial sheet survived for at least 34 months. There were five eyes with small but long-standing persistent epithelial defects; three of those eyes healed spontaneously and two required re-grafting. In 10 eyes, postoperative visual acuity was improved by more than two lines. All eyes showed some peripheral corneal neovascularization. Thus, we established a successful tissue-engineering technique to generate cultivated autologous oral mucosal epithelial sheets and succeeded in reconstructing the ocular surface using cultivated non-ocular mucosal epithelium. This mid-term study demonstrates the effectiveness of cultivated autologous oral mucosal epithelial sheet transplantation and supports our initial report by documenting multiple successful clinical results. We suggest that this surgical modality may be safe and effective, especially in younger patients with the most severe OSD.

PHENOTYPIC INVESTIGATION OF THE TRANSPLANTED CULTIVATED ORAL MUCOSAL EPITHELIAL SHEETS

Our initial and mid-term clinical assessments of COMET yielded favorable results from the perspective of corneal surface stabilization;[4,5] longevity and phenotypic analyses of the cultivated oral mucosal epithelial sheets to the corneal surface needs to be performed. Since it had not been confirmed what happens to failed and successful grafts on the corneal surface, we compared our clinical observations with the results of the cellular phenotype analysis of autologous COMET.[6]

In the clinically failed transplants, electron microscopy (EM) and immunohistochemical analysis showed only small areas where the original cultivated oral mucosal epithelial sheets persisted. Surrounding conjunctival epithelial cells had apparently invaded a large portion of the corneal surface (oral mucosal epithelial marker keratin 3(−), goblet cell marker Muc5ac (+)). Our clinical, ultrastructural, and cell biological findings revealed that the process of graft failure was responsible for the loss of cultivated oral mucosal epithelial sheets, due to postoperative bacterial infections and that this event was followed by neighboring conjunctival invasion onto the corneal surface (Fig. 45.8).

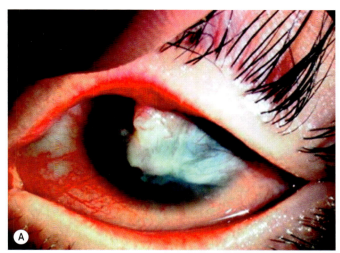

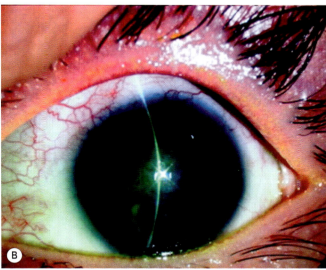

Figure 45.7 Clinical photographs of a patient with Stevens – Johnson syndrome before (**A**) and after (**B**) cultivated oral mucosal epithelial cell transplantation. (**A**) Before transplantation, the patient had a total corneal epithelial defect, including limbus accompanied severe inflammation on the conjunctiva. (**B**) Eleven months after transplantation, the corneal surface was covered by a clear cultivated oral mucosal epithelial sheet. (Modified from Nakamura T, Inatomi T, Sotozono C, Amemiya T, Kanamura N, Kinoshita S. Transplantation of cultivated autologous oral mucosal epithelial cells in patients with severe ocular surface disorders. Br J Ophthalmol 2004;88:1280–4.)

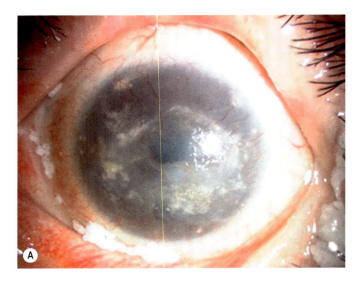

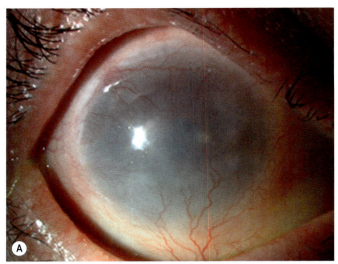

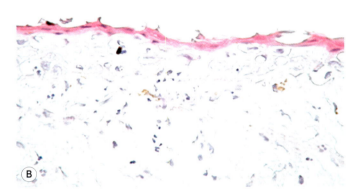

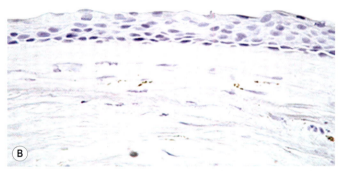

Figure 45.8 Clinical photograph of failed case after cultivated oral mucosal epithelial transplantation (**A**). Light microscopically, the removed cultivated oral mucosal epithelial grafts showed 2–5 stratified cell layers and disorganized epithelium (**B**). In these areas, the amniotic membrane could not be observed. (Modified from Nakamura T, Inatomi T, Cooper LJ, Rigby H, Fullwood NJ, Kinoshita S. Phenotypic investigation of human eyes with transplanted autologous cultivated oral mucosal epithelial sheets for severe ocular surface diseases. Ophthalmology 2007;114:1080–8.)

Figure 45.9 Clinical photograph of successful case after cultivated oral mucosal epithelial transplantation (**A**). Light microscopically, the removed cultivated oral mucosal epithelial grafts showed 5–6 stratified cell layers and cornea-like (oral mucosal sheet) epithelial cells (**B**). The amniotic membrane substrate was clearly observed throughout the epithelium and there were no inflammatory cells. (Modified from Nakamura T, Inatomi T, Cooper LJ, Rigby H, Fullwood NJ, Kinoshita S. Phenotypic investigation of human eyes with transplanted autologous cultivated oral mucosal epithelial sheets for severe ocular surface diseases. Ophthalmology 2007;114:1080–8.)

In the clinically successful transplants, the cultivated oral mucosal epithelial sheets survived and had adapted well to the host corneal tissues (oral mucosal epithelial marker keratin 3 (+), goblet cell marker Muc5ac (−)). In the course of postoperative follow-up, their distinctive fluorescein staining patterns made it easy to distinguish transplanted cultivated oral mucosal epithelial sheets from surrounding conjunctival epithelium. The staining pattern of cultivated oral mucosal epithelial cells is more like that of superficial punctate keratopathy than of conjunctival epithelium. This set of findings confirmed that transplanted cultivated oral mucosal epithelial cells can survive on the ocular surface and maintain ocular surface integrity (Fig. 45.9).

Thus, we demonstrated that the process of graft failure after COMET is responsible for the loss of transplanted cultivated oral epithelial sheets and that this is followed by invasion of the surrounding conjunctival epithelial cells onto the corneal surface. We confirmed that in clinically successfully transplanted eyes, cultivated oral mucosal epithelial cells survived on the corneal surface and maintained ocular surface integrity. Our findings have important clinical implications and provide valuable insights into the mechanisms of both graft failure and graft integrity after COMET.

LONG-TERM CLINICAL RESULTS IN THE SCAR PHASE OF SEVERE OSDS

More recently, our experimental and serial clinical studies demonstrated the efficacy and usefulness of COMET for the treatment of severe OSD. Even though initial and mid-term clinical results of COMET have been reported from several groups worldwide,[7,8] the long-term clinical assessments of COMET are entirely unknown and the feasibility of this technique still requires detailed investigation.

Finally, we present the long-term clinical data on 19 eyes that received COMET, for which the mean follow-up period was 55 months; the longest follow-up period being 90 months.[9] The study included 19 eyes of 17 patients in the scar phase of severe OSD who underwent OSR with COMET and who could be followed up for more than 36 months. In this study, to precisely examine the long-term clinical results of COMET for OSR, we excluded the patients who received penetrating keratoplasty (PKP) after the initial COMET, as well as patients who received COMET for con-junctival fornix reconstruction. Clinical efficacy was evaluated in terms of the patients' postoperative visual acuity. The clinical results were evaluated and graded on a scale from 0 to 3 according to their severity. Clinical safety was evaluated in terms of persistent epithelial defects, ocular hypertension, and infections. During the postoperative follow-up, best-corrected visual acuity was improved by more than two lines in 15 eyes, and visual acuity at the postoperative thirty-sixth month was improved in eight eyes. During the long-term follow-up period, postoperative clinical conjunctivalization was significantly inhibited (Fig. 45.10). Moreover, corneal opacification tended to improve during the long-term follow-up period. All eyes manifested various degrees of superficial corneal vascularization, but it gradually abated and its activity was comparatively stable from 6 months after transplantation. During the long-term follow-up period, postoperative symblepharon formation was also significantly inhibited; seven of the 19 eyes manifested persistent epithelial defects at least once during the follow-up. Postoperative ocular hypertension was observed in a total of three eyes during the follow-up periods. The occasional increase in intraocular pressure was mainly managed by the administration of carbonic anhydrase inhibitor. Corneal infection was mainly observed within 6 months after transplantation, and methicillin-resistant *Staphylococcus aureus* was found to be the only cause the infection.

We found that COMET permits sustained reconstruction of the ocular surface epithelium in many eyes with severe OSD. The management of postoperative persistent epithelial defects and neovascularization may further increase the efficacy of this type of surgery. Thus, this study has important clinical implications and provides new information regarding the long-term clinical results and survival of transplanted cultivated cells for the treatment of the scar phase of severe OSD.

Development of the Next Generation of COMET

THE USE OF AUTOLOGOUS SERUM IN THE DEVELOPMENT OF CULTIVATED EPITHELIAL SHEETS

The currently preferred method of cultivating epithelial sheets requires the use of xenobiotic materials in the culture system, such as fetal bovine serum (FBS) and

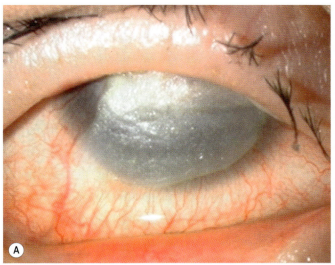
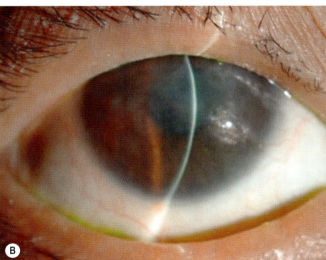

Figure 45.10 The clinical progress of one representative patient with Stevens – Johnson syndrome. Before transplantation, all eyes manifested severe destruction of the ocular surface with limbal stem cell deficiency (**A**). The postoperative appearance at 50 months shows a relatively smooth, epithelialized corneal surface with minimal corneal neovascularization, scarring, and inflammation (**B**). (Modified from Nakamura T, Takeda K, Inatomi T, Sotozono C, Kinoshita S. Long-term results of autologous cultivated oral mucosal epithelial transplantation in the scar phase of severe ocular surface disorders. Br J Ophthalmol 2011;95:942–6.)

mouse-derived 3T3 feeder cells. However, the use of FBS in the culture system is a major concern, as bovine spongiform encephalopathy cannot be detected by any known in vitro assay. Various serum-free culture systems, developed to delete the FBS from the culture system, have mainly been used to study the roles of various growth factors.[10] The clinical use of these serum-free culture systems has been limited because of their lower efficacy for cell proliferation, compared to FBS-supplemented medium. In the development of a cultivated oral mucosal epithelial sheet for clinical application, the ideal culture system is one that is free from disease transmission, as well as being able to support cell proliferation and differentiation. Therefore, the use of autologous serum (AS) as an alternative to FBS is significantly advantageous, as it eliminates the need for bovine material in the culture process. We wanted to determine if AS from patients with severe OSD was similarly useful in supporting the cell proliferation and differentiation of cultivated oral mucosal epithelial sheets, compared to conventional FBS-supplemented culture methods. Here, we demonstrate that the AS-supplemented culture system derived from severe OSD patients was able to support epithelial cell proliferation, as well as the development of transplants showing morphological and ultrastructural characteristics that are similar to normal tissues.[11]

First, AS was obtained from Stevens – Johnson syndrome (SJS) patients. Venesection was then performed at the antecubital fossa under aseptic conditions; 30 mL of blood was collected into a sterile container, centrifuged, and filtered, and the resultant serum was then purified and stored in sterile tubes at $-30°C$ for clinical use. Oral mucosal epithelial cells were cultivated in medium supplemented with either AS or FBS.

BrdU cell proliferation assay and colony-forming efficiency analysis showed that oral mucosal epithelial cells cultivated in AS-supplemented media had comparable proliferative abilities, compared to cells cultivated in FBS-supplemented media. The cultivated oral mucosal epithelial sheets in AS- and FBS-supplemented media were morphologically similar, and showed the normal expression of tissue-specific keratins and basement membrane assembly. These findings demonstrate the ability of the AS-supplemented culture system to support the continued proliferation and differentiation of cultivated oral mucosal epithelial sheets, which is of paramount importance when considering its use in clinical applications. The presence of a well-formed stratified epithelium, a basement membrane, and hemidesmosomal attachments was confirmed by EM. These findings are important in ensuring graft integrity during surgical manipulation, as well as following transplantation.

Thus, AS-supplemented cultures were effective in supporting the proliferation of human oral mucosal epithelial cells, as well as the development of transplantable cultivated oral mucosal epithelial sheets. The use of AS is of clinical importance in the development of autologous xenobiotic-free bioengineered transplants for clinical transplantation. These findings bring us one step closer to the development of a safe and effective xenobiotic-free bioengineered cultivated transplant for clinical application.

AS-DERIVED COMET

We previously demonstrated the use of COMET for treating severe OSD using the FBS culture system, which is particularly useful in bilateral severe OSDs.[4,5] However, the use of FBS may be associated with the risk of transmission of zoonotic infection and other unknown pathogens. As bovine spongiform encephalitis cannot be detected by any known in vitro assay, the use of bovine-derived products is a major health concern in many parts of the world. We previously showed that human AS was able to support epithelial cell proliferation,[11] which raises the possibility of using the patient's own serum as an alternative to FBS in the culture

system. The use of AS is advantageous, as it eliminates the need for bovine material and reduces the risk of disease transmission. In this clinical study, we compared the efficacy of AS supplementation with conventional FBS supplementation in developing cultivated oral mucosal epithelial sheets, and evaluated the usefulness of AS-derived COMET for the treatment of severe OSD.[12]

This AS clinical study included 10 eyes of 10 patients with severe OSD who underwent autologous COMET. The preoperative diagnosis was SJS in seven patients, thermal and chemical injury in ttwo patients, and mucous membrane pemphigoid in one patient. These patients demonstrated a reasonable reflex tear function and tear meniscus level. All patients were followed up for a minimum period of 6 months after transplantation, with the longest follow-up being 19 months (mean follow-up: 12.6 months).

It has been reported that a high concentration of serum soluble Fas (sFas) ligand at the onset of SJS may play a crucial role in keratinocyte apoptosis and in the pathophysiology of the disease. Therefore, we analyzed the serum sFas ligand levels of the severe OSD patients to determine if AS could be safely used as a cell-culture supplement. In our study, we found that serum sFas ligand levels were too low to be detected in severe OSD subjects and healthy controls, indicating that this would not be an impediment in our oral mucosal epithelial cell culture system.

Cultivated oral mucosal epithelial sheets using AS- and FBS-supplemented media were found to be similar in histology and morphology, and formed basement membrane assembly proteins important for maintaining graft survival. Complete corneal epithelialization was achieved within 2–5 days postoperatively. The ocular surface remained stable without major complications in all eyes during the mean follow-up of 12.6 months. The visual acuity improved by more than two lines in nine of the 10 eyes, with the transplanted oral mucosal epithelial sheet surviving up to 19 months. During the follow-up period, four eyes developed small, persistent epithelial defects which eventually healed over from the adjacent oral mucosal epithelium. All eyes manifested some degree of superficial peripheral neovascularization. This gradually reduced with time and did not interfere with visual acuity or cause any serious postoperative complications.

Therefore, we describe the successful clinical use of cultivated oral mucosal epithelial sheets that are derived almost entirely from autologous tissue and material. This study has important clinical implications and represents an important advancement in the pursuit of completely autologous xenobiotic-free bioengineered transplants for clinical application, as it reduces the risks of allograft rejection and the transmission of infection, as well as the need for long-term immunosuppressive therapy.

Potential Diversity of COMET

COMBINATION OF COMET AND PENETRATING KERATOPLASTY

Severe OSD is sometimes accompanied by severe corneal stromal scarring and opacity and/or corneal endothelial dysfunction. Therefore, most patients require PKP for visual

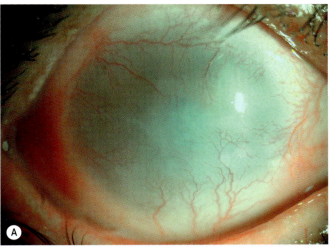

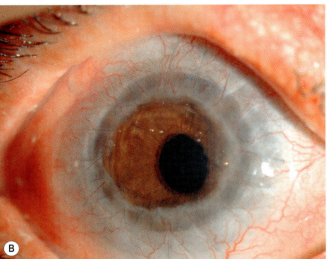

Figure 45.11 Clinical appearance before and after ocular surface reconstruction using cultivated oral mucosal epithelial transplantation (COMET) and penetrating keratoplasty (PKP). Two months after the initial surgery with COME (**A**). Status at 3 months after PKP (**B**).

recovery. To improve the clinical outcome and long-term prognosis of these patients, their reconstructed cornea must be provided with a more stable epithelial supply, such as cultivated epithelial transplantation. Therefore, a two-step surgical strategy that utilizes a combination of COMET and PKP has been developed.[13]

The initial COMET for OSR may be performed as described in previous reports (Fig. 45.11).[4,5] PKP is then performed 5–6 months after the initial COMET. PKP with cataract surgery was also performed according to the usual clinical procedures. In brief, a 7-mm diameter trephination was performed on the host cornea, followed by continuous circular capsulorrhexis using micro-forceps. The lens was removed through the cornea using the regular phacoemulsification and aspiration technique. After inserting the intraocular lens, a fresh donor cornea was transplanted and then fixed with interrupted and continuous sutures. Finally, the ocular surface was covered with a medical-use soft contact lens.

COMBINATION OF COMET AND AUTOMATED LAMELLAR THERAPEUTIC KERATOPLASTY

Combined surgical modalities, such as lamellar keratoplasty and cataract surgery are commonly required at the time of COMET. However, these procedures are not easy, compared with the single surgical procedure for a non-ocular-surface disease. In particular, corneal opacity prevents the corneal transparency that is essential for intraocular surgery. Therefore, special surgical modifications that increase visibility and reduce reflected light are necessary for safe cataract surgery. Lamellar keratoplasty and deep lamellar keratoplasty are effective procedures to remove scarred corneal opacity. Automated lamellar therapeutic keratoplasty (ALTK) is a newly developed surgical procedure based on microkeratome-assisted keratoplasty that provides a smooth and sharp corneal stromal excision. This surgical procedure is also very useful to improve intraoperative visibility at the time of cataract surgery in patients with a hazy cornea. Once the cornea was excised by microkeratome following removal of the conjunctivalized tissue, corneal clarity improved well enough for cataract surgery to be performed. Staining the anterior lens capsule with indocyanine green and surgical slit lamp illumination are effective and useful procedures when performing cataract surgery in conditions of poor visibility. A corneal graft of the same size was then created using the Moria ALTK manual microkeratome system and sutured with 10-0 nylon. The corneal surface was then covered with cultivated oral mucosal epithelium, resulting in improvement of visual acuity. Not only the new cultivated epithelial transplantation, but also the combined surgery using new instruments, has dramatically improved clinical results and postoperative visual quality.[14]

COMBINATION OF COMET AND EYELID SURGERY

In severe OSD, the corneal epithelial stem cells in the corneal limbus are destroyed and coverage of the corneal surface by invading neighboring conjunctival epithelium results in the ingrowth of fibrous tissue, chronic inflammation, neovascularization, and stromal scarring. In specific, various degrees of pathologic symblepharon formation and entropion frequently occur in patients with severe OSD and disturb the integrity of the ocular surface. Furthermore, an abnormal eyelid can often make a severe OSD worse, due to the fact that the eyelid margin rotation or structural abnormalities disturb tear spreading and corneal wetting. Malfunction of the conjunctival fornix by symblepharon can cause severe OSDs, such as dry eye and an inflamed ocular surface resulting from cicatricial entropion and restriction of ocular motility. Therefore, it was recently reported that the selection of the proper surgical procedure depends upon the severity of pathogenic symblepharon formation. Moreover, it was also recommended that the eyelid and fornix abnormalities be reconstructed prior to performing OSR. Therefore, it is necessary to reconstruct not only the ocular surface but also the formation of the eyelid in patients with severe OSD. (Fig. 45.12).[15]

The surgical procedure is as follows: First, the conjunctivalized scarred tissue of each patient was completely removed by performing a thin superficial keratectomy.

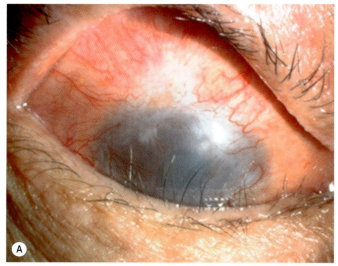

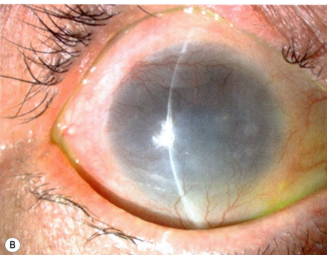

Figure 45.12 Clinical appearance before and after reconstruction using cultivated oral mucosal epithelial transplantation and eyelid surgery. Preoperatively, there was total conjunctivalization with symblepharon and lower-eyelid entropion (**A**). Seven months after surgery, the cultivated oral mucosal epithelial sheet showed no epithelial defect and the ocular surface was stable (**B**). (Modified from Takeda K, Nakamura T, Inatomi T, Sotozono C, Watanabe A, Kinoshita S. Ocular surface reconstruction using the combination of autologous cultivated oral mucosal epithelial transplantation and eyelid surgery for severe ocular surface disease. Am J Ophthalmol 2011;152:195–201.)

Subconjunctival spaces were then treated with 0.04% mitomycin C for 5 minutes, followed by AM being transplanted over the ocular surface. All three cases required an additional surgical procedure to address existing entropion of either the upper or lower eyelid. In that procedure, a 6-0 nylon suture was first passed through the eyelid from the tarsus side to the skin side, followed by the second needle of that same suture being passed through in the same manner. The two ends of that suture were then tied off and implanted under the skin. This was repeated two or three times at the appropriate positions in relation to the first suture, with the number of additional sutures needed being determined by the severity of the entropion of each

particular case. Finally, the cultivated oral mucosal epithelial sheet was transferred onto the corneal surface, and the ocular surface was then protected with a medical-use contact lens.

Future Challenges of OSR: a Novel Cell Origin for OSR

In view of the previous clinical trial pertaining to COMET, the above-described surgical procedures stand as currently established procedures in the field of OSR. In an aim to further develop these surgical methods, several groups worldwide have recently reported the use of cell sources obtained from a novel cell origin.

MESENCHYMAL STEM CELLS

Mesenchymal stem cells (MSCs) have been used in an attempt to treat a variety of diseases based on the theory that MSCs could become functional cells in host tissues. Using an animal model, Ma et al. investigated whether the transplantation of MSCs could successfully reconstruct the corneal surface, and also whether transplanted MSCs could transdifferentiate into corneal epithelial cells.[16] In that study, after growth and expansion on AM, MSCs were transplanted onto a rat corneal surface 7 days after chemical injury. The results of that study showed that the transplantation of MSCs, like corneal limbal epithelial stem cells, successfully reconstructed the damaged corneal surface. Interestingly, the therapeutic effect of MSC transplantation may be associated with the inhibition of postoperative inflammation and angiogenesis rather than with corneal epithelial differentiation from the MSCs. Thus, that study provided the novel findings that MSCs can be used for OSR in the treatment of severe OSD.

EPIDERMAL STEM CELLS

It is well known that the epidermal and corneal keratinocytes are derived from ectoderm during embryogenesis. The keratinocyte stem cells of these two biological systems share several important attributes, such as expression of the same markers and transdifferentiation from corneal to epidermal. Yang et al. recently reported a new surgical strategy for OSR using an autologous transplantation of epidermal adult stem cells (EpiASCs) in a goat model.[17] The goats in that report were treated by the transplantation of tissue-engineered cell sheets composed of EpiASCs, leading to the restoration of corneal transparency and improvement of postoperative visual acuity in 80% of the experimental eyes. The authors also showed that the reconstructed corneal epithelium expressed keratins 3/12, which are both thought to be cornea-specific markers, and that it had the function of secreting glycocalyx-like material. These findings not only indicate that EpiASCs can reconstruct the damaged corneal surface of goats with severe OSD, but also that EpiASCs can transdifferentiate into corneal epithelial cell types in vivo. However, further studies are needed to elucidate whether these experimental results hold true for humans.

IMMATURE DENTAL-PULP STEM CELLS

Searching for a source of epithelial stem cells that have characteristics similar to those of corneal limbal epithelial stem cells, Monteiro et al. recently reported that human immature dental-pulp stem cells (hIDPSCs) share similar characteristics with corneal limbal epithelial stem cells and might be used as a potential alternative cell source for OSR.[18] Interestingly, the authors showed that hIDPSCs display all of the unique characteristics of multipotent adult stem cells, expressing human embryonic stem cell markers (OCT4, SSEA-3/4, and NANOG) and several MSCs (SH2/3/4). Interestingly, hIDPSCs were also shown to express markers that are in common with corneal limbal epithelial stem cells, such as p63, ABCG2, and keratins 3/12. In that study, transplantation of a tissue-engineered hIDPSC sheet using a temperature-responsive culture dish was shown to be successful for the OSR in an animal model of severe OSD.

NASAL MUCOSA

Kim et al. reported that transplantation of autologous nasal mucosa is a useful surgical procedure for achieving OSR in cases of severe OSD.[19] In that report, they showed that nasal mucosal epithelium expressed an abundance of p63 and keratin 3. Moreover, goblet cells and MUC5AC expression were also observed in the nasal mucosal epithelium. In all patients, ocular surface integrity recovered with no major postoperative complications and an increase of goblet cells was apparently observed on the ocular surface. In view of those clinical findings, they concluded that transplantation of nasal mucosa may be an ideal surgical method for the treatment of severe OSD.

HAIR FOLLICLE BULGE-DERIVED STEM CELLS

It has been reported that hair follicle bulge-derived stem cells (HFSCs) have a high degree of tissue plasticity and can cross cell lineage boundaries and differentiate into a different cell phenotype. Most recently, Meyer-Blazejewska et al. reported the therapeutic potential of murine vibrissae HFSCs as an autologous stem cell source for OSR.[20] That study is an expansion of their previously studies showing transdifferentiation of HFSCs into a corneal epithelial cell phenotype, and their findings showed that the HFSC transplant successfully reconstructed the ocular surface in 80% of the transplanted eyes. These experimental data, including the use of a mouse model of severe OSD, highlight the therapeutic potential of using HFSCs to reconstruct the ocular surface.

Future Goals

In view of the basic research and developments in the field of regenerative medicine for OSR, both past and present, great progress has been made in the fundamental understanding and development of a new therapeutic modality, such as the transplantation of cultivated oral mucosal epithelial sheets using tissue engineering techniques. Greater knowledge regarding epithelial stem cell behavior from non-ocular sources and the surrounding extracellular matrix will provide a foundation for the further development of treatments for severe OSD.

References

1. Nakamura T, Endo K, Cooper LJ, et al. The successful culture and autologous transplantation of rabbit oral mucosal epithelial cells on amniotic membrane. Invest Ophthalmol Vis Sci 2003;44:106–16.
2. Ballen PH. Mucous membrane grafts in chemical (lye) burns. Am J Ophthalmol 1963;55:302–12.
3. Gipson IK, Geggel HS, Spurr-Michaud SJ. Transplant of oral mucosal epithelium to rabbit ocular surface wounds in vivo. Arch. Ophthalmol 1986;104:1529–33.
4. Nakamura T, Inatomi T, Sotozono C, et al. Transplantation of cultivated autologous oral mucosal epithelial cells in patients with severe ocular surface disorders. Br J Ophthalmol 2004;88:1280–4.
5. Inatomi T, Nakamura T, Koizumi N, et al. Mid-term results on ocular surface reconstruction using cultivated autologous oral mucosal epithelial transplantation. Am J Ophthalmol 2006;141:267–75.
6. Nakamura T, Inatomi T, Cooper LJ, et al. Phenotypic investigation of human eyes with transplanted autologous cultivated oral mucosal epithelial sheets for severe ocular surface diseases. Ophthalmology 2007;114:1080–8.
7. Nishida K, Yamato M, Hayashida Y, et al. Corneal reconstruction with tissue-engineered cell sheets composed of autologous oral mucosal epithelium. N Engl J Med 2004;351:1187–96.
8. Satake Y, Dogru M, Yamane GY, et al. Barrier function and cytologic features of the ocular surface epithelium after autologous cultivated oral mucosal epithelial transplantation. Arch Ophthalmol 2008;126:23–8.
9. Nakamura T, Takeda K, Inatomi T, et al. Long-term results of autologous cultivated oral mucosal epithelial transplantation in the scar phase of severe ocular surface disorders. Br J Ophthalmol 2011;95:942–6.
10. Kruse FE, Tseng SCG. Growth factors modulate clonal growth and differentiation of cultured rabbit limbal and corneal epithelium. Invest Ophthalmol Vis Sci 1993;34:1963–76.
11. Nakamura T, Ang LPK, Rigby H, et al. The use of autologous serum in the development of corneal and oral epithelial equivalents in patients with Stevens-Johnson syndrome. Invest Ophthalmol Vis Sci 2006;47:909–16.
12. Ang LPK, Nakamura T, Inatomi T, et al. Autologous serum-derived cultivated oral epithelial transplants for severe ocular surface disease. Arch Ophthalmol 2006;124:1543–51.
13. Inatomi T, Nakamura T, Kojyo M, et al. Ocular surface reconstruction with combination of cultivated autologous oral mucosal epithelial transplantation and penetrating keratoplasty. Am J Ophthalmol 2006;142:757–64.
14. Inatomi T, Nakamura T, Koizumi N, et al. Current concepts and challenges in ocular surface reconstruction using cultivated mucosal epithelial transplantation. Cornea 2005;24(8 Suppl):S32–8.
15. Takeda K, Nakamura T, Inatomi T, et al. Ocular surface reconstruction using the combination of autologous cultivated oral mucosal epithelial transplantation and eyelid surgery for severe ocular surface disease. Am J Ophthalmol 2011;152:195–201.
16. Ma Y, Xu Y, Xiao Z, et al. Reconstruction of chemically burned rat corneal surface by bone marrow-derived human mesenchymal stem cells. Stem Cells 2006;24:315–21.
17. Yang X, Moldovan NI, Zhao Q, et al. Reconstruction of damaged cornea by autologous transplantation of epidermal adult stem cells. Mol Vis 2008;14:1064–70.
18. Monteiro BG, Serafim RC, Melo GB, et al. Human immature dental pulp stem cells share key characteristic features with limbal stem cells. Cell Prolif 2009;42:587–94.
19. Kim JH, Chun YS, Lee SH, et al. Ocular surface reconstruction with autologous nasal mucosa in cicatricial ocular surface disease. Am J Ophthalmol 2010;149:45–53.
20. Meyer-Blazejewska EA, Call MK, Yamanaka O, et al. From hair to cornea: toward the therapeutic use of hair follicle-derived stem cells in the treatment of limbal stem cell deficiency. Stem Cells 2011;29:57–66.

Box 46.1   Schedule for Standard Investigations before and after Ocular Surface Stem Cell Transplantation (OSST) to Assess a Patient's Baseline Health Status and to Monitor for Adverse Events

Before OSST

- Medications list, previous medical history, transplant immunologist assessment
- Physical exam completed by primary care physician within 30 days of surgery
- Blood pressure
- Weight
- Lab investigations (CBC, BMP, liver function panel, UA with urinary protein, culture and sensitivities)
- Serology testing (Hepatitis A, B, C, HIV, EBV, CMV)
- Tuberculosis exposure (TB skin test or chest x-ray)
- Up to date mammogram, pap smear, colonoscopy
- Pregnancy status (beta HCG)
- Cardiac stress test if > 50 year old or history of heart problems or blood pressure

First Three Visits after OSST

- Tacrolimus levels (target 8–10 ng/mL)

6 months after limbal allograft surgery, target serum tacrolimus trough levels should be between 8 and 10 ng/mL. Thereafter, a trough level of 5 to 8 ng/mL is targeted for 12–18 months after surgery.

INDIVIDUALIZATION OF THE PROTOCOL

There are local factors innate to the diseased eye and donor and recipient immunological factors involved in tailoring a patient's systemic immunosuppression regimen. High-risk eyes are those with stage 2B or 2C disease: total limbal stem cell deficiency and conjunctival inflammation with associated conjunctival scarring, decreased aqueous tear production, and high likelihood of ocular surface keratinization.[4] Examples of ocular conditions in this category would be severe Stevens–Johnson syndrome, ocular cicatricial pemphigoid, and severe chemical injuries. Risk stratification also includes ABO blood type, donor type (living relative versus cadaver), tissue human leukocyte antigen (HLA) type, panel reactive antigen (PRA) percentage, donor-specific antigen (DSA) detection, repeat transplantation failure, or need for repeat OSST (Table 46.2). The primary antigens recognized by the immune system include blood type and HLA proteins. Blood type ABO antigens have

Table 46.2   Tissue Selection Factors for the Individualization of the Systemic Immunosuppression Protocol in Ocular Surface Stem Cell Transplantation Once ABO-Matching Between a Living Relative Donor and Recipient is Established

Donor Type	Living Relative Donor						Cadaveric Donor		
HLA Typing	HLA identical			Non-HLA identical			Not applicable		
PRA %	0	0–50	>50	0	0–50	>50	0	0–50	>50
Induction	None			None	Basiliximab[1]		None	Basiliximab[1]	
Maintenance[2]	Standard			Standard			Standard		
Initiation of maintenance regimen	Day of surgery	1 week before surgery	2 weeks before surgery	2 weeks before surgery			2 weeks before surgery		
Goals	Begin Prograf taper at 3 months, Cellcept monotherapy at 6 months			Taper Prograf at 1 year, Cellcept monotherapy at 6 months			Taper Prograf at 2 years, Cellcept monotherapy at 2 years		
Repeat transplant	OK			OK if DSA is negative			OK if PRA = 0, otherwise use living donor vs. Kpro		

[1]Basiliximab (Simulect) 20 mg IV is given 30 minutes prior to transplantation with a second dose given 4 days after transplantation.
[2]Standard maintenance protocol includes oral prednisone 1 mg/kg, tacrolimus (FK-506 or Prograf) 4 mg twice daily, MMF (Cellcept) 1 g twice daily, oral valganciclovir (Valcyte) 225 mg daily, and trimethoprim/sulafamethoxazole (Bactrim single strength) 1 tablet on Mondays, Wednesdays, Fridays, or dapsone 100 mg orally daily if the patient has a sulfa allergy. The higher the percentage of PRA, panel reactive antibodies, the harder it is to find a match and the patient is more likely to reject. Transplants are at higher risk of failure if DSA, donor-specific antibodies, is positive.
(Modified from Holland EJ, Mogilishetty G, Skeens HM, et al. Systemic immunosuppression in ocular surface stem cell transplantation: Results of a 10-year Experience. Cornea 2012;31:655-61.)

attempted until later: the tacrolimus dosage is decreased

Table 46.3   Adverse Events Reported in 136 Patients

medications. An understanding of the methodology in tailoring immunosuppression regimens to each patient can assist the ocular surgeon in achieving an ideal balance between too little immunosuppression, which can lead to allograft rejection, versus too much, which can lead to medication side effects and patient adverse events.

Many ophthalmologists are hesitant to approach the prevention of rejection in OSST with the same rigor as solid organ transplant specialists. Therefore, collaboration with a transplant specialist can be essential to provide adequate systemic immunosuppression to patients undergoing OSST to achieve better results. Transplant physicians are also well trained to recognize and manage medical complications that may be introduced by the immunosuppressive medications.

With appropriate long-term monitoring by a cornea specialist and transplant specialist, the long-term risk of irreversible toxicity from modern systemic immunosuppression in these patients can be minimized, which would alleviate the fears associated with the use of systemic immunosuppression therapy in limbal allograft transplantation.

References

1. Holland EJ. Epithelial transplantation for the management of severe ocular surface disease. Trans Am Ophthalmol Soc 1996; 94:677–743.
2. Biber JM, Skeens HM, Neff KD, et al. The cincinnati procedure: technique and outcomes of combined living-related conjunctival limbal allografts and keratolimbal allografts in severe ocular surface failure. Cornea 2011;30:765–71.
3. Niederkorn JY. Effect of cytokine-induced migration of Langerhans cells on corneal allograft survival. Eye 1995;9(Pt 2):215–8.
4. Holland EJ, Schwartz GS. The evolution of epithelial transplantation for severe ocular surface disease and a proposed classification system. Cornea 1996;15:549–56.
5. Holland EJ, Djalilian AR, Schwartz GS. Management of aniridic keratopathy with keratolimbal allograft: a limbal stem cell transplantation technique. Ophthalmology 2003;110:125–30.
6. Liang L, Sheha H, Tseng SC. Long-term outcomes of keratolimbal allograft for total limbal stem cell deficiency using combined immunosuppressive agents and correction of ocular surface deficits. Arch Ophthalmol 2009;127:1428–34.
7. Holland EJ, Mogilishetty G, Skeens HM, et al. Systemic immunosuppression in ocular surface stem cell transplantation: Results of a 10-year Experience. Cornea 2012;31:655–61.
8. Rao SK, Rajagopal R, Sitalakshmi G, et al. Limbal allografting from related live donors for corneal surface reconstruction. Ophthalmology 1999;106:822–8.
9. Donnenfeld ED. Difluprednate for the prevention of ocular inflammation postsurgery: an update. Clinical Ophthalmology 2011;5: 811–6.
10. Ekberg H, Tedesco-Silva H, Demirbas A, et al. Reduced exposure to calcineurin inhibitors in renal transplantation. N Engl J Med 2007; 357:2562–75.
11. Vanrenterghem YF. Which calcineurin inhibitor is preferred in renal transplantation: tacrolimus or cyclosporine? Curr Opin Nephrol Hypertens 1999;8:669–74.
12. Mycophenolate mofetil in renal transplantation: 3-year results from the placebo-controlled trial. European Mycophenolate Mofetil Cooperative Study Group. Transplantation 1999;68:391–6.
13. Chapman TM, Keating GM. Basiliximab: a review of its use as induction therapy in renal transplantation. Drugs 2003;63:2803–35.
14. Alloway R, Mogilishetty G, Cole L, et al. Ocular surface transplant recipients experience minimal immunosuppression complications: implications for composite tissue transplants. Am J Transplant 2007;1058:419b.

47 Ocular Surface Transplantation: Outcomes and Complications

ANDREA Y. ANG and EDWARD J. HOLLAND

Introduction

The development of ocular surface stem cell transplantation (OSST) has greatly improved our ability to treat ocular surface disorders arising from limbal stem cell deficiency (LSCD). However, there is still a significant failure rate due to complications, such as stem cell rejection and concurrent disease, such as cicatrizing eyelid pathology and severe tear film abnormalities. This chapter will evaluate the reported success rates of conjunctival limbal autograft (CLAU), keratolimbal allograft (KLAL), living-related conjunctival limbal allograft (lr-CLAL), and ex vivo cultured limbal epithelial transplantation (CLET). We will discuss the complications that may arise and potential strategies to improve outcomes.

Outcomes

When evaluating success rates with different surgical techniques it is important that we compare 'apples with apples.' Factors that affect success rates include length of follow-up, preoperative diagnosis and severity of disease, and the immunosuppression (IS) regimen used. Most studies evaluating OSST outcomes are small retrospective case series, and care must be taken in comparing outcomes between studies, due to marked variation in the factors listed above. Most studies use ocular surface stability and improvement in visual acuity as outcome measures.

The length of follow-up should be at least 1 year to ensure that the surface stability is due to repopulation by transplanted stem cells and not from the donor corneal epithelium that can survive up to 13 months postoperatively.[1] Evaluation of shorter-term results may reveal a falsely high success rate initially. For example, an aniridic with conjunctivalization of the cornea and stromal scarring who undergoes a penetrating keratoplasty alone will initially experience dramatic improvement in vision. However, the ocular surface will inevitably fail when the donor epithelium sloughs and is replaced by conjunctivalization.

The preoperative diagnosis and severity of disease will affect outcomes. Schwartz et al.[2] classified ocular surface disease based on the extent of limbal stem cell loss and the presence or absence of conjunctival inflammation. Patients with partial limbal stem cell deficiency and no conjunctival inflammation (e.g. contact-lens induced keratitis) will be easier to treat and have better outcomes than patients with total limbal stem cell deficiency and active conjunctival inflammation (e.g. Stevens–Johnson syndrome). The preoperative diagnosis will also affect the visual acuity achieved postoperatively. For example, an aniridic with foveal hypoplasia will not have the potential to achieve the same vision postoperatively as a chemical injured eye with a normal retina. Thus improvement in visual acuity is important, but cannot be the sole factor used to compare outcomes between studies.

Studies utilize varying definitions of ocular surface stability. Most describe "failure" as the presence of a combination of the following signs of abnormal corneal epithelium: late fluorescein staining, persistent epithelial defects, neovascularization, conjunctivalization, and inflammation. Most describe "success" as the absence of the above signs and the presence of healthy transparent corneal epithelium. Between stability and failure is another category of 'improved' surface, defined as partial failure with areas of healthy corneal epithelium and areas of abnormal conjunctival epithelium on the cornea either in a mosaic or sectoral pattern. Figure 47.1 demonstrates partial limbal stem cell failure in a mosaic pattern.

CLAU

In unilateral LSCD, CLAU from the healthy fellow eye remains the procedure of choice, since rejection is not an issue and outcomes are excellent. Rao et al.[3] described stable ocular surfaces in 15/16 (93.8%) eyes that underwent CLAU for ocular surface burns. Similarly, Yao et al.[4] achieved a stable ocular surface in 32/34 (94.1%) of eyes with severe chemical or thermal burns who underwent

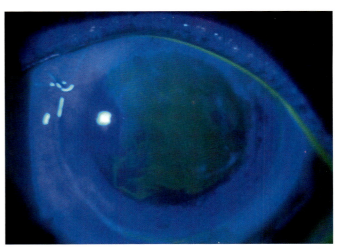

Figure 47.1 Partial stem cell failure. Note the mosaic pattern of late fluorescein staining of abnormal epithelium.

simultaneous CLAU and deep lamellar keratoplasty with 27 ± 15.4 months of follow-up.

KLAL

The reported success rates of KLAL surgery vary widely, due to differences in preoperative diagnoses, length of follow-up, and immunosuppressive regimens used. Solomon et al.'s study[5] of 39 eyes undergoing KLAL and amniotic membrane transplantation (AMT) illustrates how length of follow-up affects success rates. They describe a progressive attrition in the survival of KLAL: $76.9\%\pm6.7\%$ at 1 year, $47.4\%\pm11.7\%$ at 3 years, and only $23.7\%\pm17.7\%$ at 5 years. Similarly, in Ilari and Daya's study[6] of 23 eyes undergoing KLAL, graft survival was 54.4% at 1 year, 33.3% at 2 years, and 27.3% at 3 years and only 21.2% at 5 years. Both studies had a similar mix of preoperative diagnoses with 30/39 eyes in Solomon's study and 20/23 eyes in Ilari's study having stage b or c disease (conjunctival involvement). The worse results in Ilari's study may possibly be attributable to differing immunosuppressive regimens. Oral cyclosporine A (CSA) was used only in high-risk cases (9/20 patients), compared to Solomon's study in which all patients received oral CSA indefinitely. In comparison, in Holland's study[7] of 31 eyes with aniridia, 74.2% achieved a stable ocular surface at 35.7 months of follow-up. They noted the effect of IS with 90.5% of eyes receiving systemic IS obtaining a stable ocular surface, whereas only 40.0% of eyes receiving systemic IS achieving surface stability. The higher success rate in this study may possibly be attributable to all cases being aniridic and thus having no conjunctival involvement (stage a disease).

LR-CLAL

There are few studies that describe the success rates of lr-CLAL. In a study by Gomes et al.[8] of 10 eyes undergoing combined lr-CLAL and amniotic membrane transplantation, six eyes had successful ocular surface reconstruction with 19 months (range 8–27 months) follow-up. Only patients with less than 75% HLA compatibility between recipient and donor received oral immunosuppression with CSA. In a study by Javadi et al.[9] 32 eyes had lr-CLAL and 40 eyes had KLAL performed for mustard gas-induced LSCD. They found that the rejection-free graft survival rate was 39.1% in the lr-CLAL group and 80.7% in the KLAL group 40 months postoperatively. This result may be explained by the different IS regime used in their two groups: the lr-CLAL group received 1 year of oral CSA, compared to the KLAL group receiving oral CSA for 1.5 to 2 years in addition to mycophenolate mofetil for at least 6 months. Also, they did not use HLA-matching for their lr-CLAL group. The results of their study emphasize the importance of preoperative HLA-matching and postoperative IS in lr-CLAL. At the authors' institute, combined lr-CLAL and KLAL, 'the Cincinnati procedure,' is used to treat patients with the most severe ocular surface failure, having both severe LSCD and conjunctival deficiency, such as in Stevens – Johnson syndrome. In our study[10] of 19 eyes undergoing combined lr-CLAL/KLAL, the ocular surface was stable in 54.2%, improved in 33.3%, and failed in 12.5% of eyes with follow-up of 43.4 months (range 12.2 to 125.5 months).

CLET

Shortt et al.[11] performed a review of 17 papers of CLET techniques using autograft, allograft, or oral mucosal sources of stem cells. A total of 131 of 170 eyes (77%) treated for partial or total LSCD reported improvement in clinical parameters, with little difference in the rate of improvement between autografts (86/114, 75.4%) and allografts (45/56, 80%). However, the authors warned against interpretation of these results as the outcome measures used to define successful treatment were poorly described by most studies, and lacked objectivity, as there was no comparison of defined pre- and post-treatment parameters.

Complications

IMMUNOLOGIC REJECTION

Immunologic rejection of allograft OSST is the most important cause of stem cell failure. In contrast to corneal transplants that have relative immune privilege, limbal tissue is highly vascularized and rich in antigen-presenting cells and Langerhans cells. Pathologic findings in rejected KLAL specimens indicate that rejection is a T-cell mediated phenomenon.[12] Rejection may present clinically as severe or low grade, as shown in Table 47.1 and Figure 47.2. In the authors' study[13] of 222 eyes with mean follow-up of 62.7 months (range 12.0–158.3 months), rejection occurred in 31.1% (69/222) of patients at a mean of 19.3 months postoperatively (range 0.2–93.1 months). This demonstrates that rejection is a long-term concern, due to the perpetuation of donor epithelial cells within the donor limbus. Risk factors for rejection were younger age, KLAL alone (versus lr-CLAL or combination of lr-CLAL/KLAL), and noncompliance with IS. Patients who rejected had a worse outcome despite treatment with increased immunosuppression and repeat OSST if necessary: at the final follow-up visit only 36.6% (26/69) of patients had a stable ocular surface, compared to 71.9% (110/153) of those that did not reject. Even though the transplant may not immediately fail at the time of rejection, these patients have a higher rate of ocular surface failure in the long term.

Patients should be adequately immunosuppressed to prevent rejection. At the authors' institution, immunosuppression is managed in conjunction with the renal transplant team, using a regimen of short-term oral prednisone

Table 47.1 Clinical Features of Severe and Low-Grade Rejection

Severe Rejection	Low-Grade Rejection
Moderate-to-severe pain	Mild discomfort
Intense sectoral or 360° injection	Mild limbal injection
Edema and neovascularization of KLAL or lr-CLAL segments	Neovascularization of KLAL segments
Epithelial rejection line	Epithelial rejection line
Signs of abnormal epithelium: Late fluorescein staining, irregular thickened epithelium, neovascularization	Signs of abnormal epithelium: Late fluorescein staining, irregular thickened epithelium, neovascularization

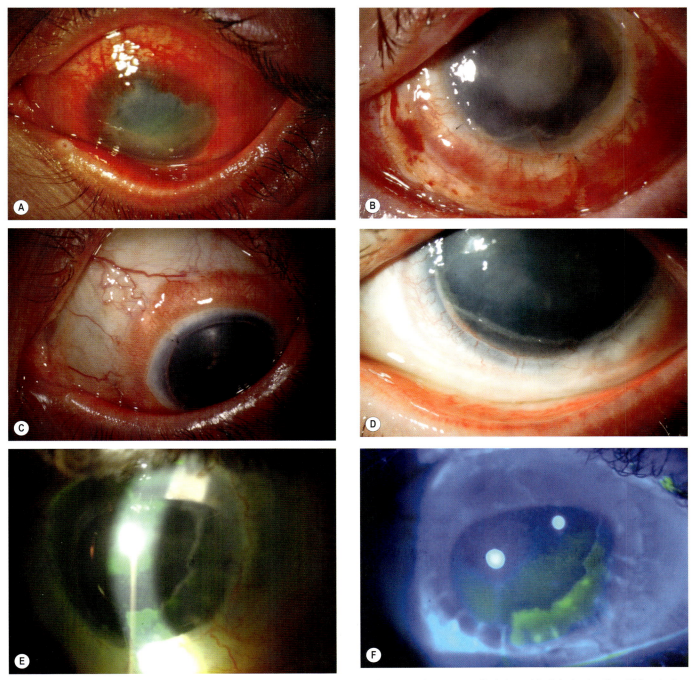

Figure 47.2 Severe Rejection: (**A**) Severe limbal injection. (**B**) Lenticule edema and neovascularization and inferior epithelial rejection line. (**C**) Lenticule edema and injection. Low-grade rejection: (**D**) Relatively quiet eye with inferior epithelial rejection line. (**E**) Epithelial rejection line with associated late fluorescein staining of failed area (**F**).

(tapered over 1 to 3 months) and longer-term tacrolimus and mycophenolate mofetil (tapered over 2 to 3 years).[14] Patients' tacrolimus levels are monitored to ensure therapeutic effect and compliance, and patients are educated preoperatively regarding the necessity and importance of immunosuppression for a successful transplant. If rejection is suspected, the patient should be treated aggressively with increased topical and systemic immunosuppression. Patients with a prior history of rejection should be

maintained on low-dose immunosuppression indefinitely if systemically tolerated.

PERSISTENT EPITHELIAL DEFECTS

Persistent epithelial defects (PED) may result from OSST failure but can also occur with a successful OSST. PED may occur in OSST patients from a variety of causes: micro-trauma from eyelid abnormalities, such as trichiasis and entropion; exposure keratopathy from ectropion and lagophthalmos; aqueous and mucin deficiency from conjunctival inflammation and scarring; neurotrophic effects from keratoplasty; and irregular epithelium and breakdown that occur after failure of OSST. Strategies to prevent PED include correction of eyelid abnormalities prior to or at the time of OSST, and aggressive treatment of tear film abnormalities. The authors advocate a low threshold for performing a lateral tarsorrhaphy at the time of OSST and for placing a bandage contact lens until the surface has completely healed. Other options include punctal occlusion and the use of amniotic membrane or autologous serum.

MICROBIAL KERATITIS

Patients with OSST and keratoplasty are particularly susceptible to microbial keratitis. The combination of the presence of epithelial defects and the use of immunosuppression (both topical and systemic) sets the environment for opportunistic infections, especially fungal keratitis. Figure 47.3 illustrates a fungal keratitis in an eye that had undergone OSST. In Solomon's study[5] of 39 eyes undergoing KLAL, three of 24 eyes that had also undergone PK developed microbial keratitis. Two corneal grafts that were severely infected by *Candida* species required therapeutic keratoplasty, and one eye had coagulase negative *Staphylococcus*. In the authors' experience, fungal keratitis is difficult to eradicate medically and often requires an early therapeutic keratoplasty. Medical treatment consists of aggressive topical and oral antifungals, cessation of all topical steroids, and reduction of the systemic immunosuppression. If the infection cannot be controlled medically, an early therapeutic keratoplasty should be performed before the infiltrate reaches the graft – host interface.

GLAUCOMA

Glaucoma is often a pre-existing co-morbidity with ocular surface diseases and can be further exacerbated by OSST,

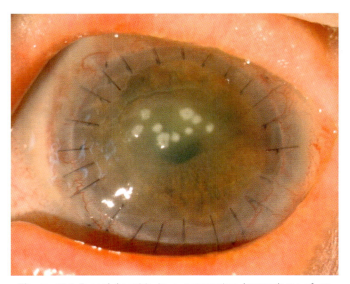

Figure 47.3 Fungal keratitis in a penetrating keratoplasty of an SJS patient with combined living-related conjunctival allograft/keratolimbal allograft.

subsequent keratoplasty, and the long-term topical steroids required to prevent rejection. Many patients with aniridia and conditions with chronic inflammation, such as chemical injuries require glaucoma drainage devices (GDD) to control intraocular pressure. All patients should be assessed by and managed in conjunction with a glaucoma specialist. If a GDD is required, we recommend that this is performed prior to OSST if possible. Our clinical impression is that there is an increased risk of sectoral stem cell failure if the GDD is placed after OSST.

Etiology of Failure

Immunologic rejection, both severe and low grade, is the leading cause of OSST failure in allograft procedures. As discussed above, systemic immunosuppression is crucial in preventing immune rejection, and patients should be monitored regularly and treated aggressively if they have rejection episodes. Non-immunologic inflammation is another contributing factor to OSST failure. Chronic background inflammation and recurrent episodes of inflammation may occur in diseases, such as Stevens – Johnson syndrome and ocular cicatricial pemphigoid and may further stress the transplanted limbal stem cells.

Concurrent cicatrizing eyelid pathology that occurs in these diseases contributes to OSST failure and should be addressed prior to or at the time of OSST surgery. Disorders of the lid – lash complex may cause microtrauma and perpetuate chronic inflammation through the mechanical rubbing of lashes against the ocular surface. Ectropion or lagophthalmos can cause exposure keratopathy and delay healing after OSST. Conjunctival involvement may result in aqueous and mucin deficiency, and in the most severe cases keratinization of the surface. Holland's study[15] found that keratinization of the conjunctiva was a risk factor of OSST failure, as was a Schirmer test of 2 mm or less at 5 minutes without anesthesia.

After an initially successful OSST, late failure may occur, due to chronic exhaustion of the donor limbal stem cell pool. The etiology of stem cell exhaustion is not well understood, but is likely due to chronic inflammation depleting stem cells that may already be reduced in number from surgical trauma. The added mitotic demand of penetrating or deep anterior lamellar keratoplasty may further exhaust the limbal stem cell population. In some cases, chronic low-grade immune rejection that is asymptomatic and undiagnosed may cause limbal stem cell exhaustion. Some also hypothesize that it may be due to loss of mitotic activity of the transplanted stem cells over time.

Conclusion

The reported success rates of various OSST procedures differ between studies. In general, it appears that success rates decrease with increasing length of follow-up, with more severe ocular surface diseases, such as stage IIc disease, and with weaker immunosuppression regimens. Patients need to be monitored regularly and long term for complications, such as immune rejection, epithelial defects, microbial keratitis, and progression of glaucoma.

References

1. Krachmer JH, Alldredge OC. Subepithelial infiltration. A probable sign of corneal transplant rejection. Arch Ophthalmol 1978;96:2234–7.
2. Schwartz GS, Gomes JAP, Holland EJ. Preoperative staging of disease severity. In: Holland EJ, Mannis MJ, editors. Ocular surface disease: medical and surgical management. New York: Springer-Verlag; 2002.
3. Rao SK, Rajagopal R, Sitalakshmi G, et al. Limbal autografting: comparison of results in the acute and chronic phases of ocular surface burns. Cornea 1999;18:164–71.
4. Yao YF, Zhang B, Zhou P, et al. Autologous limbal grafting combined with deep lamellar keratoplasty in unilateral eye with severe chemical or thermal burn at late stage. Ophthalmology 2002;109:2011–7.
5. Solomon A, Ellies P, Anderson DF, et al. Long-term outcome of keratolimbal allograft with or without penetrating keratoplasty for total limbal stem cell deficiency. Ophthalmology 2002;109:1159–66.
6. Ilari L, Daya SM. Long-term outcomes of keratolimbal allograft for the treatment of severe ocular surface disorders. Ophthalmology 2002; 109:1278–84.
7. Holland EJ, Djalilian AR, Schwartz GS. Management of aniridic keratopathy with keratolimbal allograft: a limbal stem cell transplantation technique. Ophthalmology 2003;110:125–30.
8. Gomes JA, dos Santos MS, Cunha MC, et al. Amniotic membrane transplantation for partial and total limbal stem cell deficiency secondary to chemical burn. Ophthalmology 2003;110:466–73.
9. Javadi MA, Jafarinasab MR, Feizi S, et al. Management of mustard gas-induced limbal stem cell deficiency and keratitis. Ophthalmology 2011;118:1272–81.
10. Biber JM, Skeens HM, Neff KD, et al. The Cincinnati procedure: technique and outcomes of combined living-related conjunctival limbal allografts and keratolimbal allografts in severe ocular surface failure. Cornea 2011;30:765–71.
11. Shortt AJ, Secker GA, Notara MD, et al. Transplantation of ex vivo cultured limbal epithelial stem cells: a review of techniques and clinical results. Surv Ophthalmol 2007;52:483–502.
12. Daya SM, Dugald Bell RW, Habib NE, et al. Clinical and pathologic findings in human keratolimbal allograft rejection. Cornea 2000; 19:443–50.
13. Ang AY, Chan CC, Biber JM, et al. Ocular surface stem cell transplantation rejection: incidence, characteristics, and outcomes. Cornea 2013;32:229–36.
14. Holland EJ, Mogilishetty GM, Skeens HM, et al. Systemic immunosuppression in ocular surface stem cell transplantation: Results of a 10-year experience. Cornea 2012;31:655–61.
15. Holland EJ. Epithelial transplantation for the management of severe ocular surface disease. Trans Am Ophthalmol Soc 1996;19: 677–743.

48 *Keratoplasty in Ocular Surface Disease*

J. STUART TIMS and W. BARRY LEE

Introduction

Ocular surface disease can range from mild keratoconjunctivitis sicca to severe conditions that damage limbal stem cells. Severe cases of stem cell deficiency may require limbal stem cell transplantation and ultimately penetrating or lamellar keratoplasty to clear the visual axis. Optimization of the ocular surface prior to keratoplasty is essential to achieve success and includes maximizing tear function, restoring normal lid anatomy and function, and ensuring an adequate supply of limbal stem cells. These vital steps help enhance survival and clarity of the corneal graft.

Approximately 50% of ocular surface reconstruction procedures will require keratoplasty for visual rehabilitation.[1] The outcome of the corneal graft is dependent on several important factors, including the extent of the limbal stem cell deficiency (largely determined by the underlying etiology) and the presence or absence of conjunctival inflammation (Fig. 48.1).[2] It is also important to consider whether other components of the ocular surface, besides limbal stem cells, are involved in the pathologic process. The consequences of ignoring any one of these items may result in non-healing epithelial defects, secondary ulceration, infectious keratitis, corneal vascularization, conjunctivalization of the cornea, and ultimate graft rejection or corneal melting. Even with perfect surgical technique and the best

tissue available, poor outcomes may result without an adequate stem cell reserve, optimal tear function, and anatomically functional lids.[1]

In this chapter, the authors review the relevant literature that describes methods and results for keratoplasty in the setting of ocular surface and limbal stem cell dysfunction, and discuss a logical approach for managing these very challenging patients.

Preoperative Considerations

Prior to keratoplasty, all patients should undergo evaluation for ocular co-morbidities, such as eyelid malposition, eyelid disorders and glaucoma. In addition, the ocular surface should be screened for dry eye and dysfunctional tear syndrome states, limbal stem cell deficiency, conjunctival dysfunction, scarring and keratinization of the cornea, corneal vascularization, corneal sensation, and the status of the corneal epithelium (Fig. 48.2). If the conditions mentioned above are not addressed prior to keratoplasty, postoperative outcomes can be disappointing and potentially devastating.

Preoperative punctal occlusion, punctal cautery, entropion or ectropion repair, treatment of lagophthalmos, and trichiasis correction remain important preoperative treatment options for patients with concurrent eyelid disorders

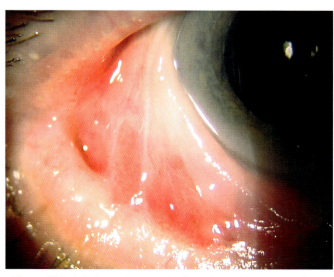

Figure 48.1 A slit lamp photograph of a patient with severe conjunctival inflammation and symblepharon formation in ocular cicatricial pemphigoid.

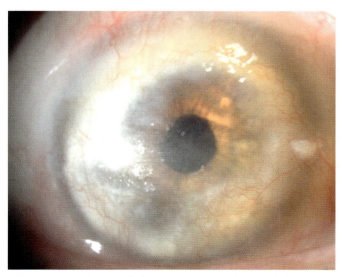

Figure 48.2 A photograph showing a patient with a guarded prognosis for keratoplasty alone, due to limbal stem cell deficiency manifest as dense vascularization, scarring and lipid deposition at the limbus.

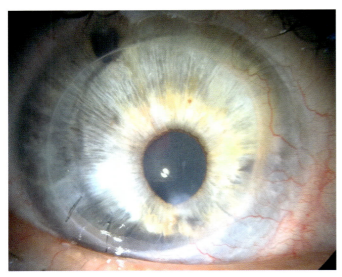

Figure 48.3 A postoperative photograph 18 months after a keratolimbal allograft (KLAL) and 1 year after a sequential PK for a severe alkaline corneal keratitis and central corneal scarring.

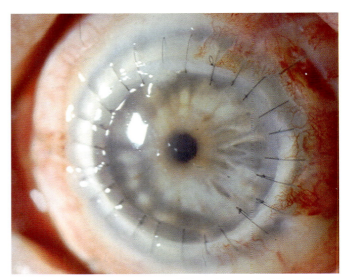

Figure 48.4 A slit lamp photograph depicting a KLAL followed by a sequential combined PK, cataract removal and intraocular lens placement. Note the presence of interrupted sutures to provide a secure wound and potential for future selective suture removal to improve post-keratoplasty astigmatism.

and dry eye conditions. Preservative-free artificial tears, gels, and lubricant ointments, as well as use of topical anti-inflammatory agents can also be important adjuncts to management of preoperative conditions. Anterior and posterior blepharitis must also be controlled prior to keratoplasty in ocular surface disease, as detailed in Chapter 10. Glaucoma can also impact the outcome of keratoplasty, whether from the toxicity of glaucoma drops, high pressure exerting optic nerve damage and poor visual outcomes, or compromised endothelial dysfunction from certain glaucoma drops, high intraocular pressure or prior glaucoma surgery.[3,4] Intraocular pressure must be managed prior to keratoplasty, with care to minimize corneal complications from glaucoma treatment.

Once the tear film and lid function have been optimized and ocular co-morbidities addressed, the limbal stem cell reserve must be replenished in the presence of limbal stem cell deficiency. Chapters 40–45 detail surgical techniques for limbal stem cell transplantation. Given the scientific evidence and clinical experience, the authors prefer to perform keratoplasty as a staged procedure at least 3 months following stem cell transplantation (Fig. 48.3).

Surgical Technique and Considerations

Penetrating keratoplasty (PK) in conjunction with or following stem cell transplant is performed with several unique considerations, compared to routine keratoplasty. Larger-diameter grafts are preferred to provide better apposition to the keratolimbal graft segments and lessen the risk of epithelial ingrowth.[5] Same-size recipient trephination is often performed to prevent overlap between the peripheral donor cornea and stem cell segments. One important exception to same size trephination is chemical injury patients, who are oversized 0.5–0.75 mm, because the recipient bed in chemical burn cases often contracts following trephination. Because there is often asymmetric wound healing at the

graft–host junction, interrupted sutures are preferred over running sutures to allow for selective removal to manage astigmatism (Fig. 48.4). Interrupted sutures also allow for easier suture removal and better wound stability after removal with a decreased risk of dehiscence, compared to running suture removal.[6,7] Ocular surface disease patients must be watched closer for loose or vascularized sutures after keratoplasty as they are at increased risk of developing suture-related complications (Fig. 48.5).

In terms of donor tissue selection, some authors prefer to use pediatric or neonatal limbal tissue to allow for the greatest density of limbal stem cells for transplantation.[8] Since pediatric donor corneal tissue is not commonly available, performing staged procedures allows for use of adult donor cornea tissue at a later date for keratoplasty. Optimizing keratoplasty donor tissue quality, especially relative to the donor ocular surface, can help prevent postoperative epithelial defects that could become persistent.[9]

Another consideration with keratoplasty in ocular surface disease is the choice of technique. The majority of reports in the literature on keratoplasty in ocular surface disease discuss PK; however, advances in deep anterior lamellar keratoplasty (DALK) and keratoprosthesis (KPro) make these procedures advantageous in selected circumstances. Femtosecond lasers and Anwar's big bubble technique allow for deeper tissue dissections with DALK and decreased risk of interface haze/opacity, compared to lamellar techniques abandoned in the mid-twentieth century.[10–13] The main advantages of DALK over PK include elimination of endothelial tissue rejection, extraocular rather than intraocular surgery, minor endothelial cell damage, faster potential suture removal, and the potential for increased tectonic wound strength (Fig. 48.6).[10–14]

The keratoprosthesis provides another viable alternative to limbal stem cell rehabilitation and cadaveric keratoplasty in this patient population. The advantages of a KPro over cadaveric tissue include elimination of endothelial tissue

Simultaneous limbal allograft transplantation with PK was first described by Tsubota et al.[32] in 1995 in eight patients, utilizing the same donor tissue for the stem cell transplant and the keratoplasty. Patients received oral and topical cyclosporine A, as well as intravenous dexamethasone postoperatively. Five of the eight grafts remained clear for a mean of 12.3 months. Although there were two episodes of graft rejection that were managed medically and two patients required a second limbal graft, all eight patients had an improvement in visual acuity.[32]

In 1997, Tseng and Tan[33] presented a case report of simultaneous KLAL and PK in a patient with severe thermal burns. Again, a single donor was used for both tissues. Postoperative medication included oral cyclosporine A 5 mg/kg, topical prednisolone acetate 1% and topical tobramycin 0.3%. The cornea reepithelialized within 24 days, and the cornea remained clear for the brief follow-up period of 21 weeks.[33]

In 1998, Tseng et al.[34] reported, as part of a larger series, 14 eyes that received combined KLAL and PK from a single donor, following a previously performed amniotic membrane transplant. Nine of 14 eyes (64%) developed corneal graft rejection, with two eyes requiring repeat PK, due to irreversible endothelial rejection and three developing persistent corneal epithelial defects. None experienced limbal graft rejection.[34]

Tsubota et al.[35] (1999) described a series of 43 eyes of 39 patients that underwent keratolimbal allograft, of which 28 eyes had simultaneous PK. Similar to previous reports, the KLAL and the donor cornea tissue were obtained from the same donor, limiting antigenic challenge. Cyclosporine A was used systemically preoperatively and for 1 month postoperatively, along with IV dexamethasone, which was used for 4 days postoperatively. Fifty-four percent (15 of 28) of the penetrating grafts survived, while 46% (13 of 28) rejected. Nine of those 13 that rejected were regrafted, and seven of those rejected again. Four patients required a third PK. Etiology of stem cell deficiency had an effect on epithelialization and rejection, as patients with Stevens–Johnson syndrome or ocular cicatricial pemphigoid epithelialized only 41%, compared to 71% of patients with chemical or thermal burns. On the other hand, chemical and thermal burns had a 69% rejection rate, compared to 27% of pemphigoid and Stevens–Johnson patients. Thirty-seven percent developed significant ocular hypertension following simultaneous surgery.[35]

In 2001, Shimazaki et al.[36] published a case series of 45 eyes of 43 patients that had simultaneous KLAL and PK. Endothelial rejection occurred in 16 eyes (35.6%), of which 10 eyes (62.5%) were clear following treatment. Overall, there was no evidence of clinical rejection in the limbal grafts during the periods of corneal graft rejection, and all corneas re-epithelialized following rejection episodes. The authors theorized different mechanisms of rejection for the two types of tissue, with no effect on limbal stem cell function associated with corneal graft rejection.[36]

Solomon et al.[37] performed combined KLAL and PK in 23 eyes and published the results in 2002. Patients received topical corticosteroids and antibiotics postoperatively, as well as systemic cyclosporine A 5 mg/kg, with a taper to appropriate trough levels. Central corneal graft survival was 47.8% after the first year and only 13.7% after 3 years.

Grafts with Stevens–Johnson syndrome had significantly worse outcomes, with only 20% surviving at 1 year, and none surviving after 3 years.[37]

More recently, two case series have highlighted simultaneous limbal stem cell transplantation with DALK. In 2005, Fogla and Padmanabhan[38] reported a series of 7 eyes of 7 patients that underwent combined conjunctivo-limbal autograft and DALK for unilateral severe chemical injury. All eyes achieved successful re-epithelialization and retained a stable ocular surface for a mean of 16.5 months. Average best-corrected final visual acuity was 20/50 and all but one eye had remarkable improvement in visual acuity.[38] In 2010, Omoto and colleagues[39] published a series of six eyes of five patients that had simultaneous KLAL and DALK for various etiologies, including Stevens–Johnson syndrome, aniridia, and gelatinous drop-like dystrophy. Four of five eyes (80%) retained a smooth epithelial surface and had improvement in visual acuity of more than two lines.[39]

DALK has the advantage of eliminating the risk of endothelial rejection and limits the antigenic challenge when combined surgery requires multiple donors. In addition, it avoids the risks of penetrating intraocular surgery, particularly in aniridia patients who are more prone to anterior movement of the lens during open-sky keratoplasty. However, DALK is a more technically challenging procedure, which adds to the complexity when performing simultaneous surgery. It also may be less advantageous to perform DALK simultaneously because of the difficulty evaluating the health of the host corneal endothelium through scarred and vascularized epithelium and stroma prior to surgery. If the intention is to perform DALK for keratoplasty, sequential surgery should be considered.

To date, only two published studies have compared staged versus simultaneous surgery. In 2004, Shimizaki et al.[8] reported 32 eyes of 32 patients with limbal stem cell deficiency from chemical burns (27 eyes) and thermal burns (5 eyes). Twenty-one eyes received KLAL transplantation, of which 15 had simultaneous PK and six had staged keratoplasty at a mean of 7.7 months. Although not statistically significant, corneal epithelialization and clarity were better in the staged group. Endothelial rejection was significantly greater in the simultaneous group than in the staged group (53.3% versus 0%, $p = 0.019$), and the need for a repeat limbal stem cell transplant was more common in the simultaneous group (66.7% versus 16.7%, $p = 0.06$).[8] Most recently, in 2011, Basu described 12 eyes with combined autologous cultivated limbal epithelial transplantation and PK, compared to 35 eyes performed in two stages.[40] Corneal allograft survival at 1 year was significantly higher in the staged group versus the simultaneous group (80% versus 25%, $p = 0.0003$). Recurrence of limbal stem cell deficiency was significantly higher in the simultaneous group than the staged group (58.3% versus 14.3%, $p = 0.008$).[40]

Conclusion

Severe ocular surface disease poses a difficult challenge to the corneal surgeon. To rehabilitate the ocular surface and provide an optimal optical outcome requires patience, perseverance and careful surgical strategic planning. Understanding the specific etiology of the stem cell deficiency will allow the physician to prepare the eye adequately and to maintain a healthy surface following keratoplasty. At present, based on the scientific literature, it appears that performing limbal stem cell transplantation followed at a later date by keratoplasty, either penetrating or deep anterior lamellar, will lower the likelihood of endothelial rejection and of failure of limbal grafts, although larger studies with longer follow-up are needed. With careful detail in monitoring for surface breakdown and inflammation, these challenging patients can have successful outcomes and experience remarkable improvements in quality of life.

References

1. Biber JM, Neff KD, Holland EJ, et al. Corneal transplantation in ocular surface disease. In: Krachmer JH, Mannis MJ, Holland EJ, editors. Cornea: fundamentals, diagnosis, and management. vol. 2, 3rd ed. Philadelphia: Elsevier; 2010.
2. Holland EJ, Schwartz GS. The Paton Lecture: ocular surface transplantation: 10 year's experience. Cornea 2004;23:425–31.
3. Ayyala RS. Penetrating keratoplasty and glaucoma. Surv Ophthalmol 2000;45:91–105.
4. Alvarenga LS, Mannis MJ, Brandt JD, et al. The long-term results of keratoplasty in eyes with a glaucoma drainage device. Am J Ophthalmol 2004;138:200–5.
5. Skeens HM, Holland EJ. Large-diameter penetrating keratoplasty: indications and outcomes. Cornea 2010;29:296–301.
6. Abou-Jaoude ES, Brooks M, Katz DG, et al. Suture-related complications following keratoplasty: a 5-year retrospective study. Ophthalmology 2002;109:1291–6.
7. Lee WB, Mannis MJ. Corneal suturing techniques. In: Macsai MS, editor. Ophthalmic microsurgical suturing techniques. New York: Springer; 2006. Ch. 6.
8. Shimazaki J, Shimmura S, Tsubota K. Donor source affects the outcome of ocular surface reconstruction in chemical or thermal burns of the cornea. Ophthalmology 2004;111:38–44.
9. Kim T, Palay DA, Lynn M. Donor factors associated with epithelial defects after penetrating keratoplasty. Cornea 1996;15:451–6.
10. Yoo SH, Kymionis GD, Koreishi A, et al. Femtosecond laser-assisted anterior lamellar keratoplasty. Ophthalmology 2008;115:1303–7.
11. Anwar M, Teichmann KD. Big bubble technique to bare Descemet's membrane in anterior lamellar keratoplasty. J Cataract Refract Surg 2002;28:398–403.
12. Anwar M, Teichmann KD. Deep lamellar keratoplasty: surgical techniques for anterior lamellar keratoplasty with and without baring of Descemet's membrane. Cornea 2002;21:374–83.
13. Lee WB, Mannis MJ. The return of lamellar keratoplasty. Vision Panamerica 2009;8:164–7.
14. Reinhart WJ, Musch, DC, Jacobs DS, et al. Deep anterior lamellar keratoplasty as an alternative to penetrating keratoplasty. Ophthalmology 2011;118:209–18.
15. Zerbe BL, Belin MW, Ciolino JB, et al. Results from the multicenter Boston Type 1 keratoprosthesis study. Ophthalmology 2006;113:1779–84.
16. Bradley JC, Hernandez EG, Schwab IR, et al. Boston Type 1 Keratoprosthesis: the University of California Davis experience. Cornea 2009;28:321–7.
17. Biber JM, Skeens HM, Neff KD, et al. The Cincinnati procedure: technique and outcomes of combined living-related conjunctival limbal allografts and keratolimbal allografts in severe ocular surface failure. Cornea 2011;30:765–71.
18. Sayegh RR, Ang LPK, Foster S, et al. The Boston keratoprosthesis in Stevens–Johnson syndrome. Am J Ophthalmol 2008;145:438–44.
19. Fernandes M, Sridhar MS, Sangwan VS, et al. Amniotic membrane transplantation for ocular surface. Cornea 2005;24:639–42.
20. Seitz B, Das S, Sauer R, et al. Simultaneous amniotic membrane patch in high-risk keratoplasty. Cornea 2011;30:269–72.
21. Lee WB. Therapeutic hydrogel bandage lenses. In: Tasman W, Jaeger EA, editors. Duane's clinical ophthalmology. Vol 4. Philadelphia: Lippincott Williams & Wilkins; 2007. Chapter 11.
22. Schrader S, Wedel T, Moll R, et al. Combination of serum eye drops with hydrogel bandage contact lenses in the treatment of persistent epithelial defects. Graefes Arch Clin Exp Ophthalmol 2006;244:1345–9.
23. Matsumoto Y, Dogru M, Goto E, et al. Autologous serum application in the treatment of neurotrophic keratopathy. Ophthalmology 2004;111:1115–20.
24. Lambiase A, Manni L, Bonini S, et al. Nerve growth factor promotes corneal healing: structural, biochemical, and molecular analyses of rat and human corneas. Invest Ophthalmol Vis Sci 2000;41:1063–9.
25. Mannis MJ. Penetrating keratoplasty in ocular stem cell disease. In: Holland EJ, Mannis MJ, editors. Ocular surface disease: medical and surgical management. New York: Springer; 2002. p. 253–6.
26. Kenyon KR, Tseng SCG. Limbal autograft transplantation for ocular surface disorders. Ophthalmology 1989;96:709–22.
27. Frucht-Pery J, Siganos CS, Solomon A, et al. Limbal cell autograft transplantation for severe ocular surface disorders. Graefe's Arch Clin Exp Ophthalmol 1998;236:582–7.
28. Croasdale CR, Schwartz GS, Malling JV, et al. Keratolimbal allograft: recommendations for tissue procurement and preparation by eye banks, and standard surgical technique. Cornea 1999;18:52–8.
29. Sangwan VS, Fernandes M, Bansal AK, et al. Early results of penetrating keratoplasty following limbal stem cell transplantation. Indian J Ophthalmol 2005;53:31–5.
30. Baradaran-Rafii A, Ebrahimi M, Kanavi MR, et al. Midterm outcomes of autologous cultivated limbal stem cell transplantation with or without penetrating keratoplasty. Cornea 2010;29:502–9.
31. Biber JM, Skeens HM, Neff KD, et al. The Cincinnati procedure: technique and outcomes of combined living-related conjunctival limbal allografts and keratolimbal allografts in severe ocular surface failure. Cornea 2011;30:765–71.
32. Tsubota K, Toda I, Saito H, et al. Reconstruction of the corneal epithelium by limbal allograft transplantation for severe ocular surface disorders. Ophthalmology 1995;102:1486–96.
33. Theng JT, Tan DT. Combined penetrating keratoplasty and limbal allograft transplantation for severe corneal burns. Ophthalmic Surg Lasers 1997;28:765–8.
34. Tseng SCG, Prabhasawat P, Barton K, et al. Amniotic membrane transplantation with or without limbal allografts for corneal surface reconstruction in patients with limbal stem cell deficiency. Arch Ophthalmol 1998;116:431–41.
35. Tsubota K, Satake Y, Kaido M, et al. Treatment of severe ocular-surface disorders with corneal epithelial stem-cell transplantation. N Engl J Med 1999;340:1697–703.
36. Shimazaki J, Maruyama F, Shimmura S, et al. Immunologic rejection of the central graft after limbal allograft transplantation combined with penetrating keratoplasty. Cornea 2001;20:149–52.
37. Solomon A, Ellies P, Anderson DF, et al. Long-term outcome of keratolimbal allograft with or without penetrating keratoplasty for total limbal stem cell deficiency. Ophthalmology 2002;109:1159–66.
38. Fogla R, Padmanabhan P. Deep anterior lamellar keratoplasty combined with autologous limbal stem cell transplantation in unilateral severe chemical injury. Cornea 2005;24:421–5.
39. Omoto M, Shimmura S, Hatou S, et al. Simultaneous deep anterior lamellar keratoplasty and limbal allograft in bilateral limbal stem cell deficiency. Jpn J Ophthalmol 2010;54:537–43.
40. Basu S, Mohamed A, Chaurasia S, et al. Clinical outcomes of penetrating keratoplasty after autologous cultivated limbal epithelial transplantation for ocular surface burns. Am J Ophthalmol 2011;152:917–24.

49 Indications for the Boston Keratoprosthesis

KATHRYN A. COLBY and ANITA N. SHUKLA

Introduction

In the past, keratoprosthesis implantation was considered a surgery of last resort, fraught with complications and generally poor outcomes. There has been a dramatic increase in the use of the type I Boston keratoprosthesis (Boston KPro) over the last decade as design modifications to the device itself and changes to the postoperative regimen have improved outcomes and reduced postoperative complications (Fig. 49.1). Graft failure remains the most common indication for the Boston KPro (Table 49.1)[1]. However, in recent years, the Boston KPro has been used successfully as the primary corneal surgery in conditions in which standard penetrating keratoplasty (PKP) has a poor prognosis, including neurotrophic or vascularized host beds (Fig. 49.2), congenital or acquired limbal stem cell deficiency, autoimmune ocular disorders, and pediatric corneal opacities. Cicatricial and inflammatory autoimmune conditions remain the most challenging KPro cases, and need further advances with immunomodulation and improved biologic materials before the Boston KPro will find widespread acceptance as a treatment for these devastating ocular surface diseases.[2]

Use of the Boston KPro in Herpetic Keratitis

The 5-year success rate of corneal grafts in patients with herpetic keratitis is significantly less than that in other corneal diseases, such as keratoconus and corneal dystrophies.[3] Anesthesia of the host corneal bed, frequent graft rejection episodes, corneal vascularization and poor wound healing all contribute to the suboptimal outcomes of PKP in the setting of herpetic disease.[1] In contrast, case reports and small case series suggest the Boston KPro can be successful in patients with herpes simplex or herpes zoster, even in the setting of corneal anesthesia and active inflammation.[3–5]

The Boston KPro was used in 17 eyes of 14 patients who had repeatedly failed traditional PKP.[3] Twelve patients had herpes zoster or herpes simplex as the initial diagnosis, while two patients had keratoconus and developed herpetic keratitis in the corneal graft. Visual acuity improved from light perception to 20/200 preoperatively to 20/25 to 20/70 in 15 of 17 eyes. No complications were reported in 10 patients over a follow-up period that ranged from 7 to 39 months. The remaining patients experienced complications from pre-existing glaucoma or new-onset sterile vitritis.[3]

The Boston KPro in Congenital Aniridia

The keratopathy associated with congenital aniridia results from corneal epithelial stem cell deficiency and corneal

Table 49.1 Surgeon-supplied Diagnoses for Type I Boston KPros 2010–2011

Diagnosis	Number of KPros	%
Graft failure	903	50.30
Corneal scar	175	9.70
Endothelial failure	139	7.70
Chemical injury	139	7.70
Aniridia	74	4.10
Stevens–Johnson syndrome	53	3.00
Limbal stem cell failure	43	2.40
Infection	37	2.00
Pemphigoid	36	2.00
Herpes/neurotrophic keratitis	31	1.70
KPro replacement	31	1.70
Corneal neovascularization	24	1.30
Corneal melt	20	1.10
Miscellaneous	91	5.10
Total	1796	

2040 KPros were ordered from 1/1/2010 to 12/31/2011. Diagnoses were supplied for 1796 cases.
Miscellaneous includes any diagnosis with fewer than 20 cases.

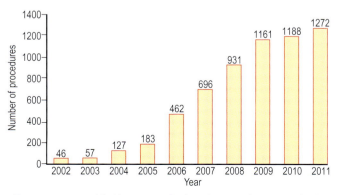

Figure 49.1 Worldwide use of the Boston keratoprosthesis, 2002–2011.

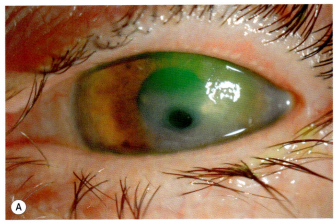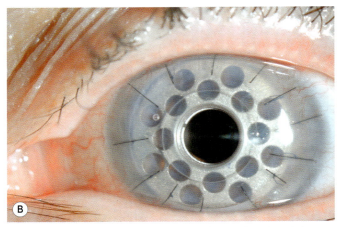

Figure 49.2 (**A**) Preoperative appearance of a 42-year-old woman with a chronic descemetocele in an anesthetic cornea from trigeminal nerve damage following neurosurgery. Prior attempts at ocular surface reconstruction with amniotic membrane had been unsuccessful. Preoperative vision was 20/200. (**B**) Postoperative appearance 1 week following type I Boston KPro, cataract removal and intraocular lens placement. Uncorrected vision was 20/20. The patient is now more than 2 years after the KPro placement with maintenance of excellent vision and without complications.

invasion by conjunctival stem cells causing recurrent erosions, chronic pain, corneal ulceration, scarring, and vascularization.[6] Treatment with PKP provides short-term visual rehabilitation, but long-term outcomes are poor, due to underlying stem cell deficiency. Keratolimbal allograft can provide visual rehabilitation but requires systemic immunosuppression.[7] The Boston KPro offers another option for the visual rehabilitation of aniridic keratopathy and has the advantage of not requiring immunosuppression.

In a retrospective multicenter study of the Boston KPro in aniridia, 14 of 15 patients experienced improved visual acuity from a median of counting fingers to 20/200.[6] No KPro extrusions were reported throughout a follow-up period ranging from 2 to 85 months. Preoperative optic nerve and foveal hypoplasia limited the final postoperative vision. Further investigation of the Boston KPro as a standard treatment approach to aniridic keratopathy is underway, and results thus far are encouraging.

Use of the Boston KPro in Children

In pediatric PKP, surgically induced astigmatism hinders visual rehabilitation and amblyopia management.[1] In addition, the robust immune response in children leads to an increased risk of immunologic rejection and visually significant corneal neovascularization. The Boston KPro provides rapid visual rehabilitation, thus facilitating amblyopia management in children, and has the additional advantage that there is no risk of rejection.

Very few reports of pediatric KPro have been published. Following the initial report of two cases,[8] a multicenter case series reported outcomes of 21 Boston KPro procedures in pediatric patients (age 1.5 to 136 mo).[9] The most common preoperative diagnoses were failed grafts (55%, mean 3.25 prior grafts) and primary congenital corneal opacity (45%, from Peter anomaly, congenital glaucoma, spontaneous corneal perforations, or dermoid tumor). In patients older than 4 years of age, postoperative visual acuity ranged from

counting fingers to 20/30; all infants were able to follow light, fingers, and objects. The Boston KPro was retained in all cases without dislocation, infection or extrusion, although the reported follow-up was limited, ranging from 1 to 37 months with a mean of 9.7 months. Refraction was stable (and without astigmatism) within days of surgery, facilitating amblyopia management. The rapid refractive stability is one of the main theoretic advantages of this device in children.[9] Refractive error can be managed by changing the power of the bandage contact lens, thus allowing optimal visual acuity to be maintained as the eye grows. However, some pediatric ophthalmologists have expressed concern that limitation of light exposure to the peripheral retina through the 3-mm aperture of the Boston KPro may have untoward effects, such as progressive high myopia in very young children.

The decision to implant a Boston KPro in a child should not be made lightly, but rather must be made with adequate consideration to the many factors that are required for successful long-term outcomes. Most important is parental commitment to regular follow-up with a surgeon experienced with both keratoprosthesis and pediatric corneal surgery, and to the permanent use of a bandage contact lens, topical antibiotics and steroids. One must also weigh the risk of glaucoma and other postoperative complications. While standard keratoplasty is challenging in children, failure to maintain compliance with postoperative medications or follow-up generally only results in failure of the graft. In contrast, with a Boston KPro, failure to have adequate follow-up or use appropriate medications can result in loss of the eye, through devastating infection, or loss of light perception through progression of glaucoma. Adequate follow-up is essential for all Boston KPro patients, but it especially vital for the youngest patients.

Although early reports have shown that the Boston KPro can provide rapid visual recovery in children, further long-term follow-up of children already implanted with this device is essential to determine if the Boston KPro truly represents an advantage over standard keratoplasty in this patient population.

The Boston Keratoprosthesis in Autoimmune Diseases

Patients with ocular autoimmune disorders are typically poor candidates for a traditional PKP, due to concurrent limbal stem cell deficiency and ongoing ocular surface inflammation. Autoimmune diseases, such as Stevens–Johnson syndrome and mucous membrane pemphigoid (MMP) are well established to have the least favorable prognosis for long-term Boston KPro success.[2,10] The high incidence of donor tissue melt and retraction surrounding the central stem of the prosthesis make the use of the Boston KPro in autoimmune eye diseases very challenging, although results have improved over the last 10 years.[11] Corneal melting is thought to be due to the heightened inflammatory response intrinsic to the pathogenesis of these diseases. These patients also have a reduced tear film that allows increased microbial activity and proliferation, which may also contribute to ongoing inflammation and subsequent corneal melt.[11]

In a case series of 15 patients (16 eyes) with SJS who underwent either type I (6 eyes) or type II (10 eyes) Boston KPro surgery, 12 eyes achieved a visual acuity of 20/200 or better after surgery, with eight eyes attaining vision of 20/40 or better. Visual acuity was maintained at 20/200 or better over a mean period of 2.5 years for these 12 eyes. Pre-existing glaucoma was found to be a significant risk factor for visual loss. There were no cases of KPro extrusion or endophthalmitis in this series, which included the addition of topical vancomycin to the postoperative medication regimen.[12]

The Boston KPro has also been used in other autoimmune diseases, including toxic epidermal necrolysis, MMP, and autoimmune polyendocrinopathy–candidiasis–ectodermal dystrophy.[11] Visual acuity can be improved with the Boston KPro, although re-operation is common in patients with underlying autoimmune disease.[11] Further understanding of the pathogenesis of corneal melting in these most challenging conditions and advancements in the use of systemic immunomodulators are necessary before widespread use of the Boston KPro in autoimmune ocular surface diseases can be recommended.

Other Indications for the Boston KPro

The Boston KPro has been successfully used following ocular trauma, including chemical, mechanical, and thermal injury. A recent series of 30 trauma patients with preoperative visual acuity ranging from counting fingers to light perception reported postoperative visual acuity ranging from 20/20 to no light perception.[13] Postoperative complications, including glaucoma continue to be a challenge, especially following chemical injury.

A recent case report showed short-term anatomical and functional success of the type I Boston Kpro for severe vernal keratoconjunctivitis and Mooren's ulcer. The keratoprosthesis was retained in both eyes at 1 year postoperatively with a best corrected visual acuity of 20/30 in both patients.[14]

The Boston KPro can also be used to treat chronic hypotony and corneal opacification.[15–17] Dohlman et al.[15] reported the initial case of bilateral phthisis secondary to alkali burn with visual acuity improving from LP to 20/60 in both eyes over a 5-month period following Boston KPro implantation. Utine et al.[16] reported three monocular patients with chronic hypotony who received a Boston KPro in conjunction with pars plana vitrectomy and silicone oil injection. Functional vision was achieved in two of the three patients. At a follow-up of 11 to 13 months, all three KPros were still in place without retroprosthetic membrane or epithelial defects and with a quiet anterior chamber. A recent retrospective study of patients with silicone oil–induced keratopathy who underwent Boston KPro implantation demonstrated anatomic retention and visual improvement in 7 of 8 eyes.[17] The visual acuity improved to 20/200 or better in six eyes, suggesting that eyes that otherwise were likely to fail another corneal graft and eventually progress to phthisis bulbi might be salvaged with some improvement in visual function.

Outcomes of Boston Keratoprosthesis in Ocular Surface Disease compared with Graft Failure

No studies have specifically compared KPro outcomes in patients with ocular surface disease with those done in patients with failed grafts. Zerbe et al.[18] in the largest series to date showed a retention rate of 97% in non-cicatrizing graft failure (97 cases) and 89% in chemical burn (19 cases), although the follow-up period of this study was limited. Visual acuity of at least 20/200 was maintained in 90% of the graft failure eyes and in 94% of the chemical injury eyes. A more recent study[19] demonstrated more favorable visual outcomes in a small series of type I Boston KPro's done for limbal stem cell failure (23 eyes) when compared with outcomes in KPro's done for other indications at all time points of up to 3 years, possibly due to fewer ocular co-morbidities in this group. In addition, KPro retention was better for the limbal stem cell deficient eyes than those done for other conditions, when cases of Stevens–Johnson syndrome were excluded. The most common complication following KPro in the setting of ocular surface disease was persistent epithelial defects in 56% of cases. Corneal melt was also more common (30%), likely secondary to the high rate of persistent epithelial defect. Further work is needed to better characterize the long-term outcomes and complication rates for Boston KPro in ocular surface diseases, but preliminary data suggest that device retention and visual recovery is favorable in non-cicatrizing ocular surface diseases.

Conclusion

Much progress has been made in the use of the Boston KPro over the last 20 years. The current device is safe and effective for a wide variety of conditions besides graft failure. Selected patients, such as those with anesthetic or vascularized corneas or those with limbal stem cell dysfunction, may benefit from the use of the Boston KPro as a primary procedure, rather than being subject to multiple traditional keratoplasties that have little chance of success. Further research is needed to improve outcomes and reduce complications in the most challenging cases, including children and patients with autoimmune ocular surface diseases.

References

1. Colby KA, Koo EB. Expanding indications for the Boston keratoprosthesis. Curr Opin Ophthalmol 2011;22:267–73.
2. Yaghouti F, Nouri M, Abad JC, et al. Keratoprosthesis: preoperative prognostic categories. Cornea 2001;20:19–23.
3. Khan BF, Harissi-Dagher M, Pavan-Langston D, et al. The Boston keratoprosthesis in herpetic keratitis. Arch Ophthalmol 2007;125:745–9.
4. Todani A, Gupta P, Colby K. Type I Boston keratoprosthesis with cataract extraction and intraocular lens placement for visual rehabilitation of herpes zoster ophthalmicus: the "KPro Triple". Br J Ophthalmol 2009;93:119.
5. Pavan-Langston D, Dohlman CH. Boston keratoprosthesis treatment of herpes zoster neurotrophic keratopathy. Ophthalmology 2008;115(Suppl. 2):S21–3.
6. Akpek EK, Harissi-Dagher M, Petrarca R, et al. Outcomes of Boston keratoprosthesis in aniridia: a retrospective multicenter study. Am J Ophthalmol 2007;144:227–31.
7. Biber JM, Skeens HM, Neff KD, et al. The Cincinnati procedure: technique and outcomes of combined living-related conjunctival limbal allografts and keratolimbal allografts in severe ocular surface failure. Cornea 2011;30:765–71.
8. Botelho PJ, Congdon NG, Handa JT, et al. Keratoprosthesis in high-risk pediatric corneal transplantation: first 2 cases. Arch Ophthalmol 2006;124:1356–7.
9. Aquavella JV, Gearinger MD, Akpek EK, et al. Pediatric keratoprosthesis. Ophthalmology 2007;114:989–94.
10. Dohlman CH, Terada H. Keratoprosthesis in pemphigoid and Stevens–Johnson syndrome. Adv Exp Med Biol 1998;438:1021–5.
11. Ciralsky J, Papaliodis GN, Foster CS, et al. Keratoprosthesis in autoimmune disease. Ocul Immunol Inflamm 2010;18:275–80.
12. Sayegh RR, Ang LP, Foster CS, et al. The Boston keratoprosthesis in Stevens-Johnson syndrome. Am J Ophthalmol 2008;145:438–44.
13. Harissi-Dagher M, Dohlman CH. The Boston keratoprosthesis in severe ocular trauma. Can J Ophthalmol 2008;43:165–9.
14. Basu S, Taneja M, Sangwan VS. Boston type 1 keratoprosthesis for severe blinding vernal keratoconjunctivitis and Mooren's ulcer. Int Ophthalmol 2011;31:219–22.
15. Dohlman CH, D'Amico DJ. Can an eye in phthisis be rehabilitated? A case of improved vision with 1-year follow-up. Arch Ophthalmol 1999;117:123–4.
16. Utine CA, Gehlbach PL, Zimmer-Galler I, et al. Permanent keratoprosthesis combined with pars plana vitrectomy and silicone oil injection for visual rehabilitation of chronic hypotony and corneal opacity. Cornea 2010;29:1401–5.
17. Iyer G, Srinivasan B, Gupta J, et al. Boston keratoprosthesis for keratopathy in eyes with retained silicone oil: a new indication. Cornea 2011;30:1083–7.
18. Zerbe BL, Belin MW, Ciolino JB. Results from the multicenter Boston Type 1 Keratoprosthesis Study. Ophthalmology 2006;113:1779 e1–e7.
19. Sejpal K, Yu F, Aldave AJ. The Boston keratoprosthesis in the management of corneal limbal stem cell deficiency. Cornea 2011;30:1187–94.

50 *Boston Keratoprosthesis Surgical Technique*

CHRISTINA R. PRESCOTT and JAMES CHODOSH

Background

Pellier de Quengsy first proposed the idea of a synthetic or partly synthetic cornea in 1789.[1] Dr. Claes Dohlman began development of the Boston keratoprosthesis in 1965; since then, over 7000 have been implanted.[2] The Boston keratoprosthesis, when constructed, includes four parts (Fig. 50.1). As configured for implantation, the most anterior component is the optic, which is lathed from a single piece of polymethyl methacrylate (PMMA) to form the front plate and its stem. A corneal carrier button (allograft or autograft) permits suturing of the device to host cornea and sits between the front plate and the back plate, which is also made of PMMA. Finally, a C-shaped, titanium locking ring encircles the posterior optic stem and prevents disassembly once the keratoprosthesis is implanted in the eye. Incremental improvements in the device since its inception include a snap-in, rather than screw-in, assembly; the addition of back plate perforations to improve nutrition to the corneal carrier and reduce keratolysis; inclusion of the titanium locking ring (Fig. 50.2); and, currently awaiting approval from the U.S. Food and Drug Administration, a change in back plate material from PMMA to titanium.[3,4] Other advances include the long-term use of antibiotics and soft

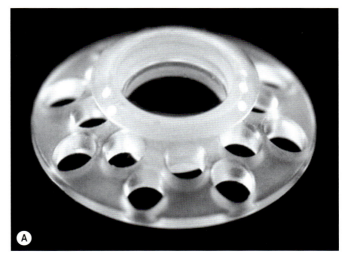

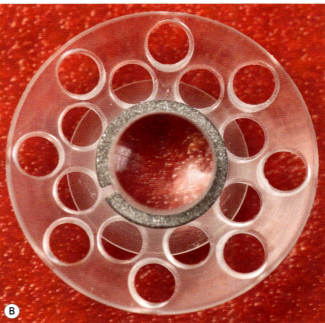

Figure 50.2 (**A**) An assembled Boston Keratoprosthesis type I with a PMMA back plate, without the donor cornea. (Photo courtesy of Claes H. Dohlman, MD, Ph.D.) (**B**) Posterior view of an assembled Boston keratoprosthesis type I shows the PMMA back plate with 16 holes and the titanium locking ring.

Front plate/optic

Back plate

Locking ring

Figure 50.1 Schematic of the Boston keratoprosthesis type I components. The type II design differs only by an anterior extension of the front plate to protrude through closed eyelids.

contact lenses.[5] The Boston keratoprosthesis type I is likely the most commonly implanted artificial cornea worldwide. The Boston keratoprosthesis type II, a modified version of the type I designed to fit through closed eyelids, is used less often.

Once the decision is made to proceed with implantation (see Chapter 49: Keratoprosthesis Indications), a choice must be made whether to implant a type I or type II design. Underlying pathology, as well as completeness of eyelid closure, quality and quantity of preocular tear film, and depth of conjunctival fornices must be determined. The type II device is only utilized in cases of corneal blindness in which damage to the ocular surface and adnexa is extensive enough to make successful retention of the type I device unlikely.[6] Candidate patients for a type II keratoprosthesis typically have ocular surface keratinization, severe aqueous tear deficiency, symblephara, and foreshortening of the fornices.[7]

A detailed preoperative discussion of the risks and benefits of keratoprosthesis implantation is extremely important. Patients must understand that they will need continuous treatment, including daily antibiotics, bandage contact lens wear (for the type I keratoprosthesis), and lifelong follow-up care with a qualified corneal specialist. Long-term follow-up is necessary to maintain patient compliance with medications, recognize and treat indolent infection and early keratolysis, and diagnose new-onset or worsening of pre-existing glaucoma, any of which may compromise the visual gains from the initial surgery and lead to loss of the keratoprosthesis and/or the eye. Patients should also be aware that the cosmetic appearance of the eye will change with keratoprosthesis surgery (Fig. 50.3A), quite notably with the keratoprosthesis type II (Fig. 50.3B). To improve cosmesis following type I keratoprosthesis, some patients choose to wear a painted contact lens. After type II surgery, the cosmetic options are limited to the use of tinted glasses, so patients must receive complete preoperative counseling and be willing to accept this limitation prior to undergoing surgery. For best outcomes in patients with underlying inflammatory and autoimmune conditions, such as Stevens–Johnson syndrome/toxic epidermal necrolysis or mucous membrane pemphigoid, attempts should be made to minimize ocular surface inflammation prior to surgery. This may require use of a systemic immunosuppressive agent, such as mycophenolate mofetil. For chronically immunosuppressed patients, collaboration with a rheumatologist, or other similarly qualified physician, is critical to the long-term preservation of the keratoprosthesis.

Prior to surgery, choices must be made about the specific keratoprosthesis to be ordered and what adjunctive procedures will be performed at the time of surgery. In phakic and aphakic patients, keratoprosthesis power is chosen based on the axial length of the eye. If the patient is already pseudophakic, and the surgeon intends to leave the intraocular lens in place, a pseudophakic keratoprosthesis should be used. If the patient is phakic, lens extraction must be performed at the time of keratoprosthesis surgery. Other procedures performed concurrently with keratoprosthesis implantation may include insertion of a plano intraocular lens, insertion of a glaucoma valve, and possible performance of a pars plana vitrectomy or other retina procedure.

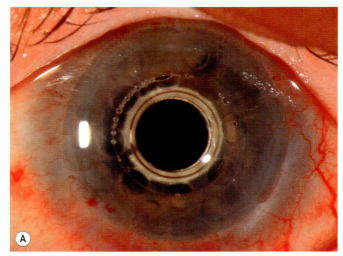

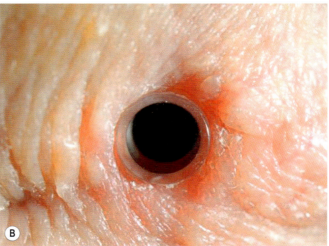

Figure 50.3 Physical appearance after Boston keratoprosthesis type I and type II surgery. (**A**) Clinical photograph of a 37-year-old male patient with a severe alkali burn to both eyes 4 years after type I keratoprosthesis surgery following a failed penetrating keratoplasty. Vision is 20/25 in the keratoprosthesis eye and no light perception in the other eye. (**B**) Close-up clinical photograph of a 57-year-old female with cicatricial corneal blindness following toxic epidermal necrolysis, affecting both eyes, who at the time of the photograph was 5 months post Boston keratoprosthesis type II insertion, with 20/25 vision (from preoperative best vision of hand movements).

In phakic patients, the authors typically plan for implantation of a plano, posterior chamber, intraocular lens at the time of lens extraction, so that the keratoprosthesis power will be appropriate even if capsular support is inadequate to support intraocular lens placement.

Special Considerations for the Boston Keratoprosthesis Type I

As with a standard corneal transplants, the choice of anesthesia for a Boston keratoprosthesis type I depends on both the patient's ocular condition and general health. For most patients, retrobulbar anesthesia is adequate. Patients are prepped and draped in the standard fashion for ophthalmic surgery, using a povidone-iodine 5% preparation in the eye and 10% preparation to the skin. Prior to the first incision, graft size must be chosen based on the corneal pathology and size. The standard keratoprosthesis back plate is 8.5 mm in diameter, although a 7.0-mm back plate is available for pediatric patients and patients with smaller eyes. Because the keratoprosthesis front plate is 5 mm in diameter, the donor graft diameter should never be less than 7 mm, lest the donor corneal rim be insufficient to allow suture fixation. The donor graft diameter is typically trephined to a size 0.5 mm greater than the host trephination diameter, which should be no less than 8 mm when using an 8.5-mm back plate.

Preparation of the Boston Keratoprosthesis Type I

After creation of a sterile field, the presence of all keratoprosthesis components should be verified by visual inspection prior to proceeding with surgery (front plate, back plate, locking ring, and locking pin, the latter used to assemble the device). The donor cornea is then trephined twice: the inner opening is made with a 3.0-mm skin biopsy punch (packaged by the manufacturer with the keratoprosthesis), and the outer trephination is created with a standard corneal donor trephine after diameter selection, as described above. The decision as to which trephination is performed first depends on individual surgeon preference. If eccentric keratoprosthesis placement is indicated, creation of the central corneal trephination should be correspondingly eccentric, thus ensuring proper positioning of the optic at the visual axis.

The keratoprosthesis is then assembled by positioning the optic with the front plate facing down. This can be done on a manufacturer-provided double-sided adhesive, which secures the prosthesis and thus may make assembly easier. The donor cornea's 3-mm opening is then positioned over the stem, endothelial side up, and the cornea is lowered over the stem until the epithelial side contacts the back of the front plate. The back plate is then positioned over the stem, with the concave side up, and is pushed down the stem onto the donor cornea using the locking pin. It is unclear whether healthy corneal endothelium is necessary for successful keratoprosthesis implantation,[8] but a small amount of viscoelastic may be placed on the endothelial surface to minimize trauma. The prosthesis components are then locked into place by placement of the titanium locking ring over the stem. An audible snap, appreciated with gentle downward pressure by the locking pin, indicates proper positioning of the locking ring, although proper positioning of the device should always be confirmed by careful inspection, under magnification, prior to implantation. The fully assembled keratoprosthesis is then placed in corneal preservation medium and kept covered in a sterile container until needed.

Boston keratoprosthesis Type I Surgery

Once the keratoprosthesis is constructed, the patient's cornea is removed using a trephine and corneal scissors, as in traditional penetrating keratoplasty, and is sent for pathologic assessment. The iris is inspected through the corneal opening, and, if corectopia resulting in iris obstruction of the visual axis through the keratoprosthesis optic is present, an iridoplasty is performed. If the patient is phakic, cataract extraction must also be performed. The need for placement of a glaucoma drainage implant at the time of surgery (or later) provides rationale for implantation of a posterior chamber intraocular lens, although surgeon preference dictates whether an intraocular lens is placed or the patient is left aphakic. If the patient is pseudophakic, the intraocular lens is stable, and the surgeon has chosen the pseudophakic-powered keratoprosthesis, the intraocular lens is left in place.[9]

The assembled keratoprosthesis is brought to the operative field, is placed back plate down in the wound and is secured with 12 interrupted 9-0 nylon sutures or 16 interrupted 10-0 nylon sutures. It is particularly important to place and retain a 2–3-mm corneal shield over the keratoprosthesis optic, once the first four cardinal sutures are placed, to avoid phototoxicity to the retina. All corneal sutures are buried in the host tissue, and the wound is checked for leakage.

The authors' standard intraoperative medications include peribulbar vancomycin, 25 mg in 0.5 mL, ceftazidime 100 mg in 0.5 mL, and triamcinolone 20 mg in 0.5 mL, all given at the conclusion of surgery. These must be injected in a peribulbar fashion to avoid ballooning of the conjunctiva and subsequent difficulty in placing a contact lens. The Boston keratoprosthesis is provided with a 16 mm diameter, 9.8 base curve Kontur™ contact lens (Hercules, CA), which is placed over the eye at the conclusion of surgery and remains in place postoperatively. A semi-pressure patch is then placed, followed by a Fox shield. Ophthalmic ointment is unnecessary and should not be used so as to avoid displacement of the contact lens.

Most patients tolerate the procedure very well and have minimal postoperative pain, similar to the nominal pain experienced after penetrating keratoplasty. On the first postoperative day, topical prednisolone acetate 1%, and a topical fluoroquinolone, both administered four times daily, are initiated. Patients also begin topical vancomycin, 14 mg/mL with benzalkonium chloride preservative, administered once daily within the first week of surgery. The prednisolone and fluoroquinolone are tapered to once-daily administration over 2–3 months following surgery. The authors recommend use of at least one drop per day of a broad-spectrum topical antibiotic long term, and for those cases in which secondary infection risk is of particular concern, additionally one drop of topical vancomycin daily. The long-term use of topical corticosteroid is unnecessary in many cases. More frequent use of topical antibiotics is also unnecessary in the long term and may encourage fungal contamination of the contact lens and/or front plate, with subsequent infection.

Special Considerations for the Boston Keratoprosthesis Type II

The Boston keratoprosthesis type II design is comparable to the type I design, with the exception of an anterior extension of the optic to allow implantation through surgically closed eyelids. The device is prepared similarly to the type I keratoprosthesis, and the corneal component of type II surgery is analogous to type I surgery. However, the remainder of the surgical procedure is much more extensive. General anesthesia is indicated in type II implantation, due to the longer duration of the surgery and the extent of periocular tissue dissection involved.

Boston keratoprosthesis Type II Surgery

Because implantation of the Boston keratoprosthesis type II requires complete closure of the eyelids, avoidance of encystment requires removal of all ocular surface epithelium. Prior to trephination of the cornea, existing symblephara are divided, and conjunctival mucosal epithelium is removed with sharp dissection, including bulbar, foniceal, and tarsal conjunctiva. The upper and lower eyelid margins are infiltrated with 1% lidocaine containing epinephrine, and the eyelid margins are excised, with care taken to fully excise all eyelash follicles. After the host corneal trephination diameter has been chosen, the cornea is marked with the appropriate trephine, and the limbal and corneal epithelium peripheral to the marked area are removed using sharp dissection. The host cornea is trephined and removed as above. If the eye has not previously undergone intraocular surgery, it may be reasonable to minimize additional procedures inside the eye (although, the crystalline lens must always be removed). However, since most patients receiving a type II keratoprosthesis have had prior surgery, an aggressive approach is recommended in order to prevent postoperative glaucoma. These patients might benefit from total iridectomy, removal of the lens and its capsule, pars plana vitrectomy, and posterior placement of an Ahmed valve. Such additional procedures often require involvement of both a vitreoretinal and a glaucoma surgeon. The prepared keratoprosthesis is typically secured with 12 interrupted 9-0 nylon sutures. Knots are rotated posteriorly but need not be buried. However, as in keratoprosthesis type I surgery, it is important to keep a cover over the anterior keratoprosthesis optic throughout the surgery to prevent light toxicity to the retina (Fig. 50.4A).

After implantation of the keratoprosthesis, peribulbar antibiotics and corticosteroid are administered as above, and the eyelids are surgically closed around the optic. Two or three interrupted 6-0 Vicryl sutures are placed on each side of the keratoprosthesis (medial and lateral) using partial-thickness tarsal bites. Once the upper and lower tarsi are brought together on either side of the keratoprosthesis stem, the eyelid margins can be gently closed in mattress style with bolsters and 8-0 nylon sutures. Finally, a notch in the upper lid is fashioned with Vannas scissors (Fig. 50.4B) to allow the keratoprosthesis nub to protrude between the eyelids. It is important that this notch be positioned with the eye in primary gaze so that the keratoprosthesis and eyelid opening are properly aligned.

Prior to reversal of general anesthesia, retroseptal antibiotics and corticosteroid are administered as above, and a retrobulbar anesthetic may be injected to reduce postoperative discomfort. Antibiotic ointment is administered over

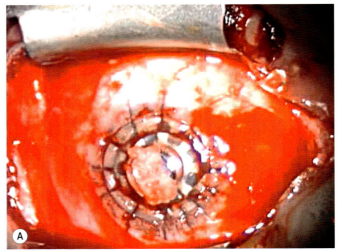

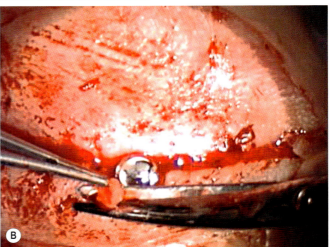

Figure 50.4 Type II keratoprosthesis surgery. (**A**) Appearance of the eye immediately following implantation of the keratoprosthesis and conjunctival dissection. Note the corneal shield. (**B**) Eyelids are closed around the optic and skin is removed with scissors to create a notch for the optic.

the skin closure prior to placement of a gentle patch and Fox shield. Postoperatively, the same eye drop regimen described after type I keratoprosthesis placement is utilized. Antibiotic ointment to the eyelid margins is discontinued 2 weeks postoperatively, at which time the skin sutures and bolsters are removed. If present, elevated intraocular pressure is treated with oral acetazolamide or methazolamide. Topical fluoroquinolones and vancomycin are tapered to twice-daily administration after several weeks, and continued indefinitely to reduce microbial contamination of the skin around the keratoprosthesis optic. Once the eyelid skin has fully healed around the keratoprosthesis, usually by 2–3 weeks postoperatively, topical medications do not penetrate to the eye. Topical glaucoma drops are therefore ineffective in reducing intraocular pressure.

Conclusion

Boston keratoprosthesis implantation is a procedure that can be performed by any experienced corneal transplant surgeon, and an important treatment option for patients with severe corneal pathology, who are motivated to improve their vision. Recipient eyes require lifelong care and follow-up.

References

1. deQuengsy GP. Precis au cours d'operations sur la chirurgie des yeux. Paris: Didot; 1789.
2. Klufas MA, Colby KA. The Boston keratoprosthesis. Int Ophthalmol Clin 2010;50:161–75.
3. Khan BF, Harissi-Dagher M, Khan DM, et al. Advances in Boston keratoprosthesis: enhancing retention and prevention of infection and inflammation. Int Ophthalmol Clin 2007;47:61–71.
4. Todani A, Ciolino JB, Ament JD, et al. Titanium back plate for a PMMA keratoprosthesis: clinical outcomes. Graefes Arch Clin Exp Ophthalmol 2011;249:1515–8.
5. Dohlman CH, Dudenhoefer EJ, Khan BF, et al. Protection of the ocular surface after keratoprosthesis surgery: the role of soft contact lenses. CLAO J 2002;28:72–4.
6. Ciralsky J, Papaliodis GN, Foster CS, et al. Keratoprosthesis in autoimmune disease. Ocul Immunol Inflamm 2010;18:275–80.
7. Pujari S, Siddique SS, Dohlman CH, et al. The Boston keratoprosthesis type II: the Massachusetts Eye and Ear Infirmary experience. Cornea 2011;30:1298–303.
8. Robert MC, Biernacki K, Harissi-Dagher M. Boston Keratoprosthesis type 1 surgery: use of frozen versus fresh corneal donor carriers. Cornea 2012;31:339–45.
9. Utine CA, Tzu JH, Dunlap K, et al. Visual and clinical outcomes of explantation versus preservation of the intraocular lens during Boston type I keratoprosthesis implantation. J Cataract Refract Surg 2011;37:1615–22.

Boston Keratoprosthesis Complications

MARK A. GREINER, JENNIFER Y. LI, and MARK J. MANNIS

Introduction

Many of the complications associated with the Boston type 1 and type 2 keratoprosthesis (KPro) have been addressed successfully through design alterations, surgical technique modifications, and medical therapy. Despite this, KPro implantation remains a surgery of last resort, in part because the complications can result in permanent vision loss (Table 51.1). Although the use of a donor cornea improves the biocompatibility and ease of implantation, complications related to implant integration after Boston KPro surgery remain of significant concern, including implant extrusion, periprosthetic tissue necrosis, and infection. The ocular surface is the gateway to many of these complications. In this chapter, the authors describe the complications associated with the Boston keratoprosthesis, with special emphasis on the role of the ocular surface in the pathology.

Epithelial Defects and Contact Lens Related Complications

Epithelial defects on the donor or recipient cornea can be problematic after Boston KPro implantation and, as expected, occur more frequently in dry eye, inflammatory, and stem cell deficiency states. Given the elevated profile of the KPro's anterior plate relative to the donor cornea, the surrounding ocular surface is more vulnerable to evaporative forces and dellen formation,[1] and the area adjacent to the anterior plate in particular has been associated with persistent epithelial defects.[2] In addition to this mechanical disadvantage, chronic ocular surface dryness and an inhospitable ocular surface related to the preoperative diagnosis can also lead to epithelial defects. Frequently, one or more of the common mechanisms contributing to KPro related epithelial defects – diminished aqueous production from

Table 51.1 Postoperative Complications after Boston Type 1 Keratoprosthesis Implantation

Study Group No. Keratoprosthesis Eyes Average Follow-up	NYEE 2011 n = 58 22 mon	UC Davis 2011 n = 40 34 mon	JSEI 2009 n = 50 17 mon	WEI 2009 n = 37* 16 mon	Multicenter 2006 n = 141 8.5 mon
Postoperative Complications			**No. Eyes (%)**		
Retroprosthetic membrane	29 (50)	22 (55)	22 (44)	24 (65)	35 (25)
YAG membranotomy	17 (29)	10 (25)	17 (34)	8 (22)	26 (18)
Surgical membranectomy		5 (13)	5 (10)	1 (3)	4 (3)
Glaucoma	44 (76)	34 (85)	38 (76)	32 (86)	
Elevated intraocular pressure	15 (26)	16 (40)	9 (18)	14 (38)	21 (15)
New diagnosis postoperatively		11 (28)		5 (14)	
Progression		9 (23)		5 (14)	
End-stage		7 (18)			
GDD erosion		9 (23)		2 (5)	
ECP		3 (8)			
CPC	1 (2)	2 (5)			
New GDD implant	2 (3)	2 (5)	1 (2)	2 (5)	11 (8)
Endophthalmitis	1 (2)	5 (13)		4 (11)	
Corneal melt	2 (3)	6 (15)	8 (16)	3 (8)	1 (1)
Keratoprosthesis extrusion	2 (3)	6 (15)		1 (3)*	1 (1)
Keratoprosthesis replacement	4 (7)	7 (18)	5 (10)	1 (3)*	
Keratoprosthesis removal	3 (5)	4 (10)			7 (5)
Retinal detachment	6 (10)		4 (8)	1(3)	5 (4)
Other posterior segment	10 (17)		14 (28)	7 (18)	21 (15)

*= Includes one type II Boston keratoprosthesis.
NYEE: New York Eye and Ear Infirmary. See manuscript text reference no. 8.
UC Davis: University of California Davis Health System Eye Center. See manuscript text reference no. 3.
JSEI: Jules Stein Eye Institute. See manuscript text reference no. 2.
WEI: Wills Eye Institute. See manuscript text reference no. 6.
Multicenter: Boston Type 1 Keratoprosthesis Study Group. See manuscript text reference no. 7.

conjunctival scarring, evaporative dysfunction from meibomian gland scarring, exposure keratopathy from lagophthalmos, and trichiasis from cicatricial entropion – is associated with the pathology prompting KPro surgery. Occult microbial keratitis without corneal infiltrate can prevent epithelialization, and positive fungal and bacterial cultures of persistent epithelial defects with resolution after appropriate antimicrobial treatment have been documented.[2] Regardless of the cause, epithelial defects place the donor cornea at risk for further tissue destruction from collagenases, as well as other enzymes released from polymorphonuclear leukocytes in the tear film.[1] These defects can ultimately lead to keratolysis, implant extrusion, microbial keratitis, and endophthalmitis.

Treatment of a persistent epithelial defect after KPro implantation is approached as one would after penetrating keratoplasty (PK), with copious lubrication, emollient ointments or consideration of bandage soft contact lens (SCL) placement and lateral tarsorrhaphy. Medial tarsorrhaphy may be necessary if lateral tarsorrhaphy does not cover the area of concern sufficiently. Procedures to provide additional coverage of the defective area with a conjunctival flap or mucosal grafts may be required and performed at the time of tarsorrhaphy. Additionally, a lamellar patch graft using donor corneal tissue may be needed with or without conjunctival, mucosal or amniotic membrane graft coverage. Attention should also be paid to the toxicity profile of topical eye drops required for treatment, with an attempt to minimize toxic preservative-containing agents when possible.

The routine use of a wide-diameter contact lens, typically a Kontur™ hydrogel SCL of 16-mm diameter or larger (Kontur Kontact Lens Co., Inc., Hercules, CA), helps prevent and treat epithelial defects and reduces the risk of corneal infection and melting. A suitable contact lens fit maintains a thin tear meniscus, especially around the anterior plate, and diminishes evaporative forces to achieve better hydration of the corneal surface. In the presence of an epithelial defect, the SCL promotes epithelialization by acting as a mechanical barrier protecting the vulnerable corneal surface from the shear forces of blinking and may limit access of polymorphonuclear leukocytes to the underlying tissue, thereby retarding stromal keratolysis.[1] Postoperative use of a SCL may also provide improved comfort for patients bothered by the anterior plate edge, correction of spherical refractive error, and in the case of tinted lenses, diminished glare and photophobia with improved cosmesis.[1] Typically, KPro surgeons replace the SCL on a periodic basis and/or whenever there is debris build-up on the lens surface, since the deposits can adversely affect vision and represent a nidus for attachment of microbes (Fig. 51.1).

SCL use after Boston KPro surgery has improved outcomes, but bandage contact lens use per se is not free of complications. Difficulty retaining the SCL can be problematic, and patients with multiple contact lens dislocations require particular attention. Replacement requires additional office visits and contributes significantly to the real cost of the prosthesis. As with any SCL, infection can occur and has been reported with the Kontur™ SCL used in conjunction with KPro surgery, although the majority of reported Kontur™ SCL-related infections have occurred in patients with a history of glaucoma surgery.[1,3,4] Kontur™

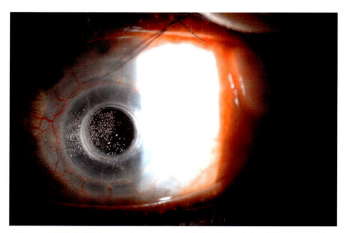

Figure 51.1 Soft contact lens with debris limiting vision in an eye with a Boston keratoprosthesis.

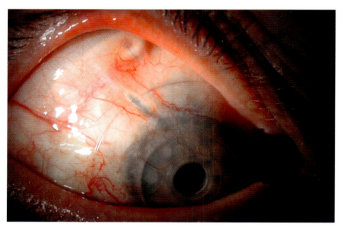

Figure 51.2 Erosion of glaucoma drainage device after Boston keratoprosthesis surgery. Focal mechanical trauma of the bandage contact lens edge and ocular surface dysfunction contributes to the erosion of these devices.

SCLs have been associated, in particular, with glaucoma drainage tube erosion (Fig. 51.2).[5,6] In the series reported by Li et al., one-third of patients with glaucoma drainage device (GDD) erosion incurred conjunctival breakdown at the edge of contact lens. In that series, the erosion event was implicated in the development of endophthalmitis and periprosthetic infection leading to extrusion in two eyes, despite daily prophylaxis with vancomycin. Presumably, the focal mechanical trauma of the contact lens edge on top of the GDD, in combination with a dysfunctional ocular surface, contributes to the erosion of these devices. Although an SCL is needed to protect the ocular surface, careful attention must be paid at each follow-up visit to the status of all hardware in KPro eyes and, in particular, to glaucoma surgical sites to detect erosion and infection.

The initial strategy to promote retention of the SCL is lateral tarsorrhaphy, although some patients will experience recurrent contact lens dislocation despite this and may require medial tarsorrhaphy or further lid surgery to address any underlying lid malposition. A promising

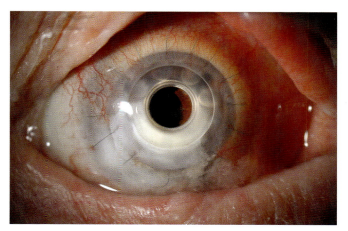

Figure 51.3 Periprosthetic infiltrate on the donor tissue after Boston keratoprosthesis surgery. The suspicion for microbial keratitis should be very high.

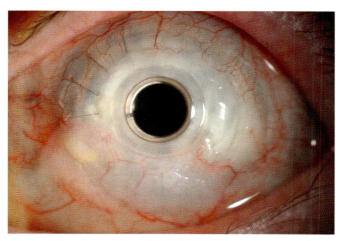

Figure 51.4 Fungal keratitis after Boston keratoprosthesis implantation.

approach to the problem of SCL retention, especially in KPro patients with a dry ocular surface, is refitting with a scleral rigid gas-permeable (RGP) contact lens. Scleral RGP lenses are an underappreciated option in the treatment of patients with ectasia, irregular astigmatism, and ocular surface disease. Design features of modern scleral RGP lenses allow for successful fitting of eyes with challenging contours, including GDDs and foreshortened fornices. Modern fluid-ventilated scleral RGP lenses create an expanded pre-corneal tear film over the ocular surface, and some designs do not contact the ocular surface at all. Although expensive, this device appears to be well tolerated and may prove to be useful in ocular surface management after KPro surgery.

Corneal Infiltrates

Infiltrates can occur on the donor or recipient cornea, and although the location of the infiltrate relative to the implant is important for structural integrity, an etiology may not be presumed based on location alone. Donor corneal infiltrates may be inflammatory and sterile, but with bacterial and fungal isolates recovered in all of the major series in the KPro literature,[2,3,6–8] the suspicion for microbial keratitis should be very high (Fig. 51.3). Risk factors for bacterial keratitis after KPro surgery include significant blepharitis, noncompliance with the postoperative chronic antibacterial eye drop regimen, lid abnormalities, and the presence of other surgical hardware in the eye, including GDDs.[5] Risk factors for fungal keratitis after KPro surgery include use of a contact lens and topical vancomycin,[9] and similar to PK, topical steroid administration. Corneal infiltrates may be diagnosed clinically as infectious, but a corneal scraping for Gram stain and bacterial and fungal cultures typically is performed. Persistent epithelial defects may also be considered for culture, given the possibility of occult microbial keratitis.[2] Although the ocular surface is commonly colonized with Gram-positive organisms, it is important to ensure that antibacterial treatment of a corneal infiltrate covers both Gram-negative and Gram-positive microbes,

since most patients will already have been receiving daily vancomycin prophylaxis, and a selection pressure is placed on an eye with administration of topical vancomycin alone.[3]

Fungal keratitis is of particular concern after KPro surgery for its morbidity and increased incidence in this era of routine SCL and topical vancomycin use (Fig. 51.4). As Barnes and colleagues reported,[9] *Candida* species colonize and can cause devastating infections after KPro surgery. However, since none of the eyes in which surveillance cultures were performed developed fungal keratitis or endophthalmitis, surveillance cultures do not appear to be useful predictors of fungal infection. It is also imperative to consider treatment with topical and possibly oral antifungal agents when suspicion for fungal infiltrates is high.

Corneal Melts and Implant Extrusion

Corneal melting may result from desiccation of the ocular surface and erosion into the donor stroma, immune-related inflammation, keratolysis, and infection. More frequently, corneal melts are an inflammatory rather than an infectious complication. Preoperative diagnoses associated with corneal melting include Stevens–Johnson syndrome (SJS), ocular cicatricial pemphigoid (OCP), and aniridia, all of which predispose the prosthesis to an inhospitable, poorly hydrated and stem cell-deficient ocular surface (Fig. 51.5).[10] When assessing the status of the implant at postoperative examination, it is of particular importance to examine the area of cornea adjacent to the anterior plate carefully because of its vulnerability to chronic desiccation, persistent epithelial defects, and consequent melting. Seidel testing should be performed routinely to look for aqueous leaks, with special attention paid to areas adjacent to hardware and any regions of thinning and erosion. Regardless of etiology, progression of an erosion through Bowman's layer into stroma – and through the stroma – can occur quickly, and extrusion of implant hardware may occur spontaneously (Fig. 51.6).

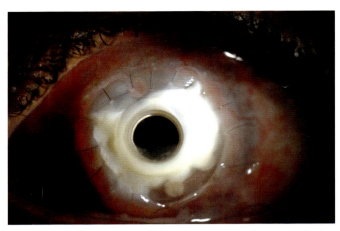

Figure 51.5 Corneal melt and necrosis after Boston keratoprosthesis surgery in a patient with a history of rheumatoid arthritis.

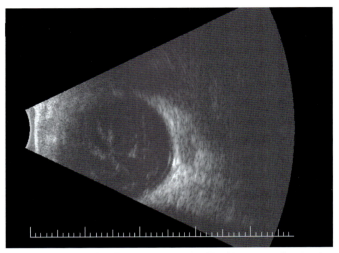

Figure 51.7 B-scan concerning for endophthalmitis after Boston keratoprosthesis surgery. Prior glaucoma surgery is one of several risk factors for this complication.

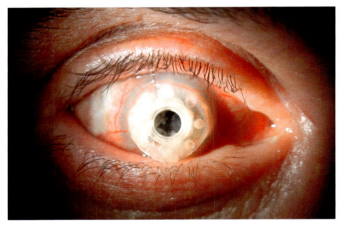

Figure 51.6 Extrusion of Boston keratoprosthesis implant.

Although corneal melting typically leads to further morbidity and intervention, it does not always lead directly to vision loss – even in high-risk patients with as SJS[11] and rheumatoid arthritis.[3] Treatment of corneal melts can extend the life of the implant and maintain useful ambulatory vision. Initial treatment of a corneal melt is fundamentally similar to treatment of a persistent epithelial defect. Copious lubrication, SCL placement, and early consideration of tarsorrhaphy are cornerstones of the approach to this difficult problem. Additionally, patients may be treated with oral doxycycline to help inhibit matrix metalloproteinase activity. In cases of aqueous leak, anatomic stability needs to be achieved either with cyanoacrylate glue application to temporize, followed by wound revision, KPro replacement if warranted, or explantation with PK.

Endophthalmitis

Although endophthalmitis after KPro surgery can be bacterial or fungal in origin, infection typically occurs with Gram-positive bacteria, reflecting the central role of commensal organisms of the ocular surface in this devastating

complication (Fig. 51.7). In their landmark study of bacterial endophthalmitis prevention and the Boston KPro, Durand and Dohlman[12] found that the addition of vancomycin eye drops (14 mg/mL) to a fluoroquinolone eye drop was effective in preventing bacterial endophthalmitis in KPro eyes. That study included 255 eyes with type I and type II Boston KPros, noted a reduction in the rate of endophthalmitis from 4.13% without vancomycin to 0.35% with vancomycin per patient-year, and has influenced the practice of most KPro surgeons. However, it is imperative to pay particular attention to the possibility of Gram-negative and fungal infections, due to selection pressure from inclusion of vancomycin in the antibiotic regimen. Of the five eyes that developed endophthalmitis at UC Davis, all were using vancomycin eye drops at the time of infection; three developed Gram-negative infections and one developed a fungal infection. Clearly, there is a need for long-term treatment with antibiotics that cover for Gram-negative in addition to Gram-positive organisms in the postoperative treatment regimen.

Several risk factors have been associated with endophthalmitis after KPro surgery. Most significantly, prior glaucoma surgery appears to be a risk factor, with reports of endophthalmitis developing in eyes with prior trabeculectomy and GDD implants.[1,3,4] Given that the conjunctiva has been violated surgically, and glaucoma drainage hardware is often present, there may be a greater risk for infection with virulent organisms that do not typically grow on the ocular surface in these eyes. Other risk factors include preoperative SJS, OCP, and chemical burns, although a substantial number of endophthalmitis cases have occurred in eyes with prior graft failures. Treatment noncompliance, keratitis, aqueous leak, and hardware exposure are also clear risk factors for endophthalmitis.

In cases of a sudden onset of pain, intraocular inflammation and decreased vision suspected of endophthalmitis, samples of aqueous, vitreous or both are obtained and submitted for culture. Treatment typically includes vitreous aspirate or vitrectomy plus intraocular injection of antibiotics as soon as possible. When exposed hardware is present in the setting of infection, irrigation of the affected site, explantation of affected and possibly nonaffected hardware, closure of the globe, and repeat KPro implantation or PK may all be considered, depending on the clinical findings and anatomical status of the infected eye. The sequelae of endophthalmitis generally include intraocular membrane formation, and the prognosis for vision recovery is guarded.

Sterile Vitritis

Sterile vitritis may occur after KPro surgery, with clinical features that can masquerade as endophthalmitis. An incidence of approximately 5% was documented in the definitive study of this complication by Nouri et al.[13] Hallmark characteristics – and distinguishing findings that separate this entity from endophthalmitis – include sudden-onset vision loss with little to no discomfort or conjunctival injection, massive 'snowflake' vitritis, and anterior chamber reaction. The etiology is unclear, and no clear associations with preoperative conditions have been discerned, due to its low incidence, but it is generally thought to represent an immune-related uveitis. Although the diagnosis is clinical, the work-up typically involves vitreous aspiration or vitrectomy for culture to rule out infection. Treatment generally includes injection of broad-spectrum antibiotics, as well as corticosteroids. Unlike in endophthalmitis, visual acuity typically recovers to pre-episode levels within weeks with appropriate treatment.

Retroprosthetic Membranes

Retroprosthetic membrane (RPM) formation is the most common complication after Boston KPro implantation. These membranes develop in the early postoperative period,[6] can be refractory to initial treatment with yttrium–aluminum–garnet (YAG) laser capsulotomy, and can limit vision significantly (Fig. 51.8). The histopathology of membranes refractory to initial YAG capsulotomy reveal compact, fibrous, multilayered membranes comprising host stroma admixed with multiple cellular and extracellular components, including iris stroma, metastatic lens epithelium, lens capsule, myofibroblasts and collagen.[14] In addition to stromal downgrowth from the host cornea, epithelial downgrowth from the ocular surface has been implicated in RPM formation.[15] Factors contributing to RPM formation include inflammation, as well as breaks in Descemet's membrane induced by contact with the back plate, which allows a pathway for migration of stroma.[14] The use of a back plate constructed from titanium rather than polymethyl methacrylate may reduce the frequency of RPM formation,[16] a difference that appears to be significant both statistically and clinically. However, widespread incorporation of the titanium back plate has not yet occurred at the time of writing, and the clinical impact of this design modification remains to be seen.

Although YAG laser membranotomy is successful in many cases, early treatment is warranted because of the progressive nature of these membranes. RPMs that recur after laser present a substantial problem to patients and physicians and generally require surgical intervention, via either a pars plana membranectomy or possibly replacement of the KPro (Fig. 51.9). One concern with YAG laser membranotomy is the risk of pitting or cracking of the PMMA optic within the KPro device during the laser procedure. This occurrence may ultimately affect visual acuity regardless of complete membrane removal, and care must be taken to avoid this complication, if possible.

Glaucoma

Glaucoma represents the most significant complication of Boston KPro surgery. Glaucoma after KPro is often resistant to treatment and may lead to permanent vision loss. It is frequently present prior to KPro surgery and, as with PK, may develop or worsen after KPro surgery, due to progressive angle closure from peripheral anterior synechiae or anterior segment crowding, trabecular meshwork collapse, forward rotation of a residual iris stump, or steroid response. The current method of monitoring intraocular pressure (IOP) palpation is inaccurate and can lead to a loss of IOP

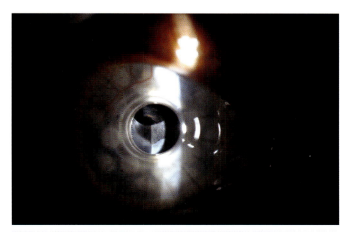

Figure 51.8 Retroprosthetic membrane after Boston keratoprosthesis surgery.

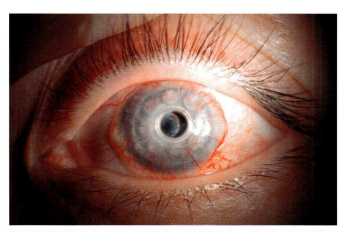

Figure 51.9 Persistence of retroprosthetic membrane after YAG membranotomy, requiring surgical membranectomy.

control, although promising developments in tonometry technology are on the horizon. Humphrey and Goldmann visual fields and retinal nerve fiber layer analysis of the optic nerve head are useful for monitoring the health of the optic nerve, but a compromised view in to the posterior pole may not allow for adequate perimetry, optic nerve examination or imaging. Moreover, the small optical entrance of the KPro can produce generalized constriction of the visual field. Together, limitations in both tonometry and optic nerve imaging/assessment complicate postoperative monitoring and increase the probability of glaucoma progression (Fig. 51.10). Progressive nerve dysfunction and end-stage glaucomatous optic neuropathy can occur despite close monitoring.[3,6] Awareness of other glaucoma-related events that cause vision loss, including branch retinal vein occlusion and loss of fixation, should be high.

Given that a significant number of patients are diagnosed preoperatively with glaucoma and postoperatively with glaucoma progression, some authors have advocated for implantation of GDDs in eyes with marginal IOP control. Although these devices can achieve IOP control and prevent glaucoma progression, they have been associated with complications that can cause vision loss. Li and colleagues recently evaluated the long-term safety and efficacy of GDDs, including Ahmed glaucoma valves and Baerveldt glaucoma implants, in this patient population.[5] The authors found that glaucoma drainage tube erosions occurred in 10 of 40 eyes and led to endophthalmitis in at least two cases. Risk factors for GDD erosion include GDD implantation prior to KPro surgery (older tubes are more likely to erode), localized trauma of the contact lens edge on top of the tube, and the presence of hardware known to be associated with erosions, such as Hoffman elbows. In addition to avoiding hardware known to be associated with erosions, their study recommended considering an approach to GDD implantation that minimizes contact between the tube and contact lens and maximizes coverage of the tube with tissue and/or graft reinforcement. Alternatives, such as trans-scleral or endoscopic cyclophotocoagulation should be considered carefully in glaucoma management with the Boston KPro. The authors also concluded that pre-surgical evaluation for glaucoma and involvement of the glaucoma specialist in the pre-surgical assessment of all KPro patients is mandatory. The UC Davis group commonly places a stage I Baerveldt GDD at the time of the initial KPro surgery for hook-up at a later date if necessary.

Retinal Detachment

The incidence of retinal detachment (RD) was reported at 12% in the largest study of posterior segment complications after KPro surgery (Fig. 51.11).[17] In that series, RDs that occurred in isolation or with treatable vitreous opacities (including RPM and hemorrhage) had some recovery in vision, but RDs that were associated with other retinal pathology (including proliferative vitreoretinopathy and subretinal fibrosis) had no improvement or a decline in vision after surgery. Due to the presence of foreshortened anterior segment anatomy, modifications to standard trans-conjunctival pars plana vitrectomy approaches are required, including placement of incisions as anteriorly as possible.

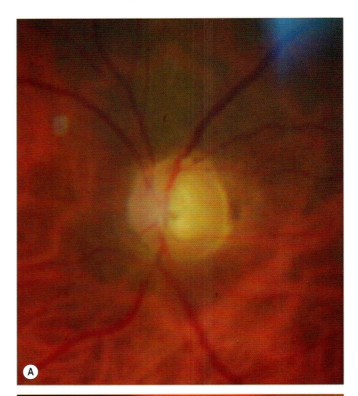

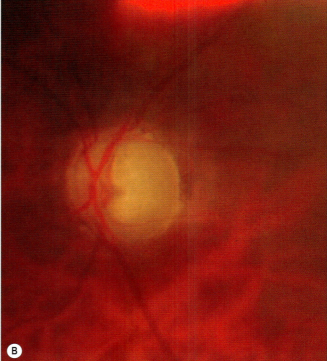

Figure 51.10 Early glaucomatous cupping of the optic nerve after Boston keratoprosthesis surgery (**A**). Advanced glaucomatous cupping of the optic nerve after Boston keratoprosthesis (**B**).

Retinal and choroidal detachments occur more frequently after type II Boston KPro implantation, which has been speculated to result from chronic inflammation causing vitreoretinal traction and subsequent RD in this population enriched with SJS and OCP patients.[18] Retinal surgeons are

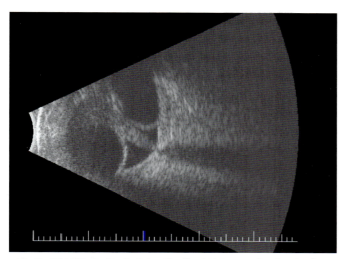

Figure 51.11 Funnel retinal detachment and serous choroidal detachment in an eye with a type 1 Boston keratoprosthesis.

hampered by limitations in visibility of the retinal periphery when faced with the need for performing pars plana vitrectomy or RD repair in the KPro patient. In patients who are at high risk for post-surgical retinal pathology, collaborative evaluation of the patient by the retina surgeons preoperatively is important.

Conclusion

The decision to undertake keratoprosthesis surgery in a patient should be based on careful consideration of the likelihood of postoperative complications. This will require a careful assessment of the viability and function of the ocular surface, the ocular adnexa, the presence or absence of glaucoma, anatomic risk factors for developing glaucoma, and predisposition to accompanying retinal pathology. For this reason, KPro surgery should be undertaken only when visual dysfunction is significant enough to warrant the associated risks of complication and when collaborating subspecialists (glaucoma, retina, and oculoplastics) are available to the cornea surgeon in a team approach.

References

1. Dohlman CH, Dudenhoefer EJ, Khan BF, et al. Protection of the ocular surface after keratoprosthesis surgery: the role of soft contact lenses. CLAO J 2002;28:72–4.
2. Aldave AJ, Kamal KM, Vo RC, et al. The Boston type I keratoprosthesis: improving outcomes and expanding indications. Ophthalmology 2009;116:640–51.
3. Greiner MA, Li JY, Mannis MJ. Longer-term vision outcomes and complications with the Boston type 1 keratoprosthesis at the University of California, Davis. Ophthalmology 2011;118:1543–50.
4. Tsui I, Uslan DZ, Hubschman JP, et al. *Nocardia farcinica* infection of a Baerveldt implant and endophthalmitis in a patient with a Boston type 1 keratoprosthesis. J Glaucoma 2010;19:339–40.
5. Li JY, Greiner MA, Brandt JD, et al. Long-term complications associated with glaucoma drainage devices and Boston keratoprosthesis. Am J Ophthalmol 2011;152:209–18.
6. Chew HF, Ayres BD, Hammersmith KM, et al. Boston keratoprosthesis outcomes and complications. Cornea 2009;28:989–96.
7. Zerbe BL, Belin MW, Ciolino JB. Boston Type 1 Keratoprosthesis Study Group. Results from the multicenter Boston Type 1 Keratoprosthesis Study. Ophthalmology 2006;113:1779.e1–e7.
8. Patel AP, Wu EI, Ritterband DC, et al. Boston type 1 keratoprosthesis: the New York Eye and Ear experience. Eye 2011;26:418–25.
9. Barnes SD, Dohlman CH, Durand ML. Fungal colonization and infection in Boston keratoprosthesis. Cornea 2007;26:9–15.
10. Yaghouti F, Nouri M, Abad JC, et al. Keratoprosthesis: preoperative prognostic categories. Cornea 2001;20:19–23.
11. Sayegh RR, Ang LP, Foster CS, et al. The Boston keratoprosthesis in Stevens–Johnson syndrome. Am J Ophthalmol 2008;145:438–44.
12. Durand ML, Dohlman CH. Successful prevention of bacterial endophthalmitis in eyes with the Boston keratoprosthesis. Cornea 2009;28:896–901.
13. Nouri M, Durand ML, Dohlman CH. Sudden reversible vitritis after keratoprosthesis: an immune phenomenon? Cornea 2005;24:915–9.
14. Stacy RC, Jakobiec FA, Michaud NA, et al. Characterization of retrokeratoprosthetic membranes in the Boston type 1 keratoprosthesis. Arch Ophthalmol 2011;129:310–6.
15. Dudenhoefer EJ, Nouri M, Gipson IK, et al. Histopathology of explanted collar button keratoprostheses: a clinicopathologic correlation. Cornea 2003;22:424–8.
16. Todani A, Ciolino JB, Ament JD, et al. Titanium back plate for a PMMA keratoprosthesis: clinical outcomes. Graefes Arch Clin Exp Ophthalmol 2011;249:1515–8.
17. Ray S, Khan BF, Dohlman CH, et al. Management of vitreoretinal complications in eyes with permanent keratoprosthesis. Arch Ophthalmol 2002;120:559–66.
18. Pujari S, Siddique SS, Dohlman CH, et al. The Boston keratoprosthesis type II: the Massachusetts Eye and Ear Infirmary experience. Cornea 2011;30:1298–303.

52 Boston Keratoprosthesis Outcomes

JENNIFER Y. LI, MARK A. GREINER, and MARK J. MANNIS

Introduction

The Boston Keratoprosthesis™ (Boston KPro) was developed at the Massachusetts Eye and Ear Infirmary for the treatment of corneal blindness in patients who otherwise have a poor prognosis for a standard penetrating keratoplasty (PKP). Since its approval by the FDA in 1992, the Boston KPro has become the most commonly used keratoprosthesis device in the United States. Over 3500 Boston keratoprosthesis devices have been implanted worldwide, with the vast majority having been implanted since 2006.[1]

The Boston type I KPro is the more commonly used model and has been studied more extensively. Several groups in the United States have evaluated outcomes of the Boston type I keratoprosthesis, and we now have both short-term and long-term outcome data for these patients. We review these results and discuss outcomes for specific groups of patients undergoing keratoprosthesis surgery.

Advances in the Boston Keratoprosthesis to Improve Outcomes

Several advances in both the design of the Boston type I keratoprosthesis and in our understanding of the postoperative management of these patients have led to improved outcomes and contributed to the popularity of the surgery.[1] Major postoperative complications, such as corneal melting, keratoprosthesis extrusion, and endophthalmitis can lead to removal of the keratoprosthesis and significant vision loss. However, even retroprosthetic membranes, which are the most common postoperative complications after keratoprosthesis surgery, may lead to vision decline.

Current design features of the Boston keratoprosthesis that have helped to improve retention of the KPro include holes in the back plate of the KPro, a threadless design, and a titanium locking ring.[2-4] The holes in the back plate of the KPro allow nutrients, such as glucose to pass from the aqueous to the corneal carrier tissue.[2] An early study showed a statistically significant decrease in tissue necrosis or melt around a keratoprosthesis from 51% of eyes with a solid PMMA back plate to 10% of eyes of eyes with a back plate with holes.[2] The threadless design of the stem of the KPro prevents misthreading or inadequate threading of the back plate, a design that previously led to gaps between the front plate and the cornea carrier tissue and resulting anterior protrusion of the front.[3] Anterior protrusion of the KPro was associated with tissue melting around the stem.[3] The titanium locking ring helps prevent intraocular loosening of the KPro postoperatively.[4]

Postoperatively, the use of a bandage contact lens and long-term vancomycin drops has been instrumental to reducing vision-threatening complications of keratoprosthesis surgery. Bandage contact lenses improve outcomes by decreasing the risk of corneal melting from desiccation of the ocular surface.[5]

Long-term topical vancomycin eye drops (14 mg/mL) help decrease the risk of bacterial endophthalmitis.[6] Bacterial endophthalmitis is a devastating complication associated with a very poor visual outcome.[6] In their retrospective review of bacterial endophthalmitis in KPro eyes between 1990 and 2006, Durand and Dohlman. found that only two of 18 eyes regained useful vision.[6] Eight of 18 eyes in their review lost light perception vision entirely, with five eyes retaining only hand motions or light reception vision.[6] Fortunately, they also found a statistically significant lower incidence of bacterial endophthalmitis in patients on topical vancomycin prophylaxis, compared with those on a single commercially available antibiotic agent alone (0.35% versus 4.13% per patient-year, $p=0.001$).[6] Keratoprosthesis surgeons now routinely use topical vancomycin in combination with another commercially available broad-spectrum antibiotic agent. although the precise regimen varies among surgeons.[1]

Finally, decreasing the frequency of retroprosthetic membrane formation may also help improve long-term visual outcomes after KPro surgery. Although visually significant retroprosthetic membranes can typically be treated with a simple YAG membranotomy, some membranes may be refractory to laser treatment, causing a decline in vision and necessitating more aggressive surgical removal.[7-9] In some instances, the retroprosthetic membrane may be recalcitrant even to surgical removal.[9] A titanium back plate for the Boston keratoprosthesis is currently being evaluated at the Massachusetts Eye and Ear Infirmary. The preliminary findings are encouraging, with a trend towards decreased postoperative inflammation and less frequent formation of retroprosthetic membranes in patients with a titanium back plate.[10]

Early Postoperative Outcomes of the Boston Type 1 Keratoprosthesis

Early postoperative outcomes for the Boston type 1 keratoprosthesis are generally excellent. Table 52.1 highlights

Table 52.1 Shorter-term Outcomes of Boston Keratoprosthesis Surgery: Average Follow-up Period Less than 12 Months

Author, Year	Number of Eyes	Average Follow-up Period (Range)	Visual Acuity	Retention Rate at Last Follow-up Visit
Zerbe et al., 2006[7]	136	8.5 months (0.03–24 months)	Pre op : 3.6% ≥ 20/200 Post op: 57% ≥ 20/200 19% ≥ 20/40	95.2% in 62 eyes with a least 1 year follow-up
Robert et al., 2011[12]	47	10 months (3–18.5 months)	Pre op: 6% > 20/200 Post op: 66% > 20/200 11% > 20/40	100%
Dunlap et al., 2010[11]	126	6 months	Pre op: 29% > 20/400 Post op: @ 3 months: 54% ≥ 20/200 18% ≥ 20/40	100%

studies looking at shorter-term outcomes (average follow-up period < 12 months). Within the first few months after surgery, visual improvement is often drastic. Dunlap et al. reported short-term visual outcomes of the Boston type I keratoprosthesis and found that in their series of 126 eyes, 82.5% (104 eyes) had improved visual acuity within the first 6 months.[11] Of those 104 eyes, 31 eyes (30%) achieved best-corrected vision within 1 week of surgery.[11] By postoperative month 1, 59 eyes (54%) had achieved their best-corrected visual acuity.[11] The 22 eyes which did not have an improvement in visual acuity postoperatively had co-morbid conditions limiting visual potential.[11]

Robert and Harissi-Dagher reported similar outcomes in their patients.[12] In a group of 47 eyes, they observed that 84% had an improvement of best-corrected visual acuity, with the median visual acuity improving from hand motions preoperatively to 20/150 by postoperative month 3.[12] There was 100% anatomic retention of the keratoprosthesis in these patients.[12]

Zerbe et al. also reported positive outcomes in the United States multicenter study.[7] Postoperatively, 57% of eyes had a best-corrected vision of 20/200 or better, compared to just 3.6% preoperatively.[7] There was a 95% rate of KPro retention in this study.[7]

However, when evaluating outcomes for the Boston type I keratoprosthesis, it is important to consider more than just the best-corrected visual acuity postoperatively. Short-term improvement in visual acuity is only one measure of success. Postoperative complications related to the KPro, such as recalcitrant retroprosthetic membranes, endophthalmitis, device extrusion, and glaucoma often lead to vision loss over time, especially as the cumulative risk of developing a vision-threatening complication increases. Therefore, a second outcome measure to consider in these patients is long-term retention of postoperative visual acuity improvements.

Interestingly, even in their relatively short follow-up period (average, 10 months; range, 3–18.5 months), Robert and Harissi-Dagher had four patients (8%) who had progressively worsening vision.[12] One patient lost vision from phthisis; three patients lost vision from progression of glaucoma.[12] Similarly, Zerbe et al. reported that in 62 eyes with at least 1 year follow-up (average, 14.5 months; range, 12–27 months), 12.9% (eight eyes) had decreased vision at the final follow-up visit, compared to 1 month postoperatively.[7] The reasons cited for vision loss included end-stage glaucoma, retinal detachment, and age-related macular degeneration.[7]

Long-Term Outcomes of the Boston Type 1 Keratoprosthesis

An analysis of the long-term outcomes of the Boston KPro suggests the need for continued research and development in this field of keratoprosthesis surgery. Table 52.2 summarizes the KPro outcomes from the published literature.

For the most part, outcomes remain positive for the first 2 to 3 years after keratoprosthesis surgery.[13–15] Aldave et al. reviewed a series of 57 keratoprosthesis surgeries that were performed in 50 eyes. Seventy-nine percent (38/48 eyes) had improved vision at the final postoperative visit, compared with preoperative vision.[14] They found it encouraging that the percentage of eyes with a visual acuity of 20/200 or better increased over time.[14] Of the eight eyes with at least 3 year follow-up data, all eight eyes (100%) had a visual acuity of 20/200 or better.[14] The authors speculate that many of the complications of keratoprosthesis surgery which affect vision, such as retroprosthetic membrane formation, cystoid macular edema and posterior capsular opacification, appear and are managed in the first postoperative year, allowing for better vision later in the postoperative course.[14] These are by far the best results reported in the literature to date. However, despite these encouraging results, long-term retention of the keratoprosthesis shows a downward trend with a 90% retention rate (35/39) at 1 year decreasing to 61% (14/23) at 2 years.[14]

Chew et al. also demonstrated an overall improvement of visual acuity in their patients with an improvement from a preoperative mean best-corrected visual acuity (BCVA) of count fingers to a mean best BCVA at any point postoperatively of 20/50.[15] However, even during the follow-up period ranging from 6 to 28 months, 25% patients did not maintain their best postoperative visual acuity, and the mean BCVA at the final follow-up visit for these patients was 20/90.[15] The most common causes of vision loss after keratoprosthesis surgery in this series were progression of glaucoma and endophthalmitis.[15]

Concerns regarding long-term visual acuity loss and late complications are echoed in studies of KPro patients from the New York Eye and Ear Infirmary and the University of California, Davis.[8,9] Patel et al. observed a trend of worsening visual acuity over time.[9] At the last follow-up, 43.1% of eyes had attained a BCVA ≥ 20/200 and 55.2% of eyes had improved vision, compared to preoperative vision.[9] This is comparable to the study by Zerbe et al. but worse than what Aldave et al. had reported.[7,14] However, over time, the

Table 52.2 Longer-term Outcomes of Boston Keratoprosthesis Surgery: Average Follow-Up Period Greater than 12 Months

Author, Year	Number of Eyes	Average Follow-up Period (Range)	Visual Acuity	Retention Rate at Last Follow-up Visit
Aldave et al., 2009[14]	50	18 months (4–49 months)	Pre op: 0% ≥20/200 Post op: @ 6 months, 67% (30/45) ≥20/100 @ 1 year, 75% (21/28) ≥20/100 @ 2 years, 69% (9/13) ≥20/100 @ 3 years, 100% (7/7) ≥20/100	84% @ 1 year: 90% (35/39 eyes) retention rate @ 2 years: 61% (14/23 eyes) retention rate
Chew et al., 2009[15]	37 (36 type 1, 1 type 2 Boston KPro)	16 months (6–28 months)	Pre op: Mean BCVA count fingers Post op: 81% ≥20/200 43% ≥20/50	100% of type 1 Kpros
Patel et al., 2011[9]	58	21.5 months (3–47 months)	Pre op: 12.1% >20/400 Post op: @ 1 year, 74.5% (35/47) ≥20/200 @ 2 years, 50% (16/32) ≥20/200 @ 3 years 36.3% (4/11) ≥20/200	87.9%
Greiner et al., 2011[8]	40	33.6 months (5–72 months)	Pre op: 5% ≥20/400 Post op: @ 1 year, 59% (19/32) ≥20/200 @ 2 years, 59% (16/27) ≥20/200 @ 3 years, 50% (7/14) ≥20/200 @ 4 years, 29% (2/7) ≥20/200	80%
Verdejo-Gomez et al., 2011[13]	12	23 months (6–42 months)	Pre op: 8.3% ≥20/400 Post op: 41.7% ≥20/400	100%

percentage of eyes with BCVA ≥20/200 visual acuity decreased from 74.5% (35/47) at 1 year, 50.0% (16/32) at 2 years and 36.3% (4/11) at 3 years.[9] Additionally, the incidence of complications increased with time: 19.0% of eyes had at least one adverse event by 1 month, 65.5% by 6 months, and 75.9% by 1 year.

Greiner et al. reported very similar results with visual acuity worsening over time.[8] Although 89% of eyes achieved a BCVA ≥20/200 at some point during the postoperative period, only 59% retained this level of vision at 1 year and 2 years postoperatively, 50% at 3 years, and only 29% at 4 years postoperatively.[8] They found that the most common cause for progressive vision loss was progression of glaucoma.[8] Other causes for vision loss included retroprosthetic membranes, endophthalmitis, and recurrent corneal melts with KPro extrusion.[8]

Eventual outcomes for the Boston keratoprosthesis are variable. For the most part, visual acuity seems to improve rapidly after surgery; however, there appears to be a trend towards long-term vision loss. Understanding how to prevent complications, such as progressive glaucoma and retroprosthetic membrane formation will be key to addressing the issue of preserving vision and keratoprosthesis retention in the long term.

Preoperative diagnosis may provide prognostic indications of ultimate postoperative outcomes.[16] In the next section, we will review outcomes for individual indications for Boston keratoprosthesis placement.

Aniridia and Keratoprosthesis Surgery

Congenital aniridia is a bilateral, panocular disease which may affect cornea, iris, lens, macula and optic nerve. These patients develop a limbal stem cell deficiency which may

lead to conjunctivalization, vascularization and opacification of the cornea, requiring limbal stem cell transplantation and corneal transplantation.[17,18]

Keratoprosthesis surgery has been used as an alternative to immunosuppressive therapy that is required in patients undergoing limbal stem cell transplantation. Two retrospective studies have looked at keratoprosthesis surgery specifically in patients with congenital aniridia.

In the study by Akpek et al., 16 eyes in 15 patients with aniridia underwent Boston type I keratoprosthesis surgery.[19] Visual acuity improved in 15 patients and was maintained in 14 patients at their last follow-up visit.[19] Postoperative visual acuity ranged from 20/60 to hand motions (median 20/200), compared to preoperative visual acuities which ranged from 20/300 to light perception (median count fingers).[19] Postoperative visual acuity was limited by factors related to the underlying congenital aniridia, such as foveal hypoplasia, optic nerve hypoplasia, nystagmus and glaucomatous optic nerve damage.[19] Postoperative complications did occur in several patients, including three patients with choroidal detachments of which one progressed to retinal detachment, hypotony and vision loss.[19] All devices were retained at the last follow-up visit for the study (range 2–85 months, median 17 months), but there was one case of a tissue melt requiring a scleral patch graft.[19]

Bakhtiari et al. describe nine cases of Boston type I keratoprosthesis surgery in eyes with aniridic fibrosis syndrome, a condition in which progressive anterior chamber fibrosis occurs in a patient with congenital aniridia who had had multiple intraocular surgeries.[20] After keratoprosthesis surgery, vision improved in all eyes, ranging from hand motions to count fingers preoperatively to 20/200 to 20/500 postoperatively.[20] Successful outcomes in these challenging cases were achieved with intraocular lens explantation, removal of the fibrotic membrane and placement of a Boston KPro.[20]

Autoimmune Disease, Corneal Limbal Stem Cell Deficiency and Keratoprosthesis Surgery

Autoimmune diseases affecting the ocular surface and leading to corneal opacification present a significant challenge for the corneal surgeon. Patients with diseases, such as Stevens–Johnson syndrome (SJS), toxic epidermal necrolysis syndrome (TENS), and mucous membrane pemphigoid (MMP) frequently have corneal limbal stem cell deficiency or tear dysfunction resulting in failure with traditional corneal transplantation. Similarly, corneal limbal stem cell deficiency in the setting of chemical injuries may render traditional penetrating keratoplasty ineffective. The Boston keratoprosthesis has been used as an alternative in these difficult cases.[21–23]

Unfortunately, in these patients, the prognosis for keratoprosthesis surgery is extremely guarded.[16] In an early study from Massachusetts Eye and Ear Infirmary, keratoprosthesis surgery in SJS patients had the worst visual outcome with no eyes retaining 20/200 vision or better at 5 years.[16] Postoperative complications requiring operative repair was also far higher in the SJS group of patients with 71% requiring some type of postoperative surgical intervention.[16] Noncicatricial diseases had the most favorable prognosis with MMP and chemical burns, falling into a middle prognostic category.[16] Sixty-four percent of eyes of chemical burns and 43% of eyes with MMP had 20/200 vision or better at 5 years.[16]

Subsequent retrospective case reviews have supported these initial observations by Yaghouti et al.[16] Despite improvements in design and management of the Boston keratoprosthesis with use of vancomycin prophylaxis, chronic soft contact lens use and holes in the back plate of the keratoprosthesis,[2–6] SJS continues to have a less favorable outcome with the device than in patients with non-autoimmune diseases. In 15 patients with SJS who underwent KPro surgery (both type I and type II KPro) between 2000 and 2005, seven eyes (44%) retained 20/70 vision or better postoperatively.[21] Five eyes that had initial improvement of vision postoperatively had subsequent deterioration of vision long term, with four of these five eyes ultimately losing light perception.[21] In this series of patients, however, there were no cases of KPro extrusion.[21] Four eyes (25%) did develop tissue melt and aqueous leakage.[21]

Sejpal et al. reviewed 23 eyes in 22 patients with limbal stem cell deficiency, including seven eyes (30.4%) with chemical injury, six eyes (26.1%) with SJS, and one eye (4.3%) with OCP.[23] Seven keratoprostheses were removed over the duration of the postoperative follow-up period.[23] Five of seven were removed in patients with SJS, one was removed in a patient with OCP and one from a patient with a chemical injury.[23] Visual acuity results in this case series were more favorable than in other series with similar patient populations, with improvement of corrected distance visual acuity in 19 of 21 (90.5%) eyes with a retained keratoprosthesis at the final follow-up visit.[23] The most common postoperative complication in these patients was persistent epithelial defect, which was a risk factor for infectious keratitis.[23] Persistent epithelial defects were found to be significantly more common in these eyes with limbal stem cell deficiency than in those without (56.5% versus 23.2%, $p=0.008$).[23]

Finally, in a sobering reminder of the challenges of managing patients with autoimmune disease affecting the cornea, Ciralsky et al described two patients, one with TEN and the other with MMP, who both required multiple repeat Boston keratoprosthesis implantations, due to recurrent corneal melts.[22]

The outcomes for keratoprosthesis surgery in patients with autoimmune disease and, in particular, Stevens–Johnson syndrome and toxic epidermal necrolysis, is extremely guarded. An improved understanding of the pathogenesis of these diseases and the immune response after keratoprosthesis implantation may ultimately help to target appropriate immunomodulating therapies to better the outcomes in these patients.[22]

Pediatric Keratoprosthesis

Pediatric corneal opacities are a particularly challenging situation for the corneal surgeon. Penetrating keratoplasty surgery in the pediatric population is associated with a higher rate of graft rejection, complications and failure.[24,25] A review of the literature on keratoprosthesis surgery in children is relatively sparse with only a few scattered case reports and one retrospective review.[26,27] In their retrospective review of 21 cases of Boston keratoprosthesis placement in children ranging from 1.5 months of age to 136 months of age, Aquavella et al. had no intraoperative complications.[27] All keratoprostheses were retained for the duration of their follow-up period (range 1–30 months).[27] Postoperative complications included five cases of retroprosthetic membrane formation requiring intervention and two cases of hypotony with glaucoma drainage device and subsequent retinal detachment in each case.[27] In the seven eyes in which visual acuity could be measured, visual acuity ranged from 20/30 to light perception.[27] The remaining eyes in pre-verbal children demonstrated fix and follow vision.[27]

There are theoretical advantages of keratoprosthesis surgery in children, including rapid postoperative recovery with a stable refraction and a clear visual axis. These conditions allow for more rapid visual rehabilitation and amblyopia management without the risk of allograft rejection.[28] It has also been observed that placement of a Boston KPro in children causes less photophobia, epiphora, and blepharospasm than traditional penetrating keratoplasty.[28] Similar postoperative complications can be expected in children undergoing keratoprosthesis surgery as in adults and will likely affect the long-term outcomes in these children.

Graft Failures and Keratoprosthesis Surgery

Surgical outcomes in patients with non-cicatrizing ocular surface conditions carry the best prognosis after keratoprosthesis surgery.[16] These are patients who have failed traditional penetrating keratoplasty and have underlying diseases ranging from corneal dystrophies or degenerations to bacterial and viral keratitis. They tend to have a better visual outcome at 5 years and are less likely to lose best-corrected visual acuity of 20/200 or better after surgery.[16]

Patients who are at particularly high risk of corneal allograft failure are those with underlying herpes simplex keratitis.[29,30] In a series of 17 failed traditional penetrating keratoplasties in 14 patients with underlying herpetic keratitis, the outcomes were quite favorable after placement of a Boston keratoprosthesis.[31] The authors found that 15 eyes (88%) achieved a best-corrected visual acuity between 20/25 and 20/70 during the postoperative period, and 11 eyes (73%) were able to maintain that level of visual acuity at the last follow-up visit (median, 17 months; range 6–72 months).[31] There were no device extrusions observed during the follow-up period.[31]

The Boston keratoprosthesis may be a very viable option for patients who have failed prior penetrating keratoplasty for these non-cicatrizing corneal diseases. Given the increased risk of graft failure with each subsequent regraft and the decreased time of survival of each subsequent regraft, the Boston keratoprosthesis should be considered in patients motivated to obtain visual rehabilitation.[32]

Other Indications for Boston Keratoprosthesis Surgery and Outcomes

The Boston type I keratoprosthesis has been used successfully for a wide variety of indications, including herpes zoster neurotrophic keratopathy,[33] severe vernal keratoconjunctivitis,[34] Mooren's ulcer,[34] and ocular trauma.[35] These case reports demonstrate both successful anatomic outcomes and improved visual function after keratoprosthesis surgery in patients with an otherwise poor prognosis for standard penetrating keratoplasty.

References

1. Klufas MA, Colby KA. The Boston keratoprosthesis. Int Ophthalmol Clin 2010;50:161–75.
2. Harissi-Dagher M, Khan BF, Schaumberg DA, et al. Importance of nutrition to corneal grafts when used as a carrier of the Boston keratoprosthesis. Cornea 2007;26:564–8.
3. Dohlman C, Harissi-Dagher M. The Boston keratoprosthesis: a new threadless design. Digital J Ophthalmol 2007;13.
4. Khan BF, Harissi-Dagher M, Khan DM, et al. Advances in Boston keratoprosthesis: enhancing retention and prevention of infection and inflammation. Int Ophthalmol Clin 2007;47:61–71.
5. Dohlman CH, Dudenhoefer EJ, Khan BF, et al. Protection of the ocular surface after keratoprosthesis surgery: the role of soft contact lenses. CLAO J 2002;28:72–4.
6. Durand ML, Dohlman CH. Successful prevention of bacterial endophthalmitis in eyes with the Boston keratoprosthesis. Cornea 2009; 28:896–901.
7. Zerbe BL, Belin MW, Ciolino JB, et al. Results from the multicenter Boston type 1 keratoprosthesis study. Ophthalmology 2006;113: 1779–84.
8. Greiner MA, Li JY, Mannis MJ. Longer-term vision outcomes and complications with the Boston type 1 keratoprosthesis at the University of California, Davis. Ophthalmology 2011;118:1543–50.
9. Patel AP, Wu EI, Ritterband DC, et al. Boston type 1 keratoprosthesis: the New York Eye and Ear experience. Eye 2012;26:418–25.
10. Todani A, Ciolino JB, Ament JD, et al. Titanium back plate for a PMMA keratoprosthesis: clinical outcomes. Graefes Arch Clin Exp Ophthalmol 2011;249:1515–8.
11. Dunlap K, Chak G, Aquavella JV, et al. Short-term visual outcomes of Boston type 1 keratoprosthesis implantation. Ophthalmology 2010; 117:687–92.
12. Robert MC, Harissi-Dagher M. Boston type 1 keratoprosthesis: the CHUM experience. Can J Ophthalmol 2011;46:164–8.
13. Verdejo-Gónez L, Peláez N, Gris O, et al. The Boston type I keratoprosthesis: an assessment of its efficacy and safety. Ophthalmic Surg Lasers Imaging 2011;42:446–52.
14. Aldave AJ, Kamal KM, Vo RC, et al. The Boston type I keratoprosthesis: improving outcomes and expanding indications. Ophthalmology 2009;116:640–51.
15. Chew HF, Ayres BD, Hammmersmith KM, et al. Boston keratoprosthesis outcomes and complications. Cornea 2009;28:989–96.
16. Yaghouti F, Nouri M, Abad JC, et al. Keratoprosthesis: preoperative prognostic categories. Cornea 2001;20:19–23.
17. Ramaesh K, Ramaesh T, Dutton GN, et al. Evolving concepts on the pathogenic mechanisms of aniridia related keratopathy. Int J Biochem Cell Biol 2005;37:547–57.
18. Holland EJ, Djalilian AR, Schwartz GS. Management of aniridic keratopathy with keratolimbal allograft: a limbal stem cell transplantation technique. Ophthalmology 2003;110:125–30.
19. Akpek EK, Harissi-Dagher M, Petrarca R, et al. Outcomes of Boston keratoprosthesis in aniridia: a retrospective multicenter study. Am J Ophthalmol 2007;144:227–31.
20. Bahktiari P, Chan C, Welder JD, et al. Surgical and visual outcomes of the type I Boston keratoprosthesis for the management of aniridic fibrosis syndrome in congential aniridia. Am J Ophthalmol 2009; 153:967–71.
21. Sayegh RR, Ang LPK, Foster CS, et al. The Boston keratoprosthesis in Stevens–Johnson syndrome. Am J Ophthalmol 2008;145:438–44.
22. Ciralsky J, Papaliodis GN, Foster CS, et al. Keratoprosthesis in autoimmune disease. Ocul Immunol Inflamm 2010;18:275–80.
23. Sejpal K, Yu F, Aldave AJ. The Boston keratoprosthesis in the management of corneal limbal stem cell deficiency. Cornea 2011;30: 1187–94.
24. Dana MR, Moyes AL, Gomes JA, et al. The indications for and outcome in pediatric keratoplasty. A multicenter study. Ophthalmology 1995; 102:1129–38.
25. Huang C, O'Hara M, Mannis MJ. Primary pediatric keratoplasty: indications and outcomes. Cornea 2009;28:1003–8.
26. Botelho PJ, Congdon NG, Handa JT, et al. Keratoprosthesis in high-risk pediatric corneal transplantation: first 2 cases. Arch Ophthalmol 2006;124:1356–7.
27. Aquavella JV, Gearinger MD, Akpek EK, et al. Pediatric keratoprosthesis. Ophthalmology 2007;114:989–94.
28. Nallasamy S, Colby K. Keratoprosthesis: procedure of choice for corneal opacities in children? Semin Ophthalmol 2010;25:244–8.
29. Epstein RJ, Seedor JA, Dreizen NG, et al. Penetrating keratoplasty for herpes simplex keratitis and keratoconus. Allograft rejection and survival. Ophthalmology 1987;94:935–44.
30. Ficker LA, Kirkness CM, Rice NS, et al. The changing management and improved prognosis for corneal grafting in herpes simplex keratitis. Ophthalmology 1989;96:1587–96.
31. Kahn BF, Harissi-Dagher M, Pavan-Langston D, et al. The Boston keratoprosthesis in herpetic keratitis. Arch Ophthalmol 2007;125: 745–9.
32. Bersudsky V, Blum-Hareuveni T, Rehany U, et al. The profile of repeated corneal transplantation. Ophthalmology 2001;108:461–9.
33. Pavan-Langston D, Dohlman CH. Boston keratoprosthesis treatment of herpes zoster neurotrophic keratopathy. Ophthalmology 2008; 115(Suppl. 2):S21–3.
34. Basu S, Taneja M, Sangwan VS. Boston type 1 keratoprosthesis for severe blinding vernal keratoconjunctivitis and Mooren's ulcer. Int Ophthalmol 2011;31:219–22.
35. Harissi-Dagher M, Dohlman CH. The Boston keratoprosthesis in severe ocular trauma. Can J Ophthalmol 2008;43:165–9.

53 Modified Osteo-Odonto-Keratoprosthesis: MOOKP

GUILLERMO AMESCUA and VICTOR L. PEREZ

Introduction

Corneal transplantation has revolutionized the treatment of corneal blindness. Corneal allografts into non-inflamed recipients with a healthy ocular surface (e.g. keratoconus) offers a survival rate of > 80% at 5 years under optimal conditions.[1] This high anatomical allograft survival doesn't apply to patients with corneal blindness that is associated with an inflamed ocular surface and/or vascularized cornea, such as autoimmune disease (ocular cicatricial pemphigoid, Stevens–Johnson syndrome) and limbal stem cell deficiency (aniridia, severe chemical burns). Corneal allografts in these situations have a poor prognosis, with graft survival rates of less than 25%.[2] According to the World Health Organization, corneal blindness is the fourth most common cause of blindness in the industrialized world and the second most common cause of blindness in the developing world. The majority of these cases occur in the setting of end-stage ocular surface disease.[3] There has been a need for a safer and effective alternative to corneal allografts. Guillaume Pellier de Quengsy initiated the idea of designing a keratoprosthesis as an alternative to corneal allograft.[4] Currently, the three most common keratoprosthetic devices are the Boston Keratoprosthesis (KPro™), the AlphaCor™ artificial cornea and the osteo-odonto-keratoprosthesis (OOKP).[5]

The OOKP was developed more than 45 years ago. The basic concept of this keratoprosthesis is to use the patient's own tissue (heterotopic autograft of patient's own tooth root and alveolar bone) to support an optical cylinder of polymethyl methacrylate (PMMA), thereby significantly reducing the possibility of an immunogenic response against foreign tissue. Having autologous living material supporting the optical cylinder decreases the chance of prosthesis extrusion and offers long-term stability to the optical cylinder. The OOKP is conformed by the patient's own tooth root and alveolar bone that are fashioned into a lamina that supports a PMMA optical cylinder. The device is covered by mucosa (preferably buccal mucosa) to offer a layer of protection from a hostile environment, such as a keratinized ocular surface (Fig. 53.1). Currently, the OOKP designed by Strampelli and modified by Falcinelli (MOOKP) is the keratoprosthesis with best visual outcomes and proven long-term follow-up to restore sight in patients with end-stage ocular surface disease.[6]

MOOKP Indications and Preoperative Considerations

The MOOKP is indicated for patients with bilateral corneal blindness and associated end-stage ocular surface disease, severe vascularization of the cornea and/or end-stage limbal stem cell deficiency (Box 53.1). Relative and absolute contraindications for the OOKP surgery are listed in Table 53.1.

Surgical candidates for MOOKP need to have an extensive ophthalmic and medical evaluation. Evaluation includes the estimation of potential visual acuity, detailed slit lamp examination, ultrasound biomicroscopy, A-scan biometry and digital or mechanical estimation of intraocular pressure. The cornea surgeon should evaluate the eye in

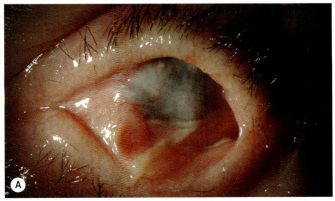
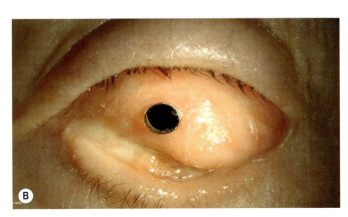

Figure 53.1 (A) Patient with history of SJS and multiple graft failures in the contralateral eye, including a limbal stem cell allograft. (B) The same patient 8 months after OCKP in the left eye with BCVA of 20/20.

Box 53.1   Indications for OOKP Surgery

Stevens–Johnson syndrome
Toxic epidermal necrolysis
Ocular cicatricial pemphigoid
Trachoma
Ocular surface burns (chemical, thermal)
Severe exposure keratopathy from eyelid malfunction
    (e.g. craniosynostosis)
End-stage autoimmune drye eye (e.g. Sjogren syndrome)
Iatrogenic complete stem cell loss with vascularized cornea
    (e.g. cryotherapy, radiation)
Multiple corneal graft failures with associated advanced ocular
    surface disease

Table 53.1   Contraindications for OOKP

Absolute Contraindications	Relative Contraindications
Pediatric patients, due to the high rate of bone reabsorption	Defective light perception, especially in the setting of known advanced glaucoma.
Phthisis bulbi	Patient unable or refusing to have close clinical follow-up
Eyes with no light perception	
Eyes with inoperable retinal detachment or a severely damaged posterior segment.	
Unrealistic visual and/or cosmetic expectations	

collaboration with a glaucoma surgeon to detect the possibility of preoperative glaucoma, and to determine a medical and/or surgical treatment strategy for either current or future glaucoma management. Approximately 50% of all patients who require a keratoprosthesis have a pre-existing diagnosis of secondary glaucoma and progressive optic nerve damage from glaucoma, which is the most common cause of vision loss in patients with MOOKP.[7]

Visual evoked potential (VEP) and electroretinography (ERG) can be used in the preoperative evaluation to obtain a more objective estimate of the potential visual acuity. The use of these tests is not absolutely necessary, but studies have shown that eyes demonstrating normal ERG or VEP achieved better visual outcomes than those with abnormal test results.[8]

The preoperative evaluation also needs to include a detailed psychological evaluation of the patient. The majority of patients that are candidates for MOOKP surgery have a history of years of poor visual acuity and also a history of multiple failed surgical efforts to rehabilitate vision. It is important to explain in detail the risk involved with this procedure to the patient, the patient's family, and support staff involved in the care. Even though visual outcomes of MOOKP surgery are good, they often can differ from the patient's expectations. Patients need to understand that after a successful operation, the field of vision will still be limited and that the prosthesis will require long-term care. Also, the cosmetic results may interfere with social interactions with those unfamiliar with this procedure.

A detailed evaluation of the patient's oral mucosa and the overall oral cavity health needs to be performed prior to the MOOKP. Orthopantomography and X-ray of the tooth are mandatory, and the use of spiral computerized tomography (CT) is helpful. The healthiest tooth with the largest root is chosen for the harvesting step. According to Falcinelli et al.,[6,9] the preferred choice for the tooth, in descending order of usefulness, is the upper canine, inferior canine, bother upper incisors, first or second upper premolar, first and second inferior premolar and inferior incisors. In cases of poor oral health, where it is not possible to harvest a healthy tooth, an allograft from a living relative is considered. This will mandate the use of systemic immunosuppression. Before making the decision to proceed with an allograft, the patient needs to understand the risk of immunosuppressive treatment and know that the long-term outcomes are not equal to the standard procedure.

Surgical Technique

The Rome–Vienna Protocol was published under the leadership of Professor Falcinelli in 2005. This surgical protocol serves as the gold standard for OOKP surgery and provides a detailed description of the surgical technique.[9] Our group strictly follows this protocol (Fig. 53.2).

The MOOKP has two major surgical stages. Stage 1 involves the preparation of the globe, mucosa and the osteo-odonto lamina. Stage 2 involves the implantation of the osteo-odonto lamina. Both surgical stages require general anesthesia. It is an absolute requirement that the patient receives a pre-anesthetic evaluation. Patients with Stevens–Johnson syndrome (SJS) frequently suffer from oropharyngeal mucosal erosions, scarring, and strictures, all of which can cause a difficult intubation. Surgical stage 1 can be managed with nasotracheal or orotracheal intubation and stage 2 with orotracheal intubation.[10]

STAGE 1

The goal of this stage is to obtain an ocular surface covered with healthy buccal mucosa and having the osteo-odonto lamina placed in the subcutaneous space, preferably in the orbitozygomatic area. The main roll of the mucosa is to protect the ocular surface from desiccation, support the osteo-odonto-acrylic lamina (OOAL), serve as a barrier against infection and provide blood supply to the bone. Surgical stage 1 can be separated into two different surgical days. The buccal mucosa placement can be performed first in cases where the reconstruction of the anterior segment is expected to be a long surgical operation or when there is significant risk of non-survival of the buccal mucosal graft (e.g. poor blood supply or extreme dryness). The OOAL can only stay in the subcutaneous space for around 3 to 5 months, so timing of the various stages remains extremely important. Keeping the OOAL in the subcutaneous space for a longer time may cause significant reabsorption of the bone.

Preparation of the Mucosa

Mucosa from the buccal area is the preferred area for harvesting. Lip, palatine or vaginal mucosa can also be used.

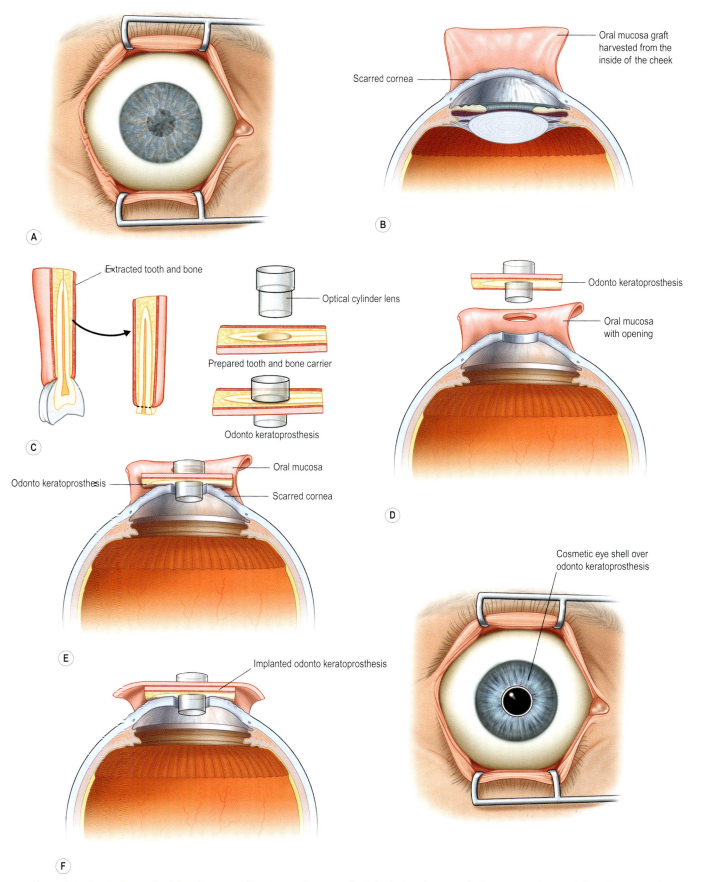

Figure 53.2 Surgical steps for OOKP. (Courtesy of University of Miami-Miller School of Medicine, Media Department, Bascom Palmer Eye Institute.)

Under general anesthesia, the oral cavity is opened with a speculum and cleaned with povidone-iodine. A diameter of 3 to 4 cm of buccal mucosa is excised, being careful to respect the parotid duct. Most of the submucosal fat is excised. The mucosa is stored in antibiotic solution.

Preparation of the Globe

The anterior surface of the globe needs to be well prepared before it is covered with the buccal mucosa. A conjunctival peritomy is performed with extension to the insertion of the recti muscles. The corneal epithelium, Bowman's membrane and limbal stem cells are also removed. Bleeding is controlled with gentle cautery. Tenon's capsule should be used to cover the cornea in cases where there is no significant corneal neovascularization. If there is significant corneal thinning (e.g. previous perforation) a lamellar or full-thickness keratoplasty is typically performed in conjunction with this step. Once the anterior surface of the globe is ready, the mucosal graft is removed from the antibiotic solution and rinsed with balanced salt solution. The mucosa is extended over the ocular surface and sutured to the episclera using interrupted absorbable sutures close to the insertion of the recti muscles. When possible, the conjunctiva should be attached with sutures to the edge of the mucosa.

Preparation of the Lamina

This step should be done in collaboration with an oral and maxilofacial surgeon (OMFS). Under general anesthesia, the oral cavity is rinsed with povidone-iodine. Using a bone saw, the root and surrounding alveolar bone are removed. It is important to preserve the periosteum of the bone as this will cover the bone of the implant in a later stage. The recommended size of the dento–alveolar lamina is about 15 mm in length and 10 mm of the former labiopalatinal dimension. After removing half of the root, the lamina should have a thickness of 3.5 mm (no less than 3.0 mm). During the grinding procedure, the lamina should be irrigated. In order to avoid damage to the dento-alveolar ligament, manipulation of the lamina is achieved by grasping the crown. The next step is to remove half of the root from the former temporal or medial side of the alveolar bone with a diamond-coated flywheel. The drilling of the hole for the cylinder should be centered on the dentine, leaving at least 1 mm of dentine on either side of the cylinder. The hole should be perpendicular to the plane of the dentine to avoid tilting of the optical cylinder. The dimensions of the optical cylinder can vary.[11] Our group follows the recommendations by Falcinelli and his team. In order to hold the cylinder in position during cementing, the diameter of the posterior part should be around 0.3 mm larger than the anterior part. It is crucial that the cementing is done with a dry surface. Using the flywheel, the crown of the tooth is removed and the implant is rinsed in povidone-iodine. Next, the crown is soaked in antibiotic solution and inserted into a subcutaneous pouch (Fig. 53.3). The implant will remain there for approximately 3 months, allowing enough time to promote revascularization of the implant and growth of the periosteum. The OOAL should be inserted with the dentine facing the orbit and the bone toward the periorbital muscle. The wound healing process involves careful monitoring for any signs of infection (Fig. 53.4).

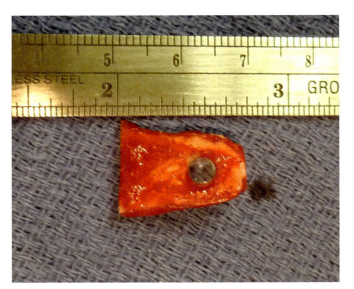

Figure 53.3 Osteo-odonto-acrylic-lamina ready to be implanted in the subcutaneous space. (Courtesy of Dr. Victor L. Perez and Dr. Yoh Sawatari, Univeristy of Miami-Miller School of Medicine.)

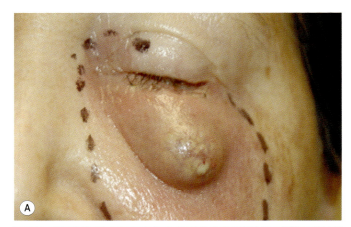

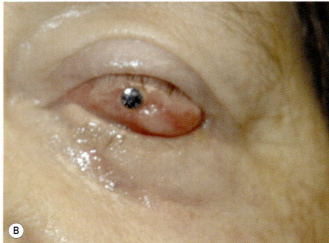

Figure 53.4 (**A**) Skin cellulitis following subcutaneous implantation of the OOAL. (**B**) The same patient 12 months later; the OOAL was removed and implanted under the subcutaneous tissue of the left breast.

STAGE 2

This stage of the procedure is scheduled 3 months after the implantation of the OOAL. The mucosal graft should be completely integrated to the ocular surface with no signs of necrosis. Under sterile conditions, the lamina is removed from the subcutaneous space and carefully inspected for any signs of significant bone reabsorption. The OOAL is explanted and the connective tissue is removed. Next, the mucosa covering the ocular surface is excised superiorly and lifted from the ocular surface with creation of a partial flap that remains attached inferiorly. A Flieringa ring is sutured to the sclera and traction sutures are placed 180° apart. These sutures are used to lift the ring at the time of insertion of the lamina. The center of the cornea is located and then trephined. Facinelli et al. recommend complete removal of the iris, lens and anterior vitreous if still present.[6,9] Three radial incisions of the cornea are performed to give exposure. For the lens removal an intracapsular or extracapsular technique can be performed.[5] The implant is placed by pulling of the traction sutures attached to the Flieringa ring. The radial incisions are sutured for closure. Filtered air or balanced salt solution can be injected to pressurize the eye. The implant is fixed with interrupted nylon sutures. The back part of the implant should be in contact with the cornea and no connective tissue should be left within the area. With the use of indirect ophthalmoscopy, the centration of the cylinder in relation to the fovea is carefully examined. The Flieringa ring is removed. The final step is to reflect back the mucosa and perform a central trephination to expose the anterior surface of the optical cylinder. The mucosa is then sutured to the episclera and conjunctiva.

POSTOPERATIVE CARE

A scleral shield should be used after surgical stage 1 to avoid shrinking of the fornix and to prevent desiccation of the mucosa. Topical and systemic antibiotics are used immediately after stages 1 and 2. Low-dose systemic corticosteroids can be used for a week after each surgical stage. To avoid infection of the mucosal area after stage 1 surgery, antiseptic mouthwashes are used until the buccal mucosa defect closes. The mucosa and prosthesis are cleaned daily with sterile balanced salt solution and a sterile cotton-tipped stick. Close follow-up is required during the first postoperative month, and then the patient has a life-long follow-up every 4 months. During follow-up visits, visual acuity and digital palpation of the globe are checked. Automated visual fields and standardized photography of the optic nerve is recommended every 6 months. If there is suspicious of bone reabsorption (e.g. changes in the refraction), a spiral CT scan with three-dimensional reconstructions should be obtained.

Visual and Anatomical Outcomes after MOOKP

Facinelli's group has the largest series of patients with the longest follow-up.[9] Their latest report included 224 patients with an anatomical success of 94% with a median follow-up of 9.4 years, with some patients with over 25 years of follow-up. This report offers the longest follow-up available for any type of keratoprosthesis. From another report, Facinelli et al. showed that from the 224 patient series a total of 181 patients were chosen because these patients follow the exact same surgical protocol. Survival analysis estimated that 18 years after the surgery, the probability of retaining an intact prosthesis was 85%. Mean best-corrected visual acuity (BCVA) varied from 0.41 Log Mar (patients with bullous keratopathy following glaucoma surgery) to 0.8 Log Mar (patient with corneal burns and dry eye syndrome).[6]

Another report from India of 50 cases with a mean follow-up of 15.38 months (range of 1 to 58 months) showed an anatomical success similar to the group in Italy with a mean BCVA of > 20/60 in 66% of the patients. Only five patients had a decrease in vision after the OOKP surgery.[12] The Asian MOOKP group reported the results of 16 patients with a mean follow-up of 19.1 months (range 5–31 months). The anatomical success was favorable in 15 of the 16 patients. One patient with a history of multiple glaucoma procedures had an expulsive choroidal hemorrhage at the time of stage 2. Eleven of the 15 patients with anatomical success obtained a BCVA of at least 20/40.[13] The first MOOKP performed in the United States was in 2009, on a patient blinded by Steven–Johnson syndrome.[14,15] The surgical procedure was a success and the clinical outcome after 2 years of follow-up is comparable to other published series, with a BCVA of 20/25. No complications have developed to date. Three additional patients have undergone one of more stages of MOOKP to date at the same facility.

Surgical Complications of MOOKP

MOOKP STAGE 1 INTRAOPERATIVE AND EARLY POSTOPERATIVE COMPLICATIONS

The complications related to the harvesting of the tooth include damage to the adjacent teeth and to the maxillary sinus. If the maxillary cavity is entered, this defect should be fixed by closing the surrounding mucosa in order to avoid a fistula formation. The OMFS on the team should be the one dealing with these types of complications. The tooth needs to be manipulated carefully to avoid a crack on the bone or dentine because this cannot be repaired and a second tooth will need to be harvested if a crack does develop. The site of implant of the OOAL is also monitored during the early postoperative period for any signs of infection. If an infection develops, the OOAL is removed, and the wound is cultured and cleaned. The lamina is also cleaned, rinsed with antibiotic solution and re-implanted at a different subcutaneous location. Any patient with infection should be treated with systemic antibiotics.

During the process of harvesting the buccal mucosa, there is a risk of damaging the parotid duct. Excessive bleeding from the mucosal defect is another potential complication. Bleeding can be controlled with cautery and packing the wound with a haemostatic agent. Significant fibrosis can develop during the healing of the mucosal defect.

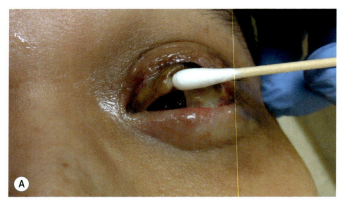
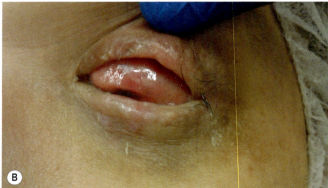

Figure 53.5 (A) Necrosis of oral mucosa with positive culture for *P. aeruginosa.* **(B)** The same patient a month later after antibiotic treatment excision of necrotic mucosa and implantation of new mucosal graft.

Complications related to the preparation of the globe include the possibility of perforation of the globe during the suturing process. If the perforation cannot be repaired with sutures, a patch graft should be performed in order to avoid hypotony and endophthalmitis. Close observation of the mucosa during the early postoperative period is important to identify cases of necrosis. If a high suspicion for necrosis develops, the mucosa should be cultured in order to rule out an infectious process (Fig. 53.5).

MOOKP STAGE 2 INTRAOPERATIVE AND EARLY POSTOPERATIVE COMPLICATIONS

After removing the implant from the subcutaneous pocket it is carefully examined for any signs of chronic infection, damage to the dentine and dentoalveolar ligament. The cylinder should be strongly attached to the haptic block.

As with any open-sky surgery, there is a risk that an expulsive hemorrhage may develop as in intraoperative complication during the preparation of the globe. Significant intraoperative bleeding may occur after a complete iridectomy. A vitreous hemorrhage may develop as a result of the intraoperative bleeding. Anterior vitrectomy and a potential of intravitreal cautery may be needed. The blood should be cleaned as much as possible with anterior vitrectomy. High intraocular pressure is common during the early postoperative period and patients should be treated with systemic carbonic inhibitors or an osmotic diuretic agent for at least 1 week after surgery.

LATE POSTOPERATIVE COMPLICATIONS

Endophthalmitis

The OOAL and the mucosa function is an excellent barrier against microorganisms, and this explains the low rate of endophthalmitis, compared to other keratoprosthetic devices.[16,17] Falcinelli et al. reported endophthalmitis in 2.2% of a series of 181 patients.[6,17] The Brighton series reported two cases of endophthalmitis in a retrospective review of 35 consecutive MOOKP surgeries.[17] In cases of endophthalmitis, the recommendation is to lift the mucosa, remove the implant, perform a full vitrectomy, and deliver intravitreal antibiotic injections with broad-spectrum antibiotics. The treatment requires the use of a temporary keratoprosthesis. The eye should then be closed with a corneal graft and refixation of the mucosa with sutures.

Glaucoma

As previously mentioned, a high number of patients who require MOOKP surgery for visual rehabilitation have already had the diagnosis of glaucoma. For this reason, the intraocular pressure should be optimized when possible before stage 1 or stage 2 surgeries. The use of glaucoma drainage devices (GDD) is the preferred surgical technique. Endoscopic cyclophotocoagulation (ECP) has also been used as an alternative to GDD. There are no long-term reports of safety in the use of ECP for MOOKP surgery and serious complications have already been reported.[18] It is the recommendation of the Rome–Vienna protocol to use GDD as the first option in the management of high intraocular pressure and to avoid placing the GDD during stage 2 surgery. Due to the significant changes in the anatomy of the anterior segment after stage 2 surgery there is a potential for secondary glaucoma. The intraocular pressure should be monitored closely with digital palpation. If the intraocular pressure increases and cannot be controlled with topical or systemic medication or if optic nerve damage is confirmed (visual field testing or optical coherence tomography (OCT) of the nerve fiber layer), a GDD should be implanted.[19]

Retinal Detachment

The risk of retinal detachment (RD) according to Falcinelli's group is around 5%.[6,9] In 2008, the Brighton group reported a rate of 14% with five of 35 patients developing RD in their case series. Three were rhegmatogenous RD and two were secondary to endophthalmitis.[17] Successful repair is possible with the use of a BIOM system or lifting the mucosa and placing a temporary keratoprosthesis. A scleral buckling procedure can be useful for repair, but additional intraocular retinal surgery is likely required, including the need for gas tamponade and/or silicone oil placement.[20]

Retroprosthetic Membranes (RPM)

This is a rare complication of the MOOKP surgery. In the rare event of RPM formation, the membrane can be removed with a YAG laser procedure. If the laser does not adequately remove the RPM or if recurrence develops, a surgical excision of the RPM may be required to clear the visual axis.

Conclusion

The MOOKP surgical procedure is a long, difficult and challenging surgical technique that requires cooperation between multiple medical and surgical services. The long-term stability of the prosthesis and the proven good visual outcomes make it the keratoprosthesis of choice for patients with bilateral corneal blindness secondary to severe autoimmune corneal disease or end-stage ocular surface pathology.

References

1. Rahman I, Carley F, Hillarby C, et al. Penetrating keratoplasty: indications, outcomes and complications. Eye (Lond) 2009;23: 1288–94.
2. Tugal-Tutkun I, Akova YA, Foster CS. Penetrating keratoplasty in cicatrizing conjunctival diseases. Ophthalmology 1995;102: 576–85.
3. Whitcher JP, Srinivasan M, Upadhyay MP. Corneal blindness: a global perspective. Bull World Health Organ 2001;79:214–21.
4. Mannis MJ. Corneal transplantation. Western J Med 1984;140:270.
5. Liu C, Paul B, Tandon R, et al. The osteo-odonto-keratoprosthesis (OOKP). Semin Ophthalmol 2005;20:113–28.
6. Falcinelli G, Falsini B, Taloni M, et al. Modified osteo-odonto-keratoprosthesis for treatment of corneal blindness: long-term anatomical and functional outcomes in 181 cases. Arch Ophthalmol 2005;123:1319–29.
7. Netland PA, Terada H, Dohlman CH. Glaucoma associated with keratoprosthesis. Ophthalmology 1998;105:751–7.
8. de Araujo AL, Charoenrook V, de la Paz MF, et al. The role of visual evoked potential and electroretinography in the preoperative assessment of osteo-keratoprosthesis or osteo-odonto-keratoprosthesis surgery. Acta Ophthalmol 2011;19.
9. Hille K, Grabner G, Liu C, et al. Standards for modified osteo-odontokeratoprosthesis (OOKP) surgery according to Strampelli and Falcinelli: the Rome–Vienna Protocol. Cornea 2005;24:895–908.
10. Garg R, Khanna P, Sinha R. Perioperative management of patients for osteo-odonto-kreatoprosthesis under general anaesthesia: a retrospective study. Indian J Anaesth 2011;55:271–3.
11. Hull CC, Liu CS, Sciscio A, et al. Optical cylinder designs to increase the field of vision in the osteo-odonto-keratoprosthesis. Graefes Arch Clin Exp Ophthalmol 2000;238:1002–8.
12. Iyer G, Pillai VS, Srinivasan B, et al. Modified osteo-odonto keratoprosthesis – the Indian experience–results of the first 50 cases. Cornea 2010;29:771–6.
13. Tan DT, Tay AB, Theng JT, et al. Keratoprosthesis surgery for end-stage corneal blindness in Asian eyes. Ophthalmology 2008;115:503–10, e3.
14. Parel JM, Sweeney D. OOKP. Cornea 2005;24:893–4.
15. Sawatari Y, Perez VL, Parel JM, et al. Oral and maxillofacial surgeons' role in the first successful modified osteo-odonto-keratoprosthesis performed in the United States. J Oral Maxillofac Surg 2011;69: 1750–6.
16. Nouri M, Terada H, Alfonso EC, et al. Endophthalmitis after keratoprosthesis: incidence, bacterial causes, and risk factors. Arch Ophthalmol 2001;119:484–9.
17. Hughes EH, Mokete B, Ainsworth G, et al. Vitreoretinal complications of osteoodontokeratoprosthesis surgery. Retina 2008;28: 1138–45.
18. Lee RM, Al Raqqad N, Gomaa A, et al. Endoscopic cyclophotocoagulation in osteo-odonto-keratoprosthesis (OOKP) eyes. J Glaucoma 2011;20:68–9.
19. Kumar RS, Tan DT, Por YM, et al. Glaucoma management in patients with osteo-odonto-keratoprosthesis (OOKP): the Singapore OOKP Study. J Glaucoma 2009;18:354–60.
20. Ray S, Khan BF, Dohlman CH, et al. Management of vitreoretinal complications in eyes with permanent keratoprosthesis. Arch Ophthalmol 2002;120:559–66.

54 Treatment Paradigms for the Management of Severe Ocular Surface Disease

EDWARD J. HOLLAND, W. BARRY LEE, and MARK J. MANNIS

Introduction

The management of patients with severe ocular surface disease requires a systematic and stepwise approach to treatment. Choosing the most appropriate management option for the patient is of utmost importance in providing optimal results in rehabilitation of the ocular surface. In addition, tear dysfunction, abnormal eyelids, and other significant ocular co-morbidities must be addressed prior to surgical treatment of the ocular surface for successful postoperative results. Examples would include the correction of lagophthalmos, trichiasis, severe dry eye disease, or glaucoma prior to undertaking any form of ocular surface transplantation. Important considerations in the choice of a treatment regimen include the nature of any underlying pathology; the extent and severity of ocular surface disease, including the degree of stem cell damage; unilaterality or bilaterality of the pathology; the presence or absence of conjunctival inflammation; whether tear production is normal, significantly altered or absent; the age of the patient; and systemic co-morbidities that may be relevant to the use of systemic immunosuppression.

The options for ocular surface stabilization using medical treatment are outlined in Box 54.1. While medical therapy can be both helpful and often necessary for restoration of the integrity of the ocular surface, it may not be suitable as a long-term treatment option, especially if there is severe stem cell damage. In conditions resulting from severe stem cell deficiency, management options shift to surgical alternatives. The flow diagrams outline our approach to

---

Box 54.1 Medical or Office-Based Treatment Strategies for Ocular Surface Disease

- Frequent preservative-free artificial tears, gels, or lubricant ointment
- Temporary or permanent punctal occlusion
- Amniotic membrane
- Tarsorrhaphy
- Oral omega-3 fatty acid supplements
- Topical vitamin A
- Topical autologous serum
- Topical albumin
- Topical anti-inflammatory agents (cyclosporine, corticosteroid)
- Systemic immunomodulators
- Therapeutic contact lens wear
  - Bandage soft contact lens (temporary)
  - Scleral contact lens (long term)

---

decision-making in the surgical treatment of ocular surface disease based on whether the pathology is unilateral (Fig. 54.1) or bilateral (Fig. 54.2).

Surgical Treatment Options

The primary considerations for decision-making in the surgical management of ocular surface disease from stem cell deficiency include: (1) the laterality of disease, (2) the degree of stem cell involvement, (3) the level of tear production/baseline tear status, and (4) whether or not there is conjunctival inflammation. The presence of conjunctival inflammation is a particularly important finding and may have significant bearing on the surgical planning for repair of the damaged ocular surface. Treatment strategies are outlined in the flowcharts for unilateral disease (Fig. 54.1).

UNILATERAL DISEASE

Unilateral Conjunctival Disease

In a patient with unilateral ocular surface disease, preoperative planning should include careful evaluation of the status of the conjunctiva in *both* eyes. A patient with unilateral disease limited to the conjunctiva does not require limbal stem cell transplantation. Conditions in this category would include primary and recurrent pterygium and unilateral focal conjunctival tumors, such as squamous cell carcinoma or conjunctival intraepithelial neoplasia (CIN). These conditions may benefit from a conjunctival autograft from the same eye or from the contralateral eye. The autograft can be harvested from the superior or inferior bulbar conjunctiva, taking into consideration that symblepharon formation remains a slightly higher risk for inferior conjunctival grafts. Limbal tissue is not needed when harvesting an autologous conjunctival graft. Figure 54.1 provides a flow diagram for surgical treatment options.

If conjunctiva cannot be harvested from the same or contralateral eye, amniotic membrane can serve as an adjunct to close the conjunctival defect. Amniotic membrane by itself carries slightly higher risk for recurrence, compared to conjunctival grafts, but can be used when viable conjunctiva is not available.[1,2] Conjunctival autograft or amniotic membrane fixation is performed with either suture or fibrin glue and requires local immunosuppression with corticosteroids. Systemic immunosuppression is not required with these techniques.

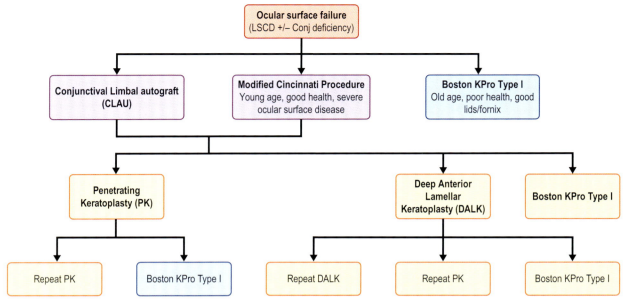

Figure 54.1 Ocular surface surgical treatment options for unilateral disease.

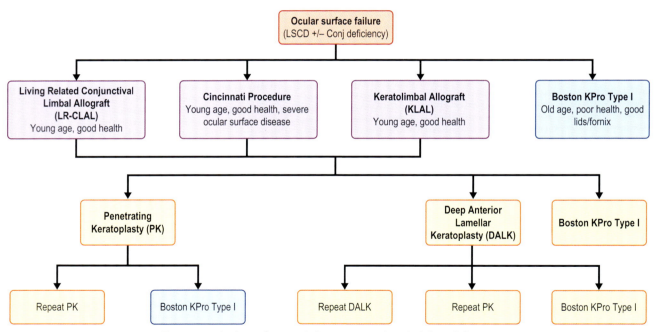

Figure 54.2 Ocular surface surgical treatment options for bilateral disease.

Unilateral Limbal Disease

When the ocular surface disease is unilateral and involves limbal tissue, as well as conjunctiva, assessment of the extent of limbal involvement in the affected eye is paramount to the clinical management decision. In this setting, the ophthalmologist should carefully assess the contralateral eye to determine if early limbal disease has occurred. An example of unilateral limbal insult would include a chemical injury or severe contact lens-induced stem cell damage to the ocular surface. If the disease involvement is localized to a small area (less than 50%), a sequential conjunctival epitheliectomy can be performed. If the area is more extensive, a conjunctival/limbal autograft (CLAU) can be taken from the contralateral eye. Options might include ex vivo stem cell expansion with either limbal autograft or allograft tissue. These techniques call for local immunosuppression with corticosteroids and/or cyclosporine, or in the case of the living-related or cadaveric donor tissue, systemic immunosuppression is required as well.

Unilateral Combined Conjunctival and Limbal Disease

When the ocular surface disease is unilateral, but involves both conjunctiva and limbal tissue, the extent of damage is an important preoperative consideration. Conjunctival inflammation must be controlled prior to consideration of any surgical techniques. The prognosis in this situation remains more guarded when compared to either unilateral conjunctival or limbal ocular surface disease alone. Clinical situations would include more extensive chemical ocular surface injury such as a severe alkaline burn. The same treatment strategies can be implemented as with limbal disease alone and include stem cell transplantation techniques such as CLAU or the modified Cincinnati procedure. In cases where the conjunctival and limbal stem cell damage is extensive, with severe ocular surface failure and broad symblepharon, it is felt that the 'modified Cincinnati procedure' is a more appropriate treatment option over CLAU alone. The 'modified Cincinnati procedure' utilizes lr-CLAL segments to the superior and inferior limbus in combination with cadaveric KLAL along the nasal and temporal limbus. Alternatively, a keratoprosthesis could be used in this setting, especially in the elderly patient with multiple systemic co-morbidities who are poor candidates for systemic immunosuppression.

BILATERAL DISEASE

Bilateral ocular surface disease has a more guarded prognosis and the surgical options are more limited. Both the extent of disease and the presence of conjunctival inflammation are important considerations in the preoperative evaluation. In bilateral disease, use of tissue from the contralateral eye is not feasible. Figure 54.1 provides a flow diagram for surgical treatment options.

Bilateral Limbal Disease with Normal Conjunctiva

When the ocular surface disease is bilateral and involves significant portions of the limbus but spares the conjunctiva, a limbal stem cell procedure will ultimately be needed for ocular surface restoration. Accurate assessment of the extent of limbal involvement is crucial to surgical planning. Congenital stem cell deficiencies, such as aniridia or bilateral severe contact lens-induced deficiency are examples of this disease situation. When limbal disease is partial (less than 50%), sequential conjunctival epitheliectomy can be an effective treatment strategy. When the limbal involvement is greater than 50%, the treatment options are limbal stem cell transplantation with a keratolimbal allograft (KLAL) or living-related conjunctival limbal allograft (lr-CLAL) The KLAL procedure provides an abundant source of stem cells and utilizes readily available cadaveric tissue. The lr-CLAL has the potential for an excellent tissue match between the donor and recipient and thus, a significant reduction in the risk of graft rejection. Patients undergoing KLAL or lr-CLAL will require topical and systemic immunosuppression for successful ocular surface rehabilitation. Keratoprosthesis surgery is another option for elderly patients or patients with significant systemic co-morbidities who cannot tolerate systemic immunosuppression.

Many of the ocular surface disease states are complicated by corneal scarring and opacification and will ultimately require subsequent keratoplasty. In such situations, deep anterior lamellar keratoplasty (DALK) may be advantageous over penetrating keratoplasty (PK) with elimination of potential endothelial rejection and improved tectonic wound stability.[3] Keratoprosthesis surgery may also be useful after failed keratoplasty in lieu of DALK or PK in conditions where repeat cadaveric tissue transplantation has little to no chance of survival. Patients with bilateral limbal disease should not undergo DALK or PK prior to an ocular surface transplantation procedure, because the graft will not survive functionally if a significant amount of the limbal stem cells have been damaged.

Bilateral Limbal Disease with Prior Conjunctival Disease

This category of ocular surface disease involves conditions which cause bilateral limbal disease with previous but now subsided or controlled conjunctival inflammation. Box 54.1 lists the treatments that might be used to treat such inflammation. This category includes eyes with past injuries to the conjunctiva or previous episodes of inflammation from conjunctival inflammatory conditions. In these patients, KLAL or lr-CLAL, or a combination of the two (Cincinnati Procedure) are potential options for surgical treatment. Keratoprosthesis surgery is an additional option. If minimal conjunctival damage is present and/or no living-related donors are present, KLAL is the best option unless the patient is elderly or has systemic disease that would contraindicate the systemic immunosuppression needed with KLAL. If conjunctival damage is significant and a living-related donor is available, lr-CLAL remains the best options in a young and otherwise healthy patient as conjunctiva and limbal cells are provided to the ocular surface and a tissue match may be possible. In severe cases with large amounts of symblepharon and ocular surface failure, the preferred treatment option would be the Cincinnati procedure. This procedure combines lr-CLAL segments to the superior and inferior limbus in combination with cadaveric KLAL along the nasal and temporal limbus. Keratoprosthesis surgery may be the best option if systemic immunosuppression is contraindicated.

Bilateral Limbal Disease with Active Conjunctival Inflammation

Bilateral limbal disease with concurrent active conjunctival inflammation represents the most challenging situation for surgery of the ocular surface. This category of diseases includes conditions such as Stevens–Johnson syndrome, ocular cicatricial pemphigoid, and autoimmune inflammatory conditions. These disease states carry the poorest prognosis of diseases of the ocular surface. Prior to any surgical intervention, every effort must be made to mitigate conjunctival inflammation. The authors typically utilize topical, as well as systemic immunosuppressive therapy, including a number of additional adjunct medical treatments listed in Box 54.1. Autologous serum drops can be a particularly useful adjunct to topical and systemic immunosuppression, due to its constituents of vitamins, anti-inflammatory factors and growth factors that promote stabilization of the ocular surface.[4] Any surgery should be delayed if possible until there is either resolution or significant improvement in conjunctival inflammation.

Once conjunctival inflammation is controlled, the best surgical treatment options include lr-CLAL, KLAL or a combination of the two (Cincinnati Procedure). Amniotic membrane may be used as an adjunct to this technique in an attempt to limit conjunctival fibrosis and inflammation. These techniques require intensive topical and systemic immunosuppression. Ex vivo stem cell expansion with autologous or living-related stem cells is another potential surgical treatment option for limbal disease with conjunctival inflammation and also requires both topical and systemic immunosuppression.

Ocular surface transplantation performs poorly in conditions with keratinized bulbar and palpebral conjunctiva, keratinized corneal surface, and/or little to no aqueous tear production. In these situations, keratoprosthesis surgery could be considered, but is also at high risk for failure. An osteo-odonto-kertoprosthesis (OOKP) may be the best option in these patients. Regardless of the procedure utilized, this clinical situation has a guarded prognosis and remains the most challenging of all ocular surface diseases for surgical treatment and surface rehabilitation.

While ocular surface disease, particularly limbal stem cell deficiency, often requires surgical treatment, medical therapies are important and useful adjuncts in stabilizing the ocular surface before, during, and after ocular surface transplantation. Although every ocular surface disease should be treated on an individual basis, this chapter presents the thought process the authors use in developing a treatment paradigm. Preoperative assessment of the laterality and extent of disease, as well as the degree of inflammation significantly enhances the surgical decision-making process. Moreover, any consideration of surgical rehabilitation of patients with ocular surface disease must first take into account ocular co-morbidities (e.g. glaucoma) and the anatomy and function of the ocular surface, including the eyelids, conjunctiva, and tear film. Consideration of patient age and systemic co-morbidities should also be taken into account, since many ocular surface transplant techniques require systemic immunosuppression which has potential side effects. Topical and systemic immunosuppression adds another layer of complexity to the successful management of ocular surface transplantation. While these situations can provide substantial surgical challenges, ocular surface transplant techniques enable the surgeon to convert some of the most challenging and debilitating conditions into rewarding and gratifying outcomes for both patient and surgeon.

References

1. Luanratanakorn P, Ratanapakorn T, Suwan-Apichon O, et al. Randomised controlled study of conjunctival autograft versus amniotic membrane graft in pterygium excision. Br J Ophthalmol 2006;90: 1476–80.
2. Kaufman SC, Lee WB, Jacobs DS, et al. Options and adjuvants in surgery for pterygium: A Report by the American Academy of Ophthalmology. Ophthalmology 2013;120:201–8.
3. Reinhart WJ, Musch, DC, Jacobs DS, et al. Deep anterior lamellar keratoplasty as an alternative to penetrating keratoplasty. Ophthalmology 2011;118:209–18.
4. Quinto GG, Campos M, Behrens A. Autologous serum for ocular surface diseases. Arq Bras Oftalmol 2008;71:47–54.

olopatadine
  allergic eye disease, 119–120
  vernal keratoconjunctivitis, 101
omega 3 fatty acid supplementation, 4, 277–278
  dry eye disease, 88
  meibomian gland disease, 71–74
omega 6 fatty acid supplementation, 277–278
  dry eye disease, 88
ophthalmic artery, 14, 26
ophthalmic (VI) nerve, 14
optical coherence tomography (OCT) of the anterior segment, 3–4
optic nerve examination, 417–418, 418f
oral contraceptives, 186
oral mucosal epithelial stem cells
  culture of, 348, 350
  ocular surface transplantation, 9
orbicularis oculi, 11, 11f
orbital fat, 13
orbital septum, 12–13
oropharynx in ligneous conjunctivitis, 185
osmolarity, 3–4, 19–20, 20f, 52
osteo-odonto-acrylic lamina (OOAL), 428
osteo-odonto-keratoprosthesis (OOKP)
  bilateral disease, 438
  see also modified osteo-odonto-keratoprosthesis (MOOKP)
Oxford Scheme, ocular surface staining grading, 48t
oxidative stress, 130

P

p53, 132
p63, 29–30, 256–257
pain in pterygium surgery, 136
palisades of Vogt, 6, 23, 29–30, 35
palpebral conjunctival epithelium, 3
panel reactive antigen (PRA), 387
Papanicolaou smear cytology, ocular surface squamous neoplasia, 146
papillary hypertrophy in seasonal and perennial allergic conjunctivitis, 92, 93f
papillary resection, atopic keratoconjunctivitis, 109
pathogen-associated molecular patterns (PAMPs), 26
patient education, anterior blepharitis, 64
patient questionnaire, diagnostic techniques, 49–51, 49f–50f
PAX6 gene, 253
Pearson, R. M., 283
pedicle conjunctival flaps, 304, 305f
Pellegrini, G., 8
penetrating keratoplasty (PK)
  after keratolimbal allograft, 341, 346
  bilateral disease, 437
  in bullous skin diseases, 239
  in chemical injury, 227, 227f
  combined with COMET, 380–381, 381f
  with conjunctival limbal allograft, 401
  with conjunctival limbal autograft, 331
  in ectrodactyly-ectodermal dysplasia-cleft lip syndrome, 257
  with keratolimbal allograft, 401
  surgical technique and considerations, 398
perennial allergic conjunctivitis *see* seasonal allergic conjunctivitis (SAC)/perennial allergic conjunctivitis (PAC)
perforin, 232
periorbital skin, toxic keratoconjunctivitis, 189–190, 189f–190f
peripheral arcade, 14

peripheral light focusing, 133–134, 133f
Permalens, 284
persistent corneal epithelial defect (PED)
  after ocular surface stem cell transplantation, 393–394
  therapeutic contact lenses, 288–289, 288f
petroleum-mineral oil-based ointments, 87
phospholipase A2, 122–123, 272
phototherapeutic keratectomy (PTK), 295–298, 296f
  adjunct therapy, 297–298
  advantages, 295
  complications, 298
  contraindications, 296
  corneal epithelial adhesion disorders, 202
  disadvantages, 295
  examination, 297
  history, 295
  iatrogenic limbal stem cell deficiency following, 265
  imaging, 297
  indications, 295–296
  key points, 298
  outcomes, 298
  patient history, 297
  preoperative assessment, 296–297
  procedure, 297
  vernal keratoconjunctivitis, 122
Phthrisis pubis blepharitis, 62, 63f, 65
phylectenular keratitis, 57
pilocarpine
  delivery system, 276
  doses, 276
  dry eye disease, 88–89
  mechanism of action, 276
  side effects, 276
  toxicity, 192
pimecrolimus
  atopic keratoconjunctivitis, 121
  vernal keratoconjunctivitis, 121
pinguecula, 128
Plano T, 284
plasma, dry eye disease, 89
plasma cells in giant papillary conjunctivitis, 111
plasmin, 183
plasminogen deficiency, 183–185
plasminogen substitution, 186
plica semilunaris, 25, 35
polyacrylic acid, 87, 271
polyclonal bodies, 9
polyethylene glycol (PEG), 271
polymethyl methacrylate (PMMA), 283, 407–408, 421
Polyquad, 271
polyunsaturated fatty acids (PUFA), 88
polyvinyl alcohol (PVA), 271
postmitotic cell (PMC), 256–257
prednisolone
  following Boston keratoprosthesis, 409
  following living-related conjunctival limbal allograft, 335–337
prednisolone acetate, 272–273
  following keratolimbal allograft, 345
prednisolone sodium phosphate, 272–273
prednisone
  mucous membrane pemphigoid, 245–246
  systemic immunosuppression, 386
preoperative staging, 317–321
  non-ocular factors, 320–321
    age, 320
    personality factors, 320–321
    systemic health, 320
  ocular factors, 317–320
    conjunctival involvement, extent of, 317–319, 318f–319f, 318t

    extent of stromal scarring, 319–320
    glaucoma, 320
    laterality, 317
    limbal stem cell deficiency, extent of, 317, 318f
    mechanical eyelid problems, 320, 320f
    retinal disease, 320
preservatives
  in artificial tears, 271
  toxicity of, 191
prick test, 93–94
primary acquired melanosis, 151–153, 151f, 151t, 153f, 263
procerus muscle, 11, 11f
progenitor cells, 348–350
Prokera, 309, 310f, 311–312
Propionibacterium acnes, 57
prosthetic replacement of the ocular surface ecosystem (PROSE), 286–287, 287f
  dry eye disease, 89
  graft-versus-host disease, 289
  limbal stem cell deficiency, 289
  ocular graft-versus-host disease, 181–182, 181f
  persistent corneal epithelial defect, 288–289
  Stevens-Johnson syndrome, 289, 290f
protease inhibitors, 17, 18t
pseudogerontoxon
  atopic keratoconjunctivitis, 104–105
  vernal keratoconjunctivitis, 98, 98f
pseudoglands of Henle, 25, 25f
pseudopterygium, 128
pterygium, 3–4, 125–143
  aberrant methylation in, 132
  abnormal proliferation, 132
  amniotic membrane transplantation, 313
  anti-apoptotic mechanisms, 132
  appearance, 126, 126f
  bilateral, 126
  clinical features, 126, 126f
  complications of, 125–126
  definition, 41, 125
  differential diagnosis, 126–128
  double, 126f
  epidemiology, 125, 128
  extracellular matrix remodeling, 131
  fibroangiogenic growth factors, 130–131
  future advances, 139–140
  genetic and epigenetic changes, 132
  grading scale, 139
  growth factor receptor signaling, 130
  histopathology, 126, 127f
  inflammation, 134
  inherited factors, 131, 131b
  management, 133–139
    medical, 134
    prevention, 133–134, 133f
    surgical, 134–139, 136f–138f
  matrix metalloproteinases, 131
  neovascularization, 134–136
  neurogenic inflammation, 133
  ocular associations of, 125b
  oxidative stress, 130
  pathogenesis, 128–133, 128f
  primary, 126, 126f, 134–136
  pro-inflammatory cytokines and immunological mechanisms, 130, 130b
  public health campaigns, 139–140
  recurrent, 126, 134–136, 135f
  stem cells, 132–133, 133f
  surgical treatment, 8
  symptoms, 126
  ultraviolet light, 129–130, 129f
  unilateral, 126